Diagnosis and Management of Endocrine-related Tumors

Cancer Treatment and Research

WILLIAM L MCGUIRE, *series editor*

Livingston RB (ed): Lung Cancer 1. 1981. ISBN 90-247-2394-9.

Bennett Humphrey G, Dehner LP, Grindey GB, Acton RT (eds): Pediatric Oncology 1. 1981. ISBN 90-247-2408-2.

DeCosse JJ, Sherlock P (eds): Gastrointestinal Cancer 1. 1981. ISBN 90-247-2461-9.

Bennett JM (ed): Lymphomas 1, including Hodgkin's Disease. 1981. ISBN 90-247-2479-1.

Bloomfield CD (ed): Adult Leukemias 1. 1982. ISBN 90-247-2478-3.

Paulson DF (ed): Genitourinary Cancer 1. 1982. ISBN 90-247-2480-5.

Muggia FM (ed): Cancer Chemotherapy 1. ISBN 90-247-2713-8.

Bennett Humphrey G, Grindey GB (eds): Pancreatic Tumors in Children. 1982. ISBN 90-247-2702-2.

Costanzi JJ (ed): Malignant Melanoma 1. 1983. ISBN 90-247-2706-5.

Griffiths CT, Fuller AF (eds): Gynecologic Oncology. 1983. ISBN 0-89838-555-5.

Greco AF (ed): Biology and Management of Lung Cancer. 1983. ISBN 0-89838-554-7.

Walker MD (ed): Oncology of the Nervous System. 1983. ISBN 0-89838-567-9.

Higby DJ (ed): Supportive Care in Cancer Therapy. 1983. ISBN 0-89838-569-5.

Herberman RB (ed): Basic and Clinical Tumor Immunology. 1983. ISBN 0-89838-579-2.

Baker LH (ed): Soft Tissue Sarcomas. 1983. ISBN 0-89838-584-9.

Bennett JM (ed): Controversies in the Management of Lymphomas. 1983. ISBN 0-89838-586-5.

Bennett Humphrey G, Grindey GB (eds): Adrenal and Endocrine Tumors in Children. 1983. ISBN 0-89838-590-3.

DeCosse JJ, Sherlock P (eds): Clinical Management of Gastrointestinal Cancer. 1984. ISBN 0-89838-601-2.

Catalona WJ, Ratliff TL (eds): Urologic Oncology. 1984. ISBN 0-89838-628-4.

Santen RJ, Manni A (eds): Diagnosis and Management of Endocrine-related Tumors. 1984. ISBN 0-89838-636-5.

Costanzi JJ (ed): Clinical Management of Malignant Melanoma. 1984. ISBN 0-89838-656-X.

Wolf GT (ed): Head and Neck Oncology. 1984. ISBN 0-89838-657-8.

Diagnosis and Management of Endocrine-related Tumors

edited by

RICHARD J. SANTEN, M.D. & ANDREA MANNI, M.D.

The Milton S. Hershey Medical Center
The Pennsylvania State University
Hershey, Pennsylvania, U.S.A.

1984 **MARTINUS NIJHOFF PUBLISHERS**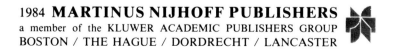
a member of the KLUWER ACADEMIC PUBLISHERS GROUP
BOSTON / THE HAGUE / DORDRECHT / LANCASTER

Distributors

for the United States and Canada: Kluwer Boston, Inc., 190 Old Derby Street, Hingham, MA 02043, USA
for the UK and Ireland: Kluwer Academic Publishers, MTP Press Limited, Falcon House, Queen Square, Lancaster LA1 1RN, England
for all other countries: Kluwer Academic Publisher Group, Distribution Center, P.O. Box 322, 3300 AH Dordrecht, The Netherlands

Library of Congress Cataloging in Publication Data

```
Main entry under title:

Diagnosis and management of endocrine-related tumors.

   (Cancer treatment and research)
   Includes index.
   1. Endocrine glands--Tumors.  I. Santen, Richard J.
II. Manni, Andrea.  III. Series.  [DNLM: 1. Neoplasms--
Diagnosis.  2. Neoplasms--Therapy.  3. Endocrine diseases
--Diagnosis.  4. Endocrine diseases--Therapy. W1 CA693 /
QZ 200 D367]
RC280.E55D5   1984    616.99'44        84-1557
```

ISBN 0-89838-636-5 (this volume)

Contents

VI

Foreword to the series

Where do you begin to look for a recent, authoritative article on the diagnosis or management of a particular malignancy? The few general oncology textbooks are generally out of date. Single papers in specialized journals are informative but seldom comprehensive; these are more often preliminary reports on a very limited number of patients. Certain general journals frequently publish good indepth reviews of cancer topics, and published symposium lectures are often the best overviews available. Unfortunately, these reviews and supplements appear sporadically, and the reader can never be sure when a topic of special interest will be covered.

Cancer Treatment and Research is a series of authoritative volumes which aim to meet this need. It is an attempt to establish a critical mass of oncology literature covering virtually all oncology topics, revised frequently to keep the coverage up to date, easily available on a single library shelf or by a single personal subscription.

We have approached the problem in the following fashion. First, by dividing the oncology literature into specific subdivisions such as lung cancer, genitourinary cancer, pediatric oncology, etc. Second, by asking eminent authorities in each of these areas to edit a volume on the specific topic on an annual or biannual basis. Each topic and tumor type is covered in a volume appearing frequently and predictably, discussing current diagnosis, staging, markers, all forms of treatment modalities, basic biology, and more.

In Cancer Treatment and Research, we have an outstanding group of editors, each having made a major commitment to bring to this new series the very best literature in his or her field. Martinus Nijhoff Publishers has made an equally major commitment to the rapid publication of high quality books, and world-wide distribution.

Where can you go to find quickly a recent authoritative article on any major oncology problem? We hope that Cancer Treatment and Research provides an answer.

WILLIAM L. McGUIRE
Series Editor

Preface

Patients with a variety of tumors present to the physician because of clinical manifestations of hormones secreted in excess. This phenomenon attracted the investigative interest of such pioneers as Harvey Cushing who recognized that pituitary tumors may cause acromegaly and Charles Mayo who associated hypertension with adrenal medullary neoplasms. Current interest in endocrine-related tumors has intensified because of the explosive development of newer methodology for their study. Specific measurements of secretory products, hybridization assays to identify products of genomic translation and quantitative assessment of tissue hormone receptors have provided means of characterizing and precisely following patients with endocrine-related tumors. Treatments based upon these advances are rapidly proliferating. The current volume attempts to synthesize much of this recent information with the goal of providing a sound basis for making clinical judgements regarding diagnosis and management.

Tumors of endocrine glandular tissues commonly confront practicing physicians with difficult management problems. Several unique features of these tumors necessitate collaboration among various specialty disciplines in order to resolve these problems and to provide a high level of clinical care. For example, endocrine neoplasms secrete active hormones or hormone precursors which produce clinical manifestations most familiar to endocrinologists. Certain therapies such as radioactive iodine for thyroid cancer take advantage of the hormone-responsiveness of these tumors to facilitate treatment. These aspects require individuals trained in endocrinology to implement complex diagnostic and therapeutic maneuvers. The use of C-peptide, proinsulin and insulin assays in the diagnosis of insulinoma involves specialists in the area of diabetes/metabolism in the management of these patients. The characteristic physiologic effects of certain tumors necessitate the participation of specialists in other areas. The multilevel influences of gastrointestinal transport on gastrin release and of gastrin on acid output requires the participation of trained gastroenterologists in the management of the Zollinger-Ellison syndrome. The physiologic effects of the catecholamines on blood pressure involve hypertension subspecialists in the diagnosis and management of pheochromocytoma. A high level of specific expertise is required for surgical management of patients with islet cell adenomas, hyperparathyroidism, thyroid carcinoma, especially when near total thyroidectomy is required, and for micro and macroadenomas of the pituitary. The special skills required necessitate the involvement of endocrine surgeons and neurosurgeons with expertise in the management of these entities. Radiologists are required to place catheters supraselectively to allow hormone measurements in veins draining certain hormone-secreting tumors. Finally, medical and surgical oncologists and radiation therapists participate in the planning and implementation of strategies to reduce tumor bulk and eradicate anatomically or physiologically important metastases. Taken together, these considerations serve to emphasize the importance of a multidisciplinary approach to diagnosis and management of endocrine-related tumors. However, a firm understanding of basic endocrinologic principles must provide a conceptual framework for management of each of these clinical disorders and serves as the theme of this book. To accomplish this aim and also to provide a broad perspective, the authors in this volume were chosen to represent a variety of disciplines including gastroenterology, endocrinology, surgery, metabolism, neurosurgery and physiology.

The organization of this volume reflects an anatomic orientation. The first 4 chapters consider pituitary tumors from a global standpoint and then according to specific secretory and non-secretory lesions. The emphasis of each is upon precise documentation of anatomy, physiology and clinical manifestations prior to and after treatment approaches. A large body of original data accumulated by the investigative group at Case Western Reserve University in Cleveland allows a number of sound conclusions based upon their extensive expertise. Three subsequent chapters address the diagnostic, medical and surgical management of patients with thyroid cancer. Two of these review primary data and utilize this material to make recommendations regarding overall management. These chapters, taken together, illustrate the lack of uniformity of treatment approaches adapted at various centers in the United States with respect to thyroid cancer.

The medical and surgical management of hyperparathyroidism provided a major field for vigorous debate in the 1970's. More recently, these controversies have been largely resolved. The development of more precise assays for PTH, the identification and follow up without surgery of a large number of patients with asymptomatic disease, and the anatomic/microscopic classification of adenomatous vs. hyperplastic forms of hyperparathyroidism provided a sound basis for resolution of several previously controversial issues. These concepts are explored in the two chapters which address parathyroid tumors. Finally, neoplasms of the adrenal cortex are reviewed with primary attention to their clinical characteristics in an additional chapter.

The spectrum of islet cell tumors of the pancreas either as isolated entities or as part of the multiple endocrine neoplasia Type I syndrome has attracted considerable attention recently. A new discipline of gastroenterologic endocrinology evolved because of the myriad of hormones made by these tumors. Recent observations regarding the molecular heterogeneity of circulating GI hormones, the neural crest derivation of several of them, and the pluripotential of their secretory capacity have stirred intensive investigative interest in this field. Chapters by the investigators at the University of Michigan provide a provocative conceptual background and detailed clinical information upon which to base therapeutic recommendations. The chapter by Dr. Denis McCarthy provides a unique perspective to the discussion of the treatment of the Zollinger-Ellison syndrome. At the NIH and later at the University of New Mexico, this author has carefully studied a large cohort of patients undergoing intensive medical therapy with histamine H_2 receptor blockers. The necessity for surgical intervention in many of these patients at some time in their treatment course has provided a rational basis of information upon which to recommend individual therapy tailored to each patient's needs. The in-depth discussion of the physiologic mechanisms which control the release of gastrin provides a framework for evaluating gastrin elevations in patients with disordered gastrointestinal function in association with gastric hyper- and hyposecretory states. The companion chapter on multiple endocrine neoplasia-type I provides a compendium of basic and clinical, detailed information regarding these commonly encountered syndromes. Finally, a comprehensive approach to the diagnosis and management of pheochromocytoma, based upon a broad personal experience, is presented.

In many areas of clinical management, insufficient prospective data exist to provide sound scientific support for particular treatment approaches. This applies to two particular areas covered by this volume, namely, prolactinomas and thyroid cancer. With respect to functioning pituitary tumors, the development of radioimmunoassays and of potent dopamine agonists for treatment has been too recent to allow prospective comparison of various medical and surgical approaches. Thyroid cancer, on the other hand, is sufficiently uncommon and indolent that no one center can accumulate adequate prospectively collected information. As a consequence, the treatment of thyroid cancer and of functioning pituitary tumors is controversial. The last chapter attempts to identify differing recommendations among various authors covering these topics. The Editors have attempted to reconcile this diversity and to provide a middle ground regarding the management of both of these clinical problems. This chapter is intended only as a working construct to provide guidelines for management until more definitive information becomes available.

List of contributors

Baha'Uddin M. Arafah, M.D.
Assistant Professor of Medicine
Division of Endocrinology
Case Western Reserve School of Medicine
University Hospitals – Cleveland
2074 Abington Rd.
Cleveland, OH 44106

William H. Beierwaltes, M.D.
Professor of Medicine
Physician-in-Charge, Division of Nuclear
  Medicine
University of Michigan Medical School
1405 E. Ann Street
Ann Arbor, MI 48109

Jerald S. Brodkey, M.D.
Professor of Neurosurgery
St. Luke's Hospital
11311 Shaker Blvd.
Cleveland, OH 44104

Stefan S. Fajans, M.D.
Professor of Internal Medicine
Chief, Division of Endocrinology and
  Metabolism
Director, Michigan Diabetes Research and
  Training Center
Department of Internal Medicine
University of Michigan Medical School
Ann Arbor, MI 48109

Allan Fredland, M.D.
Research Associate, Department of Surgery
University of Chicago Pritzker School of
  Medicine
5841 S. Maryland Avenue
Chicago, IL 60637

Joel I. Hamburger, M.D.
Clinical Endocrinologists
Associated Endocrinologists
4400 Prudential Town Center
Southfield, MI 48075

Timothy S. Harrison, M.D.
Professor of Surgery and Physiology
Department of Surgery
The Milton S. Hershey Medical Center
The Pennsylvania State University
P.O. Box 850
Hershey, PA 17033

Edwin L. Kaplan, M.D.
Professor of Surgery
Department of Surgery
University of Chicago Pritzker School of
  Medicine
5841 S. Maryland Avenue
Chicago, IL 60637

Sudha R. Kini, M.D.
Pathologist
Director, Cytology Laboratory
Department of Pathology
Henry Ford Hospital
2799 W. Grant Blvd.
Detroit, MI 48202

Andrea Manni, M.D.
Associate Professor of Medicine
Division of Endocrinology
The Milton S. Hershey Medical Center
The Pennsylvania State University
P.O. Box 850
Hershey, PA 17033

J. Martin Miller, M.D.
Clinical Associate Professor
Division of Endocrinology
Henry Ford Hospital
2799 W. Grand Blvd.
Detroit, MI 48202

Denis M. McCarthy, M.D.
Professor of Medicine
University of New Mexico School of Medicine
Chief, Gastroenterology Division
Veterans Administration Medical Center-111
2100 Ridgecrest Dr. SE
Albuquerque, NMEX 87108

Thomas M. O'Dorisio, M.D.
Professor of Medicine
Division of Endocrinology
Ohio State University Medical Center
Columbus, OH 43210

Robert B. Page, M.D.
Professor of Surgery
Division of Neurosurgery
The Milton S. Hershey Medical Center
The Pennsylvania State University
P.O. Box 850
Herhsey, PA 17033

Olof H. Pearson, M.D.
Professor of Medicine
Case Western Reserve School of Medicine
University Hospitals-Cleveland
2065 Adelbert Road
Cleveland, OH 44106

Richard J. Santen, M.D.
Professor of Medicine
Chief, Division of Endocrinology
The Milton S. Hershey Medical Center
The Pennsylvania State University
P.O. Box 850
Hershey, PA 17033

O. Peter Schumacher, M.D.
Clinical Professor
Department of Endocrinology
Cleveland Clinic Foundation
2020 E. 93rd St.
Cleveland, OH 44106

Louis M. Sherwood, M.D.
Professor and Chairman
Department of Medicine
Albert Einstein College of Medicine
1300 Morris park Ave.
Bronx, NY 10461

Justin Silver, M.D.
Visiting Professor (from Israel)
Division of Endocrinology
Department of Medicine
Albert Einstein College of Medicine
1300 Morris Park Ave.
Bronx, NY 10461

William E. Strodel, M.D.
Assistant Professor of Surgery
University of Michigan Hospital
SACB 2226
Ann Arbor, MI 48109

Johannes D. Veldhuis, M.D.
Associate Professor of Medicine
Division of Endocrinology
University of Virginia Medical Center
Charlottesville, VA 22908

Aaron I. Vinik, M.D.
Professor of Internal Medicine
Department of Internal Medicine/Surgery
University of Michigan Hospital
SACB 2226
Ann Arbor, MI 48109

1. Approach to the pituitary tumor: anatomic, diagnostic and surgical considerations

ROBERT B. PAGE and RICHARD J. SANTEN

1. Introduction

Patients harboring putative pituitary tumors reach neurosurgeons through three lines of referral. Neurologists refer patients with symptoms and signs of intracranial mass such as dulled affect, lethargy, hemiparesis, seizures or failing vision [1]. Their goal of therapy is total removal of the intracranial mass which has arisen from the sellar region and restoration of brain function. Ophthalmologists refer patients with specific visual disturbances. Their goal is decompression of the visual or oculo-motor pathways with restoration of normal vision [2]. Endocrinologists refer patients with symptoms and signs of endocrine dysfunction. These may be manifestations of pituitary hypofunction with gonadal, adrenal, and/or thyroid underactivity or even, in the case of children, failure to grow at a normal rate [1, 2]. Endocrine abnormalities may also be caused by hyperfunction of adenomatous pituitary tissue with oversecretion of prolactin (PRL) [3, 4, 5], of luteinizing hormone (LH) [6, 7], or of follicle stimulating hormone (FSH) [8, 9] causing inferility, of growth hormone (GH) causing acromegaly [10, 11, 12], of adrenocorticotrophic hormone (ACTH) causing Cushing's disease [13, 14] or of thyroid stimulating hormone (TSH) causing hyperthyroidism [15, 16]. The endocrinologists' goal is complete tumor removal and restoration of pituitary function.

The goal of the neurosurgeon is to localize the tumor as precisely as possible, to approach it by the most direct route, to remove all or as much of the tumor as possible and to withdraw causing little or no disturbance and leaving little evidence of entry. Four approaches to pituitary tumors are commonly employed by neurological surgeons: from below by the transphenoidal route, from the front by the subfrontal route, from the side by the temporal route and from above by the transventricular route. The approach chosen by a surgeon to manage a particular patient will be dictated by the anatomy of the pituitary gland, the tumor, and the brain in that patient; the objective of treatment and the experience of the surgeon. A clear understanding of the anatomic interrelationships of the pituitary with neural, vascular and osseous structures is required to develop safe and effective treatment.

Santen, R.J. and Manni, A. (eds.), Diagnosis and management of endocrine-related tumors. ISBN 0-89838-636-5.
© *1984, Martinus Nijhoff Publishers, Boston. Printed in the Netherlands.*

2. Correlative anatomy

2.1 *Pituitary*

2.1.1 *Neurohypophysis.* The pituitary gland lies beneath the brain and is comprised of neural and glandular tissue. Its neural portion, the neurohypophysis, is a diverticulum of brain [17] made up of axon terminals, fenestrated capillaries, and glial cells [18, 19, 20] (Fig. 1). The neurohypophysis is subdivided into three regions [21]. The *median eminence* (infundibulum) is its most rostral region and forms the floor of the third ventricle. The *neural lobe* (infundibular process) is its most caudal region and lies within the sella turcica at the base of the skull. The *infundibular stem* passes from the median eminence through the subarachnoid space and diaphragma sellae to the neural lobe and forms the neural component of the pituitary stalk [22].

The primate *median eminence* is divided into an external and an internal zone [23, 24, 25]. The external zone is the terminus of aminergic and peptidergic neuronal systems which originate in the hypothalamus [26]. The dopaminergic tubero-infundibular tract originates in the hypothalamic arcuate (tuberal) nuclei and terminates in the perivascular space of fenestrated median eminence capillaries [27]. Peptidergic neuronal systems containing gonadotropin releasing hormones (GNRH), corticolibrin (CRF), somatostatin (SOM), thyrotropin releasing hormone (TRH), oxytocin (OXY), and vasopressin (AVP) also terminate in the perivascular space of external plexus capillaries [28, 29, 30]. On the basis of anatomic studies in rats, GnRH fibers have been found to originate in the medial preoptic region and pass anteriorly to the median eminence. CRF, TRH, and SOM systems have been found to originate in the hypothalamic periventricular nucleus and in the parvocellular division of the paraventricular nucleus. These fiber systems, with systems containing oxytocin and vasopressin which also

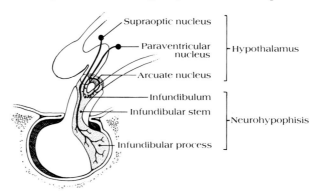

Figure 1. Schematic representation of the human pituitary gland. The neurohypophysis and its neural connections with the hypothalamus are emphasized. The terminology (infundibulum, infundibular stem and infundibular process) emphasizes the unity of the neurohypophysis. Note that infundibulum is a synonym for median eminence and infundibular process for neural lobe.

originate in the paraventricular nucleus, pass ventrolaterally to the lateral preoptic region and then course ventromedially to terminate in the median eminence external zone [31]. Peptidergic neuronal systems terminate in the perivascular space of median eminence capillaries. Their neurosecretions regulate adenohypophyseal function [for review see 28, 32]. The internal zone is made up of fibers of the supraoptico-hypophyseal tract. These fibers contain oxytocin and vasopressin and they pass through the median eminence and infundibular stem to terminate in the neural lobe [29].

The *infundibular stem* is comprised of at least two neuronal fiber tracts: the supraoptico-hypophyseal tract [29] and the dopaminergic tubero-hypophyseal tract [33]. Both these fiber tracts pass through the infundibular stem to terminate in the neural lobe. Terminals of the peptidergic neurosecretory system containing TRH and SOM are also present in this region.

The *neural lobe* is the terminus of the supraoptico-hypophyseal and of the tubero-hypophyseal tracts. In this region of the neurohypophysis magnocellular neurons of the supraoptico-hypophyseal tract terminate in the perivascular space of fenestrated capillaries [34, 35]. Their neurosecretions regulate the function of distant target organs such as the kidney, uterus, and breast.

2.1.2 *Adenohypophysis*. The glandular portion of the pituitary is called the adenohypophysis (Fig. 2). It is generally believed to arise from the primitive foregut – the stomodeum. A diverticulum of ectodermal tissue (Rathke's pouch) migrates cranially from the roof of the primitive mouth to become applied to the evaginating neurohypophysis [36]. The posterior wall of this ectodermal pouch becomes adherent to the neural lobe to form the pars intermedia. In humans, this region of the adenohypophysis is identifiable only in fetal stages and in adult pregnant females. The anterior wall of the Rathke's pouch enlarges greatly to become the pars distalis which lies within the sella turcica with the neurointer-

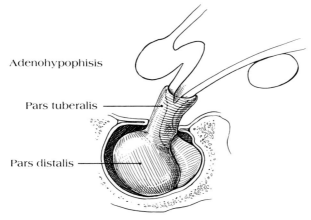

Adenohypophisis

Pars tuberalis

Pars distalis

Figure 2. Schematic representation of the human pituitary gland from the same perspective as in Fig. 1. The pars tuberalis lies above the sella turcica. The pars distalis lies within it.

4

mediate lobe but is separated from it by Rathke's (hypophyseal) cleft. Tissue from Rathke's pouch also migrates cranially to become applied to the infundibular stem and median eminence as the pars tuberalis [37]. The median eminence with the pars tuberalis makes up the tuber cinereum [38]. Thus, the adenohypophysis, like the neurohypophysis, is subdivided into three regions: the pars tuberalis, the pars intermedia, and the pars distalis.

Within the adenohypophysis there is a regional segregation of glandular cells along functional lines [39, 40] (Fig. 3). In the pars tuberalis, only gonadotrophs and thyrotrophs can be identified by immunohistochemical techniques [41]. Immunohistochemical studies have demonstrated cells containing alpha-melanocyte stimulating hormone (aMSH) in the portion of the pars distalis apposed to the neural lobe of the human pituitary – that region corresponding to the pars intermedia of lower species [42]. Within the pars distalis, gonadotrophs, thyrotrophs, and corticotrophs lie mostly in the central mucoid wedge whereas lactotrophs and somatotrophs predominate in the lateral wings [43].

2.1.3 *Pituitary vasculature*. The adenohypophysis does not possess a direct arterial supply (Fig. 4). Its pars distalis is not innervated from the central nervous system [19]. Both nutrient blood flow and regulatory signals come from the neurohypophysis. The neurohypophysis receives arterial blood at its rostral pole (the

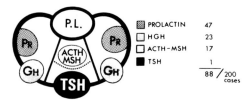

Figure 3. Schematic drawing illustrating the preferential localization of pars distalis epithelial cells and sites of various pituitary adenomas. (Reprinted from Hardy J., Diagnosis and Treatment of Pituitary Tumors. Amsterdam: Excerpta Medica 1973, pp 179, with permission of the publisher).

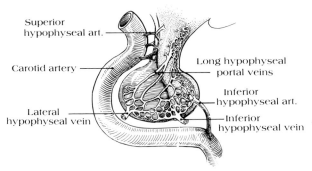

Figure 4. Schematic representation of the blood supply to the human pituitary gland with same perspective as Fig. 1.

median eminence) from superior hypophyseal arteries and at its caudal pole (the neural lobe) from inferior hypophyseal arteries. In some species, including man, a third supply to the junction of the lower infundibular stem with the neural lobe is present. In man, this middle hypophyseal artery is called 'the trabecular artery' [44]. Blood flow between regions of the neurohypophysis occurs with the infundibular stem forming a 'watershed zone' between sources of arterial supply [45, 46].

The neural lobe is drained by paired inferior hypophyseal veins which course to the posterior aspect of the cavernous sinus on either side of the midline [47]. Some blood passes from the neural lobe by capillary and short portal connections to the adjacent pars distalis allowing neural secretions from the neural lobe to influence function in the adjacent adenohypophysis [46].

The median eminence is drained by a restricted system of capillaries and portal vessels which course from the median eminence down the pituitary stalk and break up into a secondary capillary plexus within the pars distalis [48, 49, 50]. Blood containing hypothalamic releasing and inhibiting hormones, which have been released from neurosecretory terminals in the median eminence, is carried by these routes to the pars distalis to control its function [28, 46, 51]. The pars distalis in turn drains to the cavernous sinus [52]. A small region in the lateral wings of the pars distalis drains by lateral hypophyseal veins to the adjacent cavernous sinus [48]. The bulk of the pars distalis drains into the adenohypophyseal limbs of Y-shaped inferior hypophyseal veins [47] which course to the posterior aspect of the cavernous sinus lateral to the midline [46].

2.2 Sellar anatomy and pituitary relationships

2.2.1 The intra-sellar pituitary gland. Most, but not all, of the pituitary lies within the sella turcica – a depression in the sphenoid bone at the base of the skull [22] (Fig. 5). The neural lobe and pars distalis lie within its confines. The median eminence and pars tuberalis (the tuber cinerum) lie outside the sella turcica at the base of the brain. The infundibular stem and pars tuberalis (the pituitary stalk) pass through the subarachnoid space at the base of the brain and connect the tuber cinereum with the intrasellar pituitary.

2.2.2 Sellar boundaries. The sella turcica is bounded superiorly by a dural membrane, the diaphragma sellae, through which passes the pituitary stalk. The orifice in the diaphragma sellae through which the pituitary stalk passes has been measured in postmortem series. Its diameter is variable and is greater than 5 mm in about half the specimens examined [22, 53].

The anterior, inferior and posterior boundaries of the sella turcica are osseous [54]. Anteriorly, the sella is defined by the tuberculum sella and the anterior clinoids. Inferiorly, it is defined by the lamina dura. The lamina dura varies

6

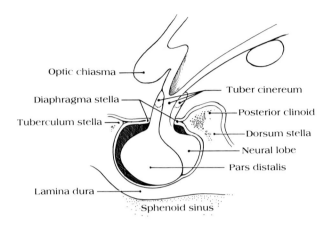

Optic chiasma

Diaphragma stella

Tuberculum stella

Tuber cinereum

Posterior clinoid

Dorsum stella

Neural lobe

Pars distalis

Lamina dura

Sphenoid sinus

Figure 5. Schematic representation of the osseous relationships of the neural and glandular pituitary with same perspective as Fig. 1.

considerably in thickness from approximately 1 mm (in 76% of specimens) to 2 cm [22]. It is the floor of the sella turcica and the roof of the sphenoid sinus. Posteriorly the sella is defined by the dorsum sellae and the posterior clinoids.

The lateral boundaries of the sella turcica, like its superior boundary, are not osseous. They are formed by the cavernous sinuses (Fig. 6) which, like other major intracranial sinuses, are intradural spaces lined by endothelium [55]. The cavernous sinuses receive blood from the pituitary gland via lateral and inferior hypophyseal veins [46, 47, 48, 52], from the eyes via the superior and inferior ophthalmic veins, from the brain via the superior middle, cerebral and inferior cerebral veins, and variably from the dura via the middle meningeal vein. They drain to the jugular vein via the superior and inferior petrosal sinuses, and into the pterygoid plexus [55]. The paired cavernous sinuses are interconnected by the anterior and posterior intercavernous plexuses which lie within the sella turcica. The anterior intercavernous plexus lies in the dura interposed between the pars distalis and the lamina dura. The posterior intercavernous sinus lies rostral to the junction of the neural lobe and the dura of the dorsum sella. The basilar plexus, which lies outside the sella turcica on the dorsal aspect of the dorsum sellae and the clivus, also provides a route of communication between the two cavernous sinuses. The relative sizes of these interconnections are variable [53].

2.2.3 *Parasellar structures.* Important neural and vascular structures surround the pituitary (Fig. 6). The internal carotid artery passes through the cavernous sinus. Its cavernous segment enters the sinus posteriorly from the petrous temporal bone. It passes forward to the anterior limit of the sinus and then bends to form a loop and proceeds rostrally and posteriorly to enter the skull beneath the anterior clinoids [56]. The carotid artery in this region thus resembles a siphon – a bent tube or pipe having legs of unequal length. The carotid artery is the most medial structure within the cavernous sinus and is separated from the intrasellar pituitary gland by only a layer of dura [56, 57]. Within the cavernous sinus it lies in the carotid sulcus of the sphenoid bone. This sulcus is seen as the carotid prominence when the roof of the sphenoid sinus is inspected from below. The carotid prominences lie in the superior lateral corners of the cuboidal sphenoid sinus. The prominences frequently bulge below the level of the sellar floor. The layer of bone separating the horizontal segment of the cavernous carotid arteries from the sphenoid sinus was less than 0.5 mm in thickness, in 88% of cases, and absent in 8% of cases in one recent study [56]. The distance between the paired carotid siphons averaged 14 mm in another study with a range of 4–23 mm [22].

The 3rd, 4th, 5th and 6th cranial nerves also lie in the cavernous sinuses but are more laterally located than the carotid arteries [58]. The 3rd and 4th cranial nerves lie in the superior aspect of the lateral wall, whereas the first division of the 5th cranial nerve and the 6th cranial nerve lie in its inferior aspect. There is at present controversy as to whether these nerves lie within the cavernous sinus surrounded by blood or within the leaves of its lateral wall [59, 60, 61, 62]. Preganglionic sympathetic fibers arising from the superior cervical ganglion pass with the internal carotid artery through the cavernous sinus [55]. The cavernous sinus thus contains within it efferent nerves which control oculomotor and pupillary function, sympathetic nerves which innervate the pupillodilator muscle and Mueller's muscle of the eyelid, and sensory nerves which mediate sensation over the periorbital region of the face.

2.3 Supra-sellar anatomy

2.3.1 *The supra-sellar pituitary gland.* The tuber cinereum lies at the base of the brain within the confines of the Circle of Willis (Fig. 7). It protrudes into the subarachnoid space at the base of the brain. It lies between the optic chiasm (anteriorly) and the mammillary bodies (posteriorly). Above the supra-sellar pituitary lies the third ventricle and the hypothalamus. The vessels comprising the Circle of Willis (the intracranial internal carotid arteries, the anterior cerebral arteries, the anterior communicating artery and the posterior cerebral artery) give rise to superior hypophyseal arteries which supply the rostral neurohypophysis (the median eminence of the tuber cinereum). These same vessels supply the medial basilar hypothalamus. The optic chiasm receives its blood supply from the same superior hypophyseal vessels which supply the anterior median eminence, the anterior hypothalamus and the preoptic region.

2.3.2 *Chiasmal relationships.* The optic chiasm lies in front of the tuber cinereum and pituitary stalk and overlies the diaphragma sella. Its relationship to the tuber cinereum and pituitary stalk is fixed but its relationship to the tuberculum sella is variable. This finding is of considerable importance to surgeons as the distance

8

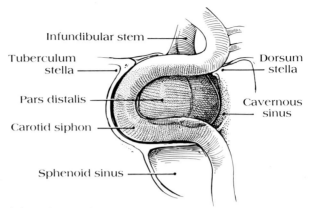

Figure 6a. Lateral view – the carotid artery and cavernous sinus have been superimposed upon Fig. 5.

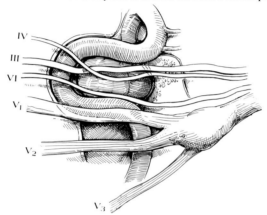

Figure 6b. Lateral view – the cranial nerves within the cavernous sinus have been superimposed on Fig. 6a.

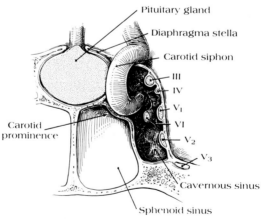

Figure 6c. Schematic representation of the vascular relationships of the human pituitary gland as seen by the surgeon performing a transphenoidal operation. Perspective similar to that observed in a coronal view of a CT scan (e.g. Fig. 14a).

between the back of the tuberculum sellae and the front of the chiasm determines the available space through which the surgeon may gain access to the sella turcica and its contents. In 9% of 225 autopsy specimens, this prechiasmal space was less than the length of the tuberculum sellae and these chiasms were defined as prefixed. In 11% of the specimens, the optic chiasm lay over the dorsum sellae and the length of the prechiasmal space was 6 mm or greater than the length of the tuberculum sellae. In such specimens the chiasm was judged to be postfixed. The remainder (80%) were regarded as normal [22].

2.3.3 *Vascular relationships*. Each suprasellar carotid artery enters the cranium beneath the anterior clinoid processes and courses posteriorly beneath and lateral to the optic nerves and lateral and superior to the diaphragma sellae. It then turns rostrally (lateral to the chiasm) to bifurcate into the middle and anterior cerebral artery. The proximal anterior cerebral artery (A_1 segment) then passes anteriorly and medially superior to the chiasm. In the midline it comes within several millimeters of the contralateral anterior cerebral artery and they are united by the anterior communicating artery. The distal (A_2) segment of each anterior cerebral artery then passes around the corpus callosum to supply the medial surface of the hemispheres (Fig. 7) [65].

3. Tumors which compromise pituitary function

Primary tumors of the neurohypophysis are rare but may arise from displaced germ cells in the median eminence (dysgerminoma, teratoma) or from glial cells in the neural lobe (infundibuloma) [66]. As the neurohypophysis has a high blood flow [67] and as blood destined for the adenohypophysis must first pass through the neurohypophysis [18, 19, 32], metastatic tumors are more frequently found in

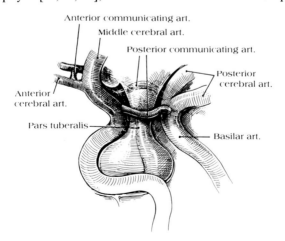

Figure 7. Schematic diagram of the pituitary and its relationship to the circle of Willis.

the neural lobe than in the pars distalis [68, 69]. However, the incidence of neurohypophyseal tumors is far less than the incidence of adenohypophyseal tumors.

Primary tumors of the adenohypophysis are common and comprise about 20% of surgically treated intracranial tumors [70] (Fig. 8). They arise from glandular epithelial cells [71, 72] to form pituitary adenomas and from ciliated epithelial cells lining Rathke's cleft to form Rathke's cleft cysts [73, 74]. The origin of craniopharyngioma, another adenohypophyseal tumor, is controversial with some proposing that it represents squamous metaplasia of the cells lining Rathke's cleft [75, 76, 77] and others proposing that it arises from squamous cell rests in the tuber cinereum and pituitary stalk which are unrelated to Rathke's cleft [66]. Timperly [78] points out histochemical similarities between cranio-pharyngioma and the primitive toothbud.

Pituitary adenomas are the most common adenohypophyseal tumor. In post-mortem series, incidental adenomas have been found in 8–22% of asymptomatic cases [79]. They usually arise in the pars distalis within the sella turcica. Rarely, a pituitary adenoma may arise below the sella turcica along the course of the craniopharyngeal canal – the tract left by the pharyngeal evagination of Rathke's pouch [80, 81]. Although they formerly classified pituitary tumors according to their tinctorial properties after staining with analine dyes (i.e., chromaphobe, acidophilic, or basophilic adenomas), pathologists now classify pituitary ade-nomas by their functional properties as demonstrated by immunohistochemical techniques [82]. Nonfunctioning adenomas do not react with antibodies to known pituitary hormones. Functioning adenomas of lactotrophs, gonadotrophs, cor-ticotrophs, somatotrophs, and thyrotrophs have been described and the syn-dromes caused by their hypersecretion have been characterized both clinically and chemically [3–16, 83]. Functioning adenomas need not secrete a biologically active hormone, but may secrete only a biologically inactive hormone fragment and thus be clinically indistinguishable from nonfunctioning pituitary adenomas [84].

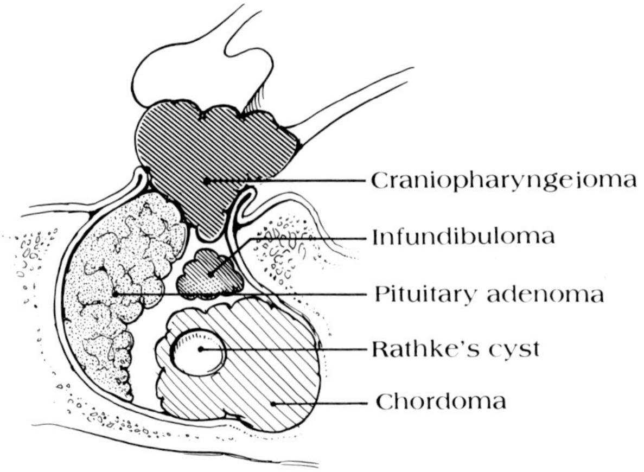

Figure 8. Schematic representation of tumors within the pituitary, both infra and suprasellar.

Tumors other than adenomas arise in the pars distalis. Rathke's cleft cysts are lined by ciliated cuboidal epithelium and apocrine cells. These cysts contain a mucinous fluid and can expand to compromise pituitary and even visual function.

Craniopharyngiomas comprise 3% of cranial tumors and usually arise above the diaphragam sellae in the pituitary stalk or tuber cinerum [66]. These tumors disturb pituitary function by disrupting the portal circulation, the neural tracts within the infundibular stem, and by destroying the median eminence; but not, as in the case of pituitary adenoma or Rathke's cleft cysts, by destroying the bulk of pituitary tissue within the pars distalis.

Lesions arising outside the pituitary in the parasellar region may masquerade as pituitary tumors. Meningiomas of the olfactory groove, planum sphenoidale or tuberculum sellae may alter pituitary, visual and cerebral function to mimic large, nonfunctioning pituitary tumor [85, 86]. In such cases the pituitary gland within the sella turcica is not directly involved with the pathologic process. Hypopituitarism results from disruption of the vascular supply to the hypothalamus or median eminence, from pressure or distortion of the hypothalamic peptidergic neurosecretory tracts passing from the periventricular area to the median eminence or from involvement of the median eminence and infundibular stem. Aneurysms of the internal carotid artery within the subarachnoid space or within the cavernous sinus can exert pressure upon the pituitary gland to alter its function. Intracranial aneurysms arising from the circle of Willis can also compromise visual function as well as pituitary function and mimic pituitary adenomas [87, 88]. Chordomas arising from the clivus or the sphenoid sinus may invade the sella turcica and destroy the pituitary gland [89, 90, 91]. Pathologic states far from the pituitary gland may also influence its function. Pituitary insufficiency, acromegaly, and precocious puberty have been reported with hydrocephalus and resultant deformation of the infundibular recess of the 3rd ventricle and hence of the median eminence [1, 92] (Table 1).

4. Diagnostic considerations

The evaluation of a patient with a suspected tumor of the pituitary gland or parasellar region should be completed prior to making a decision concerning the surgical approach to the lesion and consists of (a) a complete history and physical examination, (b) neuro-ophthalmologic examination, (c) endocrine testing, and (d) radiological testing of the patient. In practice, the focus of the initial evaluation depends upon the source of the referral. However, a team approach to patient management provides optimal care for such patients. The endocrinologist can best evaluate historical and physical findings referable to the endocrine system. The ophthalmologist can perform quantitative visual assessment. The neurologist can best uncover findings of specific neurological dysfunction and the neuroradiologist can define specific structural abnormalities. It is incumbent upon the surgeon who will operate upon the patient to correlate the findings referable to all three systems with the aid of the appropriate consultants before attempting to choose an approach to the tumor.

In evaluating a given patient, it is necessary to determine whether historical and physical findings document dysfunction solely related to the pituitary gland, to the pituitary gland with involvement of neighboring structures, or to the pituitary gland, neighboring structures, and the surrounding brain. Symptoms and signs referable only to the endocrine system suggest that the tumor is limited to the pituitary gland. However, the tumor may lie above the diaphragma sellae at the base of the brain (e.g. craniopharyngioma) or within the sella turcica (e.g. pituitary adenoma). Rarely the tumor may lie below the sella turcica in the craniopharyngeal canal.

4.1 *Endocrine dysfunction – an overview*

Pituitary disorders may be conveniently subdivided into those of hyposecretion and hypersecretion. Pituitary hypofunction can result from the presence of a nonfunctioning pituitary adenoma within the sella which expands and compromises the function of normal pituitary glandular cells. It is commonly held that the normal pituitary gland is compressed within the rigid confines of the sella turcica, and that its failure to function is due to increased pressure exerted upon the

Table 1.

PITUITARY TUMORS		
	Adenohypophysis – Pars Distalis	Adenoma Carcinoma Rathke's Cyst
Sellar		
	Neurohypophysis – Neural Lobe	Infundibuloma Metastatic
	Adenohypophysis – Pars Tuberalis	Craniopharyngioma Dermoid
Suprasellar		
	Neurohypophysis – Median Eminence	Teratoma Dysgerminoma
EXTRA-PITUITARY LESIONS		
Parasellar	Meningioma Aneurysm	
Sphenoidal Clival	Chordoma	
Distant	Hydrocephalus	

normal gland. Other mechanisms such as distortion of the portal system or alterations in portal blood flow have received little attention. Pituitary hypofunction can also be caused by tumors which invade the sella turcica (e.g. chordoma), tumors which metastasize to the pituitary (e.g. carcinomas) or by masses which compress the normal gland within the sella (e.g. aneurysms, dilated infundibular recess with hydrocephalus). Further, pituitary hypofunction can be caused by suprasellar tumors which disrupt portal blood flow, destroy the median eminence or pituitary stalk, or distant peptidergic neurosecretory tracts passing from the periventricular hypothalamic region to the median eminence. The disappearance of normal pituitary function is not a specific finding and may indicate sellar, parasellar or distant cerebral pathology.

Occasionally, disconnection of the pars distalis from the median eminence by a nonfunctioning growth such as craniopharyngioma, nonsecreting pituitary adenoma, meningioma or aneurysm may produce a positive sign – the appearance of galactorrhea with elevated PRL secretion from lactotrophs in the residual normal gland. The elevated PRL secretion occurs in such situations as the pituitary lactotrophs are under tonic inhibitory hypothalamic control.

Hyperfunction of the pituitary gland most frequently implies an adenoma comprised of secretory pituitary cells. The signs and symptoms of pituitary hyperfunction may be both positive and negative. Positive signs include (a) the appearance of acral growth; the development of diabetes mellitus, cardiomyopathy, osteoarthritis, and skin thickenig which accompany acromegaly, (b) the appearance of moon facies, truncal obesity, buffalo hump, striae, and the development of hypertension, capillary fragility, osteoporosis, and hyperkalemia which accompany Cushing's disease, (c) the appearance of tremor, tachycardia, and the development of weight loss and signs of hypermetabolism which accompany the development of TRH secreting tumors and (d) the appearance of galactorrhea in patients with PRL-secreting tumors. Although positive signs (the appearance of an abnormal function) are the hallmark of a secretory pituitary tumor, negative signs (the disappearance of normal function) may also be encountered with the hypersecretion of a pituitary hormone. Elevated PRL levels can cause amenorrhea with infertility in females and loss of libido in males [93].

In general, the appearance of signs of pituitary hypersecretion will direct attention toward the glandular contents of the sella turcica with the expectation of finding a functioning pituitary adenoma. It must be remembered that with growth of a functioning pituitary adenoma, compression of normal pars distalis tissue may also occur. A mixed endocrinologic picture will then appear with positive signs secondary to hypersecretion of one pituitary hormone and negative signs secondary to compromise of normal pituitary tissue – a state named by Cushing [1] 'dyspituitarism'.

Hormone testing usually includes an assessment of basal hormone concentrations and reserve function during provocative stimulatory tests. These procedures may be carried out during a single 4–8 h period but are preferably conducted on

14

separate days. A device such as heparin lock facilitates repeated blood sampling. As shown in *Fig. 9,* a number of provocative stimulatory tests for each hormone are available. A convenient protocol utilizes a combination of provocative stimuli, (i.e., insulin-induced hypoglycemia in combination with L-Dopa, TRH and LHRH) to test growth hormone, prolactin, TSH, LH, FSH and ACTH reserve. The pituitary 'battery of tests' is repeated serially if necessary to demonstrate improvement or deterioration and hormone reserve function following surgical intervention.

For evaluation of hypersecretory states, suppresson tests such as the inhibition of growth hormone with glucose may be required. Growth hormone is measured during a standard glucose tolerance test or in a single sample obtained one hour after ingestion of 100 g of glucose. Since stress is a potent stimulator of growth hormone and other anterior-pituitary hormones, elevated levels under basal conditions are abnormal only if non-suppressibility can be demonstrated. Indirect tests to assess hypersecretion, based upon the biologic action of the hormones, can also be used. Somatomedin C, for example, provides an indirect measure of excess GH secretion.

Posterior pituitary function may be evaluated by indirect as well as direct testing. The finding of a high plasma and low urine osmolality during basal conditions or during water deprivation strongly suggests the diagnosis of diabetes insipidus. Demonstration of a response to exogenous ADH can be used under these circumstances to exclude renal causes of urinary hypo-osmolarity and to establish the state of central antidiuretic hormone deficiency. If the study is

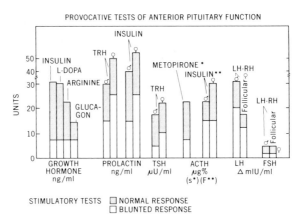

Figure 9. Overview of the tests available to stimulate various anterior pituitary hormones. The height of the shaded bars represents mean levels in normal subjects after provocative stimulation. The open bars reflect blunted responses. Growth hormone, prolactin, TSH, LH, and FSH are usually measured directly, whereas cortisol (Compound F) or 11-Desoxycortisol (Compound S) are used as an indirect marker of ACTH secretion. Note that sex differences must be considered in the interpretation of certain tests. Reprinted from Wells S., Jr. and Santen R.: The Pituitary and Adrenal Glands, Ch. 27. In: Davis-Christopher Textbook of Surgery, D. Sabistan (ed). Phila.: W.B. Saunders Co., 1981, p 747.

carried out under carefully controlled conditions, even states of partial diabetes insipidus can be demonstrated with this indirect testing procedure. Antidiuretic hormone can now be measured with commercially available radioimmunoessays. A protocol to correlate AVP levels with plasma osmolality during the infusion of hypertonic saline allows precise assessment of AVP secretory dynamics.

4.2. Neuro-ophthalmologic examination

Visual complaints, loss of visual acuity and visual field defects are common manifestations of sellar and parasellar lesions. Optic atrophy and pupillary abnormalities may accompany visual loss. Expansion of a pituitary adenoma will displace the optic chiasm superiorly [94]. Distortion of the optic chiasm by a pituitary adenoma (Fig. 10) most frequently produces a bitemporal visual loss (Fig. 11). This pattern has been reported in 70%, 84%, and 93% of patients with pituitary adenoma and visual fields defects [94, 95, 96]. Whether the visual dysfunction which accompanies rostral expansion of a pituitary adenoma is secondary to compression of neural tissue or secondary to distortion of nutrient

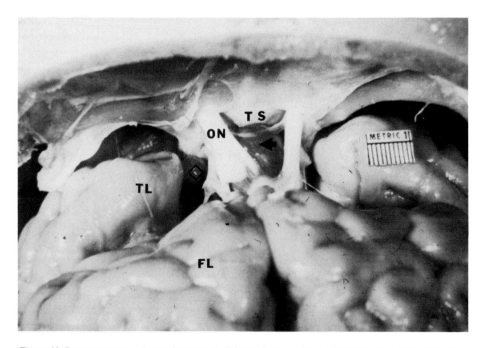

Figure 10. Postmortem specimen photographed from above. A large pituitary tumor with suprasellar extension (arrow) and escape into the left temporal fossa (diamond) between the left optic nerve (ON) and the left internal carotid artery displaces and thins the chiasm. FL – Frontal Lobe, TL – Temporal Lobe, TS – Tuberculum Sellae. Courtesy of R.M. Bergland, M.D.

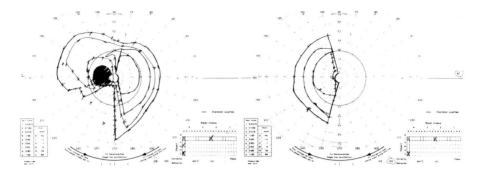

Figure 11. Visual field examination depicting ditemporal field defects secondary to chiasmal compression as in Fig. 10.

vessels is at present unsettled [64, 97]. The visual defect usually commences with the appearance of a temporal slant or cut in the upper outer quadrant [98]. Wilson and Falconer [94] believed that the finding of bitemporal scotomata indicated that the summit of the tumor lay posterior to the chiasm predominantly distorting the crossing macular fibers.

Craniopharyngiomas can displace the chiasm upward and forward as they originate from the tuber cinereum. Pressure on the posterior part of the chiasm was believed by Cushing [85] to be the cause of bitemporal central scotomata that he fequently observed in this condition. Meningiomas and interal carotid artery aneurysms can also produce a bitemporal hemianopia when they arise from a suprasellar site [85, 87, 99]. The finding of a bitemporal hemianopia in a patient with pituitary insufficiency is not of itself diagnostic of a pituitary adenoma.

A complaint of double vision in a patient with pituitary dysfunction raises the spector of an invasive pituitary adenoma [100] with direct involvement of the oculomotor nerves within the cavernous sinus. However, complaints of diplopia may be voiced by patients with bitemporal hemianopia but with normal extraocular muscle function. The double vision is secondary to a lack of overlapping fields in these patients with failure of fusion of the image from each eye. Oculomotor dysfunction with diplopia may also be caused by pressure exerted upon the cavernous sinus by a pituitary adenoma [101] and need not be indicative of cavernous sinus invasion. Facial pain has also been attributed to pressure on the cavernous sinus without invasion of it [102]. However, pituitary dysfunction with diplopia and hypalgesia over the first division of the 5th cranial nerve is highly suggestive of cavernous sinus invasion. If accompanied by a Horner's syndrome, invasion of the cavernous sinus is almost certain [100]. Signs of cavernous sinus invason should alert the physician to the possibility not only of an invasive pituitary adenoma but also of a dysgerminoma [103], an intracavernous aneurysm [59], or an invasive chordoma at the base of the skull [89, 90].

Neuro-ophthalomologic evaluation should then include testing of visual acuity and funduscopic examination. Visual fields should be screened by color confrontation [104] and tested formally by perimetry [105]. Complaints of diplopia should prompt complete examination of extraocular motions as well as tests of pupillary sympathetic function.

4.3. Neurological evaluation

A large sellar or parasellar lesion will alter brain function as well as endocrine and visual function. Mental status is altered in the presence of a large subfrontal tumor or hydrocephalus which can result from the superior growth of a sellar or suprasellar tumor with obstruction of the intraventricular foramen of Monro. Anosmia indicates the presence of a meningioma of the olfactory groove and not a pituitary adenoma as the cause of pituitary and visual dysfunction. The presence of papilledema signifies an increased intracranial pressure secondary to a large intracranial mass or hydrocephalus. Motor, sensory or reflex abnormalities indicate significant intracranial involvement.

4.4. Neuroradiologic testing

A routine series of skull x-rays is a basic first step in the radiographic evaluation of a patient suspected of harboring a pituitary or parasellar tumor. The size and configuration of the sella turcica can be determined by examination of plain x-rays as its anterior, inferior and posterior margins are osseous. The presence of an enlarged or misshapen sella turcica raises the spector of a pituitary adenoma in a patient with pituitary dysfunction. The sella is considered enlarged if its area (measured on the lateral x-ray) is greater than 130 mm^2 (Fig. 12) [106] although McLachlan et al. [107] state that maesurements of sellar areas or volume are of limited usefulness in evaluating sellar size and that the judgement of an experienced radiologist is more reliable. The configuration of the sella turcica can also be assessed on the lateral view. The presence of a 'double floor' suggests that the lamina dura is depressed on one side by an expanding tumor. However, while highly suggestive of the presence of a tumor in a patient with an enlarged sella, the presence of a 'double floor' in a patient with a normal sized sella is not diagnostic of a tumor. It may be found if there is a slight depression in the central portion of the sella turcica, if there is asymmetrial development of the lamina dura, if there is uneven development of the sphenoid sinus, or if the carotid sulcus is prominent

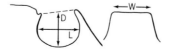

Figure 12. Measurements made to calculate the area and volume of the sella turcica. L = length, D = depth, W = width.

on one side of the sella [106]. Although interest is primarily directed at the size and shape of the sella, coned down views or tomograms are not a substitute for a skull series. From the skull series, information can be gained concerning the size, shape and consistency of the skull which the surgeon will enter.

Tomograms of the sella turcica in the postero-anterior, lateral, and base views help to clarify local bony relationships and to plan surgical therapy (Fig. 13). The floor of the sella can be better defined than with plain x-rays. In the evaluation of the enlarged sella, tomography is useful to identify marked depressions or erosions in the sellar floor, tilting of the sellar floor and herniation of the tumor into the sphenoid sinus. There is at present controversy over the role of the tomography in the diagnostic evaluation of patients with normal sized sellas who are suspected of harboring small pituitary adenomas. In patients with elevated prolactin or growth hormone levels but with sellas of normal size, the presence of thinning or blistering or slanting of the lamina dura is said to be predictive of the presence of a small (functioning) pituitary adenoma [107, 108, 109]. In patients evaluated with elevated circulating prolactin levels, Richmond et al. [110] stated

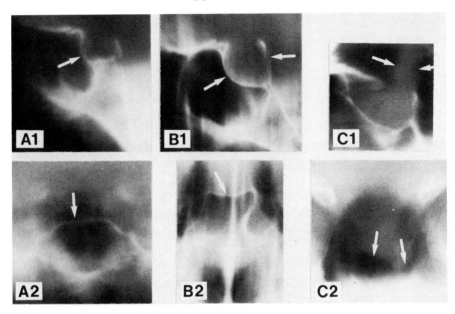

Figure 13. A microadenoma (Grade 1) of the pituitary, which has produced focal erosion (arrows) as seen in the lateral (top) and posterior anterior (bottom) tomographic views. (Note: Focal erosion is a nonspecific finding and may occur as a varient of normal. B, Macroadenoma of the pituitary (Grade II), which has produced assymmetric enlargement of the sella on the lateral (top) and posteroanterior (bottom) tomographic views. C, Invasive macroadenoma of the pituitary (Grade IIIA) which has grown superiorly into the subarachnoid space (top, arrows) as seen during pneumoencephalography and inferiorly (bottom) into the sphenoid sinus (see text for classification). Reprinted from Davis-Christopher – Textbook of Surgery – D. Sabiston (Ed.). Wells S., Jr., Santen R: The Pituitary and Adrenal Glands, Ch. 27. In: Davis-Christopher Textbook of Surgery, D. Sabistan (ed). Phila.: W.B. Saunders Co., 1981, p 746.

that subtle changes in the sellar floor are not only diagnostic of the presence of a tumor but also predictive of its site within the pituitary. However, Swanson and Deboulay [111] evaluated plain skull x-rays and tomograms taken at the time of pneumoencephalography in 85 patients with neurological disease unrelated to the neuroendocrine system. All patients had normal sized sella turcicas. 31.7% demonstrated a double floor on plain x-rays and 16.5% demonstrated 'thinning' of the lamina dura. Burrow et al. [112] examined the pituitary glands histologically, the sellas radiologically, and investigated plasma prolactin levels in 120 unselected postmortem cases. On the basis of interpretation of sella tomograms they found a false positive result in 78% and a false negative result in 81% of examinations. It seems fairly certain that in patients with a normal sized sella turcica, a tilted, thinned or blistered floor is of little significance in a patient who does not demonstrate pituitary hyperfunction [113]. In acromegaly the presence of a pituitary adenoma is almost assured even if the sella is normal size and irrespective of the sellar contour [12]. In patients of hyperprolactinemia [5] or Cushing's syndrome [14], the presence of a pituitary adenoma is not assured in a patient with a normal sized sella turcica. As the tomographic changes which purport to demonstrate small pituitary tumors may be seen in patients without pituitary disease, their presence in patients with hyperprolactinemia or Cushing's syndrome is not diagnostic of a pituitary adenoma within the sella turcica. Independent radiographic or endocrinologic testing is necessary to demonstrate the presence of a pituitary adenoma. The knowledge gained from the tomograms may be useful in establishing a diagnosis in some cases and is helpful in planning a surgical approach if the transphenoidal route is contemplated.

Computerized tomography (CT) permits visualization of the sellar contents as well as the osseous anterior, inferior and posterior margins of the sella [114] (Fig. 14A). The diaphragma sella separates the intrasellar pituitary from the subarachnoid space. As the latter is filled with cerebrospinal fluid of low attenuation and as the sella is filled with pituitary tissue of higher attenuation, the superior border of the intrasellar pituitary and the pituitary stalk can be studied by computerized tomography [115]. Small intrasellar tumors can be identified by this technique (Fig. 14B) and suprasellar tumors are obvious (Fig. 14C). Further delineation of the superior boundaries of a pituitary adenoma can be achieved by the injection of small amounts of air or iodinated contrast media into the subarachnoid space followed by CT scanning in the coronal plane [116]. If the encroachment upon the suprasellar cistern is dome-shaped, the diaphragma sella may be presumed to be stretched over the top of the tumor. If the encroachment is eccentric or irregular, subarachnoid extension of the tumor is likely. Metrizimide cisternography can also be employed to evaluate the contents of the sella turcica if an empty sella is suspected [117, 118].

Classification of pituitary adenomas on the basis of plain x-ray, tomographic and CT findings is useful in choosing an approach to the tumor and in predicting the results of surgery [119]. From a radiologic viewpoint, pituitary tumors may be

20

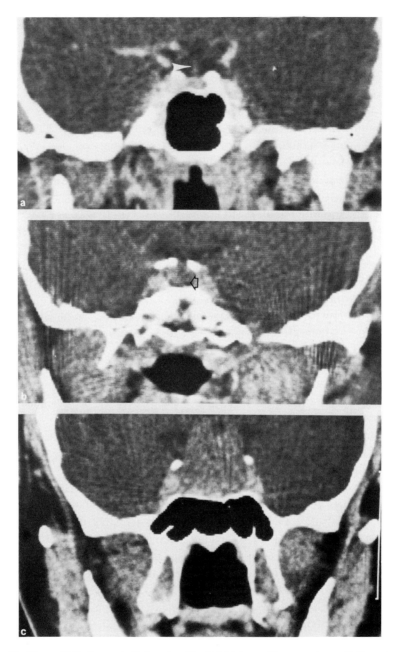

Figure 14a. Coronal CT of normal pituitary (see Fig. 6a). Note small homogeneous pituitary gland, flat diaphragm sella, water density over superior border of gland and straight vertical pituitary stalk (white arrowhead).

Figure 14b. Microadenoma of pituitary gland. Note hypodense area within pituitary at arrowhead.

Figure 14c. Macroadenoma with suprasellar extension.

placed in two groups (enclosed and invasive). Hardy [120] defined enclosed tumors as tumors which remain 'within the anatomical confines of the osteo-aponeural sheath of the sella turcica'. Within the subgroup of enclosed adenomas, the lesions may be graded. Grade 1 – normal sellar size, asymmetry of the sellar floor, tumor less than 10 mm in diameter (as documented by CT scan or at surgery). Such tumors are defined as microadenomas. Grade 2 – enlarged sella but sellar floor intact. Suprasellar extension may be present in this group and is staged. In stage A, the tumor does not extend to the floor of the infundibular recess of the 3rd ventricle. In stage B, the tumor does extend to the floor of the infundibular recess (the tuber cinereum). In stage C, the infundibular recess is elevated and distorted. Hardy [120] defined these tumors as macroadenomas. The second major subgroup – invasive adenomas – are defined as tumors which have eroded through the floor of the sella turcica with herniation of tumor tissue into the sphenoid sinus. In Grade 3 there is localized erosion of the sellar floor. In Grade 4 there is diffuse destruction of the sellar floor. Suprasellar extension of such tumors may occur and is staged A, B or C as with the enclosed adenomas.

This system of grading is extremely useful but by no means complete. The clinical usage of the term 'invasive adenoma' was coined by Jefferson [100] and refers to invasion of the cavernous sinus which is not included in this classification. However, the presence of oculomotor dysfunction, Horner's syndrome or sensory findings in the distribution of the first division of the 5th cranial nerve should alert the clinician of this possibility. If a functional tumor is present, the finding of markedly elevated plasma levels of the secreted hormone is also indicative of cavernous sinus invasion [121, 122, 123]. The classification presented also does not consider the possibility of a herniation of the tumor through the diaphragma sella with consequent subarachnoid tumor spread. However, with these limitations in mind, it has become a useful means by which to classify pituitary tumors and to correlate radiologic findings preoperatively with postoperative surgical results.

Cerebral arteriography remains the only certain means by which to study the anatomy of the cavernous and intracranial carotid arteries. The cavernous segment of the internal carotid arteries has important relationships to the roof of the sphenoid sinus, the sella turcica, and the pituitary gland [22, 53, 56, 57]. These vessels cross over the superior-lateral recess of the sphenoid sinus just lateral to the sella turcica and are covered only by a thin (1–2 mm) layer of bone. In about 8% of cases they lie exposed without a bony covering. Rarely one or both cavernous segments will course medially becoming interposed between the sella and the sphenoid sinus. The intracranial internal carotid arteries and the A_1 segment of the anterior cerebral arteries are closely related to the median eminence, optic chiasm and hypothalamus [53, 64, 65]. The A_1 segment of the anterior cerebral artery is typically elevated in the presence of a suprasellar mass. Large lesions may distort both the A_1 and proximal A_2 segments. Aneurysms are best revealed by this technique [106]. Most importantly, the location and relationships of vascular stuctures to the lesion can be appreciated so that an appropriate and safe surgical procedure can be planned. Recently, digital subtraction arteriography has become available [124–127]. This procedure produces satisfactory images of the cavernous carotid arteries and of their major intracranial branches with minimal morbidity and discomfort to the patient. The authors have employed this procedure in the preparation of patients for transphenoidal surgery. If further details of the vascular anatomy are required, formal arteriography is then undertaken.

Cavernous sinus venography [128, 129] remains the best method by which to study the lateral margins of the sella turcica. When performed by the transfemoral route, advancement of the catheter to the inferior petrosal sinus can be achieved. This procedure permits sampling of cavernous sinus blood for hormone concentration [138] to lateralize small radiologically inapparent adenomas; or,

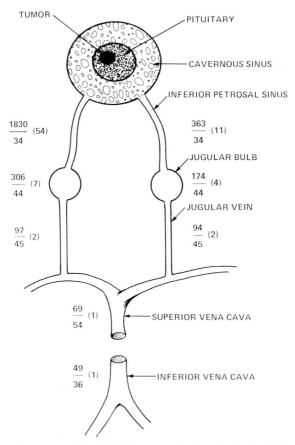

Figure 15. Schematic representation of inferior petrosal sinus, jugular bulb, jugular vein, superior vena cava, and inferior vena cava sampling for ACTH (pg/ml). The numbers in parenthesis represent the central to peripheral gradient. This study shows lateralization of the tumor to the right of the midline. Reprinted from Manni A., et al. J Clin Endocrinol Metab 57: 1070–1073, 1983.

with injection of contrast material to recognize cavernous sinus invasion in the case of larger lesions (Fig. 15).

5. Clinical and radiologic correlation

An accurate history, a physical examination, a complete visual examination, a study of plasma hormones and a skull series will establish three factors: (a) whether the sella turcica is of normal size or enlarged, (b) whether the patient demonstrates signs and symptoms of pituitary hyperfunction, hypofunction or of dyspituitarism, (c) whether vision is normal or compromised.

The presence of a normal sella turcica in a patient with pituitary hyperfunction and normal vision implies the presence of a small functioning pituitary adenoma within the pars distalis or the craniopharyngeal canal. In such patients, pituitary microadenomas can be fequently identified by CT scanning [115, 130]. The presence of a tumor may be suggested by local mass effect (e.g. convex shape of the diaphragma sella , focal erosion or sloping of the sellar floor, displacement of the pituitary stalk from the midline), or by abnormal intrasellar attenuation. Rarely (about 1%), focal calcification within the tumor is noted (Fig. 16). Following intravenous administration of contrast material, focal intrasellar regions of tumor enhancement or of relative hypodensity of the tumor may be observed. Pathological enhancement has been reported in 64 of 85 patients [130]. Selective simultaneous petrosal venous sampling may reveal a pituitary source of hypersecreted hormones, if CT scanning is negative [131].

A normal sella turcica in a patient with pituitary hypofunction and normal vision may harbor a pituitary adenoma. The CT scan will demonstrate similar findings. Cerebral arteriography plays a role in evaluation of patients with pituitary dysfunction but normal vision and a sella of normal size in whom a pituitary adenoma has been documented by CT scanning. It is not employed for diagnostic purposes [132] but to document the distance between the paired cavernous segments of the carotid artery on anterior-posterior views. As this distance varies between 4–23 mm [22], it must be known to the surgeon planning a transphenoidal approach to the pituitary lest the carotid arteries be traumatized in the approach. Arteriography is also employed to rule out an aneurysm lying within the cavernous sinus.

A normal sized sella in a patient with pituitary hypofunction, and visual failure raises the spector of a suprasellar lesion such as a craniopharyngioma or a meningioma arising from the tuberculum sella. In the former instance, suprasellar calcification will be demonstrable in the vast majority of children and in about half the adults [75, 133, 134]. In the latter instance, examination of the skull x-rays will reveal hyperostosis of the tuberculum sella with stippling and blistering of the bone [85, 106]. CT scanning can demonstrate the presence of calcium and cyst formation within craniopharyngiomas whereas meningiomas ususally

24

enhance homogeneously (Fig. 17). However, there may be overlap in these patterns [135]. Arteriography is employed to evaluate displacement of the intracranial internal carotid artery and of its major branches. Lesions arising below the chiasm and elevating it will typically also elevate the A_1 segments of the anterior cerebral arteries (Fig. 18). In the case of meningiomas, a vascular stain may be

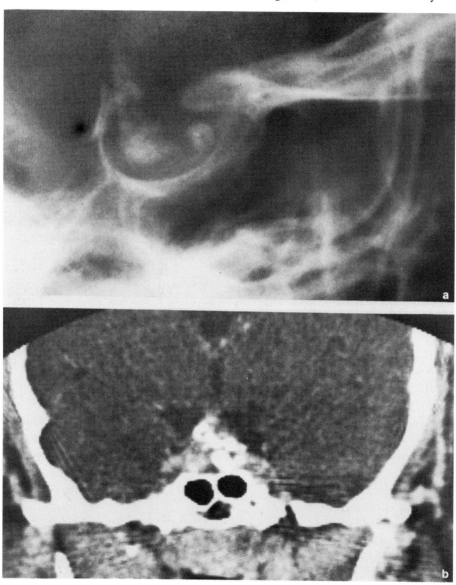

Figure 16a. Lateral x-ray of sella turcica demonstrating focal calcifications within a pituitary adenoma. Note slight enlargement of sella and presence of a 'double floor'.

Figure 16b. Coronal CT scan of same patient. Note extensive intrasellar calcifications.

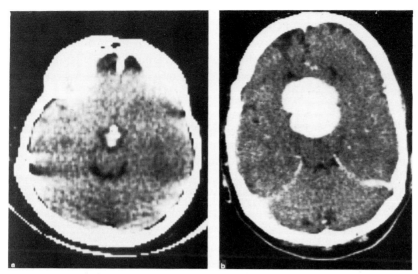

Figure 17a. Horizontal CT of a suprasellar craniopharyngioma. Note calcification.

Figure 17b. Horizontal CT of a large tuberculum sella meningioma. Enhancement is homogeneous.

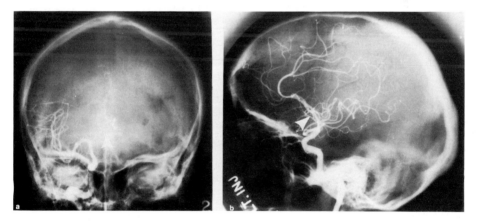

Figure 18. Cerebral arteriogram – AP (a) and lateral (b) projections demonstrates marked elevation of the A_1 segment of the anterior cerebral artery (arrowhead) in patient with a tuberculum sella meningioma. Note sella is not enlarged. Same patient as 17b.

revealed. Craniopharyngiomas are usually avascular [106]. Meningiomas may have a large extracerebral blood supply through the internal maxillary artery and its branches. Preoperative embolization of this extracerebral supply can make surgery safer by reducing blood loss.

Patients with an enlarged sella turcica and pituitary hyperfunction with or without visual failure harbor large pituitary adenomas. In such cases, CT scanning is used for operative planning and not to make a diagnosis of tumor type. Such adenomas demonstrate a heterogeneous picture following contrast enhancement homogeneous; heterogeneous or even ring enhancement; or relative hypodensity when compared to the normal gland [136]. Arteriography is employed both to evaluate the anatomy of the cavernous segments of the internal carotid arteries and to assess vascular displacements of the intracranial carotid arteries and their major branches.

Patients with an enlarged or destroyed sella turcica, pituitary hypofunction and visual failure may harbor a pituitary adenoma, craniopharyngioma, metastatic tumor, chordoma, teratoma, or cavernous aneurysm. Although pituitary adenoma is the most common lesion to produce sellar enlargement, other lesions must be considered if the patient demonstrates pituitary hypofunction on plain skull x-rays. In the craniopharyngioma series presented by Hoff and Patterson [134], 'an enlarged or eroded sella turcica suggested that a tumor was present in 31% of the children and in 51% of the adults'. Tavaras and Wood [106] note that the sella was enlarged in 46 of 64 patients with craniopharyngioma seen at the New York Neurological Institute. Sellar enlargement with destruction is also seen with dysgerminomas (teratomas) [103], metastasis to the pituitary [68, 69] and with invasion by chordoma [90]. Aneurysms arising from the cavernous carotid artery can produce enlargement and destruction of the sella turcica. These changes are usually accompanied by erosion of the ipsilateral anterior clinoid process and widening of the ipsilateral superior orbital fissure – best appreciated with optic foramen vieuws. An eggshell rim of calcification which lies in the aneurysm wall may be seen on inspection of the lateral films [59, 137]. CT scanning may be helpful at establishing a diagnosis as craniopharyngiomas frequently contains calcium, are cystic, and exhibit heterogeneous enhancement. In single cases of a teratoma of the intrasellar pituitary [103] and of an intrasellar chordoma cared for by the authors, CT scanning succesfully demonstrated the tumor which heterogeneously enhanced. Aneurysms frequently demonstrate ring enhancement [119, 134, 138]. Cerebral arteriography is again helpful to evaluate both the cavernous and intracranial carotid arteries and to rule out the presence of an aneurysm. Cavernous sinus venography is employed to rule out cavernous sinus invasion.

6. Surgical Approaches to the pituitary

6.1. The transphenoidal approach

The transphenoidal route leads the surgeon into the sella turcica and its contents (Fig. 19). The surgical approach to the sella from below was pioneered by Cushing [2] who modified existing transphenoidal techniques making surgery both simpler and safer. By 1912 he was able to report the results of 38 transphenoidal operations with four operative deaths (mortality rate 10%). These results were achieved before the routine use of endotracheal anesthesia, availability of hormonal or blood replacement or utilization of antibiotics. Vision was improved in 25 of these 38 patients (63%).

Although Cushing's results were truly remarkable they must be placed in historical perspective. He was operating on patients with pituitary tumors who demonstrated changes in visual and/or mental function and enlarged sella turcicas on lateral x-rays of the skull. These tumors were all Grade II or larger by the classification of Hardy [120]. He operated by this route to 'afford relief to neighboring symptoms' – to improve vision. With respect to endocrine dysfunction Cushing [2] stated 'hyperpituitarism, so far as glandular oversecretion is concerned, is a condition that tends to right itself (and) it must remain for the time-being a matter of uncertainty as to whether or not, in the absence of a degree of hyperplasia sufficient to cause neighboring symptoms, operative measures can hold out any promise of permanently controlling the disorder'.

Cushing abandoned the transphenoidal approach as he felt the incidence of meningitis (2/38), and cerebrospinal fluid leak (2/38) to be significant and as he felt that large lesions could best be dealt with by the transfrontal approach. However, his student Norman Dott at Edinburgh continued to employ the technique. Guiot [139] was trained in this approach by Dott and added to the technique the use of the operative microscope to improve visualization of the gland. With Hardy he developed the intraoperative use of fluoroscopy to monitor the approach and assure accurate exposure of the sella turcica. The transphenoi-

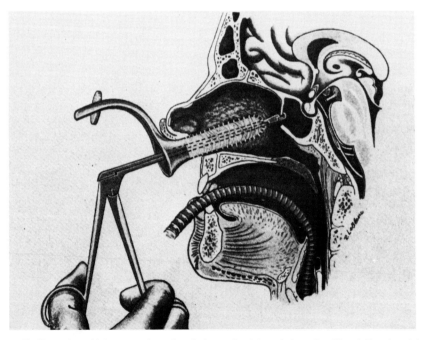

Figure 19. Transphenoidal approach to the pituitary gland from below. See Fig. 6. Reprinted from Hardy J., J. Neurosurgery 34: 582–594, 1971.

dal approach originally developed by Cushing at the beginning of the century to decompress large pituitary adenomas and restore vision reappeared 50 years later as a method to remove the normal pituitary gland from a normal sella turcica in the treatment of metastatic breast cancer or to remove microadenomas which cause hypersecretory states without significant visual dysfunction [140].

The addition of operative fluoroscopy and of the surgical operating microscope [140] to the technique described by Cushing [2] has made pituitary surgery safer and more effective. Further refinements of the approach [141, 142, 143] permit better exposure of the sellar floor and give a more cosmetic result. Operative fluoroscopy permits the surgeon to open the lamina dura accurately and not to open the skull anterior (via the floor of the frontal fossa) or posterior (into the interpeduncular cistern) to the sellar floor with disastrous consequences – a major problem in Cushing's time [2]. Its use also prevents the surgeon from inadvertently progressing into the cranial vault from the sella turcica. With the operative microscope the surgeon can identify the carotid prominences which flank the lamina dura and enter the sella turcica in the midline. The entire sellar floor can be removed without entering the cavernous sinus or injuring the carotid arteries. The dura lying in front of the pars distalis can be inspected to see if the anterior intercavernous sinus is large and bleeding from it might become troublesome or dangerous. The operative microscope also permits complete tumor removal of microadenomas as their appearance differs from the normal gland. It permits exploration of the intrasellar pituitary if the tumor does not present on the ventral surface of the gland. With knowledge of the preferential localization of specific functioning adenomas, of the tomographic and CT findings, and of the results of paired simultaneous superior petrosal venous sampling, the surgeon can intelligently explore the gland removing adenomas as small as one or two millimeters in diameter. With the operating microscope the surgeon can remove large adenomas with suprasellar extension which are capped by an intact diaphragma sella. The instillation of air into the subarachnoid space permits identification of the superior pole of the tumor by fluoroscopy. As air enters the sella turcica the diaphragma sellae becomes progressively defined with continued tumor removal until the diaphragma is identified both by direct inspection through the operating microscope and by fluoroscopy.

Although opinions vary somewhat, the following indications for transphenoidal removal of pituitary tumors are generally accepted. Intrasellar adenomas of all grades and stages can be approached by the transphenoidal route. Enclosed adenomas, even with suprasellar extension can be removed. The transphenoidal approach to the sella is thus employed to remove functioning adenomas in patients with hypersecretory states [140, 144–153] and even to relieve visual symptoms [154] – the primary surgical indication for Cushing [2]. Other intrasellar tumors such as Rathke's cyst [155] or dysgerminoma [103] may be approached successfully by the transphenoidal route. Cranopharyngiomas with a large intrasellar component may be removed by this means [156]. Tumors invading the sella such as chordomas are satisfactorily handled by this approach [91].

Contraindications to the transphenoidal route are subfrontal tumors lying outside the sella turcica such as meningiomas of the tuberculum sella, olfactory groove or planum sphenoidale; craniopharyngiomas which are entirely supra-sellar; and aneurysms. Pituitary adenomas with subarachnoid extension may be difficult to extirpate by the transphenoidal route. Subfrontal or subtemporal spread of the tumor is usually considered a contraindication to transphenoidal surgery. A large dumbbell-shaped tumor protruding out of the sella turcica into the third ventricle cannot be dealt with by the transphenoidal route alone if there is a wasp-waist constriction caused by a tight diaphragma sellae. Such tumors may require a combination of approaches to achieve a satisfactory result [139]. Clinical involvement of the nerves within the cavernous sinus or extremely high plasma levels of hormone secreted by a functioning adenoma should alert the referring physician and the surgeon to the possibility of cavernous sinus invasion and the likelihood that cure will not be obtained by surgical means alone.

The completeness of tumor removal depends upon the criteria employed. If the tumor is a functioning pituitary adenoma, the plasma level of the hypersecreted hormones serves as a tumor marker [146, 150, 152, 157]. Using these criteria, the surgical therapy of 'enclosed adenomas' is far more successful than that of 'invasive adenomas' [120, 153]. The completeness of removal of nonfunctioning tumors is more difficult to assess. CT scanning is the most reliable method at present by which to evaluate the amount of residual tumor following the ap-proach to a large tumor [158]. Reliance upon visual field testing alone is not a reliable guide to the completeness of tumor removal since in the experience with large functioning adenomas visual fields may markedly improve or return to normal but hypersecretion by the residual adenoma may persist.

In summary, if the sella is of normal size and pituitary hyperfunction is present but vision is normal, the transphenoidal route is the approach of choice. If the sella is of normal size and pituitary hypofunction is present the transphenoidal route is probably not indicated if vision is compromised. If the sella is enlarged and pituitary hyperfunction is present the transphenoidal route may be employed and is the approach of choice if the sphenoid sinus is invaded. If subarachnoid tumor spread is suspected, an alternative approach should be considered. If the sella is enlarged and pituitary hypofunction is present the transphenoidal route may be employed if the offending mass is not an aneurysm and if extensive intracranial invasion is not present.

6.2 The subfrontal approach

The subfrontal route leads the surgeon to the optic nerves and chiasm, the pituitary stalk and the roof of the sella turcica (the diaphragma sellae) (Fig. 20). This approach was pioneered by Cushing [159]. It was subsequently modified by

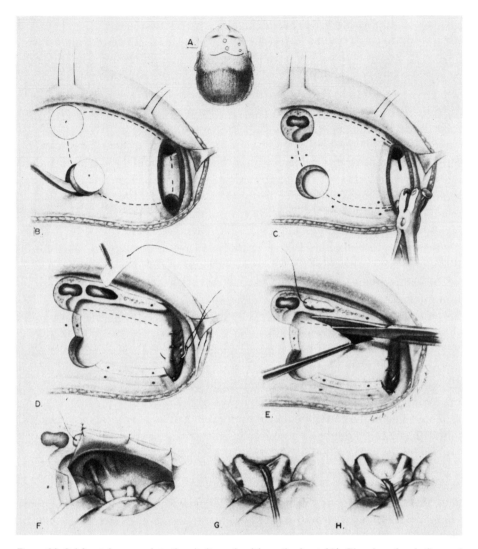

Figure 20. Subfrontal approach to the pituitary gland from the front (A). Planning of scalp flap and bony exposure (B) and (E), elevation of bone plate (D) and (E), exposure of frontal sinus and dural opening (F), (G), (H), exposure of suprasellar pituitary gland and diaphragma sella. Reprinted from Ray B., J. Neurosurg. 28: 180–186, 1968.

his pupil, Bronson Ray, and his approach is still employed today [160, 161] with the modification that the operating microscope is routinely utilized during tumor removal. In this approach, a bicoronal skin incision is made at the hairline and a skin flap with the periosteum is rolled forward in a viser fashion to expose the frontal bones bilaterally. A free bone plate is elevated on the right side for a righthanded surgeon. The base of the bone plate is low – on the floor of the frontal fossa.

The patient has previously been placed in a supine position with the head slightly elevated in order to reduce venous engorgement. Mannitol or Furosemide are administered at this point to decrease brain bulk by withdrawing water from the brain. Spinal drains which have been placed prior to the onset of the procedure are then opened and spinal fluid is removed in order to increase the slackness of the brain. The dura is then opened in a linear fashion parallel to the floor of the frontal fossa approximately 2 cm above it. The details presented above stress the point that every effort must be made to reduce brain bulk to permit access to the suprasellar region without undue retraction on the brain – a consideration not pertinent to transphenoidal surgery.

At this stage the subdural space has been entered. The brain is gently retracted to expose the floor of the frontal fossa. The frontal floor and the tuberculum sella and the right anterior clinoid process are next visualized. Self-retaining retractors are placed to maintain the exposure. Until this point the subarachnoid space has not been entered. The chiasmatic cistern is then opened under magnification and the optic nerves and carotid arteries are brought into view as is the optic chiasm [162]. If the offending lesion is a pituitary adenoma lying within the sella turcica and expanding above it, it is ususally capped by a stretched and thinned diaphragma sellae. A small needle is passed into the region of the sella turcica and aspiration is carried out to assure that the offending lesion is not an aneurysm. The diaphragma sellae is then incised and under magnification the contents of the sella are removed. The diaphragma sellae is then seen to fall away from the optic nerves and chiasm and the carotid arteries on either side. If the offending lesion is a pituitary adenoma that has burst through the diaphragma sellae, the tumor within the subarachnoid space can be well visualized by this procedure and removed from the under the optic nerves and from between the optic nerves and carotid arteries [162]. This approach may also be employed to remove craniopharyngiomas that are primarily suprasellar [133, 163, 164]. The tumor is removed by sharp dissection under operative magnification with surgical microscope. If the offending lesion is a meningioma lying above the sella turcica, it too may be approached in this fashion [85, 86]. Employing this approach the optic nerve and chiasm and the carotid arteries may be visualized during tumor removal – a benefit not afforded by the transphenoidal technique.

Modifications of this procedure may be employed under special circumstances. If the optic chiasm is prefixed, removal of the tumor emanating from the sella turcica from a space between the anterior margin of the optic chiasm and the posterior margin of the tuberculum sella may be difficult. In order to increase the amount of available room in which the surgeon may work, a pneumatic high-speed airdrill is employed to drill away the tuberculum sellae [165]. With this approach the sphenoid sinus is entered and then the sella is entered from the sphenoid sinus. The superior extension of a tumor (craniopharyngioma or pituitary adenoma) behind the chiasm into the hypothalamus and 3rd ventricle presents a more difficult problem. This situation can be foreseen as CT scanning

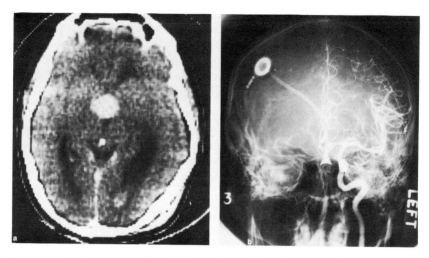

Figure 21a. CT scan demonstrates large pituitary adenoma invaginating the hypothalamus, obstructing the Foramen of Monro and causing hydrocephalus. Patient presented with headache, nausea, vomiting and papilledema requiring emergency placement of a ventriculo-peritoneal shunt.

Figure 21b. Arteriogram shows normal position of A_1 segment of anterior cerebral artery (arrowhead). Compare with Fig. 18a. Recognition of this infrequent radiologic pattern of suprasellar extension is important to planning a safe surgical approach.

will demonstrate marked suprasellar extension but the arteriographic position of the A_1 segments of anterior cerebral arteries will be normal (Fig. 21). Employing the subfrontal approach, the optic nerves and chiasm, the internal carotid arteries and the proximal anterior cerebral arteries can be visualized without undue retraction. However, the lamina terminalis and the anterior communicating artery may be hidden by the paraolfactory gyrus of the frontal lobe (e.g. the most posterior portion of the straight gyrus). It may be necessary to resect a small amount of the paraolfactory gyrus to increase exposure without undue retraction. The posterior border of the optic chiasm can then be visualized at its junction with the lamina terminalis [166]. The distal portions of the A_1 segments as well as the anterior communicating artery can be identified [65]. If the cerebral arteriograms have demonstrated good filling of each anterior cerebral artery from its ipsilateral carotid artery, the anterior communicating artery may be divided after ligation with bipolar cautery or silver clips. Excellent exposure of the lamina terminalis is thus afforded. The lamina terminals is opened gently with bipolar cautery and the tumor may be evacuated through this route [167]. More recently, it has been suggested that the tumor may be excavated first from the region of the sella turcica if it is a dumbbell tumor extending into both the hypothalamus and sella turcica. Following excavation the tumor may be gently displaced through the incision in the lamina terminalis into the excavated sella turcica and then removed from it [165]. With operative magnification, dissection of craniopharyngiomas from the hypothalamus and their removal is now possible [167, 168] but the risks and possible complications are far greater than those following transphenoidal surgery for a purely intrasellar lesion.

The subfrontal route can be employed with intrasellar lesions that exhibit suprasellar extension. It appears to the authors that pituitary adenomas lying in the sella turcica and exhibiting suprasellar extension which are capped by the diaphragma sellae can be dealt with either by a subfrontal [169, 170] or by the transphenoidal approach [154]. The relative merits of the two procedures in each case will depend upon the experience of the operating surgeon. The subfrontal approach is the approach of choice in treating patients with meningiomas arising in front of the sella turcica that have extended over its roof and with pituitary adenomas that have herniated out of the confines of the sella turcica into the subarachnoid space beneath the frontal lobe [169, 170]. In addition, it appears to be an ideal procedure to deal with suprasellar tumors arising in the pituitary stalk such as craniopharyngioma [107] or of the infundibulum such as suprasellar teratomas [171] if there is no significant intrasellar extension. The mortality rate in Dr. Ray's hands employing the subfrontal technique to treat pituitary adenomas with chiasmal compression was 1.2% with no operative deaths in 138 cases operated upon for the first time [160, 161].

6.3. *The temporal approach*

The temporal route leads the surgeon to the ipsilateral optic nerve, the optic chiasm, the pituitary stalk, and the interpeduncular fossa (Fig. 22). The subfrontal region can also be explored by this approach. An approach to pituitary tumors beneath the temporal lobe was initially attempted by Cushing [2]. This route, however, gave only limited exposure and was changed by Dandy [173] to carry it between the frontal and temporal lobes and thus gain access to the region of the sellar roof.

The procedure is carried out through a fronto-temporal bone exposure. The patient is placed on the operating room table in supine position and the head is elevated. The head turned slightly to the left for a right-handed surgeon unless the lesion is predominantly on the left side. Spinal drains are placed. A frontotemporal skin incision is then made and a bone plate is elevated that remains attached to the temporalis muscle (an osteoplastic flap). Properly performed, this exposure will reveal the dura overlying the posterior inferior frontal lobe and the temporal lobe. The pterion (the junction of the frontal bone, the greater wing of the sphenoid, and the squamous portion of the temporal bone) is then removed with a high speed air drill in order to give adequate medial exposure. The dura is then opened. With removal of the pterion and the lateral portion of the greater wing of the sphenoid, the Sylvian fissure may be easily identified as may the floor of the frontal fossa. Retractors are placed beneath the frontal lobe to gently elevate it. The Sylvian fissure is then identified and its arachnoid incised. It is then

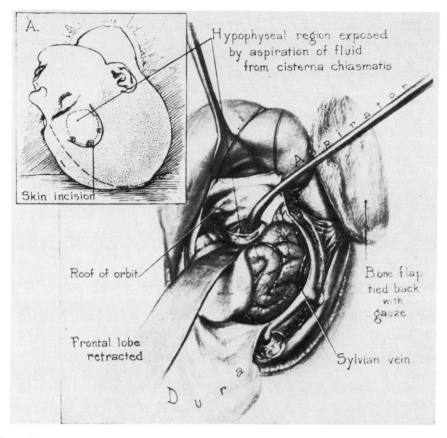

Figure 22. Temporal exposure of the pituitary gland from the side. Reprinted from Dandy W.D., The Brain, p 461. Hoeker Medical Division. New York: Harper & Row Publishers, 1969.

opened widely both medially and posteriorly permitting the frontal and temporal lobes to fall away from each other like the leaves of an open book. In this fashion the frontal lobe is gently elevated off the floor of the frontal fossa and the temporal lobe is reflected posteriorly and inferiorly. A wide view of the floor of the frontal fossa and of the ipsilateral anterior clinoid and optic nerve can be obtained. The optic chiasm can be visualized and visualization can be carried back as far as the interpeduncular fossa [174]. Having exposed the region, tumors may be handled as described under the subfrontal approach. This approach is ideal for posteriorly presenting cranopharyngiomas and for pituitary adenomas which have escaped from the diaphragma sellae and have spilled into the temporal fossa or have protruded posteriorly into the interpeduncular cistern. It permits excellent exposure of the ipsilateral optic nerve and carotid artery and tumors herniating between these two structures can be dissected safely after proper exposure has been obtained. The use of the operating microscope facilitates tumor removal [175]. The exposure is not ideal for tumors which have invaginated into the hypothalamus. Tumors with a broad base which have extended widely to the contralateral side present difficult technical problems with this approach as safe dissection around the contralateral optic nerve and carotid artery is limited by inadequate exposure.

6.4 *The transventricular approach*

The transventricular route leads the surgeon to the roof of the hypothalamus (Fig. 23). It is employed to remove hypothalamic tumors and pituitary tumors which have invaginated into the hypothalamus with obstruction of the foramen of Monro and resultant hydrocephalus. The patient is placed in the supine position. The skin incision is usually made on the right side and a skin flap is raised which extends slightly across the midline and parallel to the sagittal sinus. The surgeon may elect to enter the ventricular system through the superior frontal gyrus [173] or through the corpus callosum [176]. Significant neurologic deficits from either of these approaches are seldom encountered [177, 178, 179]. Having entered the ventricular system by either route, the surgeon identifies the foramen of Monro and its anterior border, the fornix. The roof of the third ventricle (velum interpositum) is then identified as is the ipsilateral internal cerebral vein. The vein of

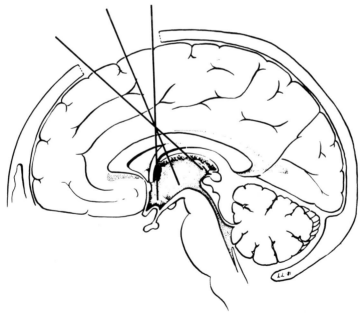

Figure 23. Transcallosal exposure of the hypothalamus and pituitary gland from above. Lines indicate the planes of visual access that may be achieved by retractor angle variation in the midline. Reprinted from Apuzzo, M.: Transcollosal interfornical exposure of lesions of the third ventricle. In: Operative Neurosurgical Techniques, Schmidek H. and Sweet W. (eds). Ch. 39, p 589. New York: Grune & Station, 1982.

the septum pellucidum and the strio-thalamic vein are identified and the strio-thalamic vein is followed into the region of the foramen of Monro and velum interpositum as it forms the internal cerebral vein [166].

Usually the tumor has herniated sufficiently high into the hypothalamus to be visualized through the foramen as monro which is enlarged and there is no need to transect either the fornix which may lead to memory deficits, or the strio-thalamic vein which may lead to infarction of ipsilateral caudate nucleus. If exposure is limited, it may be carried posterior to the strio-thalamic vein. In this region the tinea choroidea may be incised without damage to the internal cerebral vein and the third ventricle may be entered posterior to the foramen of Monro [176]. The tumor may then be removed. Often with large tumors the strio-thalamic vein is stretched and thinned and collateral drainage routes have developed. Under these conditions the vein may be cauterized and divided permitting wide exposure of the uppermost portion of the third ventricle [168]. The operating microscope is employed during these maneuvers and in the subsequent removal of the tumor through the roof of the 3rd ventricle.

The use of this procedure in dealing with pituitary tumors is limited to the special circumstance where the tumor has invaded the region of the hypothalamus. This condition may occur with huge pituitary adenomas as well as with cranopharyngiomas [180] The procedure is a difficult one if hydrocephalus is not present as the proper entry to the ventricle through the corpus callosum or through the superior frontal gyrus is not easy under this condition. Complete tumor removal in the case of craniopharyngiomas has been reported employing this method [180].

7. Summary

Patients with signs and symptoms of hyperpituitarism, normal vision and a sella of normal size should be operated on by the transphenoidal route. Patients with hyperpituitarism, visual dysfunction and an enlarged sella may be operated on by the transphenoidal, subfrontal or temporal approach. It appears that the transphenoidal approach offers the best chance of cure of these patients if the tumor is capped by an intact diaphragma sellae. If there is significant intracranial tumor spread, the subfrontal or subtemporal approaches are preferred.

Patients with signs and symptoms of hypopituitarism, visual failure, and a sella turcica of normal size most likely harbor a lesion other than a pituitary adenoma. Every effort should be made to arrive at a correct diagnosis preoperatively and the subfrontal or temporal route to the tumor should be employed. Patients with signs and symptoms of hypopituitarism, visual failure and an enlarged sella may be approached by the transphenoidal, subfrontal or temporal route. If the offending lesion is a chordoma or a metastatic tumor to the intrasellar pituitary, the transphenoidal route is preferable. If the offending lesion is an aneurysm, the transphenoidal route is contraindicated. If the tumor is a pituitary adenoma invading the cranial vault, the subfrontal or temporal routes are preferred. If extension has occurred within the subarachnoid space posteriorly into the interpeduncular cistern, the temporal route is the approach of choice. Patients presenting with pituitary dysfunction, an enlarged sella turcica, visual failure, and papilledema should be evaluated for hypothalamic invasion and obstruction of the ventricular system at the level of the foramen of Monro. Such patients may be candidates for a transventricular approach to the tumor after a giant aneurysm has been excluded.

References

1. Cushing H: Surgical experiences with pituitary disorders. In: Selected Papers on Neurosurgery, Matson DD, German WJ (eds). New Haven: Yale Univ. Press, 1969, pp 337–356.
2. Cushing H: The Pituitary Body and its Disorders. Philadelphia: Lippincott Co., 1912.
3. Peake GT, McKeel DW, Jarett L, Daughaday WH: Ultrastructural, histologic and hormonal characterization of a prolactin rich human pituitary tumor. J Clin Endocrin Metab 29: 1383–1393, 1969.
4. Nasr H, Mozaffarian G, Pensky J, Pearson OH: Prolactin-secreting pituitary tumors in women. J Clin Endocrin Metab 35: 505–512, 1972.
5. Kleinberg DL, Noel GL, Frantz AG: Galactorrhea: a study of 235 cases, including 48 with pituitary tumors. New Engl J Med 296: 589–600, 1977.
6. Geller S, Ayme Y, Kandelman M, Grisoli F, Scholler R: Micro-adenoma hypophysaire a LH. Ann d'Endocrin 37: 281–282, 1976.
7. Geller S, Scholler R: LH-only inappropriate secretion and pituitary LH-microadenoma. Prog Reprod Biol 2: 176–179, 1977.
8. Friend JM, Judge DM, Sherman BM, Santen RJ: FSH secreting pituitary adenomas: stimulation and suppression studies in two patients. J Clin Endocrin Metab 43: 650–657, 1976.
9. Snyder PJ, Muzyka R, Johnson J, Utiger R: Thyrotropin-releasing hormone provokes abnormal follicle-stimulating hormone (FSH) and luteinizing hormone response in men who have pituitary adenomas and FSH hypersecretion. J Clin Endocrin Metab 51: 744–748, 1980.
10. Cushing H, Davidoff LM: The pathologic findings in four cases of acromegaly with a discussion of their significance. Monograph of Rockefeller Institute for Medical Research # 22, April 23, 1927.
11. Glick SM, Roth J, Yalow RS, Berson SA: Immunoassay of human growth hormone in plasma. Nature 199: 784–787, 1963.
12. Roth J, Glick SM, Cuatrecasas P: Acromegaly and other disorders of growth hormone secretion. Ann Intern Med 66: 760–788, 1967.
13. Cushing H: The basophile adenomas of the pituitary body and their clinical manifestations. Bull Johns Hopkins Hosp 50: 137–195, 1932.
14. Krieger DT: Physiopathology of Cushing's disease. Endocrine Rev 4: 22–43, 1983.
15. Caavioto H, Fukaya T, Zimmerman EA, Kleinberg DL, Flamm ES: Immunohistochemical and electron-microscopic studies of functional and nonfunctional pituitary adenomas including one TSH secreting tumor in a thyrotoxic patient. Acta Neuropath 53: 281–292, 1981.
16. Hill SA, Falko JM, Wilson CB, Hunt WE: Thyrotropin-producing pituitary adenomas. J Neurosurg 57: 515–519, 1982.
17. Tilney F: The glands of the brain with especial reference to the pituitary gland. Res Publ Assoc Res Nerv Ment Dis 17: 3–47, 1938.

38

18. Wislocki GB, King LS: The permeability of the hypophysis and the hypothalamus to vital dyes, with a study of the hypophyseal vascular supply. Am J Anat 58: 421–472, 1936.

19. Green JD: The comparative anatomy of the hypophysis, with special reference to its blood supply and innervation. Am J Anat 88: 225–311, 1951.

20. Kobayashi H, Matsui T, Ishii S: Functional electron microscopy of the hypothalamic median eminence. Int Rev Cytol 29: 281–381, 1970.

21. Rioch D, Wislocki G, O'Leary J: A precis of preoptic, hypothalamic and hypophyseal terminology with atlas. Res Publ Nerv Ment Dis 20: 3–30, 1940.

22. Bergland R, Ray B, Torack R: Anatomical variations in the pituitary gland and adjacent structures in 225 human autopsy cases. J Neurosurg 28: 93–99, 1968.

23. Bergland RM, Torack RM: An electron microscopic study of the human infundibulum. Z Zellforsch 99: 1–12, 1969.

24. Kozlowski GP, Scott DE, Krobisch-Dudley G, Frenk S, Paull WK: The primate median eminence II. Correlative high-voltage transmission electron microscopy. Cell Tiss Res 175: 265–277, 1976.

25. Antunes JL, Carmel PW, Zimmerman EA: Projections from the paraventricular nucleus to the zona externa of the median eminance of the rhesus monkey: an immunohistochemical study. Brain Res 137: 1–10, 1977.

26. Ajika K: Relationship between catecholaminergic neurons and hypothalamic hormonecontaining neurons in the hypothalamus. In: Frontiers of Neuro-endocrinology, Vol. 6., Martini L, Ganong WF (eds). New York: Raven Press, 1980, pp 1–32.

27. Szentagothai J, Flerko B, Mess B, Halasz B: Hypothalamic Control of the Anterior Pituitary. Budapest: Akad Kiado, 1968.

28. Hokfelt T, Elde R, Fuxe K, Johansson O, Ljungdahl A, Goldstein M, Luft R, Efendic S, Nilsson G, Terenius L, Ganten D, Jeffcoate SL, Rehfeld J, Said S, Perez de la Mora M, Possani L, Rapia R, Teran L, Palacios R: Aminergic and peptidergic pathways in the nervous system with special reference to the hypothalamus. In: The Hypothalamus, Reichlin S, Baldessarini RJ, Martin JB (eds). New York: Raven Press, 1978, pp 69–135.

29. Zimmerman EA: The organization of oxytocin and vasopressin pathways. In: Neurosecretion and Brain Peptides, Martin JB, Reichlin S, Bick KL (eds). New York: Raven Press, 1981, pp 63–74.

30. Bugnon C, Fellmann D, Gouget A, Cardot J: Corticoliberin in rat brain: immunocytochemical identification and localization of a novel neuroglandular system. Neurosci Letters 30: 25–30, 1982.

31. Palkovits M: Neuropeptides in the median eminence: their sources and destinations. Peptides 3: 299–303, 1982.

32. Page RB: Pituitary blood flow. Am J Physiol 243: E427–E442, 1982.

33. Bjorklund A, Moore RY, Nobin A, Stenevi U: The organization of tubero-hypophyseal and reticulo-infundibular catecholamine neuron systems in the rat brain. Brain Res 51: 171–191, 1973.

34. Lederis K: An electron microscopical study of the human neurohypophysis. Z Zellforsch 65: 847–868, 1965.

35. Seyama S, Pearl GS, Takei Y: Ultrastructural study of the human neurohypophysis. I. Neurosecretory axons and their dilatations in the pars nervosa. Cell Tiss Res 205: 253–271, 1980.

36. Atwell WJ: The development of the hypophysis cerebri in man, with special reference to the pars tuberalis. Am J Anat 37: 159–193, 1926.

37. Green JD: The histology of the hypophyseal stalk and median eminence in man with special reference to blood vessels, nerve fibers and a peculiar neurovascular zone in the region. Anat Rec 100: 273–295, 1948.

38. Nauta WJH, Haymaker W: Hypothalamic nuclei and fiber connections. In: The Hypothalamus, Haymaker W, Anderson E, Nauta W (eds). Springfield: CC Thomas, 1969, pp 136–209.

39. Pearse AG, Noorden: The functional cytology of the human adenohypophysis. Canad Med Assoc J 88: 462–471, 1963.

40. Nakane PK: Classifications of anterior pituitary cell types with immunoenzyme histochemistry. J Histochem Cytochem 18: 9–20, 1970.

41. Baker BL: Cellular composition of the human pituitary pars tuberalis as revealed by immunocytochemistry. Cell Tiss Res 182: 151–163, 1977.

42. Visser M, Swabb DF: aMSH in the human pituitary. Frontiers Hormone Res 4: 42–45, 1977.

43. Baker B: Functional cytology of the hypophyseal pars distalis and pars intermedia. In: Handbook by Physiology, Vol 7: The Pituitary Gland and its Neuroendocrine Control, Part 1., Knobil E, Sawyer WH (eds). Baltimore: Williams & Wilkins, 1974, pp 45–80.

44. Xuereb GP, Prichard M, Daniel PM: The arterial supply and venous drainage of the human hypophysis cerebri. Am J Exp Physiol 39: 199–217, 1954.

45. Page RB, Bergland RM: The neurohypophyseal capillary bed. Part I. Anatomy and arterial supply. Am J Anat 148: 345–358, 1977.

46. Page RB: Directional pituitary blood flow: a microcinephotographic study. Endocrinol 112: 157–165, 1983.

47. Bergland RM, Page RB: Can the pituitary secrete directly to the brain? (Affirmative anatomical evidence). Endocrinol 102: 1325–1338, 1978.

48. Wislocki GB: The vascular supply of the hypophysis cerebri of the rhesus monkey and man. Res Publ Assoc Res Nerve Ment Dis 17: 48–68, 1938.

49. Duvernoy H, Koritke JG, Monnier G: Sur la vascularisation du tuber posterieur chez l'homme et sur les relations vasculaires tubero-hypophysaires. J Neuro-Visc Relations 32: 112–142, 1971.

50. Page RB, Leure-duPree AE, Bergland RM: The neurohypophyseal capillary bed. Part II. Specializations within median eminence. Am J Anat 153: 33–66, 1978.

51. Green JD, Harris GW: Observation of the hypophysio-portal vessels of the living rat. J Physiol 108: 359–361, 1949.

52. Green JD: The venous drainage of the human hypophysis cerebri. Am J Anat 100: 435–469, 1957.

53. Renn WH, Rhoton AL: Microsurgical anatomy of the sellar region. J Neurosurg 43: 288–298, 1975.

54. Warwick R, Williams PL (eds): Gray's Anatomy, 35th British ed. Philadelphia: Saunders, 1973a, pp 276, 288.

55. Warwick R, Williams PL (eds): Gray's Anatomy 35th British ed. Philadelphia: Saunders, 1973b, pp 693, 696.

56. Bull JWD, Shunk H: The significance of displacement of the cavernous portion of the internal carotid artery. Br J Radiol 35: 801–804, 1962.

57. Fujii K, Chambers SM, Rhoton AL: Neurovascular relationships of the sphenoid sinus. J Neurosurg 50: 31–39, 1979.

58. Harris F, Rhoton A: Anatomy of the cavernous sinus: a microsurgical study. J Neurosurg 45: 169–180, 1976.

59. Jefferson G: On the saccular aneurysms of the internal carotid artery in the cavernous sinus. Br J Surg 26: 267–302, 1938.

60. Parkinson D: A surgical approach to the cavernous portion of the carotid arteries. J Neurosurg 23: 474–483, 1965.

61. Patouillard P, Vannenville G: Cavernous sinus region. Neurochir 18: 551–560, 1972.

62. Umansky F, Nathan H: The lateral wall of the cavernous sinus, with special reference to the nerves related to it. J Neurosurg 56: 228–234, 1982.

63. Ambach G, Palkovits M, Szentagothai J: Blood supply of the rat hypothalmus. IV. Retrochiasmatic area, median eminence, arcuate nucleus. Acta Morph Acad Sci Hung 24: 93–119, 1976.

64. Bergland R, Ray B: The arterial supply of the human optic chiasm. J Neurosurg 31: 327–334, 1969.

40

65. Perlmutter D, Rhoton AL: Microsurgical anatomy of the anterior cerebral-anterior communicating recurrent artery complex. J Neurosurg 45: 259–272, 1976.
66. Russell DS, Rubinstein LJ: Pathology of Tumors of the Central Nervous System. Baltimore: Williams: Wilkins Co., 1972.
67. Page RB, Funsch DJ, Brennan RW, Hernandez MJ: Regional neurohypophysial blood flow and its control in adult sheep. Am J Physiol 241: R36–R43, 1981.
68. Teears RJ, Silverman EM: Clinico-pathologic review of 88 cases of carcinoma metastatic to the pituitary gland. Cancer 36: 216–220, 1975.
69. Max MB, Deck MDF, Rottenberg DA: Pituitary metastasis: incidence in cancer patients and clinical differentiation from pituitary adenoma. Neurology 31: 998–1002, 1981.
70. Cushing H: Intracranial Tumors. Springfield: CC Thomas, 1932.
71. Landolt AM: Pituitary adenomas. Clinico-morphologic correlations. J Histochem Cytochem 27: 1395–1397, 1979.
72. Slowick F, Lapis K, Takacs J: The ultrastructure of human pituitary adenomas. Acta Morph Acad Sci Hung 27: 235–249, 1979.
73. Shanklin WM: On the presence of cysts in the human pituitary. Anat Rec 104: 379–407, 1949.
74. Shanklin WM: Incidence and distribution of cilia in the human pituitary with a description of micro-follicular cysts derived from Rathke's cleft. Acta Anat 11: 361–382, 1951.
75. Love JG, Marshall TM: Craniopharyngeomas. Surg Gyn Obst 90: 591–601, 1950.
76. Northfield DWC: Rathke-pouch tumors. Brain 80: 293–312, 1957.
77. Yoshida J, Kobayashi T, Kageyama N, Kanzaki M: Symptomatic Rathke's cleft cyst. Morphological study with light and electron microscopy and tissue culture. J Neurosurg 47: 451–458, 1977.
78. Timperley W: Histochemistry of Rathke pouch tumors. J Neurol Neurosurg Psych 31: 589–595, 1968.
79. Parent AD, Bebin J, Smith RR: Incidental pituitary adenomas. J Neurosurg 54: 228–231, 1981.
80. McGrath P: The trans-sphenoidal vascular route in relation to the human pharyngeal hypohysis. J Anat 113: 383–390, 1972.
81. Warner BA, Santen RJ, Page RB: Growth horomone and prolactin secretion by a tumor of the pharyngeal pituitary. Ann Int Med 96: 65–66, 1982.
82. Bergland RM: Pathological considerations in pituitary tumors. Prog Neurol Surg 6: 62–94, 1975.
83. Martinez AJ, Lee A, Moossy J, Maroon JC: Pituitary adenomas: clinicopathological and immunohistochemical study. Ann Neurol 7: 24–36, 1980.
84. Ridgway EC, Klibanski A, Ladenson PW, Clemmons D, Beitins IZ, McArthur JW, Martorana MA, Zervas NT: Pure alpha-secreting pituitary adenomas. New Eng J Med 304: 1254–1259, 1981.
85. Cushing H: The chiasmal syndrome of primary optic atrophy and bitemporal field defects in adults with a normal sella turcica. In: Selected Papers on Neurosurgery, Matson DD, German WJ (eds). New Haven: Yale Univ Press, 1969, pp 394–438.
86. Gregorius FK, Hepler RS, Stern WE: Loss and recovery of vision with suprasellar meningiomas. J Neurosurg 42: 69–75, 1975.
87. Jefferson G: Compression of chiasms, optic nerves, and optic tracts by intracranial aneurysms. Brain 60: 444–497, 1937.
88. White JC, Ballantine HT: Intrasellar aneurysms simulating hypophyseal tumours. J Neurosurg 18: 34–50, 1961.
89. Givner I: Ophthalmologic features of intracranial chordoma and allied tumors of the clivus. Arch Ophthalm 33: 397–403, 1945.
90. Heffelfinger MJ, Dahlin DC, MacCarthy CS, Beabout JW: Chordomas and cartilaginous tumors at the skull base. Cancer 32: 410–420, 1973.
91. Mathews W, Wilson CB: Ectopic intrasellar chordoma. J Neurosurg 39: 260–263, 1974.

92. Page RB, Galicich JH, Grunt JA: Alteration of circadian temperature rhythm with third ventricular obstruction. J Neurosurg 38: 309–319, 1973.

93. Thorner MO, Fluckiger EF, Calve DB: Bromcriptine – A Clinical and Pharmacological Review. New York: Raven Press, 1980.

94. Wilson P, Falconer MA: Patterns of visual failure with pituitary tumors. Clinical and radiological correlations. Br J Ophthalm 52: 94–110, 1968.

95. Hollenhorst RW, Younge BR: Ocular manifestations produced by adenomas of the pituitary gland: analysis of 1000 cases. In: Diagnosis and Treatment of Pituitary Tumors, Kohler PO, Ross GT (eds). New York: Elsevier, 1973, pp 53–68.

96. Elkington SG: Pituitary adenoma. Preoperative symptomatology in a series of 260 patients. Br J Ophthalm 52: 322–328, 1968.

97. Kayan A, Earl CJ: Compressive lesions of the optic nerves and chiasm. Pattern of recovery of vision following surgical treatment. Brain 98: 13–28, 1975.

98. Traquair HM: Clinical detection of early changes in the visual field. Arch Ophthal 22: 947–967, 1939.

99. Ehlers N, Malmros R: The suprasellar meningioma. Acta Ophthalm Suppl 121: 1–73, 1973.

100. Jefferson G: The Invasive Adenomas of the Anterior Pituitary. (Sherrington Lectures III). Springfield: CC Thomas, 1972.

101. Robert CM, Feigenbaum JA, Stern WE: Ocular palsy occurring with pituitary tumors. J Neurosurg 38: 17–19, 1973.

102. Friedman AH, Wilkins RH, Kenan PD, Olanow CW, Dubois PJ: Pituitary adenoma presenting as facial pain: report of two cases and review of the literature. Neurosurgery 10: 742–745, 1982.

103. Page RB, Plourde PV, Coldwell D, Heald J, Weinstein J: Intrasellar mixed germ cell tumor. J Neurosurg 58: 766–770, 1983.

104. Trobe JD, Acosta PC, Krischer JP, Trick GL: Confrontation visual field techniques in the detection of anterior visual pathway lesions. Ann Neurol 10: 28–34, 1981.

105. Harrington DO: Chiasm. In: the Visual Field. A Textbook and Atlas of Clinical Perimetry Harrington DO (ed). St. Louis: CV Mosby, 1981, pp 267–321.

106. Taveras JM, Wood EH: Diagnostic Neuroradiology. Baltimore: Williams & Wilkins, 1976.

107. McLachlan MS, Wright AD, Doyle FH: Plain film and tomographic assessment of pituitary fossa in 140 acromegalic patients. Br J Radiol 43: 360–369, 1970.

108. Geehr RB, Allen WE, Rothman SGL: Pleuridirectional tomography in evaluation of pituitary tumors. Amer J Radiol 130: 105–109, 1978.

109. Robertson WB, Newton TH: Radiologic assessment of pituitary microadenomas. Amer J Radiol 131: 489–492, 1978.

110. Richmond IL, Newton TH, Wilson CB: Prolactin-secreting pituitary adenomas. Amer J Radiol 134: 707–710, 1980.

111. Swanson HA, duBoulay G: Borderline varients of the normal pituitary fossa. Br J Radiol 48: 366–369, 1975.

112. Burrow GN, Wortzman G, Rewcastle NB, Holgate RC, Kovacs K: Microadenomas of the pituitary and abnormal sellar tomograms in an uncelected autopsy series. New Engl J Med 304: 156–158, 1981.

113. Muhr C, Bergstrom K, Grimelius L, Larsson S-G: A parallel study of the roentgen anatomy of the sella turcica and the histopathology of the pituitary gland in 205 autopsy specimens. Neuroradiol 21: 55–65, 1981.

114. Brown SB, Irwin KM, Enzmann DR: CT characteristics of the normal pituitary gland. Neuroradiol 24: 259–262, 1983.

115. Syvertsen A, Haughton VM, Williams AL, Cusick JF: The computed tomographic appearance of the normal pituitary gland and pituitary microadenomas. Radiol 133: 385–391, 1979.

116. Hall K, McAllister VL: Metrizamide cisternography in pituitary and juxtapituitary lesions. Radiol 134: 101–108, 1980.

42

117. Gross CE, Binet EF, Esquerra JV: Metrizamide cisternography in the evaluation of pituitary adenomas and the empty sella syndrome. J Neurosurg 50: 472–476, 1979.

118. Ghoshhajra K: High-resolution metrizamide CT cisternography in sellar and suprasellar abnormalities. J Neurosurg 54: 232–239, 1981.

119. Miller JH, Pena AM, Segall HD: Radiological investigation of sellar region masses in children. Radiol 134: 81–87, 1980.

120. Hardy J: Transsphenoidal surgery of hypersecreting pituitary tumors. In: Diagnosis and Treatment of Pituitary Tumors, Kohler PO, Ross GT (eds). New York: Elsevier, 1973, pp 179–194.

121. Lundberg PO, Drettner B, Hemmingsson A, Stenkvist B, Wide L: The invasive pituitary adenoma (a prolactin-producing tumor). Arch Neurol 34: 742–749, 1977.

122. Shucart WA: Implications of very high serum prolactin levels associated with pituitary tumors. J Neurosurg 52: 226–228, 1980.

123. Vassilouthis J, Richardson AE: Prolactin levels in aggressive pituitary tumors. J Neurosurg 53: 131–132, 1980.

124. Kruger RA, Mistretta CA, Houck TL, Riederer SJ, Shaw CG, Goodsitt MM, Crummy AB, Zwiebel W, Lancaster JC, Rowe GG, Flemming D: Computerized fluoreoscopy in real time for non-invasive visualization of the cardiovascular system. Radiol 130: 49–57, 1979.

125. Ovitt TW, Christenson PC, Fisher HD, Frost MM, Nudelman S, Roehrig H, Sieley G: Intravenous angiography using digital venous subtraction: x-ray imaging system. Am J Neuroradiol 1: 387–390, 1980.

126. Christenson PC, Ovitt TW, Fisher HD, Frost MM, Nudelman S, Roehrig H: Intravenous angiography using digital videosubtraction: intravenous cervicocerebrovascular angiography. Am J Neuroradiol 1: 379–386, 1980.

127. Seeger JF, Weinstein PR, Carmody RF, Ovitt TW, Fisher HD, Capp MP: Digital video subtraction angiography of the cervical and cerebral vasculature. J Neurosurg 56: 173–179, 1982.

128. Shiu PC, Hanafee WN, Wilson GH, Rand RW: Cavernous sinus venography. Am J Radiol 104: 57–62, 1968.

129. Takahashi M, Tanaka M: Cavernous sinus venography by transfemoral catheter technique. Neuroradiol 3: 1–3, 1971.

130. Gardeur D, Naidich TP, Metzger: CT analysis of intrasellar pituitary adenomas with emphasis on patterns of contrast enhancement. Neuroradiol 20: 241–247, 1981.

131. Manni A, Latshaw RF, Page R, Santen RJ: Simultaneous bilateral venous sampling for ACTH in pituitary-dependent Cushing's disease. Evidence for lateralization of pituitary venous drainage. J Clin Endocrin Metab 57: 1070–1073, 1983.

132. Powell D, Baker H, Laws ER: The primary angiographic findings in pituitary adenomas. Radiol 110: 589–595, 1974.

133. Matson DD, Crigler JF: Management of craniopharyngioma in childhood. J Neurosurg 30: 377–390, 1969.

134. Hoff J, Patterson R: Craniopharyngioma in children and adults. J Neurosurg 36: 299–302, 1972.

135. Hatam A, Bergstrom M, Greitz T: Diagnosis of sellar and paraseilar lesions by computed tomography. Neuroradiol 18: 249–258, 1979.

136. Sakoda K, Mukada K, Yonezawa M, Matsumura S, Yoshimoto H, Mori S, Uozmi T: CT scan of pituitary adenomas. Neuroradiol 20: 249–251, 1981.

137. Rischbieth RHC, Bull JWD: The significance of enlargement of the superior orbital (sphenoidal) fissure. Br J Radiol 31: 125–135, 1958.

138. Numaguchi Y, Kishikawa T, Ikeda J, Fukui M, Kitamura K, Tsukamoto Y, Hasuo K, Matsuura K: Neuroradiological manifestations of suprasellar pituitary adenomas, meningiomas and craniopharyngiomas. Neuroradiol 21: 67–74, 1981.

139. Guiot G: Transphenoidal approach in surgical treatment of pituitary adenomas: general principles and indications in nonfunctioning adenomas. In: Diagnosis and Treatment of Pituitary

Tumors, Kohler PO, Ross GT (eds). New York: Elsevier, 1973, pp 159–178.

140.   Hardy J: Transsphenoidal hypophysectomy. J Neurosurg 34: 582–594, 1971.

141.   Tindall GT, Collins WF, Kirchner JA: Unilateral septal technique for transphenoidal micro-surgical approach to the sella turcica. J Neurosurg 49: 138–142, 1978.

142.   Kern EB, Pearson BW, McDonald TJ, Laws ER: The transseptal approach to lesions of the pituitary and parasellar regions. Laryngoscope 89, Suppl 15: 1–34, 1979.

143.   Fukushima T, Sano K: Sublabial rhinoseptoplastic technique for transsphenoidal pituitary surgery by a hinged-septum method. J Neurosurg 52: 867–870, 1980.

144.   Hardy J: Transphenoidal microsurgery of the normal and pathological pituitary. Clin Neuro-surg 16: 185–217, 1969.

145.   Wilson CB, Dempsey LC: Transphenoidal microsurgical removal of 250 pituitary adenomas. J Neurosurg 48: 13–22, 1978.

146.   Faria MA, Tindall GT: Transsphenoidal microsurgery for prolactin-secreting pituitary ade-nomas. J Neurosurg 56: 33–43, 1982.

147.   Laws ER, Piepgras DG, Randall RV, Abboud CF: Neurosurgical management of acromegaly. Results in 82 patients treated between 1972 and 1977. J Neurosurg 50: 464–461, 1979.

148.   Arafah BM, Brodkey JS, Kaufman B, Velasco M, Manni A, Pearson OH: Transsphenoidal microsurgery in the treatment of acromegaly and giantism. J Clin Endocrin Metab 50: 578–585, 1980.

149.   Balagura S, Derome P, Guiot G: Acromegaly: analysis of 132 cases treated surgically. Neu-rosurg 8: 413–416, 1981.

150.   Baskin DS, Boggan JE, Wilson CB: Transsphenoidal microsurgical removal of growth hor-mone-secreting pituitary adenomas. J Neurosurg 56: 634–641, 1982.

151.   Schnall AM, Brodkey JS, Kaufman B, Pearson OH: Pituitary function after removal of pituitary microadenomas in Cushing's disease. J Clin Endocrin Metab 47: 410–417, 1978.

152.   Bigos ST, Somma M, Rasio E, Eastman RC, Lanthier A, Johnston HH, Hardy J: Cushing's disease: management by transsphenoidal pituitary microsurgery. J Clin Endocrin Metab 50: 348–354, 1980.

153.   Hardy J: Cushing's disease: 50 years later. Canad J Neurol Sci 9: 375–380, 1982.

154.   Laws ER, Trautmann JC, Hollenhorst RW: Transsphenoidal decompression of the optic nerve and chiasm. J Neurosurg 46: 717–722, 1977.

155.   Martinez LJ, Osterholm JL, Berry RG, Lee KF, Schatz NJ: Transphenoidal removal of a Rathke's cleft cyst. Neurosurg 4: 63–65, 1979.

156.   Laws ER: Transphenoidal microsurgery in the management of craniopharyngioma. J Neuro-surg 52: 661–666, 1980.

157.   McLanahan CS, Christy JH, Tindall GT: Anterior pituitary function before and after trans-sphenoidal microsurgical resection of pituitary tumors. Neurosurg 3: 142–145, 1978.

158.   Muhr C, Berstrom K, Enoksson P, Hugosson R, Lundberg PO: Followup study with com-puterized tomography and clinical evaluation 5 to 10 years after surgery for pituitary adenoma. J Neurosurg 53: 144–148, 1980.

159.   Henderson WR: The pituitary adenomata – a followup study on the results of 238 patients. Br J Surg 26: 811–921, 1939.

160.   Ray B, Patterson R: Surgical treatment of pituitary adenomas. J Neurosurg 19: 1–8, 1962.

161.   Ray B, Patterson R: Surgical experience with chromophobe adenomas of the pituitary gland. J Neurosurg 34: 726–000, 1971.

162.   Gibo H, Lenkey C, Rhoton AL: Microsurgical anatomy of the supraclinoid portion of the internal carotid artery. J Neurosurg 55: 560–574, 1981.

163.   Svein H: Surgical experience with craniopharyngioma. J Neurosurg 23: 148–155, 1965.

164.   Hoffman HJ, Hendrick EB, Humphreys RP, Buncic JR, Armstrong DL, Jenkin RDT: Man-agement of craniopharyngioma in children. J Neurosurg 47: 218–227, 1977.

165.   Patterson RH, Danylevich A: Surgical removal of craniopharyngiomas by a transcranial

44

approach through the lamina terminalis and a sphenoid sinus. Neurosurg 7: 111–117, 1980.

166. Yamamoto I, Rhoton AL, Peace DA: Microsurgery of the third ventricle. Part I. Microsurgical anatomy. Neurosurg 8: 334–356, 1981.

167. Sweet WH: Radical surgical treatment of craniopharyngiomas. Clin Neurosurg 23: 52–79, 1976.

168. Rhoton AL, Tamamoto I, Peace DA: Microsurgery of the third ventricle. Part 2: Operative approaches. Neurosurg 8: 357–373, 1981.

169. Stern W, Batzdorf U: Intracranial removal of pituitary adenomas. An evaluation of varying degrees of excision from partial to total. J Neurosurg 33: 564–573, 1970.

170. Symon L, Jakubowski J: Transcranial management of pituitary tumours with suprasellar extension. J Neurol Neurosurg Psychiat 42: 123–133, 1979.

171. Symon L, Jakubowski J, Kendall B: Surgical treatment of giant pituitary adenomas. J Neurol Neurosurg Psychiat 42: 973–982, 1979.

172. Camins MB, Mount LA: Primary suprasellar atypical teratoma. Brain 97: 447–456, 1974.

173. Dandy WE: The Brain. New York: Harper & Row, 1969.

174. Kempe LG: Operative Neurosurgery. New York: Springer-Verlag, 1968.

175. Van Alphen HAM: Microsurgical fronto-temporal approach to pituitary adenomas with extrasellar extension. Clin Neurol Neurosurg 78: 246–256, 1975.

176. Apuzzo MLJ, Chikovani OK, Gott PS, Teng EL, Zee C-S, Giannotta SL, Weiss MH: Transcallosal, interfornical approaches for lesions affecting the third ventricle: surgical considerations and consequences. Neurosurg 10: 547–554, 1982.

177. Jeeves MA, Simpson DA, Geffen G: Functional consequences of the transcallosal removal of intraventricular tumours. J Neurosurg Neurol Psychiat 42: 134–142, 1979.

178. Winston KR, Cavazzuti V, Arkins T: Absence of neurological and behavioral abnormalities after anterior transcallosal operation for third ventricular lesions. Neurosurg 4: 386–393, 1979.

179. Geffen G, Walsh A, Simpson D, Jeeves M: Comparison of the effects of transcortical and transcallosal removal of intraventricular tumours. Brain 103: 773–788, 1980.

180. Long DM, Chou SN: Transcallosal removal of craniopharyngiomas within the third ventricle. J Neurosurg 39: 563–567, 1973.

2. Acromegaly

BAHA'UDDIN M. ARAFAH, JERALD S. BRODKEY
and OLOF H. PEARSON

Growth hormone (GH) secreting pituitary tumors represent approximately 15–20% of all pituitary tumors. Although acromegaly is a rare disorder, its impact may be important because of its serious complications. It is well known now that if left untreated, acromegaly is associated with a shorter life span [1, 2]. This is mostly caused by the development of diabetes mellitus, hypertension and cardiovascular complications. Despite these associated illnesses, the development of the symptoms is very gradual, so that it may take several years before patients seek medical attention. In our own series patients were diagnosed to have acromegaly 1-1/2 to 25 years after the onset of symptoms (mean 8.1, median 7.5 years). By the time patients present, they have features that are quite characteristic of acromegaly.

Although this disease is most common in the fourth decade of life, it can occur at any age. Whenever excess GH secretion occurs before epiphyseal closure in children, gigantism results. There also, the onset of the disease in insidious and the only clue to the diagnosis may be an increase in the rate of linear growth.

Until recently, it was thought that acromegaly always resulted from pituitary tumors. However, a recent report [3] has shed light on another possible pathophysiologic mechanism for the development of acromegaly and which led to the discovery of the GH releasing factor. In this report [3], a patient with classical features of acromegaly was described who had pituitary hyperplasia on histologic examination of the pituitary. Further work up led to the discovery of a pancreatic tumor which when excised resulted in a remission of the acromegaly. The hypothesis made was that the pancreatic tumor was producing a GH releasing factor which caused the pituitary hyperplasia and resulted in the clinical picture of acromegaly. A pancreatic tumor from a similar patient was used to isolate, characterize and discover the amino acid sequence of GH releasing factor [GRF, 4, 5]. The role of GRF in the initial development of pituitary tumors is not clear at the present time. Despite some speculations the general belief is that acromegaly and gigantism are caused invariably by primary GH secreting pituitary tumors. However, in an occasional patient other pathophysiologic mechanisms may be involved.

Acromegaly still remains a disfiguring and debilitating disease, primarily be-

Santen, R.J. and Manni, A. (eds.), Diagnosis and management of endocrine-related tumors. ISBN 0-89838-636-5.
© *1984, Martinus Nijhoff Publishers, Boston. Printed in the Netherlands.*

cause of its cardiovascular, rheumatic and cosmetic complications. Over the past decade, an increasing number of patients have been diagnosed early in whom appropriate treatment can correct the biochemical abnormalities which may hopefully result in reversal of all the associated abnormalities.

In treating patients which this disease, several therapeutic goals should be kept in mind: (1) symptomatic relief, (2) halting the progression of the disease, (3) return of hGH level and dynamics of secretion to normal, (4) preserving normal pituitary function, and (5) elimination of mechanical problems related to the growth of the adenoma.

Among the available therapeutic options transsphenoidal microsurgery can achieve some or all of these therapeutic goals in a large proportion of these patients. In patients with microadenomas, all of these goals can be realized by selective adenomectomy while in others with larger and more invasive tumors, aggressive treatment may lead to complete removal of the adenoma and also to hypopituitarism.

In evaluating the effectiveness of surgical therapy one of the limitations frequently encountered in the published series is a strict definition of 'cure'. In some series, this meant a serum hGH level of <10 ng/ml, while in others it was <5 ng/ml. Our current experience and previous data reported by us [6] and by others [7] have clearly shown that these definitions are not sufficient. We believe that a patient should not be labelled as cured until the serum GH level is in the normal range and responds appropriately to dynamic testing. The most commonly used dynamic tests in our institution are: oral glucose tolerance, insulin induced hypoglycemia and TRH stimulation test. The latter is extremely valuable, especially when preoperative testing has shown a rise in serum GH after its administration.

We will review our experience with 40 patients with acromegaly treated at our institution over the past 12 years. A brief description of the clinical, biochemical, radiological, pathological and surgical findings in these patients will be reviewed. The outcome of transsphenoidal microsurgery as well as subsequent treatments in some patients will be reviewed.

1. Methods

Pre- and postoperative endocrine studies were performed in the Clinical Research Center. The following dynamic studies of GH secretion were used: oral glucose tolerance (OGTT), insulin tolerance test (ITT), arginine stimulation test (AST), thyrotropin releasing hormone (TRH) test and an overnight study (blood drawn every 2 hours over 14 hours) to evaluate the nocturnal rise in GH. More recently we have utilized plasma somatomedin C level pre- and postoperatively.

The basal GH level in normals in our laboratory is less than 5 ng/ml. After an oral glucose load (75 g), serum GH is decreased in normals to less than 2 ng/ml.

Following insulin induced hypoglycemia or arginine infusion (30 g given IV over 30 min) serum GH level increased to ≥8 ng/ml. Following TRH administration (500 μg IV), there is no appreciable change in serum GH level in normal people. However, a positive response of GH to TRH seen in some patients with acromegaly is defined as an increase of ≥50% over baseline and an increment of 5 ng/ml or more. A normal response of GH to L-dopa (500 mg) is a rise in serum GH to ≥8 ng/ml. Although few patients had all these studies postoperatively, all had at least 2 of the dynamic tests performed.

Prolactin dynamic tests were done in some but not all patients. These included: overnight study (blood drawn every 2 hours for 14 hours), TRH and perphenazine (8 mg orally) stimulation as well as suppression with L-Dopa. The normal basal level of serum PRL is ≤25 ng/ml in women and ≤20 ng/ml in men. A normal response to TRH or perphenazine stimulation is ≥100% increase above the baseline with an increment of ≥8 ng/ml. Following L-dopa, serum PRL level decreases in normals to <7 ng/ml. In addition to GH and PRL dynamics, the following were measured pre- and postoperatively: T_4, T_3 resin uptake, serum cortisol and testosterone [8] level in male patients. The folowing serum hormone levels were measured by specific RIA using materials supplied by the NIAMDD: GH [9], PRL [10], FSH [11], LH [12] and TSH [13]. Somatomedin C level was measured by Nichols Laboratory, San Pedro, California. These studies were performed preoperatively and 3 to 6 months postoperatively. In some patients repeat studies were performed at varying intervals (1–6 years) after surgery.

2. Patients

The patients reported in this series include 40 patients who had clinical and biochemical features of acromegaly. All underwent transsphenoidal microsurgery by one neurosurgeon (JSB) over a period of 12 years. Our series includes 20 females and 20 males (Table 1). The mean age at the time of surgery, which is roughly the same time of diagnosis for most patients, was 42.1 with a range of 19–69 years. The onset of symptoms in all patients ranged from 1-1/2 to 24 years with a mean of 8.1 years (median 7.5 years). The signs and symptoms present at the time of surgery are outlined in Table 1. Of interest was the presence of galactorrhea in 4 women of whom 2 had elevated serum PRL levels while the other two had normal levels. Oligo/amenorrhea was present in 12 to 16 premenopausal women at the time of presentation. Four of the women with menstrual abnormalities had associated hyper prolactinemia while the others had normal PRL levels. Impotence was present in 6 men who otherwise had normal pituitary function. Of these 6 men, 3 had elevated serum PRL levels. Three patients had total hypopituitarism that was related to previous treatment (transfrontal craniotomy and radiation) given at other institutions.

Frank diabetes mellitus was present in only 5 of the 40 patients. However,

Table 1. Clinical presentation in 40 patients with acromegaly

	Males	Females		Males	Females
Total	20	20	Oligo/Amenorrhea	–	12
Acral changes	20	20	Galactorrhea	–	4
Increased soft tissue	20	20	Impotence	6	–
Hyperhydrosis	12	15	Visual field defects	4	3
Headaches	12	10	Hypopituitarism	1	2
Diabetes mellitus	3	2			

impaired glucose tolerance was diagnosed in a total of 16 patients.

None of the patients in this series had symptoms of clinically significant airway obstruction during sleep.

2.1 *Preoperative GH data.* The basal serum GH level in our patients ranged between 7 and 310 ng/ml with a mean of 68.3 ng/ml (Fig. 1). There was no sleep related rise in serum GH in 29 of 33 patients tested. Following a glucose load, 22 patients (55%) had no change in serum GH level, while 13 (37.5%) had a paradoxical rise and 5 (12.5%) had a partial suppression of serum GH level. Of 21 patients who had a TRH test performed preoperatively, 13 (62%) had a rise in serum GH during the test. Eight patients had either AST or an ITT and in no patient was there a rise in serum hGH during these tests.

Somatomedin C level measurement has been recently introduced in the evaluation of patients with acromegaly. All 10 patients on whom somatomedin C level was measured preoperatively had elevated levels ranging between 4.0 and 12 U/ml (normal <2.0 U/ml).

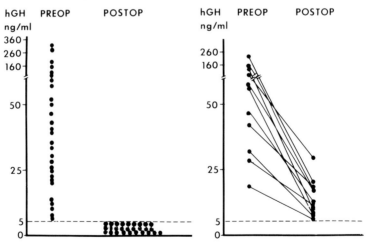

Figure 1. Pre- and postoperative basal GH levels in patients with acromegaly. The *left panel* depicts those with postop GH levels less than 5 ng/ml, while the *right panel* depicts those with postop GH levels greater than 5 ng/ml.

2.2 *Preoperative PRL data.* Serum PRL level was elevated in 11 of 38 patients (29%) in whom the level was determined. Table 2 summarizes the data on PRL dynamics pre- and postoperatively in these patients. Three additional patients had a normal basal level, but blunted responses to stimulation with TRH and perphenazine.

2.3 *Gonadal function.* Hyperprolactinemia is well known to cause decreased libido and impotence in males as well as amenorrhea and galactorrhea in females [14, 15]. On the other hand, large pituitary tumors of any type can result in secondary hypogonadism as part of a state of partial or panhypopituitarism [16]. Knowing this would help clarify the pathophysiology of hypogonadism in patients with acromegaly. Of 11 patients with hyperprolactinemia 4 were postmenopausal women. Serum gonadotropin levels were appropriately elevated in two of these 4 patients. Of 4 premenopausal women with hyperprolactinemia, 3 had amenorrhea and one had irregular menses. Amenorrhea was present in 6 additional premenopausal women who had normal PRL levels. Of great interest was the fact that two of the latter group of patients with normal PRL levels also had galactorrhea. TRH and perphenazine resulted in a blunted rise in serum PRL in these 2 patients. Whether the galactorrhea present in these 2 patients reflects the lactogenic properties of hGH or whether it is related to PRL sensitivity is not clear. In both patients the galactorrhea gradually disappeared within 3 months after surgery. Both women who had panhypopituitarism preoperatively presented with amenorrhea.

Three adult male patients who also had elevated PRL levels, complained of

Table 2. Prolactin dynamic studies in patients with acromegaly and hyperprolactinemia

Patient	Preoperative			Postoperative			Postoperative GH dynamics
	Basal (ng/ml)	Response to		Basal (ng/ml)	Response to		
		TRH	pheno-thiazines		TRH	pheno-thiazines	
1	865	–	–	45	flat	–	high GH
2	820	flat	–	80	flat	–	high GH
3	245	–	–	5	–	–	high GH
4	124	flat	flat	4	nl	nl	cure
5	55	sluggish	–	12	nl	–	nl GH; abn dyn
6	47	–	flat	8	–	nl	cure
7	40	–	flat	10	–	abn	nl GH; abn dyn
8	37	–	flat	7	nl	nl	cure
9	35	flat	flat	<1	abn	–	cure; hypopit
10	32	sluggish	flat	6	nl	–	nl GH; abn dyn
11	32	flat	–	7	flat	–	nl GH; abn dyn

nl: normal; abn: abnormal; dyn: dynamics.

impotence and decreased libido associated with low serum testosterone values and low-normal gonadotropin levels. Three other patients who had normal PRL and low serum testosterone levels presented with similar complaints. Of these 3 patients, gonadotropin levels were slightly elevated in one and normal in the remaining 2.

2.4 *Other endocrine data.* One patient had hypothyroidism associated with low serum TSH level. Three patients had panhypopituitarism from previous forms of treatment.

One patient had hyperparathyroidism 2 years before she presented with acromegaly. There was no evidence of any of the other common features of MEA-I in this patient or any of her immediate family members. The pituitary adrenal axis was impaired in 2 patients who also had hypogonadism.

2.5 *Radiological evaluation.* The size of the sella turcica was evaluated in all patients by measuring the longest anteroposterior dimension from the anterior wall to the dorsum on a 10% magnified lateral skull film. The sella turcica was considered to be minimally enlarged when the A-P dimension was greater than 15 but less than 19 mm. A grossly enlarged sella had an A-P dimension of 19 mm or greater.

Polytomography of the sella was performed in 40 patients and was abnormal in all. The abnormalities ranged from asymmetry, thinning of the wall to gross destruction of the sella (Table 3). The sella was considered to be minimally enlarged in 19 and grossly enlarged in 21. Erosion of the bone was noted on polytomography in 18 patients of whom 15 had grossly enlarged sellas (Table 3).

Prior to 1977, pneumoencephalograms were performed on 15 patients, 5 of whom had evidence of *suprasellar* extension. One patient had a coexistant extension of CSF into the sella turcica, the so-called 'empty sella'.

CT scans were performed on a total of 17 patients. The technique of scanning and resolution of each unit varied over the past few years. However, all scans were abnormal showing intrasellar masses and in some (6 of 17 patients) showing suprasellar extension.

Table 3. Abnormalities of the sella turcica seen on polytomography

	No.	No. cured	No. with extension*
Minimal enlargement, no erosion	16	12	6
Minimal enlargement, with erosion	3	1	2
Gross enlargement, no erosion	6	4	2
Gross enlargement, with erosion	15	3	13
Total	40	20	23

* Determined intraoperatively.

2.6 *Neuroophthalmological evaluation.* None of the patients had abnormalities in extraocular muscle function. Formal visual field testing was performed pre-operatively on 24 patients and was abnormal in only 7. These abnormalities ranged between quadrianopic defect to complete bitemporal hemianopsia (4 patients).

3. Surgery

Transphenoidal microsurgical exploration of the sella turcica was performed on all patients by one neurosurgeon (JSB) over a 12 year period. The surgeon usually identified the tumor and the normal tissue if the latter was seen. This was usually confirmed by intraoperative frozen section biopsy.

Our philosophy was to attempt to make every effort to remove all the tumor whenever this was feasible. In doing so, one would run the risk of the develop-ment of panhypopituitarism postoperatively. This was routinely discussed with the patient prior to surgery and a decision was usually made in advance as to whether complete hypophysectomy might be performed or not. Total hypo-physectomy was recommended whenever the tumor was invasive and normal pituitary tissue could not be left intact without the risk of leaving tumor behind. In children and in patients where fertility was of concern, the decision is individu-alized depending on the circumstances.

Patients are labelled to have extrasellar tumor extension based on the operative finding. Extension occurred infrasellar into the sphenoid sinus, laterally into the cavernous sinus or superiorly into the suprasellar region. Extension in more than one direction could be readily seen. Multiple intraoperative biopsies were done when needed to insure complete removal of the adenoma. A hemihypophysec-tomy was usually performed on the side where the tumor was whenever this procedure was feasible. This was done to insure removal of pituitary tissue just adjacent to the tumor where adenomatous cells may infiltrate without being grossly apparent.

We do not routinely give steroids to patients before, during or after trans-sphenoidal surgery. However, patients who were known to have hypopituitarism preoperatively were replaced adequately and covered with steroids during and after surgery. In patients where complete hypophysectomy was performed, intra and postoperative steroid treatment was given. In all other patients, serum cortisol levels were monitored in the first few days after surgery to ensure adequate ACTH reserve. Whenever adrenal insufficiency was suspected, ster-oids were administered immediately after blood for cortisol level determination was drawn.

Patients were up and around by the first postoperative day. Patients commonly complained about headache during the first 1 to 3 days which gradually resolved. Careful monitoring of water and electrolyte balance was done routinely. The majority of patients were discharged home in one week and were seen in follow up in 3 to 4 weeks. Antibiotics in the form of sulfa drug (Gantrisin) were administered prophylactically for 3 weeks after surgery.

After TRH became available for clinical testing, the test has been routinely performed on patients just before discharge from the hospital. Patients were readmitted in 3 to 6 months after surgery for detailed endocrine studies as described previously.

3.1 *Surgical findings.* Adenomas were easily identified at the time of surgery in all 40 patients. Extrasellar extension of the adenoma was noted intraoperatively in 23 patients (table 3). Many patients had extension into more than one area. While 11 patients had suprasellar extension, 17 had extension into the sphenoid sinus and 5 into the cavernous sinus. Total hypophysectomy was performed in 7 patients, 3 of whom had panhypopituitarism preoperatively. The remaining 33 patients had selective tumor removal as described earlier.

3.2 *Pathological findings.* Routine histological studies perfomed on the adenomas revealed that 22 were eosinophilic and 16 chromophobic in nature, using the old nomenclature. Immunoperoxidase staining [17] for GH and PRL was performed on sections of the adenomas in 21 patients. All adenomas stained positively for GH. In addition 8 of these adenomas stained positively for PRL. Serum PRL level was elevated in only 6 of these 8 patients. Two adenomas removed from other patients known to have hyperprolactinemia preoperatively showed few scattered cells positively staining for PRL. In one case we were able to demonstrate that the same cell population stained for both GH and PRL. In the other adenomas studied, different cell populations stained positively for either PRL or GH.

One patient who was considered cured of acromegaly died 23 months after surgery in an automobile accident. An autopsy was performed which showed normal pituitary tissue without any gross or microscopic evidence of an adenoma.

3.3 *Postoperative GH data.* The basal serum GH levels after surgery are shown in figure 1 in all patients. Comparison is made with the preoperative level in all patients. The basal level was measured 1 week to 6 months postoperatively. The basal GH level was normal (<5 ng/ml) in 28 patients (70%), 5–10 ng/ml in 6 patients and >10 ng/ml in the remaining 6 patients. A significant decrease in serum GH level occurred in all patients (Fig. 1). The preoperative serum GH level was not significantly different in patients who had normal as compared to those who had elevated postoperative levels. Of 28 patients with normal basal GH levels, 18 had normal dynamics of GH secretion (i.e., normal responses to suppression and stimulation, Fig. 2) as well as normal pituitary function. Two additional patients had panhypopituitarism including undetectable or low serum

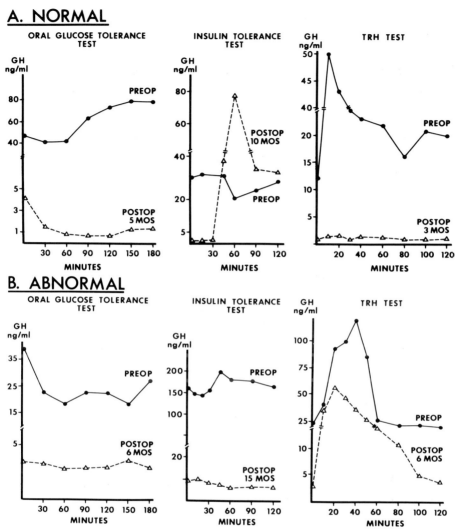

Figure 2. Pre- and postoperative GH dynamic studies in patients with acromegaly. A: Restoration of dynamics to normal. B: Persistence of abnormal GH dynamics postoperatively despite a normal serum GH basal level. (Reproduced with permission from the Journal of Clinical Endocrinology and Metabolism 50: 578–585, 1980.)

GH levels that did not change after glucose loading or TRH stimulation. These 2 patients are considered cured at the expense of being hypopituitary. Thus of the 28 patients with normal basal GH level 20 are considered cured of acromegaly. These patients have been followed for a variable period of time ranging from 9 to 140 months (mean = 78 months, median = 72 months) without any evidence of recurrence. Some of these 20 patients had repeated studies 6 to 72 months after surgery and were consistently normal. Each patient who was considered cured had a minimum of 2 dynamic tests performed postoperatively. An example of the return of GH dynamics to normal in these patients is shown in Fig. 2.

The persistence of abnormalities in GH dynamics in a group of 8 patients despite a normal basal level of GH is of great interest. Although this may represent hypothalamic or other abnormalities in GH secretion, our data strongly suggest that was not the case. During the follow up of these 8 patients, 3 had a biochemical as well as a clinical recurrence of symptoms. This occurred within one year of surgery. The remaining 5 patients had been followed up for 24 to 69 months (mean 41 months) without a significant change in biochemical or clinical evaluation. In 2 of these patients the GH response to glucose is borderline normal (suppressed to 2 to 3 ng/ml) but there was a significant rise in GH after TRH administration (Fig. 2B).

We believe that the persistence of abnormalities in GH dynamics represents in all probability an incomplete removal of the adenoma. We continue to monitor these patients clinically and biochemically for evidence of recurrence in the future.

Six additional patients had lowering of basal GH level to values between 5 and 10 ng/ml while the remaining 6 patients had levels greater than 10 ng/ml (Fig. 1). All patients had significant decrease in GH level postoperatively. The dynamics of GH secretion were abnormal in all patients with a basal level >5 ng/ml.

The importance of extrasellar extension in influencing the outcome of surgery can be appreciated if one analyzes the data in Table 4. In the absence of extrasellar extension, 16 of 17 patients had normal GH levels postoperatively. In fact 15 of these 17 patients were believed to be cured. In contrast only 5 of 23 patients with extrasellar extension were cured.

The number of patients who were treated by different modalities preoperatively is relatively small (11 patients). However, it appears that transsphenoidal surgery could be effective in these patients (Table 5). The cure rate in this group (36%) is slightly lower than in patients who never received any previous treatment (55%). However, the number of patients is relatively small to draw any

Table 4. Postoperative GH data in 40 patients

	hGH (ng/ml)				
	<5 nl dynamics	<5 hypopit	<5 abn dyn	5–10 abn dyn	>10 abn dyn
Extrasellar extension*	4	1	7	5	6
No extrasellar extension*	14	1	1	1	0
Total	18	2	8	6	6

* Determined intraoperatively.
nl: normal; abn: abnormal; dyn: dynamics.

Table 5. Postoperative GH data in patients treated previously and those who had no treatment before transsphenoidal surgery

	Total	Cure	nl GH abn dyn	GH (ng/ml)	
				5–10	>10
Previously treated*	11	4	2	2	3
No prior Rx	29	16	6	4	3
Total	40	20	8	6	6

* Radiation and/or craniotomy.

major conclusions. We advocate transsphenoidal microsurgery in patients who were treated previously as well as in those who never received any prior treatment. The outcome of surgery in either group appears to be determined by the size of the adenoma and the presence or absence of extrasellar extension and most importantly on the technical skills of the neurosurgeon.

3.4 *GH studies in the immediate postoperative period.* Changes in serum GH levels were studied in the immediate postoperative period. In 5 patients who were studied later and considered cured, the fasting serum GH level on the first postoperative day was <1 ng/ml. However, one has to be cautious in interpreting a single GH level in patients who are under the stress of surgery and receiving intravenous fluids containing glucose.

The GH response to TRH studied at one week after surgery was similar to that noted several weeks or months later. In patients who had a rise in GH in response to TRH administration preoperatively, this test provided a sensitive means of evaluating the outcome of surgery and the completeness of removal of the adenoma.

3.5 *Somatomedin C levels postoperatively.* Somatomedin C level was measured postoperatively in 16 patients. The level was normal in all patients who had normal basal GH level regardless of the responses to dynamic stimulation or suppression. Elevated somatomedin C levels to a variable degree (≥ 3 U/ml) were seen in all patients with elevated basal GH. We believe that somatomedin C level is valuable in evaluating the activity of acromegaly in patients before and after surgery. A decrease of somatomedin C level into the normal range in patients who have normalization of serum GH level was seen as early as one week after surgery.

3.6 *PRL data postoperatively.* The basal and dynamic studies of PRL secretion on 11 patients who had hyperprolactinemia preoperatively are shown in Table 2. Postoperatively, PRL levels decreased to normal in all patients who had normal basal GH levels. Of 3 patients who continued to have elevated GH levels postoperatively, one had a normal PRL level while the remaining 2 continued to have elevated PRL levels. In all patients who were considered cured of acromegaly, PRL dynamic studies became normal.

3.7 Other endocrine data. Three patients who had panhypopituitarism pre-operatively continued to be so after surgery. One patient who had a low serum T_4 and TSH levels preoperatively had normalization of both values 3 months after surgery. Of three male patients who had hyperprolactinemia and associated secondary hypogonadism, 2 recovered while one continued to have the same findings. Two patients who had low testosterone and normal PRL levels pre-operatively had normalization of testosterone values postoperatively.

Two patients who had impaired pituitary adrenal axis and hypogonadism recovered both functions postoperatively.

4. Clinical results

Symptomatic improvement occurred in all patients. A decrease in soft tissue swelling started to occur within 2–3 days after surgery in all patients. However, it was most pronounced and sustained in patients who had normal GH levels postoperatively. The improvement in soft tissue could be appreciated easily before the patient was discharged home about one week after surgery. Most patients lost approximately 2–4 kg by the time they were discharged. A decrease in soft tissue fluid could be most appreciated in the face, hands and feet. Hyperhydrosis resolved in patients who had normal GH level and improved in the remaining patients.

Improvement in the control of diabetes mellitus was seen in all 5 patients. Two patients discontinued insulin therapy immediately after surgery. Of 16 patients with impaired glucose tolerance preoperatively, 10 had normal glucose tolerance 3 months after surgery.

Libido and potency were restored in 4 of 6 patients who were not hypopituitary preoperatively. Menses resumed after surgery in 7 of 10 patients who had amenorrhea preoperatively and who were not hypopituitary.

Visual field defects resolved completely in 5 of 7 patients and persisted in the remaining 2 patients. Headaches improved in all patients with that complaint preoperatively.

4.1 Surgical complications. There was no mortality in our series. However, a few transient complications occurred. Transient diabetes insipidus developed in the immediate postoperative period in 8 patients requiring treatment for a few months in only 4 patients. One patient developed hyponatremia and inappropri-ate ADH secretion which spontaneously resolved in one week. Transient sixth nerve palsy developed in a patient who had extension of the tumor into the cavernous sinus. A 69-year-old woman had a stroke a few days after surgery from which she partially recovered in one year.

4.2 *Additional forms of treatment.* Following surgery, additional treatment was given to patients in whom surgery was not successful in restoring serum GH to normal. However, in one patient radiation therapy was given in spite of a normal postoperative GH level because his adenoma was felt to be large and invasive. Of 7 patients who received radiation to the pituitary fossa, 6 were given conventional radiation (3500–5000 rads) through a linear accelerator while one received proton beam therapy. The data on these 7 patients are presented in Table 6. Four patients had normal serum GH levels at the time of last evaluation (1 to 5 years after radiation). The other 3 patients had minimal reductions in their serum GH 12 to 30 months after receiving radiation. Total hypopituitarism developed in 4 patients 12 to 40 months after radiation.

We have used medical treatment with ergot derivative drugs in a few patients with persistent serum GH elevation. Our initial experience was with lergotrile mesylate (Eli Lilly, Indianapolis, Indiana). The dosage used range between 6 and 16 mg daily given in 4 divided doses. The side effects encountered are similar to those seen with other ergot drugs such as bromocriptine, including nausea and postural hypotension. These side effects could be avoided in most patients by administering the drug with food and escalating the dose gradually. A total of 6 patients received this drug for variable periods of time. However, treatment had to be discontinued in 2 patients within 3 months because of significant side effects. In one of these patients, serum GH level decreased promptly to normal with treatment and returned to baseline (20 ng/ml) after the treatment was discontinued. Of the remaining 4 patients 2 responded to treatment with a decrease in serum GH to normal and the remaining 2 patients did not benefit from Lergotrile treatment. Treatment with Lergotrile was discontinued on all patients in 1980 at

Table 6. Result of radiation therapy after surgery in patients

Patients	hGH (ng/ml)		Months after radiation	Complications
	Before Rx	After Rx		
1	4	<1	60	Total hypopituitarism
2	18	<1	50	Total hypopituitarism
3	7	6	30	None
4*	18	3	30	Total hypopituitarism
5	29	22	15	None
6	8	2	24	None
7	15	12	12	Total hypopituitarism

* Received proton beam therapy.

the company's (Eli Lilly) request. Of the 2 patients who responded to Lergotrile with a reduction of GH level to normal, one had elevation of serum GH to 8 ng/ml while the other had persistent decrease in serum GH level after 3 weeks of discontinuing therapy. The latter patient has been followed since then without treatment for 27 months and continued to have low serum GH levels (<1–2 ng/ml). Whether this represents a permanent effect of this treatment or infarction of the tumor is not clear. No appreciable radiologic changes were noted during Lergotrile therapy in any patient.

We have used another long acting ergot derivative developed by Eli Lilly (pergolide mesylate) in treating 4 patients with acromegaly. One of these patients responded previously to Lergotrile treatment while another did not. All 4 patients had elevated serum GH (7 to 180 ng/ml) as well as somatomedin C levels (2.5 to 12 U/ml). The dose used ranged from 0.1 to 0.5 mg of pergolide given once daily. The treatment was well tolerated by all 4 patients. Three patients had normal GH and somatomedin C level during treatment (Table 7). The fourth patient had a decrease in both serum GH (14 to 8 ng/ml) and somatomedin C (5.5 to 3.9 U/ml) (Table 7).

Two patients were treated with the well known dopaminergic drug, bromocriptine, 10–15 mg daily in divided doses. One of these patients responded with lowering of serum GH to normal within 2 months of therapy. However by 6 months early escape from the effect of bromocriptine was noted. This responded promptly to an increase in the dose from 10 to 20 mg daily.

5. Discussion

Acromegaly is a chronic disfiguring disease with many associated serious complications that should not be neglected. Optimal treatment should be provided as early as possible in the the hope of preventing further progression of the disease or reversing some of the effects.

Conventional supervoltage irradiation, heavy particle or proton beam irradia-

Table 7. Medical treatment of acromegaly with pergolide mesylate in 4 patients

Patient	Before Rx		During Rx	
	GH (ng/ml)	somato-medin c (μ/ml)	GH (ng/ml)	somato-medin c (μ/ml)
1	180	12	3	1.7
2	8	3.8	2	1.8
3	7	2.5	2	1.2
4	14	5.5	8	3.9

tion and medical treatment primarily with dopaminergic drugs are among the therapeutic options used in treating patients with this disease. However, each of these modalities has important shortcomings. Conventional supervoltage irradiation of the pituitary has a delayed onset of action such that it may take about 10 years before serum GH becomes normal in 70% of patients [18]. Furthermore, it is associated with a relatively high incidence of partial or complete hypopituitarism that develops insidiously over several years. Heavy particle irradiation can be more effective than supervoltage conventional irradiation. However, experience with this technique is limited mainly to two centers in the United States. Here also one would achieve a gradual decrease in serum GH in patients such that by 6 years about 70% of patients may have normal serum GH levels. This form of treatment is also associated with a relatively high complication rate.

Medical treatment with dopaminergic drugs can be quite effective in some patients. However, a recent report concluded that bromocriptine was not effective in treating patients with acromegaly [19]. It is evident, however, from our data as well as others reported in the literature that dopaminergic drugs can be effective in some patients.

The recent refinement of transsphenoidal microsurgical techniques in approaching the pituitary gland, has provided a new and important dimension in treating patients with acromegaly. Using this technique, an experienced neurosurgeon can in favorable cases achieve all the goals of therapy listed previously, namely immediate lowering of serum GH to normal and preservation of normal pituitary function including normal GH responses to stimulation and suppression tests. The clinical signs and symptoms can similarly improve in a short period of time (days to weeks). Symptomatic improvement can be seen as a decrease in soft tissue fluids of the face, hands, feet and tongue, disappearance of headaches, relief from hyperhydrosis and amelioration of diabetes mellitus.

Assessment of the results of surgery has in the past depended on serum GH level. However, it has become apparent recently that GH dynamic studies are important [6, 7] to assess whether patients were cured of this disease. Our definition of 'cure' in acromegaly is the achievement of a normal basal GH level that responds normally to appropriate stimulation and suppression tests. Some patients, however, may be cured of their disease at the expense of developing hypopituitarism, in which case GH dynamic tests will reveal findings of GH deficiency. Using this definition of cure, we have not seen any biochemical or clinical evidence of recurrence in any of our cured patients over a period of follow up that ranged from 9 to 140 months (mean 78 months). Measurement of plasma somatomedin C level can be helpful in evaluating patients with acromegaly before and after treatment. The somatomedin C level correlates well with the activity of the disease rather than with serum GH level [20]. Its measurement, however, will probably not be sufficient to identify patients who are cured of their disease because patients with normal GH level associated with abnormal dynamics of secretion have normal somatomedin C levels.

The success of surgery in achieving complete removal of the tumor depends not only on the skill and experience of the neurosurgeon but also on the size of the tumor and the presence or absence of extrasellar extension.

We believe that transsphenoidal surgical adenomectomy is the initial preferred treatment for patients with GH secreting adenomas. This form of treatment should be performed by an experienced surgeon and should be as extensive as necessary to achieve complete removal of the adenoma, if possible. Irradiation of the pituitary can be used in patients who are not surgical candidates or in patients whose adenomas could not be completely resected by surgery. Medical treatment with dopaminergic drugs can be helpful in some patients who respond to these drugs.

Acknowledgements

The authors wish to thank all referring physicians and the staff of the Clinical Research Center. The technical help of Mary Tupes, Beth Wilhite, Roberto Salazar, Denise Hatala, and Mary Wu is greatly appreciated.

References

1. Evans HM, Briggs JH, Dixon JS: The physiology and chemistry of growth hormone. Acromegaly. In: The Pituitary Gland, Harris GW, Donovan BT (eds), Berkeley and Los Angeles: University of California Press, 1966, p 439.
2. Wright AD, Hill DM, Lowry C, Fraser TR: Mortality in acromegaly. Q J Med 39:1–16, 1970.
3. Thorner MO, Perryman RL, Cronin MJ, Rogol AD, Draznin M, Johanson A, Vale W, Horvath E, Kovacs K: Somatotroph hyperplasia: successful treatment of acromegaly by removal of a pancreatic islet tumor secreting a growth hormone-releasing factor. J Clin Invest 70: 965–977, 1982.
4. Guillemin R, Brazeau P, Böhlen P, Esch F, Ling N, Wehrenberg WB. Growth hormone-releasing factor from a human pancreatic tumor than caused acromegaly. Science 218: 585–587, 1982.
5. Rivier J, Spiess J, Thorner M, Vale W: Characterization of a growth hormone-releasing factor from a human pancreatic islet tumor. Nature (Lond) 300: 276–278, 1982.
6. Arafah BM, Brodkey JS, Kaufman B, Velasco M, Manni A, Pearson OH: Transsphenoidal microsurgery in the treatment of acromegaly and gigantism. J Clin Endocrinol Metab 50: 578–585, 1980.
7. Schuster LD, Bantle JP, Oppenheimer JH, Seljeskog EL: Acromegaly: reassessment of the long-term therapeutic effectiveness of transsphenoidal pituitary surgery. Ann Intern Med 95: 172–4, 1981.
8. Horgan ED, Riley WJ: Protein-binding assay for plasma testosterone after purification by column partition chromatography. Clin Chem 20: 430–435, 1974.
9. Schalch DS, Parker ML: A sensitive double antibody immuno-assay for human growth hormone in plasma. Nature (Lond) 203: 1141–1142, 1964.
10. Sinha YN, Selby FW, Lewis JJ, WanderLaan WP: A homologous radioimmunoassay for human prolactin. J Clin Endocrinol Metab 36: 509–516, 1973.

11. Midgley AR: Radioimmunoassay for human follicle stimulating hormone. J Clin Endocrinol Metab 27: 295–299, 1967.
12. Midgley AR: Radioimmunoassay: a method for human chorionic gonadotropin and human luteinizing hormone. Endocrinol 79:10, 1966.
13. Pekary AE, Hersham JM, Parlow AF: A sensitive and precise radioimmunoassay for human thyroid-stimulating hormone. J Clin Endocrinol Metab 41: 676–684, 1975.
14. Kleinberg DL, Noel GL, Frantz AG: Galactorrhea: a study of 235 cases, including 48 with pituitary tumors. N Engl J Med 296: 589–600, 1977.
15. Carter JN, Tryson JE, Tolis G, Van Vliet S, Faiman C, Friesen HG: Prolactin-secreting tumors and hypogonadism in 22 men. N Engl J Med 299: 847–852, 1978.
16. Arafah BM, Brodkey JS, Manni A, Velasco ME, Kaufman B, Pearson OH: Recovery of pituitary function following surgical removal of large nonfunctioning pituitary adenomas. Clin Endocrinol 17: 213–222, 1982.
17. Sternberger LA: Immunocytochemistry, Englewood Cliffs, Prentice-Hall, 1974, pp 129–171.
18. Eastman RC, Gorden P, Roth J: Conventional supervoltage irradiation is an effective treatment for acromegaly. J Clin Endocrinol Metab 48: 931–40, 1979.
19. Lindholm J, Riishede J, Vestergaard S, Hummer L, Faber O, Hagen C: No effect of bromocriptine in acromegaly: a controlled trial. N Engl J Med 304: 1450–4, 1981.
20. Clemmons DR, Van Dyk JJ, Ridgeway EC, Kliman B, Kjellbert RN, Underwood LE. Evaluation of acromegaly by measurement of somatomedin-C. N Engl J Med 301: 1138–42, 1979.

3. Prolactin secreting pituitary adenomas in women

BAHA'UDDIN M. ARAFAH, JERALD S. BRODKEY
and OLOF H. PEARSON

1. Introduction

The introduction of a radioimmunoassay for prolactin several years ago has increased our awareness and improved our understanding of the role of PRL in reproductive function in humans. It became evident with time, that the majority of pituitary tumors that were labelled as chromophobe or nonfunctioning were in fact secreting PRL. Of all pituitary tumors those secreting PRL account for approximately 50–55%. Thus PRL secreting pituitary tumors or prolactinomas are becoming a commonly encountered disease rather than a medical curiosity.

It is important to point out that prolactinomas are not only pituitary tumors associated with hyperprolactinemia, but also those where the cells show evidence of storage and/or secretion of PRL. This can be easily demonstrated with the help of immunoperoxidase staining of the tissue using specific PRL antibodies. This distinction is important since large pituitary tumors of any cell type can be associated with hyperprolactinemia [1] through a different mechanism. Since the control of PRL secretion is under a predominantly inhibitory factor, any pressure on the pituitary stalk or interference with the portal circulation may result in elevation of PRL level. This would be one mechanism whereby large pituitary tumors can be associated with hyperprolactinemia and possibly hypopituitarism [1].

The predominant presenting symptoms in patients with prolactinomas include menstrual irregularities, infertility and galactorrhea in women and diminished libido and impotence in men. This disease seems to be diagnosed more often in women and even at an earlier stage than in men. The reasons for that are not clear but might be related to the fact that the symptoms of hyperprolactinemia in women are conceived by patients as important enough to seek medical attention at an earlier stage.

In addition to symptoms attributed to hyperprolactinemia, patients may present with signs and symptoms of mechanical effects of the tumor such as headaches and visual field defects. However, with the recent advances and sophistication in radiographic studies, many patients are presenting at an early stage with microadenomas where the mechanical effects of the adenoma are lacking.

Santen, R.J. and Manni, A. (eds.), Diagnosis and management of endocrine-related tumors. ISBN 0-89838-636-5.
© *1984, Martinus Nijhoff Publishers, Boston. Printed in the Netherlands.*

The management of prolactinomas depends primarily on the indications for treatment as well as the philosophy of the physician. With the recent refinement in transsphenoidal microsurgery in the exploration of the sella turcica, this method has gained popularity as an optimal form of treating patients with pituitary tumors. Using this approach, a tumor can be easily removed while the normal pituitary remains intact.

In this chapter we will review our experience in 105 women with prolactinomas treated over 11 years at our institution. The clinical, biochemical and radiological features will be summarized and the results of surgical treatment will be evaluated in detail.

2. Patients

Our series includes a total of 105 women who have surgically proven pituitary tumors. All patients had transsphenoidal surgery performed by one neuro-surgeon (JSB) between 1969 and 1981. The indications for treatment in these patients included hyperprolactinemia with infertility or evidence of an expanding intrasellar tumor. Two of the patients included in this series have been previously reported [2]. None of the patients had any illnesses or were on drugs known to elevate serum PRL level. None of the patients included in our series had acromegaly or Cushing's disease. One patient was diagnosed to have primary hyperparathyroidism 2 years before she presented for treatment of her pituitary tumor. Another patient had idiopathic precocious puberty diagnosed at the age of 8 years.

The age of patients at the time of diagnosis ranged between 17 and 42 years with a mean of 26.5 ± 1.0 years. The clinical features of the patients are summarized in Table 1. The majority of patients had secondary amenorrhea with galactorrhea. The duration of secondary amenorrhea ranged between 4 and 132 months with a mean of 39 ± 5 months. Galactorrhea was present for 3 to 96 months (mean 33.6 ± 4.6 months) at the time of diagnosis. Infertility was another major complaint in a total of 40 patients.

Sixty-nine women reported the use of oral contraceptive medications at some

Table 1. Clinical features of 105 women with prolactinomas

	Amenorrhea		Oligomenorrhea	Total
	Primary	Secondary		
Galactorrhea	2	89	7	98
No galactorrhea	3	2	2	7
Total	5	91	9	105

point before their presentation. The duration of use of oral contraceptives ranged between 3 and 140 months. In 48 patients, however, the onset of symptoms (amenorrhea and/or galactorrhea) was related to the discontinuation of oral contraceptive medications. In 13 patients amenorrhea and/or galactorrhea occurred postpartum. These data are in general agreement with those reported in the literature by other investigators [3–5].

Headaches were present in 31 patients of whom 2 also had visual symptoms. None of the patients had symptoms suggestive of hypothyroidism or adrenal insufficiency.

2.1. *Neuroradiologic evaluation.* The sella turcica was evaluated with thin section tomographic cuts (polytomography). Abnormalities of the sella turcica were identified in 96 patients (Table 2). The sella was considered to be normal (9 patients) when there was no asymmetry, bony erosion or increase in size. Minimal changes in the sella (64 patients) included local thinning or asymmetry without evidence of enlargement, bony erosion, displacement of the dorsum sellae or elevation of either the anterior or posterior clinoids. The anteroposterior dimension from the anterior wall to the dorsum sellae was less than 16 mm in all sellae considered to show minimal changes. Gross abnormalities of the sella turcica were detected in 32 patients. These abnormalities included gross enlargement, erosion of the lamina dura, displacement of the dorsum sellae or destruction and displacement of either of the clinoid processes [6]. Different types of CT scans were performed on 36 patients who were evaluated after 1978. The sensitivity of these scans in detecting small adenomas improved over the years. With the newest generation CT scanners microadenomas can be detected without difficulty.

2.2 *Hormone measurement and methods.* Patients were admitted to the Clinical Research Center for preoperative pituitary function tests. These studies included serum thyroxine, morning and evening serum cortisol levels. Metyrapone or insulin tolerance tests were performed to assess the pituitary adrenal axis in 42 patients. Serum FSH and LH were measured in the basal state.

The following serum hormone levels were measured employing specific radio-

Table 2. Abnormalities of the sella turcica in patients with prolactinomas

	Normal sella	Minimal changes		Gross abnormalities
		Intrasellar CSF[a]	No CSF	
Number	9	14	50	32
Extrasellar extension[b]	0	1	9	13

[a] Documented with CT scans or pneumoencephalogram.

[b] As determined during surgery.

immunoassay systems using reagents kindly supplied by NIAMDD: TSH [7], FSH [8], LH [9], PRL [10] and hGH [11]. Before the establishment of PRL RAI in our laboratory, serum PRL levels in 2 previously reported patients [2] were measured by RIA by Dr. H. Freisen.

Serum PRL levels were measured before and after stimulation with phenothiazines (perphenazine 8 mg orally or chlorpromazine 50 mg IM) or TRH (500 μg IV) and suppression with L-Dopa (500 mg orally). Serum PRL and GH levels were measured every two hours during a 14-hour overnight stay to assess the nocturnal rise in these two hormones. The highest level over this period is taken to calculate the increment and the percentage nocturnal rise over the basal (6 or 8 am) serum level. Serum GH level was also measured following the administration of L-Dopa or during insulin-induced hypoglycemia.

Preoperatively 78 patients had multiple overnight blood samples drawn to evaluate the nocturnal rise in serum PRL. Stimulation with TRH (N = 78), perphenazine or chlorpromazine (N = 88) and suppression with L-Dopa (N = 75) were performed preoperatively in the majority of patients.

The dynamics of PRL secretion (nocturnal rise, phenothiazine and/or TRH stimulation and L-Dopa suppression) were repeated 3–4 months postoperatively and at one year or more whenever feasible. Pituitary function tests were repeated on these occasions postoperatively as described earlier.

Daily serum PRL levels were measured during the first six days after surgery in 18 patients. Just before discharge from the hospital one week after surgery, a TRH test was routinely performed (N = 65). Before the availability of TRH, a thorazine stimulation test was performed at one week in 11 patients.

In 22 normal premenopausal women (normal controls), the mean $\pm$ SEM basal PRL level was 11.4 $\pm$ 1.7 ng/dl. The mean incremental rises ($\triangle$) in serum PRL after TRH (N = 22) or perphenazine (N = 20) were 38.8 $\pm$ 5 and 33.8 $\pm$ 3.8 ng/ml respectively. The mean incremental ($\triangle$) nocturnal rise in serum PRL in normal women (N = 18) was 12.8 $\pm$ 1.7 ng/ml.

The normal basal serum PRL in our laboratory is <25 ng/ml. A normal response to stimulation with either thorazine, perphenazine or TRH is defined as doubling of the basal PRL level with an increase ($\triangle$) of >8 ng/ml. A normal PRL response to L-Dopa is defined at $\geq$50% suppression of the basal level with a nadir of <8 ng/ml.

Specimens obtained at surgery were sectioned and stained using standard techniques. In addition all specimens were immunostained using the peroxidase antiperoxidase technique described by Sternberger [12] for PRL, GH and ACTH. Formalin-fixed blocks from specimens obtained prior to 1978 were sectioned and immunostained using the same technique. Nontumorous pituitary tissue obtained from unselected autopsy material served as a control.

The data are presented as mean $\pm$ SEM unless otherwise stated. Statistical analysis was done using Student-t test unless otherwise indicated.

3. Treatment

None of the patients had been previously treated surgically or with radiation therapy. Transnasal transsphenoidal microsurgical exploration of the sella turcica was performed by one neurosurgeon (J.S.B.). The diagnosis was verified by biopsy and frozen sections stained with hematoxylin and eosin as well as reticular stains [13]. A hemihypophysectomy on the side of the microadenoma was usually performed whenever that was feasible.

A microadenoma was defined at the time of surgery as an adenoma which occupied less than one half the size of the pituitary in a sella that was normal or slightly increased in size. A large adenoma was defined as an adenoma that occupied more than one half the size of the sella and showed no extrasellar extension.

3.1 *Preoperative endocrine data.* Serum PRL levels were elevated (Fig. 1) in all patients ranging between 40 and 9600 ng/ml (301 ± 109 ng/ml, mean ± SEM).

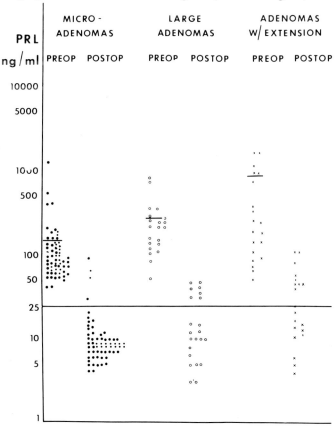

Figure 1. Pre- and postoperative serum PRL levels in 105 women with PRL secreting pituitary adenomas. The lines indicate the mean of each group.

Thorazine or perphenazine administration did not result in a significant (>100%) rise in serum PRL levels in any patient (N = 88). However, TRH administration resulted in a significant rise (>100%) in serum PRL in 5 out of 72 patients tested. Of 78 patients who had multiple overnight determinations of serum PRL, 51 (65%) did not have a nocturnal rise while 25 (32%) had <50% rise and 2 patients (3%) had a 50% rise in serum PRL. The mean percent nocturnal rise above the basal level in serum PRL in the group was $17 \pm 2.8\%$. Of 75 patients who had the L-Dopa suppression test, 7 (9%) showed no suppression, 24 (32%) had 25–50% suppression and 44 (59%) had greater than 51% suppression of serum PRL level. All patients who did not have dynamic studies done preoperatively (N = 11) had hyperprolactinemia with definite radiological abnormalities of the sella turcica.

The preoperative serum PRL levels tended to be lower in patients with microadenomas (139 ± 30 ng/ml) than in patients with large adenomas (264 ± 58 ng/ml; p = not significant). Patients with extrasellar extension had significantly higher serum PRL levels (855 ± 550 ng/ml, p<0.05) than patients with microadenomas.

Serum FSH and LH levels were in the normal range for the follicular phase. Thyroid and adrenal functions were normal in all patients.

Results

4.1 *Surgical findings*. An adenoma was identified in all patients. Sixty-two patients had microadenomas and the remaining 43 had large adenomas (Table 3, Fig. 1). Fifty patients with microadenomas underwent hemihypophysectomy while the remaining 12 had wide excision of the adenoma. Extrasellar extension was identified in 21 patients with large adenomas (18 to the cavernous and 3 to the sphenoid sinus). In only 4 patients was the adenoma located centrally while in the rest it was located in either side of the pituitary.

4.2 *Pathological findings*. The diagnosis of pituitary adenoma was confirmed histologically in 104 patients. In one patient where the tumor was identified grossly by the surgeon, the specimen was adsorbed by the cotton and was not examined histologically. Immunostaining of 101 adenomas revealed cells staining

Table 3. Postoperative serum prolactin levels in 105 patients with prolactinomas*

	Microadenomas	Large adenomas without extension	Large adenomas with extension	Total
Normal ($\leq$25 ng/ml)	58	15	11	84
Elevated (>25 ng/ml)	4	7	10	21
Total	62	22	21	105

* Measured 1–6 months postoperatively.

for PRL and not for GH or ACTH. In some adenomas occasional GH staining cells were scattered among the PRL staining cells.

4.3 Postoperative PRL studies

4.3.1 *Basal serum PRL.* Serum PRL level measured 1 to 4 months after surgery was normal in 84 (80%), 25 to 50 ng/ml in 14 (13%) and greater than 51 ng/ml in 7 (7%) patients (Fig. 1, Table 3). The importance of the adenoma size in influencing the result of surgery can be appreciated when the data are analyzed accordingly (Table 3). Of 62 patients with microadenomas, 58 (94%) had normal serum PRL postoperatively.

4.3.2 *PRL dynamic studies at 3–4 months.* Eighty-five patients (Table 4) had dynamic studies done 3–4 months postoperatively. The remaining 20 patients did not have dynamic studies done postoperatively either because they got pregnant shortly after surgery (N = 10) or because of geographical difficulties (N = 10). Of these 20 patients, 16 had normal basal serum PRL measured 1 to 84 months after surgery. The remaining 4 patients had elevated PRL levels after surgery.

Of 85 patients who had dynamic studies done 3 to 4 months postoperatively, 59 (69%) had normal basal PRL levels and dynamics (Table 4), while 10 had normal basal PRL levels but abnormal dynamics (blunted or absent responses to stimulation) and 16 had elevated basal PRL with abnormal dynamics (Table 4). All patients with normal dynamics had normal basal PRL level that increased by >100% in response to perphenazine or thorazine (N = 56) or TRH stimulation (N = 50) and had a normal nocturnal rise in serum PRL (N = 49). The administration of L-Dopa in these patients (N = 41) resulted in a >50% suppression of serum PRL with a mean nadir serum PRL level of 2.8 ± 0.9 ng/ml. All patients who had normal basal PRL and dynamics were considered cured of their disease. In such patients the responses to phenothiazines and TRH at 3 months were considered normal in each individual, i.e., a rise of >100% above baseline with an increment of >8 ng/ml. However, when one looks at the group data, the mean incremental rise (△PRL) to either stimulus was significantly less than that

Table 4. PRL dynamic studies in patients with prolactinomas 3 months after surgery

	Total*	nl PRL level nl dyn	nl PRL level abn dyn	High basal PRL abn dyn
Microadenomas	53	46	4	3
Large adenomas	17	9	2	6
Adenomas with extension	15	4	4	7
Total*	85	59	10	16

nl: normal; abn: abnormal; dyn: dynamics.

* In whom dynamic studies were performed postoperatively.

observed in the control group (Table 5). Thus the PRL response to TRH and phenothiazines seen in these patients were normal when looked at individually and subnormal when compared as a group to normal women. The reason behind this is not clear, but appears to be the delay in the recovery of lactotrophs. Further studies months to years after surgery (see below) revealed improved PRL responses that are indistinguishable from normal women.

Table 4 presents the data on the 85 patients who had dynamic studies 3 to 4 months postoperatively according to the size of their adenomas. Of 53 patients with microadenomas who had dynamic studies done 3 to 4 months postoperatively, 46 (87%) were considered cured. In contrast, only 9 of 17 (53%) patients with large adenomas and 4 of 15 patients with extrasellar extension of their adenomas were cured.

Table 6 presents the data on PRL dynamic studies in 53 patients with microadenomas according to whether a hemihypophysectomy was performed on the side of the adenoma or not. Although the p value ($p = 0.052$) is borderline, hemihypophysectomy appears to improve the cure rate in patients with microadenomas. It should be stated clearly that such a procedure did not result in any adverse effects in any of the patients.

Table 5. Basal serum PRL level and the incremental rise (Δ) after TRH and phenothiazines done 3 months after surgery in 59 patients who were considered cured and in normal women

	Basal level ng/ml	Incremental rise ($\triangle$) (ng/ml)	
		TRH	Phenothiazines
Cured patients	8.9 ± 1.9	26.1 ± 1.8[a]	19.2 ± 1.6[b]
Normal women	11.4 ± 1.7	38.8 ± 5	33 ± 3.8

[a] p<0.005 compared to normal women.
[b] p<0.001 compared to normal women.

Table 6. Results of PRL dynamic studies performed 3–4 months after surgery in 53 patients with microadenomas

	nl basal level		Elevated basal level abn dyn
	nl dyn	abn dyn	
Hemihypophysectomy[a]	38	2	2
No hemihypophysectomy	8[b]	2	1

nl: normal; dyn: dynamics; abn: abnormal.
[a] Performed on the side of the adenoma.
[b] $p = 0.052$ as compared to hemihypox (χ^2 test).

4.3.3 *PRL dynamic studies 1 to 5 years after surgery.* The dynamics of PRL secretion were studied at 3–4 months and then at one year or more after adenomectomy in 15 patients that were considered cured. Table 7 summarizes the data on these 15 patients only. The basal serum PRL level in these patients at 3 months is similar to that seen at one year or more after surgery. The results of PRL dynamic studies in these patients 1 to 5 years after surgery were similar to those obtained in normal control women (Table 7). Thus it appears that the normal lactotrophs recover gradually over several months and eventually respond to stimuli in a similar fashion to that seen in normal women.

4.3.4 *Basal PRL level in the immediate postoperative period.* Daily serum PRL levels during the first week after surgery were obtained in 11 patients that were considered cured based on the 3 months evaluation. Nine patients had undetectable PRL levels during the first 2 days after surgery while the other 2 patients had low levels (2.2 and 3.1 ng/ml). By the 6th postoperative day, only 3 patients had undetectable PRL levels while the rest had levels ranging from 2.5 to 5.6 ng/ml. Simultaneous measurement of serum GH and cortisol levels during the first few days after surgery revealed normal or elevated levels consistent with the stress of surgery. In contrast the serum PRL levels in patients who had normal PRL levels but abnormal dynamics at 3 months were higher during the first few days after surgery. In 4 such patients serum PRL level ranged from 5 to 11 ng/ml during the first 2 days after surgery. Three patients who were found to have elevated serum PRL levels in the immediate postoperative period, had similarly elevated levels 3 months later.

4.4 *Clinical results.* Of 80 patients with normal PRL postoperatively and who had amenorrhea preoperatively, 79 resumed their menses or became pregnant within 3 months after surgery. Menses resumed in 5 ± 0.2 weeks after surgery. Of 16 patients who had a postoperative PRL of >25 ng/ml, only 4 resumed their menses. Only one patient of 5 with primary amenorrhea started menstruating 2 months after surgery.

Table 7. The basal PRL level (ng/ml) and the incremental rise (Δ) in ng/ml during PRL dynamic studies in 15 patients with prolactinomas cured by surgery

	Basal[a]	TRH[a] Δ	Pz[a] Δ
3–4 months	9.7 ± 1.9	27.1 ± 4[b]	18.1 ± 3[c]
12–60 months	10.1 ± 2	36.5 ± 4.9	31.2 ± 6
Normal women	11.4 ± 1.7	38.8 ± 5	33 ± 3.8

[a] Mean $\pm$ SD.
[b] $p < 0.001$ as compared to control.
[c] $p < 0.005$ as compared to control.

Galactorrhea disappeared in 73 and significantly decreased in 6 of 79 patients who had it preoperatively and who had normal serum PRL postoperatively. The galactorrhea disappeared within 8.3 ± 0.4 weeks after surgery. Galactorrhea persisted in all patients who had a postoperative PRL of >25 ng/ml (N = 19).

Forty of 43 patients who had normal postoperative PRL levels and desired to be pregnant, became so within one year after surgery. Only one patient of 29 who were considered cured was unable to become pregnant.

Headaches disappeared in all 31 patients that had such complaints pre-operatively. Visual field defects resolved in the 2 patients who had this prior to surgery.

4.5 *Clinical follow up.* All patients who were cured continued to do well with no clinical or biochemical evidence of recurrence during the follow up period of 16 to 120 months (mean: 39.2 months). In contrast, during the follow up on 10 patients who had normal serum PRL but abnormal dynamics 3 months postoperatively, 6 showed clinical and biochemical evidence of recurrence of the adenoma. Recurrence occurred within 7 to 44 months (mean 25 months) after surgery. All 6 patients with recurrence had persistent hyperprolactinemia (33 to 180 ng/ml) associated with galactorrhea (N = 6), amenorrhea (N = 3) or irregular menses (N = 2). None of the patients complained of headaches or visual disturbances.

Recurrence could not be documented radiologically with certainty in any of the 6 patients. This is partly explained by the fact that none of the patients had radiologic studies of the sella turcica within 3 months after surgery. The presence of fascia that is usually introduced into the sella at the time of surgery makes radiological evaluation of intrasellar masses difficult unless a baseline evaluation is available for comparison.

4.6 *Other forms of treatment following surgery.* Ten patients with documented adenomas and persistent hyperprolactinemia were treated with supervoltage pituitary irradiation. Three of these patients received treatment for recurrence of symptoms and hyperprolactinemia while 7 were treated because of persistent hyperprolactinemia 3 months postoperatively. All patients received conventional radiation of 4500 to 5000 rads through a linear accelerator. Only one patient had a microadenoma at the time of surgery while 4 had large adenomas and the remaining 5 had extrasellar extension of the adenomas. The mean serum PRL in these 10 patients decreased from 75 ± 2 to 38 ± 2 ng/ml in 21 ± 1 months after irradiation. Only 2 patients achieved a normal PRL level during this period. One patient developed panhypopituitarism while another had partial hypopituitarism within 3 years of receiving irradiation. Radiation fibrosis in the temporal lobe (proven histologically) developed in one patient 4 years after receiving 5000 rads to the sella turcica.

Six patients were treated with bromocriptine (10–15 mg/day) alone following surgery. The serum PRL level decreased to normal in 5 patients within 2 months of treatment. The fifth patient had a significant decrease in serum PRL (from 2200 to 90 ng/ml) using the highest tolerable dose (10 mg/day) of bromocriptine.

Before the availability of bromocriptine, 4 patients were treated with a similar dopaminergic drug, Lergotrile mesylate (Eli Lilly, Indianapolis, Indiana). All 4 patients had normal serum PRL while on treatment and 2 became pregnant within 4 months of therapy.

4.7 Surgical complications. There was no mortality in this series. Only one patient with a large adenoma developed hypopituitarism postoperatively. Thyroid and adrenal function were normal in all remaining patients. Transient diabetes insipidus developed in 2 patients requiring treatment for about one year. One patient developed a transient episode of inappropriate ADH secretion (SIADH) lasting for 2 days. CSF rhinorrhea that spontaneously stopped developed in one patient who was the first patient in the series operated on in 1969. Sixth nerve palsy that recovered gradually over 2 months developed in a patient with a large adenoma that extended into the cavernous sinus.

5. Discussion

Over the past decade, PRL secreting pituitary tumors have become an important cause of reproductive dysfunction in humans. The vast majority of women with this disease are in the reproductive age group. Furthermore, even with increasing awareness of these tumors, there has not been a surge in the incidence of these tumors in older women. Although a clear-cut relation between oral contraceptives and prolactinomas has not been established, it is interesting to note that many women develop the symptoms of hyperprolactinemia during or after the use of oral contraceptives. These observations would at least suggest that estrogens may play a role in the development or growth of these tumors. The demonstration of specific estrogen receptors in a significant proportion of these tumors [14, 15] would strengthen this suspicion. A few recent reports have demonstrated that tamoxifen, a specific antiestrogen, has an inhibitory action on prolactinomas in vitro [16] and also in vivo [17]. However, further studies are needed to elucidate the role of estrogens in the pathogenesis of these tumors.

Recently, a few studies were reported on the natural history of these tumors [18]. Although the data reported involved a relatively small number of patients, it was evident that the majority of these tumors had a benign course with no significant progression over several years. These observations raise an important therapeutic question relating to the management of patients with this disease. Whereas the need for treatment is obvious for women with infertility and/or mechanical pressure by the adenoma, the need for therapeutic intervention is less clear in women with microadenomas who are not desirous of pregnancy. It could be argued even in that instance that such women with hyperprolactinemia may be

74

at risk for the development of premature osteoporosis [19]. It is obvious that more data are needed on untreated patients to determine whether careful follow up is sufficient in patients who have no clear indications (such as infertility) for treatment or whether instead treatment should be used in a subgroup of patients likely to show progression.

Radiation therapy, medical treatment with dopaminergic agents and surgical removal of the adenoma are the main therapeutic choices available for patients with prolactinomas. Each of these modalities has advantages and drawbacks. Irradiation of the pituitary fossa has been used in the past as the primary treatment for prolactinomas. However, with the availability of other therapeutic options such as microsurgery and dopaminergic agonist, its use has declined. Among the major drawbacks in its use as a primary treatment were the long delay in its effect and the relatively high incidence of hypopituitarism developing months or years after radiation was given.

Dopaminergic agonists such as bromocriptine have been used frequently in treating these patients. Resumption of menses, cessation of galactorrhea, and restoration of fertility have been seen in the majority of women with prolactinomas treated with such agents [20, 21]. Furthermore, a decrease in the size of existing tumors has been noted [21, 22] in 20 to 50% of these patients, especially those with large tumors. However, cessation of treatment has been frequently associated with recurrence of symptoms, elevation of serum PRL [23] and even the regrowth of adenomas that have shrunk during treatment [24]. The mechanism of action of bromocriptine and presumably other similar drugs is thought to be a decrease in the size of adenomatous cells [25, 26], although recent in vitro studies [16] suggest that an antiproliferative effect may also be present.

Transsphenoidal microsurgery is a well established therapeutic modality in the management of functioning and nonfunctioning pituitary adenomas. Using this technique, a pituitary adenoma can be selectively removed with the guidance of an operating microscope, while the normal tissue is left intact. The procedure is relatively safe with minimal morbidity and practically no mortality in good hands.

Over the past 15 years we have used transsphenoidal surgery in the treatment of functioning and nonfunctioning pituitary adenomas. The results of surgery depend on the experience of the surgeon doing the procedure as well as other important variables such as the tumor size and the presence or absence of extrasellar extension.

Our data on patients with PRL secreting pituitary adenomas confirm previous reports on the effectiveness of such treatment. Of 105 patients, 84 had normal PRL postoperatively (80%). However, when one looks at the results recorded according to the size of the adenoma, one can easily appreciate the importance of the size of the adenoma and the presence of extrasellar extension in influencing the success of surgery. Of 62 patients with microadenomas, 58 or 94% had normal serum PRL postoperatively. In contrast, 15 of 22 patients with large adenomas

(68%) and only 11 of 21 patients (52%) who had extension of the adenomas outside the sella, had normal serum PRL postoperatively. Several reports in the literature [27, 28] support our data on the importance of the size of the adenoma in influencing the outcome of surgery.

Since PRL secreting adenomas are usually located on one side of the pituitary, we have been doing a hemihypophysectomy on the side of the adenoma to ensure complete removal of the adenoma. Our data in that regard indicate that hemihypophysectomy on the side of the adenoma seems to improve the success rate of surgery, although the statistical significance ($p = 0.052$) was borderline. It must be stressed that none of the patients who had hemihypophysectomy, developed any pituitary hormone deficiency postoperatively.

Most investigators have relied on the serum PRL level and the resumption of menses, disappearance of galactorrhea and the recovery of fertility as indices in the assessment of the outcome of surgery [29, 30]. In this study we have relied on the dynamic studies performed 3 months after surgery to assess the completeness of tumor removal. Patients have had at least 2 to 3 PRL stimulation tests (nocturnal rise, TRH and thorazine or perphenazine). All patients with persistent hyperprolactinemia albeit minimal and less than preoperative levels continued to have abnormal dynamics of PRL secretion. Of 69 patients with normal serum PRL level postoperatively, PRL dynamics were normal in 59 and abnormal in 10 patients. All 59 patients with normal PRL level and dynamics are considered 'cured' of their disease. The follow up on these patients (16 to 120 months, mean 39 months), although relatively short, indicates that they are doing well without any clinical or biochemical evidence of recurrence.

The importance of performing dynamic studies following adenomectomy in these patients becomes more apparent when one looks at the follow up of patients who had normal serum PRL and abnormal dynamics 3 months after surgery. In this group of 10 patients, 6 had clinical and biochemical evidences of recurrence that were noted 7 to 44 months (mean 25 months) after surgery. Thus we believe that PRL dynamic studies performed 3 months after surgery can reliably predict recurrence in these patients. Furthermore, we believe that the reason for the persistence of abnormal dynamics in these patients is incomplete removal of the adenomas at the time of surgery.

It is important to point out that a normal rise in serum PRL following TRH should not by itself be taken as a definite evidence of a 'cure', since some patients with adenomas do respond to TRH. One patient in our series had only a TRH test done postoperatively and was thus considered unevaluable for the postoperative dynamic studies (TRH administration 10 months postoperatively resulted in >100% increase in serum PRL). However, 30 months after surgery there were clinical and biochemical evidences of recurrence.

All patients who were considered cured at 3 months had a greater than 100% rise in serum PRL following TRH or perphenazine stimulation. Furthermore the incremental rise ($\triangle$) above baseline was normal in each patient (>8 ng/ml).

However, the mean incremental rise of all the patients following these stimuli is significantly less than that obtained in normal women. Long term follow up dynamic studies of PRL secretion in patients that were considered cured were carried out in 15 patients 12 to 60 months following surgery. PRL responses to stimulation with TRH and perphenazine were normal (>100% rise) in all patients at 3 months and subsequently at the follow up studies. However, the mean incremental rise in serum PRL following provocative stimulation was significantly higher in the follow up studies. Furthermore, by this time the dynamic studies were comparable to these obtained in normal women. Although hypothalamic abnormalities cannot be excluded in these patients, the improved responsiveness to provocative stimulation after a prolonged period of time would make it an unlikely possibility. It is quite possible, however, that the improved responsiveness observed may be explained by partial suppression of the hypothalamic pituitary secretion of PRL at 3 months. Our data on PRL dynamics in the immediate postoperative period are consistent with this explanation. Recently, St. George-Tucker et al. [30] have published their data on PRL dynamics performed at 2 to 6 months and 1 to 8 years after what was considered successful surgery. In agreement with our data, they observed that although 16 of 22 patients had a >100% rise in serum PRL after TRH stimulation 2 to 6 months postoperatively, yet the mean incremental rise ($\triangle$PRL) was subnormal at that time. However, 1 to 8 years postoperatively the mean incremental rise ($\triangle$PRL) after TRH was similar to that observed in normal women. However, in contrast to our data, they found only one of 8 patients responding normally to chlorpromazine at 2–6 months and 1 to 8 years after surgery [30]. The reason for the discrepancy between our data and those of St. George-Tucker et al. is not clear.

Our data on the serum PRL levels in the immediate postoperative period are consistent with the concept of gradual recovery of lactotrophs. Serum PRL levels in the first few days after surgery were undetectable or very low (<5 ng/ml) in patients that were considered 'cured'. Simultaneous measurement of serum GH and cortisol during that period revealed normal or high values appropriate for the stress of surgery. Thus it seems that the normal lactotrophs were under chronic inhibition caused by the previously elevated serum PRL level. Such an inhibition may occur through a short loop feed back mechanism which has been shown to operate in rats [31–33], and was proposed in humans [34, 35].

Thus we believe that following complete removal of PRL secreting tumors, lactotrophs of the normal pituitary recover gradually in responding to stimuli. This recovery may take several months to occur. Our data are quite consistent with the concept that a PRL secreting tumor is a primary disease of the pituitary gland rather than a hypothalamic disease. However, one cannot totally rule out any hypothalamic involvement.

In summary, we believe that transsphenoidal microsurgey is an optimal form of treatment for PRL secreting pituitary tumors. Dynamic studies of PRL secretion done postoperatively are helpful in evaluating the outcome of surgery and identifying patients at risk of recurrence. The outcome of surgery depends not only on the experience of the surgeon, but also on the size of the adenoma and the presence or absence of extrasellar extension. In patients where complete removal is not possible, treatment with dopaminergic agonists can be effective in lowering serum PRL level and providing symptomatic relief in the majority of patients. Furthermore, a decrease in tumor size may be seen in some patients. Thus dopaminergic agonists are an important adjuvant in the management of patients with prolactinomas. Supervoltage radiation can also be used as an adjuvant in the management of these patients. However, because of the slow onset of their effect, treatment with dopaminergic agents may become necessary in many patients.

Acknowledgements

The authors thank all the referring physicians and the staff of the Clinical Research Center, where all the studies were performed. The technical help of Mary Tupes, Roberto Salazar, Edward Burkett, Carol Juzulenas, Denise Hatala, and Mary Wu is greatly appreciated.

References

1. Arafah BM, Brodkey JS, Manni A, Velasco ME, Kaufman B, Pearson OH: Recovery of pituitary function following surgical removal of large nonfunctioning pituitary adenomas. Clin Endocrinol 17: 213–222, 1982.
2. Nasr H, Mozaffarian G, Pensky J, Pearson OH: Prolactin secreting pituitary tumors in women. J Clin Endocrinol Metab 35: 505, 1972.
3. Schlechte J, Sherman B, Halmi N, VanGilder J, Chapler F, Dolan K, Granner D, Duello T, Harris C: Prolactin-secreting pituitary tumors in amenorrheic women: a comprehensive study. Endocrine Rev 1: 295–308, 1980.
4. Gomez F, Reyes F, Faiman C: Nonpuerperal galactorrhea and hyperprolactinemia, clinical findings, endocrine features and therapeutic response in 56 cases. Am J Med 62: 648, 1977.
5. VanCampenhout J, Blanchet P, Beauregard H, Papas S: Amenorrhea following the use of oral contraceptives. Fertil Steril 28: 728, 1977.
6. Ezrin C, Horvath E, Kaufman B, Kovacs K, Weiss MH: Pituitary diseases. Boca Raton, Florida. CRC Press, 1980.
7. Pekary AE, Hersham JM, Parlow AF: A sensitive and precise radioimmunoassay for human thyroid-stimulating hormone. J Clin Endocrinol Metab 41: 676–684, 1975.
8. Midgley AR: Radioimmunoassay for human follicle stimulating hormone. J Clin Endocrinol Metab 27: 295–299, 1967.
9. Raiti S, Davis WT: The principles and application of radioimmunoassay with special reference to the gonadotropins. Obstet Gynecol Surv 24: 289, 1969.
10. Sinha YN, Selby FW, Lewis JJ, Vanderlaan WP: A homologous radioimmunoassay for human prolactin. J Clin Endocrinol Metab 36: 509, 1973.
11. Schalch DS, Parker ML: A sensitive double antibody immunoassay for human growth hormone in plasma. Nature (Lond) 203: 1141–1142, 1964.

12. Sternberger LA: Immunocytochemistry. New York, John Wiley and Sons, 1979.
13. Velasco ME, Sindely SD, Roessmann U: Reticulum stain for frozen section diagnosis of pituitary adenomas. J Neurosurgery 46: 548, 1977.
14. Pichon MF, Bression D, Peillon F, Milgrom E: Estrogen receptors in human pituitary adenomas. J Clin Endocrin Metab 51: 897, 1980.
15. Takei Y, Franks Y, Pearl GS, Kurisaka M, Tandall GT: Estrogen receptors in pituitary adenomas and normal adenohypophyses. 50th Anniversary Meeting of Am Assn of Neurological Surgeons, 1981, p 57.
16. Arafah BM, Wilhite BL, Rainieri J, Brodkey JS, Pearson OH: Inhibitory action of bromocriptine and tamoxifen on the growth of human pituitary tumors in soft agar. J Clin Endocrinol Metab 57: 986–992, 1983.
17. Lamberts SWJ, Verleun T, Oosterom R: Effect of tamoxifen administration on prolactin release by invasive prolactin-secreting pituitary adenomas. Neuroendocrinology 34: 339–342, 1982.
18. March CM, Kletzky OA, Davajan V, Teal J, Weiss M, Apuzzo MLJ, Marrs RP, Mishell DR, Jr: Longitudinal evaluation of patients with untreated prolactin-secreting pituitary adenomas. Am J Obstet Gynecol 139: 835–844, 1981.
19. Klibanski A, Neer R, Beitins I, Ridgway E, McArthur J: Decreased bone density in hyperprolactinemic women. N Engl J Med 303: 1511, 1981.
20. Thorner M, McNeilly A, Hagan C, Besser G: Long-term treatment of galactorrhea and hypogonadism with bromocriptine. Br Med J 2: 419, 1974.
21. Wass JAH, Moult PJA, Thorner MO, Dacie JE, et al.: Reduction of pituitary-tumour size in patients with prolactinomas and acromegaly treated with bromocriptine with or without radiotherapy. Lancet 2: 66, 1979.
22. Chiodini P, Liuzzi A, Cozzi R, Verde G, Oppizzi G, Dallabonzana D, Spelta B, Silvestrini F, Borghi G, Luccarelli G, Rainer E, Horowski R: Size reduction of macroprolactinomas by bromocriptine or lisuride treatment. J Clin Endocrin Metab 53: 737–743, 1981.
23. Maxon W, Dudzinski M, Hammond C: Delayed return of hyperprolactinemia after bromocriptine therapy in women with pituitary prolactinomas. 63rd Ann Mtg Endocrine Society, Cincinnati, 1981, p 198 (Abstract).
24. Thorner MO, Perryman RL, Rogol AD, et al.: Rapid changes of prolactinoma volume after withdrawal and reinstitution of bromocriptine. J Clin Endocrinol Metab 53: 480, 1981.
25. Rengachary SS, Tomita T, Jeffereis BF, Watanabe I: Structural changes in human pituitary tumor after bromocriptine therapy. Neurosurgery 10: 242, 1982.
26. Tindall GT, Kovacs K, Horvath E, Thorner MO: Human prolactin-producing adenomas and bromocriptine: a histological, immunocytochemical, ultrastructural, and morphometric study. J Clin Endocrinol Metab 55: 1178, 1982.
27. Hardy J: Transsphenoidal microsurgical treatment of pituitary tumors. In: Recent Advances in the Diagnosis and Treatment of Pituitary Tumors, Linfoot JA (ed). New York: Raven Press, 1979, p 375.
28. Keye WR, Chang RJ, Monroe SE, Wilson CB, Jaffe RB: Prolactin-secreting pituitary adenomas in women. II. Menstrual function, pituitary reserves, and prolactin production following microsurgical removal. Am J Obstet Gynecol 134: 360, 1979.
29. Post KD, Biller BJ, Adelman LS, Molitch ME, Wolpert SM, Reichlin S: Selective transsphenoidal adenomectomy in women with galactorrhea-amenorrhea. J Am Med Assoc 242: 158, 1979.
30. St. George Tucker H, Becker DP: Microsurgical removal of pituitary tumors with 'cure' and retention of pituitary function. In: Pituitary microadenomas, Faglia G, Giovanelli MA, MacLeon RM (eds). London, New York: Academic Press, 1980, p 473.
31. Clemens JA, Meites J: Inhibition by hypothalamic prolactin implants of prolactin secretion, mammary gowth and luteal function. Endocrinology 82: 878, 1968.
32. Voogt JL, Meites J: Suppression of proestrous and suckling-induced increase in serum prolactin by hypothalamic implant of prolactin. Proc Soc Exp Biol Med 142: 1056, 1973.

33. Gudelsky GA, Porter JC: Release of dopamine from tuberonfundibular neurons into pituitary stalk blood after prolactin or haloperidol administration. Endocrinology 106: 526, 1980.

34. Arafah BM, Manni A, Brodkey JS, Kaufman B, Velasco M, Pearson OH: Cure of hypogonadism after removal of prolactin-secreting adenomas in men. J Clin Endocrinol Metab 52: 91–94, 1981.

35. Casper RF, Rakoff JS, Quigley ME, Gilliland B, Alksne J, Yen SSC: Changes in pituitary hormones during and following transsphenoidal removal of prolactinomas. Am J Obstet Gynecol 136: 518, 1980.

4. Anterior-pituitary function before and after transsphenoidal microsurgery for pituitary tumors

ANDREA MANNI, BAHA'UDDIN M. ARAFAH,
JERALD S. BRODKEY and OLOF H. PEARSON

1. Introduction

The introduction of transsphenoidal microsurgery represents a major improvement in the surgical management of functioning and non-functioning pituitary tumors. A distinct advantage of this technique is the ability to achieve selective tumor removal with preservation of normal pituitary tissue, especially in patients with small adenomas. Numerous reports in the literature have underscored the success of transsphenoidal surgery in correcting the hypersecretion of prolactin [1], growth hormone [2], and ACTH [3] due to a functioning pituitary adenoma. As it might be expected, the success of the surgery has been found to be inversely related to the size of the tumor, with the best results obtained in patients with microadenomas (i.e. <10 mm in diameter).

In addition to producing characteristic syndromes of hormone hypersecretion such as galactorrhea/amenorrhea, acromegaly/gigantism and Cushing's disease, pituitary tumors have also been frequently associated with partial or complete hypopituitarism. One form of hypopituitarism which has received particular attention in the literature is the hypogonadism associated with hyperprolactinemia caused by prolactin secreting adenomas. Convincing evidence has been provided that in this setting hyperprolactinemia per se induces hypogonadism primarily by inhibiting LHRH secretion by the hypothalamus [4, 5]. The clinical manifestations of the hypogonadism associated with hyperprolactinemia include oligo/amenorrhea with infertility in women [6] and impotence and azo/oligospermia in men [7]. An important aspect of this form of hypogonadism is its reversibility following correction of the hyperprolactinemic state. Transsphenoidal microsurgery has been found to be highly successful in selectively removing prolactin secreting adenomas and restoring normal gonadal function both in women [1] and men [7]. Similarly, medical treatment of the hyperprolactinemia with the dopaminergic drug bromocriptine has been found to be highly effective in correcting this form of gonadal failure [8].

In contrast to the hypogonadism associated with prolactin secreting adenomas, much less emphasis has been placed in the literature on the effect of transsphenoidal surgery on other forms of hypopituitarism associated with pituitary tumors,

Santen, R.J. and Manni, A. (eds.), Diagnosis and management of endocrine-related tumors. ISBN 0-89838-636-5.
© *1984, Martinus Nijhoff Publishers, Boston. Printed in the Netherlands.*

including hypogonadism in the absence of hyperprolactinemia. Although the mechanism involved in causing diminished pituitary reserve in such patients is not well defined, it has been thought that the hypopituitarism in this setting is probably caused by compression and destruction of the normal pituitary tissue by the expanding adenoma. Some reports describing pituitary function before and after transsphenoidal surgery have included a few patients with partial hypopituitarism preoperatively that regained normal pituitary function postoperatively [1, 9–13]. However, the data presented in this regard are frequently incomplete and consequently, the possibility of recovering normal pituitary function following adenomectomy has not been well emphasized. Thus, it is common practice among most physicians to continue indefinitely appropriate hormonal replacement after transsphenoidal microsurgery in patients who preoperatively presented with variable degrees of hypopituitarism associated with a pituitary tumor.

It is the purpose of this manuscript to first review the pertinent data available in the literature regarding the effect of transsphenoidal microsurgery on pituitary function other than gonadal function in the setting of hyperprolactinemia. We will then report our experience with 11 patients harboring large non-functioning adenomas, in whom detailed studies of pituitary function were conducted before and after transsphenoidal adenomectomy. The data clearly show that at least partial recovery of pituitary function can be expected in some patients under these circumstances. In addition, our results provide some insight into the possible mechanisms involved in the hypopituitarism associated with pituitary tumors. Based on the data to be presented, we feel that appropriate pituitary function testing should be performed postoperatively after transsphenoidal microsurgery to assess the need for continued hormonal replacement before committing a patient to a lifetime treatment.

2. Effect of transsphenoidal microsurgery on pituitary function

2.1 Review of the literature

Samaan et al. [13] carefully evaluated thyroid and adrenal function in a group of 8 acromegalic patients before and after transsphenoidal microsurgery. Preoperatively, all patients had normal serum T_4, normal TSH with adequate rise after TRH administration, and normal plasma cortisol which rose appropriately after insulin-induced hypoglycemia. When evaluated postoperatively (the time of evaluation is not specified in the report), only 3 patients had retained normal thyroid and adrenal function. The remaining 5 patients were biochemically and clinically hypothyroid and adrenal insufficient and required hormone replacement. These results are somewhat at variance with other reports in the literature where preservation of normal pituitary function is observed in the vast majority of patients after transsphenoidal microsurgery. It is likely that the high incidence of hypopituitarism which occurred postoperatively in this small series may be due to the size of the tumors and the aggressiveness of the neurosurgeon in the attempt to totally correct the hypersecretion of growth hormone. Although no details are given on radiologic findings or tumor size measured at surgery, the authors commented that some of the tumors were found to be diffuse or embedded requiring a 'more radical anterior-pituitary dissection.'

Atkinson et al. [10] evaluated thyroid and adrenal function in 16 acromegalic patients before and after transsphenoidal microsurgery. The timing of the postoperative evaluation ranged between 3 and 24 months. Of 13 patients who preoperatively had normal thyroid function, all but 2 remained euthyroid. One patient with a preoperative serum thyroxine of 3 $\mu g/100$ ml (n: 4.5–10.5) was found to have a postoperative value of 8 $\mu g/100$ ml, suggesting recovery of the pituitary-thyroidal axis. Two patients who were hypothyroid and on replacement before surgery were maintained on replacement after surgery without testing their thyroid function off thyroid hormone supplementation. Thus, a possible recovery of thyroid function could have been missed in these two patients. Of 13 patients with normal adrenal function preoperatively, 3 became adrenal insufficient after surgery. Two patients had preoperatively normal baseline adrenal function (24-hour urinary 17-hydroxycorticosteroids) but abnormal response to metyrapone. After surgery, one of these patients had regained normal adrenal reserve as shown by restoration of a normal response to metyrapone. One patient was adrenal insufficient and on replacement preoperatively. This patient was continued on replacement postoperatively without further testing of his pituitary adrenal axis. The authors emphasize that preservation of anterior-pituitary function is compatible with transsphenoidal microsurgery in the vast majority of patients. They did not emphasize, however, that recovery of previously missing pituitary functions is also possible, as reflected by their decision to continue on replacement, without postoperative testing, those patients who are hypopituitary before surgery.

Hardy et al. [11], in reporting their results with transsphenoidal surgery in 79 cases of acromegaly, emphasized the beneficial effect of this form of treatment not only on growth hormone hypersecretion but also on the remaining pituitary functions. In this latter regard they observed that 16 patients recovered from previous deficits, 52 remained unaltered and 11 were impaired by surgery. Of these 11 patients 8 were made intentionally hypopituitary by performing a total sellar 'clean out' in the attempt to achieve complete tumor removal. The data however are largely incomplete since the authors do not specify which functions actually improved and how they were assessed. In addition, no information is provided on the timing of the postoperative evaluation and the duration of follow up. Nevertheless, the results emphasize that transsphenoidal microsurgery performed by experienced neurosurgeons is highly effective in selectively removing a pituitary tumor while leaving viable normal tissue.

McLanahan ct al. [12] evaluated gonadal, thyroidal and adrenal function pre- and postoperatively in a group of 40 patients who underwent transsphenoidal microsurgery for a variety of functioning and non-functioning pituitary tumors. Of 23 patients whose pituitary function was intact preoperatively, only 2 (9%) showed evidence of impaired function postoperatively. Of 17 preoperatively impaired patients, 3 (18%) were further impaired by the surgery. Thus, it appears that pituitary failure only rarely occurs as a result of transsphenoidal microsurgery. As far as postoperative recovery of previously present hypopituitarism the authors observed that 7 of 16 patients (44%) recovered gonadal function, 2 of 6 (33%) recovered thyroid function and 2 of 4 (50%) recovered adrenal function. In addition, they observed that the likelihood of recovery of pituitary function varied inversely with the degree of preoperative impairment and the size of the tumor. Some caution should be used, however, in the interpretation of their results since the evalution of the pituitary-gonadal, thyroidal and adrenal axis was only performed with basal hormone measurements. In no case was an attempt made to evaluate the pituitary 'reserve' of the trophic hormones, i.e. LH/FSH, TSH and ACTH. Although basal measurements of serum testosterone and thyroxine are adequate in most cases to assess gonadal and thyroidal functions, a significant impairment of the pituitary-adrenal axis can be missed in some cases by simple measurement of serum cortisol or determination of 17-hydroxycortico- steroids in the urine. Finally, one cannot determine in how many patients the hypogonadism was reversed by correction of hyperprolactinemia. Since more than half of their patients had prolactin secreting tumors, this was probably the case in at least some of the 7 patients who recovered gonadal function. We feel that recovery of gonadal function following transsphenoidal microsurgery in the setting of hyperprolactinemia should be considered separate from the recovery occurring in patients with normal serum prolactin preoperatively since it involves a different mechanism.

Post et al. [1] performed detailed studies of pituitary function pre- and post- operatively in a group of 30 women with prolactin secreting adenomas who underwent transsphenoidal selective adenomectomy. The authors evaluated pituitary reserve of gonadotropins, growth hormone, ACTH and TSH after appropriate stimuli. In addition, they also assessed posterior-pituitary function by a 14-hour dehydration test. The postoperative evaluation was performed 6 to 8 weeks after surgery and the average follow up was 18.6 months. Twenty-four patients had normal pituitary function preoperatively. Of these, 8 (33%) de- veloped variable degrees of hypopituitarism after surgery. In two of these pa- tients, no attempt was made to preserve normal pituitary function but, at the request of the patient, a total sella clean out was performed. In three patients only the 'reserve' of one or more pituitary hormones (ACTH, ACTH/GH/LH, ACTH/GH) was compromised. These patients only needed supplemental corticosteroid therapy for severe stress. One patient developed partial ADH deficiency, one developed GH deficiency (clinically insignificant in an adult) and one became hypogonadal. Thus, it appears that the degree of pituitary insufficiency was quite modest whenever a selective adenomectomy was attempted. Six patients presented with variable degrees of hypopituitarism before surgery. Normal thyroid function was regained by both patients who were hypothyroid preoperatively. One of two patients with impaired pituitary adrenal axis regained normal ACTH reserve. Normal growth hormone secretion was restored in 2 of 2 patients who were initially deficient. This latter recovery, however, might have been secondary to restoration of a normal estrogen milieu following correction of the hyperprolactinemia. Estrogens, in fact, are well known to stimulate growth hormone section [14, 15]

St. George Tucker et al. [9] have reported detailed studies of anterior-pituitary function pre- and postoperatively in a group of 32 patients (16 men and 16 women) who underwent transsphenoidal microsurgery for treatment of acromegaly. The postoperative evaluation was performed 2 to 6 months after surgery. The average duration of follow up was 4 years with a range from 6 months to 7-1/2 years. Of 19 patients who had normal pituitary function preoperatively, 15 remained normal postoperatively. Two patients developed gonadal insufficiency, one patient became hypoadrenal and hypogonadal and one patient developed complete hypopituitarism. Three patients who were completely hypopituitary preoperatively, remained so after surgery. Of 9 patients who manifested only gonadal insufficiency before surgery, 2 developed complete hypopituitarism, 4 remained unchanged and 3 recovered gonadal function postoperatively. In at least one of these 3 patients, this recovery was due to correction of hyperprolactinemia. In the other 2 patients serum prolactin level was normal postoperatively but was not determined before surgery. Finally, one patient who had impaired adrenal reserve preoperatively regained normal pituitary-adrenal axis postoperatively.

In summary from this review of the literature, the following conclusions can be drawn: 1) Anterior-pituitary function is preserved in most patients in whom a selective adenomectomy is attempted, especially in the case of microadenomas; 2) Patients who present with large pituitary tumors and panhypopituitarism preoperatively are likely to remain hypopituitary after surgery; 3) In patients who present with lesser degrees of hypopituitarism, recovery of one or more pituitary functions is possible.

This last point, however, has not been satisfactorily documented for several reasons. Firstly, some authors do not specify how they assess pituitary function, thus making the interpretation of their results difficult. In some cases only 'basal' hormonal studies were performed and no attempt was made to evaluate pituitary 'reserve' with the appropriate stimulation tests. Secondly, in the vast majority of cases where gonadal function was restored, it is impossible to ascertain whether this recovery occurred as a result of correction of hyperprolactinemia or as a result of tumor removal. For reasons stated above, we believe that this distinction is important. Undoubtedly, there is ample evidence in the literature that gonadal function can be restored in hyperprolactinemic patients following normalization of serum prolactin by either surgical or pharmacologic means. The question is whether transsphenoidal microsurgery can correct hypogonadism also in patients whose preoperative serum prolactin level is normal. Virtually no information is available in the literature in this regard. Thirdly, none of the reports describing restoration of pituitary function following selective adenomectomy have included data to provide clues to the possible mechanisms involved in the hypopituitarism and subsequent recovery. In addition, in many cases, the data on recovery of pituitary function were only included in the 'tables' but only very brief and general comments, if any at all, were made by the authors in the text. Consequently, the possibility of restoring normal pituitary function with transsphenoidal microsurgery has never been adequately emphazised.

2.2 Experience at Case Western Reserve University

Over a 2-year period, 11 patients with large nonfunctioning pituitary adenomas underwent transsphenoidal adenomectomy. The nonfunctioning nature of the tumor was documented by negative immunostaining of the adenoma for PRL, GH, ACTH and HCG employing the peroxidase-antiperoxidase technique [16]. Nine patients were males and 2 were females. Their ages ranged between 49 and 72 years. The presenting complaints included signs and symptoms of hypopituitarism (8 patients), headaches (6 patients) and visual problems (2 patients). None of the patients had polyuria, polydypsia or nocturia. All patients had gross enlargement of the sella turcica. Bony erosion was evident on tomography in 8 patients. Suprasellar extension of the adenoma was documented by CT scan in 9 patients. Visual field defects were observed in 4 patients. Evaluation of pituitary function, part of which is detailed in Table 1, was performed preoperatively and repeated 3 months after surgery. Thyroid and cortisol replacement was given to all patients with documented deficiencies preoperatively. L-thyroxine replacement was discontinued 1 to 2 weeks after surgery. Cortisol replacement instead was continued for 3 months and stopped 1 to 3 days prior to the pituitary function tests.

As can be seen in Table 1, patients 1 through 8 had severe hypopituitarism preoperatively. Six of them (patients 1, 2, 5–8) were hypothyroid, hypoadrenal and hypogonadal. Patient 5, the only woman in this group, had a low serum estadiol (35 pg/ml) and low serum gonadotropism (FSH 6; LH 3 mIU/ml). In 2 patients (patients 3, 4) the thyroid and gonadal functions were compromised but the pituitary-adrenal axis was intact. In all 8 patients serum GH levels were undetectable in the basal state, throughout a 14-hour overnight monitoring or during provocative stimulation with arginine or insulin-induced hypoglycemia (data not shown). In contrast, 3 patients (patients 9–11), had entirely normal pituitary function preoperatively. Patient 9, a postmenopausal woman, had appropriately elevated serum gonadotropin levels (FSH 68, LH 47 mIU/ml).

Following surgery, thyroid function became normal in 5 patients (pts 1, 3–6),

Table 1. Pituitary function in 11 patients with non-functioning adenomas before and after adenomectomy

| | | | Free thyroxine index | | Serum testosterone (ng/dl) | | a.m. cortisol µg/dl | | Peak cortisol after hypoglycemia | | Dynamics of prolactin secretion | | | | | | | |
| | | | | | | | | | | | Basal level ng/ml | | Δ after TRH ng/ml | | Δ after perphenazine ng/ml | | Δ after hypoglycemia ng/ml | |
Patient	Age	Sex	Preop	Postop	Preop	Postop	Preop	Postop	Preop	Postop	Preop	Postop	Preop	Postop	Preop	Postop	Preop	Postop
1	65	M	4.1	5.7	55	67	4	6.6	4.3	19.2	30	12.8	19.7	8.6	1	1	1	1
2	49	M	3.3	4.6	20	55	5.1	4.3	6.3	11.9	19	12.9	25.7	26.5	–	5	–	3.2
3	55	M	2.5	5.3	193	340	22.3	11.9	–	23	12	9	10	8	1	–	–	8
4	50	M	2.1	6.5	23	69	9.3	13	–	29	18	7	24	16	7	18	–	–
5	52	F	2.0	6.1	–	–	1.5	1.5	–	4.9	41	20	22	30	–	–	–	7
6	69	M	3.6	9.0	190	340	3.4	8.7	–	19.6	35	11	13.3	13	1	12	–	16
7	68	M	1.8	1.3	50	30	1.0	<1	–	–	2.7	<1	0	0	0	0	–	–
8	49	M	1.5	1.2	25	35	1.3	<1	–	–	2	1.5	0	1.5	1	2	–	–
9	72	F	9.1	10.1	–	–	14	9	21	20	7	6	12	16	–	–	8.9	11
10	52	M	8.3	7.9	395	355	12	10.5	20.9	23	8	9	17	14	13	16	10.9	13
11	51	M	7.9	6.0	565	615	8	9	19.8	20	10	8	22	17	17	24	9	8
Normal values			5–12		300–1000 (males)		5–25		≥18.5		10±2.7*	11.4±5**	26±8*	39±19**	20±7*	33±13**		

* Mean ±SD in 19 normal men.
** Mean ±SD in 22 normal women.

was slightly below the lower limit of normal in 1 patient (pt 2) and remained low in 2 patients (pts 7, 8). The pre- and postoperative TRH test was of particular interest. As can be seen in Fig. 1, TRH administration in 3 patients before surgery resulted in a delayed and sustained rise in serum TSH consistent with hypothalamic hypothyroidism. TSH rise after TRH became normal after surgery in 2 patients (pts 1, 3) who had regained normal thyroid function but was still slightly abnormal in one patient (pt 2) who, despite some improvement in thyroid function, was still hypothyroid. Patients 7 and 8 who had the most profound hypothyroidism unaffected by surgery had undetectable TSH levels following TRH administration both pre- and postoperatively (dat not shown). These data suggest that the hypothyroidism in these two patients was due to destruction of the thyrotrophs rather than being of hypothalamic origin. Patients 9–11 who had normal thyroid function preoperatively remained euthyroid after surgery.

Of 7 men who had hypogonadism before surgery, only 2 (pts 3, 6) recovered normal gonadal function. Among the hypogonadal men these two patients had the highest preoperative serum testosterone levels. Patient 5, the woman with low serum estradiol and gonadotropins, remained unchanged after surgery. Patients 9–11, who had an intact pituitary-gonadal axis preoperatively, remained normal after surgery. Patient 9, a postmenopausal woman, retained appropriately high serum gonadotropins postoperatively (FSH 60 mIU/ml, LH 55 mIU/ml).

Of 6 patients who had low basal serum cortisol and/or impaired pituitary reserve (pts 1, 2, 5–8), 2 recovered normal function (pts 1, 6). All patients who had normal adrenal function preoperatively (pts 3, 4, 9–11) remained normal after surgery.

Serum growth hormone became measurable at low levels (1–5 ng/ml) in 6 patients but the responses to provocative stimulation with insulin induced hypoglycemia or arginine remained subnormal (<8 ng/ml) in all 8 patients (pts 1–8) who had undetectable serum growth hormone preoperatively. In contrast, serum growth hormone levels remained normal and increased appropriately (>8 ng/ml) after insulin-induced hypoglycemia in patients 9–11 who had normal growth hormone secretion before surgery.

The data on serum prolactin levels and dynamics are of particular interest (Table 1) since they provide some insight into the possible mechanism(s) of the hypopituitarism occurring in these patients. Preoperative evaluation revealed that in the group of 8 patients who were hypopituitary before surgery, basal serum prolactin levels were mildly elevated or high normal in 6 (pts 1–6) and were low in 2 (pts 7, 8). TRH administration, a direct stimulus to the lactotrophs, resulted in a normal rise in serum prolactin in the 6 patients with normal or elevated basal levels but produced no rise in the 2 patients with low basal prolactin levels. On the other hand, perphenazine administration, which induces hyperprolactinemia in normal individuals through an hypothalamic mechanism, did not cause a significant rise in serum prolactin levels in any of the six hypopituitary patients tested preoperatively. The 3 patients with normal pituitary function before surgery (pts 9–11) had normal basal serum prolactin as well as normal response to both TRH and perphenazine administration (the latter tested only in two patients). Insulin-induced hypoglycemia, another hypothalamic stimulus of prolactin secretion, also produced a significant prolactin rise in these 3 patients.

After transsphenoidal microsurgery, the basal serum prolactin levels in the 6 patients (pts 1–6) who had normal or slightly elevated levels preoperatively, were normal in all patients. In each of these cases, there was postoperatively a decrease in serum prolactin. Normal prolactin rise after TRH administration was preserved in all 6 patients. In addition, 2 of 4 patients tested (pts 4, 6) regained normal response, in terms of prolactin secretion, to perphenazine administration. In contrast, the 2 patients with low serum prolactin preoperatively (pts 7, 8) had similar levels postoperatively without any appreciable response to TRH or perphenazine administration. Finally, all 3 patients (pts 9–11) with normal pituitary function preoperatively retained normal dynamics of prolactin secretion after surgery.

It appears that preoperative serum prolactin levels is somewhat predictive of recovery of pituitary function after surgery. In 6 patients with multiple pituitary hormone deficiencies associated with normal or elevated serum prolactin levels preoperatively, 2 recovered adrenal, 2 recovered gonadal and 5 recovered thyroidal function. In contrast, in 2 patients with panhypopituitarism associated with low serum prolactin preoperatively, no recovery of any function occurred. Recovery of growth hormone response to stimulation did not occur in any of the 8 patients regardless of the preoperative serum prolactin level.

3. Discussion

Both from our data as well as review of the literature, it appears that recovery of pituitary function is possible in patients harboring pituitary tumors following transsphenoidal microsurgery. Our results compare favorably with those reported by other investigators reviewed above considering the large size of the tumors in all of our patients and the profound degree of hypopituitarism in those patients who had compromised pituitary function preoperatively. It is remarkable that of 6 patients with panhypopituitarism (pts 1, 2, 5–8) significant recovery occurred in 3 (pts 1, 5, 6). In one of them (pt 6) all three major axes, i.e. pituitary-adrenal, gonadal and thyroidal, were restored to normal after surgery. To the best of our knowledge, no other reports have described a similar degree of recovery in patients with preoperative panhypopituitarism. In addition, none of our patients lost any normal pituitary function as a result of the surgery. This finding underscores the success of transsphenoidal microsurgery in preserving normal functional pituitary tissue while selectively removing the adenoma.

In our series, none of the patients who had hypopituitarism preoperatively recovered growth hormone response to stimulation. This is somewhat at variance with at least another report in the literature previously reviewed [1] where restoration of normal growth hormone secretion was observed in some patients after transsphenoidal microsurgery. We can probably best explain this discrepancy by a difference in the patient population investigated. The patients in whom recovery of growth hormone secretion was observed were women who had undergone transsphenoidal microsurgery for treatment of prolactin-secreting tumors. Since estrogens have a positive effect on growth hormone secretion, it is possible that this recovery was due to an improved estrogen milieu following correction of the hyperprolactinemia. Such a mechanism obviously could not take place in our patients who were mostly males with nonfunctioning tumors.

Our data provide some insight into the mechanism(s) of the hypopituitarism occurring in patients with pituitary tumors. The data on serum prolactin levels and dynamics are of particular interest in this regard. Of 6 patients in whom preoperative serum prolactin was high normal or elevated, 5 had at least a partial recovery of pituitary function and one showed some improvement in thyroid function and adrenal reserve (pt 2) although neither of these axis were normalized. We believe that measurement of serum prolactin allows us to identify patients who, despite the presence of hypopituitarism, have normal pituitary tissue left, i.e. the lactotrophs, and who might then be expected to recover pituitary function once the tumor is removed. The possibility that prolactin might be secreted by the tumor itself seems unlikely in view of the fact that the serum prolactin levels were only mildly elevated and not comparable to the levels seen in prolactin secreting adenomas of large size. Furthermore, and most important, immunostaining of multiple sections of the adenomas failed to show any cells staining for prolactin. Further evidence in favor of the presence of functioning pituitary tissue in these patients is provided by the rise in serum TSH after TRH administration (Fig. 1). This finding documents that viable thyrotrophs are present and able to secrete TSH when exposed to the appropriate stimulus. Unfortunately, similar stimulation with LHRH to test the pituitary reserve of gonadotropins was not carried out in our patients.

If these patients had normal pituitary tissue, what was the cause of their hypopituitarism? We believe that at least one of the mechanisms causing deficient pituitary function in our patients may be the interruption of the hypothalamic pituitary portal circulation by the large tumor mass. The dynamic studies of pituitary function tend to support this hypothesis. The rise in prolactin levels following TRH but not perphenazine administration that was noted in our patients had been noted to occur in patients with hypopituitarism of hypothalamic origin [17, 18]. Furthermore, the pattern of TSH response to TRH is quite suggestive of hypothalamic hypothyroidism [19–21] in that the peak was delayed and the release was sustained. In a large review of the types of TSH responses to TRH administration in 108 patients with hypothalamic pituitary disorders, Faglia et al. [21] had noted that a delayed and prolonged release of TSH

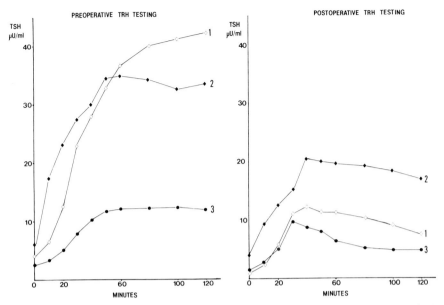

Figure 1. Serum TSH levels pre- (left panel) and postoperatively (right panel) after TRH (500 μg intravenously) administration in 3 patients.

was seen mostly in patients with craniopharyngiomas and also in patients with chromophobe adenomas associated with suprasellar extension.

Of interest in this regard is a recent report by Robinson et al. [22]. They published in an abstract form an unusual patient with carotid artery aneurysm who had panhypopituitarism associated with hyperprolactinemia. Following surgical resection of the aneurysm, complete recovery of pituitary function with normalization of serum prolactin level occurred. Based on the preoperative tests, the authors concluded that the hypopituitarism in that individual was hypothalamic in origin.

However, if interruption of the hypothalamic pituitary portal circulation was the only mechanism involved in causing hypopituitarism in our patients, one would expect recovery of all lost functions invariably to occur once the adenoma is removed. This was obviously not the case in all patients since some of them only regained normal pituitary function partially and some not at all. It seems likely that direct pressure by the tumor on the normal pituitary might destroy some of that tissue. In addition, interruption of the portal circulation may induce some focal necrosis of the normal anterior pituitary cells. Since the pituitary gland has a limited ability to regenerate [23], one would not expect the destroyed tissue to regenerate after the tumor is removed. Thus, depending on the amount of viable pituitary tissue left, one can expect variable recovery of pituitary function after adenomectomy.

The data on the 2 patients (pts 7, 8) with panhypopituitarism associated with low serum prolactin levels and absent TSH and prolactin responses to TRH, support this concept. The preoperative tests in these two patients suggest that the tumor had destroyed all viable pituitary tissue, thus preventing any recovery to occur after adenomectomy.

In summary, our data clearly show that recovery of pituitary function in patients with hypopituitarism associated with large pituitary adenomas may occur after surgical removal of the adenomas. A plausible mechanism for the hypopituitarism in such patients is the interruption of hypothalamic pituitary portal circulation by a large adenoma. A contributing factor may be ischemic destruction of normal pituitary tissue by the expanding tumor. Depending on the amount of viable pituitary tissue remaining, recovery of pituitary function may occur after adenomectomy. Finally, it is possible to identify by appropriate preoperative testing those patients who are likely to improve after surgery.

References

1. Post, KD, Biler BJ, Adelman LS, Molitch ME, Wolpert SM, Reichlin S: Selective transsphenoidal adenomectomy in women with galactorrhea-amenorrhea. JAMA 242: 158–162, 1979.
2. Arafah BM, Brodkey JS, Kaufman B, Velasco M, Manni A, Pearson OH: Transsphenoidal microsurgery in the treatment of acromegaly and gigantism. J Clin Endocrinol Metab 50: 578–585, 1980.
3. Tyrrel JB, Brooks RM, Fitzgerald PA, Cofoid PB, Forsham PH, Wilson CB: Cushing's disease: selective trans-sphenoidal resection of pituitary microadenomas. N Engl J Med 298: 753–758, 1978.
4. Franks S, Jacobs HS, Martin N, Nabarro JDM: Hyperprolactinemia and impotence. Clin Endocrinol (Oxf) 8: 277–287, 1978.
5. Bohnet HG, Dahlen HG, Wuttke W, Schneider HPG: Hyperprolatinemic anovulatory syndrome. J Clin Endocrinol Metab 42: 132–143, 1976.
6. Jacobs HS: Prolactin and amenorrhea. N Engl J Med 295: 954–956, 1976.
7. Arafah BM, Manni A, Brodkey JS, Kaufman B, Velasco M, Pearson OH: Cure of hypogonadism after removal of prolactin-secreting adenomas in men. J Clin Endocrinol Metab 52: 91–94, 1981.
8. Thorner MO, Besser GM: Bromocriptine treatment of hyperprolactinaemic hypogonadism. Acta Endocrinologica [Suppl 216] 88: 131–146, 1978.
9. St. George Tucker H, Grubb SR, Wigand JP, Watlington CO, Blackard WG, Becker DP: The treatment of acromegaly by transsphenoidal surgery. Arch Intern Med 140: 795–802, 1980.
10. Atkinson RL, Becker DP, Martins AN, Schaaf M, Dimond RC, Wartofsky L, Earll JM: Acromegaly. Treatment by transsphenoidal microsurgery 233: 1279–1283, 1975.
11. Hardy J, Somma M, Vezina JL: Treatment of acromegaly: radiation or surgery. In: Current Controversies in Neurosurgery, Moley TP (ed). W.B. Sanders, 1976, pp 377–391.
12. McLanahan CS, Christy JH, Tindall GT: Anterior-pituitary function before and after transsphenoidal microsurgical resection of pituitary tumors. Neurosurgery 3: 142–145, 1978.
13. Samaan NA, Leavens ME, Jesse RH: Serum growth hormone and prolactin response to thyrotropin-releasing hormone in patients with acromegaly before and after surgery. J Clin Endocrinol Metab 38: 957–963, 1974.
14. Frantz AG, Rabkin MT: Effects of estrogen and sex difference on secretion of human growth hormone. J Clin Endocrinol Metab 25: 1470–1480, 1965.
15. Spellacy WN, Carlson KL, Schade SL: Human growth hormone levels in normal subjects receiving an oral contraceptive. JAMA 202: 451–454, 1967.

16. Sternberger LA: Immunocytochemistry. New York: John Wiley and Sons, 1979.
17. Tolis G, Goldstein M, Friesen HG: Functional evaluation of prolactin secretion in patients with hypothalamic pituitary disorders. J Clin Invest 52: 783–788, 1973.
18. Woolf PD, Jacobs LS, Donofrio RV, Borday SZ, Schalch DS: Secondary hypopituitarism; evidence for continuing regulation of hormone release. J Clin Endocrinol Metab 38: 71–76, 1974.
19. Costom BH, Grumbach MM, Kaplin SL: Effect of thyrotropin-releasing factor on serum thyroid stimulating hormone. J Clin Invest 50: 2219–2225, 1971.
20. Foley TP, Owings J, Hayford JT, Blizzard RM: Serum thyrotropin responses to synthetic thyrotropin-releasing hormone in normal children and hypopituitary patients. J Clin Invest 51: 431–437, 1972.
21. Faglia G, Beck-Peccoz P, Ferrari C, Ambrosi B, Spada A, Travaglini P. Paracchi S: Plasma thyrotropin response to thyrotropin-releasing hormone in patients with pituitary and hypothalamic disorders. J Clin Endocrinol Metab 37: 595–601, 1973.
22. Robinson AG, Verbalis JG, Nelson PB: Reversible hypopituitarism following carotid artery aneurysm resection. 63rd Annual Meeting of the Endocrine Society, Cincinnati, Ohio, 1981, p 375.
23. Daniel PM, Treip CS: The regenerative capacity of pars distalis of the pituitary gland. In: The Pituitary Gland, vol 2, Harris GW, Donovan BJ (eds), 1966.

5. Medical treatment of thyroid carcinoma

WILLIAM H. BEIERWALTES

1. Introduction

Since this chapter is entitled the Medical treatment of thyroid carcinoma most of the emphasis will be on the treatment of papillary and follicular carcinoma of the thyroid with radioactive iodine, $Na^{131}I$. Other thyroid malignancies will be discussed primarily as they relate to the above topic. Similarly, the diagnosis and classification of thyroid malignancies will be discussed only as they relate to medical treatment.

In Chapter 6 Drs. Hamburger and Miller discuss diagnosis of thyroid nodules and in Chapter 7 Dr. Timothy Harrison discusses surgical treatment of thyroid carcinoma.

Emphasis will be centered on trying to express and document our answers on new and old controversies on medical treatment.

2. Rising incidence of well-differentiated thyroid cancer

Figure 1 shows that there was a 50% increase in the incidence of papillary and follicular carcinoma of the thyroid between 1973 and 1977 in the United States [1]. It was the third most common cancer in 15–19 year old girls, second in 20–24, and third in 30–34 year old women [2]. In the United States, papillary carcinomas outnumber follicular carcinomas about 3:1. E.D. Williams has shown a rising incidence of papillary carcinoma of the thyroid in patients on a high iodine diet [3]. In iodine deficient areas of the world, follicular carcinoma is more prevalent than papillary carcinoma [4].

3. Death rate

With modern surgery and $Na^{131}I$ therapy, rarely, should a patient die of well-differentiated thyroid cancer [5]. The major cause of death from well-differentiated thyroid carcinoma we see in patients referred to our University Hospital, is a

Santen, R.J. and Manni, A. (eds.), Diagnosis and management of endocrine-related tumors. ISBN 0-89838-636-5.
© 1984, Martinus Nijhoff Publishers, Boston. Printed in the Netherlands.

96

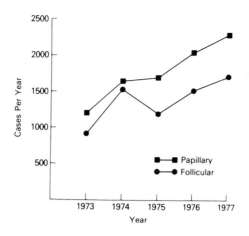

Figure 1. Graph from 1973-77 SEER Program showing a 50 increase in the incidence of papillary and follicular carcinoma of the thyroid between 1973 and 1977 in the United States. (This data is based on the Surveillance Epidemiology and End Result (SEER) Program of the National Cancer Institute from 11 population-based registries including five states and six metropolitan areas that make up approximately 10% of the U.S. population.) From Bloomer, WD: The thyroid gland, Chapter 28. Cancer of the Endocrine System; Brennan MF, Fig. 28-3, p 973, from Cancer, Principles and Practice of Oncology, DeVita VT, Jr., Hellman S, Rosenberg SA (eds). Phila.: J.B. Lippincott Co., 1982.

reluctance of the referring surgeon and physician to treat the patient aggressively while the patient is curable and a reluctance to stop treating the patient when he/she has progressed to an incurable state [5]. These attitudes appear to exist because of a lack of understanding that although well-differentiated thyroid cancer generally grows slowly in patients 16–40 years of age it grows and metastasizes aggressively in the very young (0–16 years) and in persons past 40 years of age. As a result, the physician with a thyroid cancer patient between 16 and 40 years of age may believe that the cancer may be adequately treated by local excision and the patient 'watched' in case he/she may develop recurrent growth or overt metastases.

3.1. *Children diagnosed under 16 years of age.* Winship [6] found the death rate to be 18 per cent in 546 children under 16 years of age. When the mortality rate was correlated with the patient's age at the time of diagnosis, 61.5% of 57 children diagnosed before age 7 were dead at follow-up. 12.8% of 430 children diagnosed between 7–15 years of age, were dead at follow-up [7]. In spite of these figures, there seems to be a reluctance to do a total thyroidectomy in a child with proved thyroid cancer, while it is accepted surgical practice to treat Graves' disease in children with a 95–100% 'total' thyroidectomy! [8, 9].

There is also a reluctance to treat children under 15 years of age with thyroid cancer with ^{131}I after surgery, perhaps because of the lack of the above knowledge of death rate and an undocumented fear of inducing an increased incidence of leukemia, second cancers and infertility with ^{131}I therapy.

3.2 *Adults diagnosed in the mid-decades.* 19.4% of patients we have treated with ^{131}I after surgery have had metastases of well-differentiated thyroid cancer outside the neck [5]. In these 78 patients with papillary thyroid carcinoma (mean entry age was 34–35 years) and 25 patients with follicular carcinoma (mean entry age was 50–51 years), 39.4% did not have their metastases detected at the time of the original surgery. The metastases were first detected outside the neck 7.44 years after the original surgery, with a range of 1–25 years. In the majority of patients the metastatic cancer could not be detected at the time of the original surgery because a 'nodulectomy' or subtotal thyroidectomy left sufficient thyroid gland to compete with metastases for uptake of [131]I. In many instances, ^{131}I was not used after surgery to look for metastases.

3.3 *Papillary.* Figure 2 shows our unique matching of cumulative survival rate of the 78 papillary patients with 94,751 'normals' in the State of Michigan during the mean years of 1969–71 with the mean matched entry age of 34–35 years. Of the 30 patients with papillary carcinoma who died, 21 died with residual of their thyroid carcinoma and 15 (71%) *from* their thyroid carcinoma. It is important to note that the death rate of the patients with papillary thyroid carcinoma increases with years after diagnosis over the death rate of age and sex matched controls in the same geographic areas, as shown in Table 1.

This observation indicates that the longer the follow-up of the 'young' person with thyroid cancer, the greater is the risk of death. Thus, the necessity for aggressive treatment in young people with thyroid carcinoma can not be made on

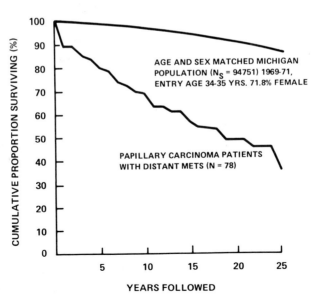

Figure 2. Cumulative survival rate of our 78 papillary thyroid cancer patients with metastases outside the neck. See text for matching of sex, age, and geographical location.

Table 1. Cumulative survival rates for distant mets patients and Michigan standardized patients

	U.M.	Mich-	Diff.
Papillary			
5 yr	.81	.99	.18
10 yr	.70	.98	.28
15 yr	.57	.95	.38
20 yr	.50	.92	.42
25 yr	.36	.87	.51
Follicular			
5 yr	.76	.96	.20
10 yr	.56	.89	.33
15 yr	.42	.81	.39
20 yr	.27	.79	.52

It is immediately obvious that there is a diverging difference between the two curves. This is a standard way for presenting this kind of data.

the basis of a 5 or 10 year follow-up experience, or the apparent presence or absence of metastases at the time of surgery.

3.4 *Follicular.* Figure 3 presents the same data for follicular carcinoma. Of the 16 dead patients with follicular carcinoma 11 (75%) died from thyroid carcinoma. Some workers have made decisions on whether to treat or not treat with ^{131}I at various ages based upon patient age and pathology type [10, 11].

We found [5], however, that when we matched the females and males under age 40 and over age 40, there was no difference in the survival between follicular thyroid carcinoma and papillary carcinoma. Thus it appears that previous statements on the apparent worse prognosis of follicular carcinomas were statistically biased because of the lack of careful age and sex matching of various study groups.

3.5 *Our surgical and ^{131}I therapeutic approach.* Our methods for selecting patients for treatment by surgery and I-131 have been described [5, 12, 13]. Routinely, the lobe of the thyroid gland containing a suspicious nodule is totally removed with the isthmus. A frozen section is done, and if the carcinoma is larger than 1.0 cm, a total extracapsular thyroidectomy is completed. If the frozen section is equivocal and the permanent histologic sections show a cancer, a total thyroidectomy is done within a few days or 6 wk later. Thyroid hormone is withheld for 6 wk after the operation.

Iodine-131 images of the neck and chest (and other areas when indicated) were done 24 h after 300 μCi of Na[131]I, using a rectilinear scanner beginning in 1954, a photoscanner in 1962, and a wide-field gamma camera with a high-energy collimator in 1979. Since 1981 we have used 2 mCi of ^{131}I with a single pin-hole

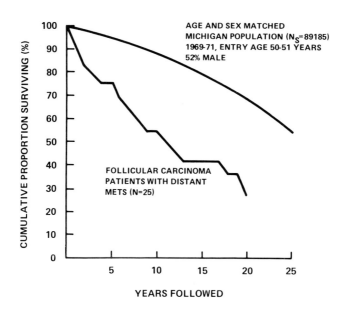

Figure 3. Same data for our 25 patients with follicular carcinoma with metastases outside the neck.

imaging of the neck and lung. If significant uptake is found in the region of the thyroidal bed, cervical lymph nodes, lungs, or bones, a therapeutic dose of Na[131]I is administered. The patient is discharged from the hospital when the total-body content of I-131 has decreased to <30 mCi. The patient is given a maintenance dose of 0.15–0.2 mg of sodium L-thyroxine. After a year, replacement thyroid hormone is discontinued for 6 weeks and the following tests are repeated: serum TSH (beginning 1974), T_4 (1971–), T_3 RIA (1976–), CBC, chest radiograph and scintigrams of the neck and chest (and other areas as indicated). If the scan shows no significant uptake, the patient resumes taking thyroid hormone and is asked to return in 2 yr. When the I-131 images are normal 3 yr after treatment, the patient is asked to return at intervals of 5 yr for life. In nine patients we have observed uptake of I-131 before recurrent neoplasms become palpable or are detected by radiographs of the chest. This has occurred as late as 15 yr after the patient is considered to be free of metastatic neoplasm.

Radioiodide is never given for ablation of remnants in the thyroidal bed unless significant uptake of I-131 (generally >2% of the dose at 25 h) is demonstrated by the scan. All possible thyroid tissue, normal or neoplastic, is excised from the neck without mutilation before treatment with I-131. It is frequently impossible to determine whether a patient has distant metastases before the removal of all normal thyroid tissue [12, 13], which effectively competes with the metastases for uptake of I-131.

Our treatment of well-differentiated thyroid carcinoma has been divided into ten procedures to determine the rate of 'conformity' to these procedures and to determine the effect of 'conformity' on survival time and 'cure' rate [5]. Lack of 'conformity' means that the procedure was not carried out because the patient had never been asked to have the procedure, or refused the procedure, or died before the procedure was carried out, etc.

In summary, these 10 procedures are:

1. Thyroidectomy done within 1 yr after a suspicious nodule has been detected.
2. Lobectomy with frozen section, and completion of total thyroidectomy within 6 mo.
3. Withholding of thyroid hormones for 6 wk before an I-131 scan of the neck is done.
4. Scintiscan done within 3 mo. after the thyroidectomy.
5. Treatment with I-131 for residual I-131 uptake.
   (a) Not less than 100 mCi for uptake in the thyroidal bed.
   (b) Not less than 150 mCi for uptake in the cervical nodes.
   (c) Not less than 175 mCi for distant metastases.
6. T_4 given between follow-up examinations.
7. Reexamination of the patient within 1 yr after treatment with I-131.
8. Reexamination of patient at 3 yr if the one-year scan in negative.
9. Reexamination of patient once every five years if patient is considered to be 'disease-free' after three years.
10. Treatment again, with more than 150 mCi of I-131, if recurrence of uptake occurs.

Using these procedures in 103 patients with well-differentiated thyroid carcinoma with metastases outside the neck, those considered to be free of their metastatic disease survived three times as long as those with persistent disease [5]. Patients freed of their metastases had a higher conformity rate with these procedures compared with patients not freed of their metastases [5].

4. 'Total' thyroidectomy vs. 'subtotal' thyroidectomy

4.1 *Risks in preparation for ^{131}I therapy*. There is general agreement that the risks of total vs. less than total thyroidectomy is dependent upon the skill and experience of the surgeon. We agree that the risks of a true total thyroidectomy for proved thyroid cancer by an *inexperienced* surgeon are unnecessary. We also believe that the risks are unnecessary for a total thyroidectomy in a child for the surgical treatment of Graves' disease by an inexperienced surgeon. We believe, however, that the solution to the problem is not inadequate surgery followed by ^{131}I ablation of uptake in the remnant for several reasons:

4.2 *Adequate surgery is more effective than ^{131}I in removing the primary cancer*. The most common cause of death from thyroid carcinoma is invasion of the structures of the superior thoracic inlet [12]. We have reviewed the literature showing that the death rates are lower after adequate surgery at the primary operation [13]. Sawyer et al. [14] found in a group of patients with papillary thyroid carcinoma that recurrences occurred in 8 of 19 patients, or 42 per cent, after nodulectomy and/or subtotal thyroidectomy. Furthermore, five, or 26 per cent of this group died from the disease. In the group of 10 patients with follicular carcinoma, similarly treated, four, or 40% developed recurrences and one patient died from the cancer.

Block [15] has also reviewed the literature showing that it is not possible to predict which lesions will respond to limited surgery. The malignancy has already spread to involve regional cervical lymph nodes in approximately 50% of patients with papillary adenocarcinoma even though metastases are not clinically evident. 'A significant number of patients with papillary and follicular adenocarcinoma of the thyroid will die of their disease. Most of the patients with these types of thyroid malignancy are young and have a long life expectancy. Thus, more radical surgery appears reasonable and justified. The more radical surgery for this disease need not be more mutilating than repeated, limited procedures [14].

4.3 *Total surgical thyroidectomy* may remove thyroid cancer that does not concentrate ^{131}I. Leeper has reported an alarming death rate from anaplastic 'transformation' of well-differentiated thyroid cancer in patients not having a total surgical thyroidectomy [11].

4.4 *There is a lower recurrence rate* after total surgical thyroidectomy than after subtotal. Recurrence of well-differentiated thyroid cancer after subtotal thyroidectomy has been found to be twice as common as after bilateral total thyroidectomy [16].

4.5 *Recurrences after inadequate surgery* result in a higher surgical morbidity from further surgeries and a 19–25% incidence of metastases that do not concentrate ^{131}I therapeutically [17, 18].

Mazzaferri reported [17] that in 576 patients in a 10 year follow-up, there were 84 recurrences. All 6 deaths from carcinoma occurred in this group. Nineteen percent of the patients with recurrences could not have their disease eradicated by any method. *Deaths in these patients began after 30 years of age. Cervical lymph node metastases were associated with increased recurrence rate.*

The M.D. Anderson group [18] in a study of 352 patients found 97 patients with recurrent disease. One fourth of these patients failed to concentrate radioiodine. Forty-four patients died of progressive thyroid carcinoma. Their deaths began after age 40 years.

It should also be remembered that recurrences occurring because the surgeon initially wishes to be 'conservative' leads to a logarithmically increasing incidence of surgical morbidity for each repeated surgery because of distorted anatomy.

5. Ablation of uptake of ^{131}I in surgical remnant

5.1 *In the presence of metastases or no detected metastases.* There appears to be no disagreement on the necessity for ^{131}I ablation of uptake in the thyroidal remnant in the presence of known metastatic disease. In our patients with known meta-stases outside the neck, however, the metastases were not detected for a mean of 7.44 years (1–25 years). The only way we can be certain that metastases are present that will concentrate ^{131}I is to ablate the competing uptake in the thyroidal remnant down to 0.5% or less of the tracer dose at 24 hours after the tracer.

Bestagno has provided quantitative information on how adequate surgery and ^{131}I ablation of uptake improve the ability of ^{131}I to detect metastases not detected by other measures [19].

In a series of 202 patients with well-differentiated thyroid carcinoma, he found that the overall incidence of functioning metastases not yet detectable by other means except at 3–5 days after an 'ablative' therapy dose of 100 mCi, was 15.8%. The incidence was 9% in those without known cervical node metastases. Sites of discovered metastases included lungs and bones. When lymph node metastases were known to be present before the ablating dose, distant metastases were discovered at 3–5 days after the ablating dose in 40% of patients with known cervical lymph node metastases not known to have distant metastases prior to this dose.

Moreover, results of ^{131}I therapy were significantly better when the metastases were detected in this manner in the 'pre-clinical' stage.

5.2 *'Normal' remnants or carcinoma in the thyroidal bed.* Advocates of the use of 29.9 mCi of ^{131}I to ablate uptake in 'normal' remnants believe that this dose will ablate the uptake in a *normal* remnant [20]. Presumably, therefore, the 39% of their patients whose remnant was not ablated with 29.9 mCi and who required an additional 100 mCi dose later had thyroid cancer in a previously judged 'normal' remnant.

Two other authors that followed their patients for longer periods to check on the 'ablative' effects of 29 mCi of ^{131}I in 'normal' remnants found that a second dose was required in 12 out of 13 patients [21] and in 16 out of 17 patients [22].

Thus we must conclude either that 29.9 mCi will not ablate uptake in the majority of 'normal' thyroid remnants, or that the majority of 'normal' thyroid remnants actually contain well-differentiated thyroid cancer that concentrates [131]I.

5.3 *Hazards of 'ablation' with 150 mCi of [131]I.* The reluctance to use a 150 mCi 'ablating' dose in such patients is difficult to understand since none of our 103 patients with distant metastases treated with ^{131}I and followed-up to 33 years from their first treatment doses died with or from leukemia, nor did they have an increased incidence of second caners [5]. Similarly, Leeper reports that the administration of far larger doses of ^{131}I than 150 mCi has not been associated with a case of leukemia at Memorial Hospital in 22 years [11].

Yet some patients who consult us for a second opinion have been started on x-ray therapy and/or cancer chemotherapy before a trial of ^{131}I therapy for well-differentiated thyroid carcinoma. Chabner has reported from the National Cancer Institute in an Editorial [23] that in ovarian cancer patients living 2 years after initiation of chemotherapy, the risk of developing acute leukemia is increased by a factor of 67–171. Similarly in patients with Hodgkin's disease the risk of developing a second cancer 4 years after lymph node irradiation and chemotherapy is increased by a factor of 21!

6. Size of therapy doses

6.1 *'Standard' doses.* We use a standard dose of 150 mCi of ^{131}I to adults for a thyroidal remnant because it is successful in 95% of patients who have had adequate surgery [24]. It commonly fails in patients who have had inadequate surgery. Freedberg et al. [25] studied 51 postmortem examinations 7 days to 11 years after administration of ^{131}I to euthyroid cardiacs. They concluded that about 50,000 rads to the normal thyroid gland was required for its total destruction; most of this delivered by the first dose.

We administer 175 mCi when there is demonstrated uptake of ^{131}I in lymph nodes after surgical lymph node extensive plucking. We administer a standard adult dose of 200 mCi for metastases outside the neck [26].

The reasons we use this 'standard' dose of 200 mCi for adults with metastases outside the neck are:

6.2 *AEC restriction on maximum single total dose.* In 1956, the Atomic Energy Commission Sub-committee on Human Use, began to include in the ^{131}I license a limit of 200 mCi on single doses for cancer [27].

6.3 *The A.E.C. Sub-committee on Human Use* based this action on a study that failed to find data to prove that single doses greater than 200 mCi were more effective than doses larger than 200 mCi. They also found that doses greater than 200 mCi were associated with an increased incidence of complications [27].

6.4 *Patients who have died from their thyroid carcinoma* have received larger total doses than patients freed of their metastases [10, 28].

6.5 Since it has been demonstrated that blood doses larger than 200 rads carry an increased risk of complications (primarily bone marrow depression), it is reasonable to do studies that allow a calculation of the dose required to deliver a blood dose of 200 rads.

The reasons we do not do this, however, are that:

a. It requires a minimum of 4 days of patient study after administering the tracer dose [10].

b. The treatment dose frequently exhibits different kinetics than the tracer dose [27].

c. The proponents of this procedure have demonstrated that treatment doses in excess of 200 mCi carry an increased risk of complications [27].

In spite of this fact the Sloan Kettering group has stated that dosimetry calculations allowing a 200 rad blood dose 'has allowed us to give an average, single therapeutic dose of 309 mCi' (range, 70–654 mCi) [11]. They have suggested that when the disease is rapidly progressive, the limits are increased to 300 rads to blood or 150 mCi body retention at 48 hours. It is our experience, however, that aggressive treatment of far advanced rapidly progressive differentiated thyroid cancer seldom if ever is successful. Usually this carcinoma is less well-differentiated and concentrates ^{131}I poorly. It has been reported that a series of doses estimated to deliver up to 500 thousand rads failed to decrease the size of the tumor [28]. Rarely if ever are bone marrow metastases cured, even when total doses reach as high as 2.5 curies.

It is for this reason that we urge more adequate surgery and ^{131}I ablative therapy in patients under 40 years of age and with well-differentiated thyroid cancer while curable, and cessation of ^{131}I therapy when the patient develops rapidly progressive, less well-differentiated and/or hopelessly advanced disease. We believe this approach is more conservative than inadequate surgery and inadequate ^{131}I therapy when the disease is curable; and aggressive therapy only when the disease is incurable.

7. Is ^{131}I after adequate surgery effective?

The effectiveness of radioiodine in the treatment of thyroid cancer remains to be determined despite 35 years of experience (1947–1987). We published [29] that a review of the literature shows that 75% of patients with all types of thyroid cancer and distant metastases die within 5 years after diagnosis. We therefore have published on this high risk group (103 patients with metastases outside their neck from well-differentiated thyroid carcinoma) followed for a period of up to 35 years to determine the effectiveness of our treatment [5].

7.1 *Our 10 'ideal' steps* in treatment that we have followed since 1947. These have been outlined on pages 7 and 8 and will not be repeated here.

7.2 *Our 1981 study.* Our study [5] consisted of 103 patients with metastases outside the neck out of 532 patients (19.4%) treated with ^{131}I after surgery, out of 1,153 patients seen at University Hospitals from November 1947 to June 1980 with a histopathologic diagnosis of any thyroid carcinoma. We have thus accrued 57 living patients and 46 dead, 52 of these patients are freed of their disease and 51 were not [5].

The questions that were asked were what 'ideal' steps appear to:
1. Free the patient of his/her disease by all criteria (including radionuclide imaging), and
2. Increase the survival time of the patient.

7.2.1 Cause of death

Papillary carcinoma – 30 dead. Twenty-one died *with* residual of thyroid carcinoma, 15 (71%) *from* their thyroid carcinoma. Four died without residual thyroid carcinoma from other cancers. When we checked out incidence of other cancers against the normal population there was no increased incidence of second cancers following radioiodine treatment.

Follicular carcinoma – 16 dead. Fifteen patients with follicular carcinoma died *with* residual of their thyroid carcinoma, 11 (73%) *from* their thyroid carcinoma. Four died from other causes.

7.2.2 Effect of ablation of uptake of radioiodine in distant metastases

Papillary carcinoma. Patients with papillary carcinoma freed of their disease by all criteria survived a mean of 16.5 years of follow-up compared to 7.6 years for those not freed of their disease, a 2.2-fold longer survival time of those freed of their disease.

Follicular carcinoma. Similarly, those freed of their disease survived 17.5 years as compared to a mean of 7.2 years of those not freed of their disease. This is a 2.4-fold longer survival time. When we compared patients freed of their disease by all criteria and alive versus those not freed of their disease and dead the survival time was three times longer in the former group.

7.2.3 Age of patient and 'cure'

Papillary carcinoma. Those freed of their disease (average age 20) were about 1/2 the age of those not freed of their disease (age 45). This constitutes a strong argument to treat young patients with papillary carcinoma of the thyroid aggressively while they are still curable.

Follicular carcinoma. Those freed of their disease (average age 36) were about 2/3 the age of those not freed of their disease (age 57). Again, this is strong evidence that younger follicular carcinoma patients should be treated aggressively while they are still curable.

7.2.4 Leukemia and second cancers.
No patient died from or with leukemia. There was no increased incidence of second cancers. This is in striking contrast to the 67–171 fold increased risk of acute leukemia at two years after the treatment of carcinoma of the ovary with cancer chemotherapy [23, 30]. It is also in striking

106

contrast to the treatment of Hodgkin's disease with x-ray therapy and cancer chemotherapy. These patients are at 21 fold increased risk of developing second cancers at four years after the onset of treatment [23, 30].

7.2.5 'Conformity' with those steps in treatment in which a trend is evident – Papillary

Step #2: Lobectomy with frozen section and second lobectomy within six months. There was an 83% conformity rate in those alive and freed of their disease by all criteria as compared to a 55% conformity rate in those dead and with their disease (P<0.05).

Step #3: Off T4 and T3 six weeks before ^{131}I scan. There was a 94% conformity rate in those alive and freed of their disease by all criteria as compared to a 63% conformity rate of those dead with their disease (P<0.05).

Step #4: Scan within three months of surgery. There was a 94% conformity rate in those alive and freed of their disease as compared to a 44% conformity rate in those dead with their disease (P<0.001).

Step #5: Treat with ^{131}I for residual carcinoma with adequate dose. There was a 71.4% conformity rate in those alive and freed of their disease as compared to a 50% and 57% conformity in those alive or dead with their disease.

7.2.6 'Conformity' in treatment of follicular carcinoma. The data was too limited to do chi square tests in two instances and not significant in the two instances where they could be tested. Nevertheless, the same trends are evident in the presentation of the data.

Step #1: Have thyroidectomy within one year of 'goiter'. There was a 71.4% conformity rate in those alive and freed of their disease as compared to a 50% conformity rate in those alive and dead not freed of their disease.

Step #3: Off T4 and T3 six weeks before scan. There was a 100% conformity rate in those alive and freed of their disease as compared to a 50% conformity rate in those alive or dead with their disease.

Step #4: Scan within three months of surgery. There was a 100% conformity rate in those alive and freed of their disease as compared to a 50% conformity rate in those alive or dead with their disease.

Step #5: Treat with ^{131}I for residual uptake. There was a 54% conformity rate in those alive and freed of their disease as compared to a 38% conformity in those dead and with their disease.

7.2.7 Question of statistical bias of age difference in the 'conformity' vs. 'non-conformity'. The only statistically significant difference in age in the two groups under #5; treat with ^{131}I for residual ^{131}I uptake in the follicular group. The 'Conformity' group had a mean age of 56.2 years vs. 40.56 years in a non-conformity group. This was to our advantage, however, because the older group (which notoriously has a worse prognosis) survived just as long (10.13 years) as the younger non-conformity group (10.22 years).

7.2.8 *Time from original surgery* (histopathological diagnosis) to first detection of metastases outside of the neck. 39.4% of the patients did not have their metastases detected at the time of the original surgery. The metastases were first detected outside the neck 7.44 years after the initial surgery with a range of 1 to 25 years.

The importance of initial adequate surgery and ^{131}I ablation in staging the patient was presented above [19]. Bestagno detected metastases with ^{131}I in 9% of those patients without 'clinical' metastases and in 40% of patients with proved cervical lymph node metastases. These 'preclinically' detected metastases after adequate surgery and ^{131}I ablation were commonly in lungs and bones. If, however, the patient has a subtotal thyroidectomy and no ^{131}I thyroidal bed ablating dose, the physician does not know if the patient has metastases because the metastases will not concentrate radioiodine as long as there is significant uptake in the thyroidal bed, with rare exceptions. Therefore, in order to be 'conservative' and 'follow' the patient, the physician is waiting until the patient has clinical evidence of cancer elsewhere, at which time statistically his/her death rate is markedly increased and there is a decreased opportunity to eradicate the patient's disease.

There is, therefore, stong evidence that radioiodine should be given to ablate uptake in the remnant after adequate surgery while the patient is still 'curable' rather than being 'conservative' and merely follow the patient.

7.2.9 *Status of dead or alive* with or without disease and location of metastases [5]. In papillary carcinoma of the thyroid, the most common location of metastases outside the neck was within the lung > mediastinum > bone. After radioiodine treatment the mediastinal metastases were easiest to 'cure' > lung > bone.

7.2.10 *Conclusions*

1. Well-differentiated thyroid carcinoma does kill.

2. Roughly 40% of patients did not have their metastases detected at the time of the initial surgery. There is now further evidence that adequate surgery and radioiodine ablation are necessary to allow 'staging'. These data also suggest that radioiodine ablation of the thyroid remnant after adequate surgery is not radical treatment but is conservative treatment.

3. Radioiodine treatment in these patients treated for distant metastases and followed to 35 years was not associated with a single incidence of leukemia or an increased incidence of second cancers.

4. Young persons with papillary or follicular carcinoma should be treated aggressively because there are no significant harmful effects from radioiodine treatment and because as they age they have a worse prognosis even with good treatment.

5. Patients with uptake ablated in the thyroidal bed have a lower death rate than those whose thyroidal bed uptake is not ablated [26].

6. Patients freed of the distant metastases with adequate radioiodine treatment after adequate surgery survive 2.2 to 3 times longer than patients not freed of their disease.

8. Why scan off all T4 and T3 in six weeks after surgery?

A delay may allow recurrence or metastases. A scan at six weeks after surgery allows treatment to ablate the remnant and treat micrometastases without delay. There is evidence in the animal model that delay increases the number of lung metastases. Prompt adequate surgery and radioiodine therapy allows immediate staging. Prompt adequate surgery and radioiodine also insures better compliance on the part of the patients.

9. Attempts to not leave the patient off thyroid hormone (to avoid hypothyroidism) while staging or treating the patient with ^{131}I.

9.1 *Does lack of T4 and T3 increase tumor growth?* The only hard data on this subject comes from experiments in animal models. We published in 1964 that well-differentiated papillary carcinoma of the thyroid grew fastest in the euthyroid rat and most slowly in the rat kept hypothyroid the longest [31]. More recently others have confirmed our observations with other cancers as well; in the sarcoma one of the Ajax mouse and Lewis fibrosarcoma in C 57BL/60 mice [32] and in mammary tumors in mice [33]. Thus the only controlled experiments indicate that lack of thyroid hormone decreases the growth rate of cancer.

9.2 *Why not continue* T4 and give TSH or TRH injections? Although this was formerly done, it is no longer done in most centers. There is a higher incidence of allergic reactions, a formation of neutralizing antibodies and TSH resistance, a rapid decline of serum TSH levels, and a lower uptake of radioiodine [34–36]. TRH injections do not produce as high TSH levels as thyroid hormone withdrawals [37].

9.3 *Why not withdraw T3* for only two weeks and thus decrease the period of fatigue and cold intolerance? We do not do this because we have had occasional patients with metastatic carcinoma of the thyroid to lung show no uptake of radioactive iodine in lung metastases after withdrawal of T3 for as long as three weeks but did show an excellent uptake for both diagnosis and treatment in the lungs when they had been off T3 for a period of six weeks.

Figure 4 illustrates this sequence of events. T.L. was a 40 year old woman when we saw her on referral from Ohio State University Hospital in January 1975. In 1947, at age 15 she had had x-ray therapy for facial acne. In 1967, at age 35, she was

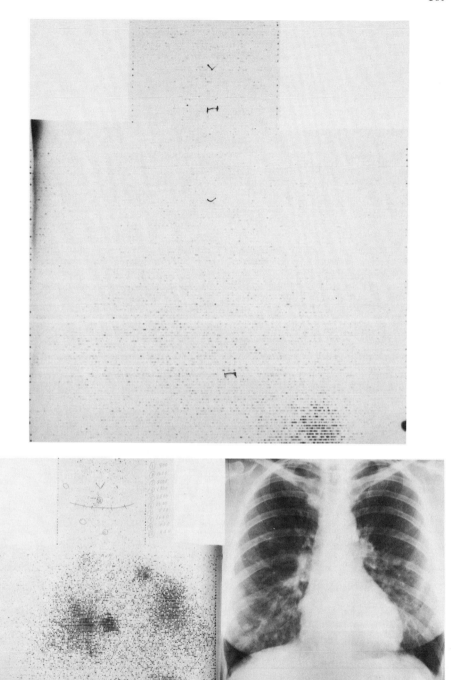

Figure 4. Lack of ^{131}I uptake in lungs of patient with lung metastases visible by chest roentgenogram, when off T3 for two weeks (4a) (1-75), but excellent uptake in lung metastases when off T3 for 7 weeks (4b) (3-11-75) (using same 300 uCi tumor dose and photoscanner settings).

noted to have a nodule in the right lobe of the thyroid gland. Because the nodule was believed to be a focus of thyroiditis, she was treated with steroids for one year. In 1968 the lump increased in size. A 'total' surgical thyroidectomy was performed and she was started on 0.2 mgm sodium-1-thyroxine/day. In 1972 she had a severe upper respiratory infection with a temperature of 100° F and a hemoptysis with a normal chest roentgenogram. Bronchoscopy with sputum exam were normal. In 1974 (at age 42) a routine chest roentgenogram showed metastases to lungs. A thyroid scan after five days of 10u TSH and 1 day after administration of isotope showed residual uptake in the pyramidal lobe but no uptake in lungs after a 20 mCi ablating dose, off thyroxine for six weeks and off triiodothyronine for two weeks. A lung biopsy was read as 'papillary adenocarcinoma of the thyroid'. She was started on 4 grains of desiccated thyroid a day. In December of 1974, she was again taken off desiccated thyroid for six weeks and triiodothyronine for two weeks. A repeat lung scan with 300 uCi of ^{131}I and a photoscanner showed no uptake of ^{131}I in lungs (Fig. 4a). In January of 1975 she was seen at our hospital and we confirmed these findings under identical circumstances. We asked her to stay off *all* medication for seven weeks.

On March 11, 1975 a repeat scan under identical circumstances showed good uptake in lungs (Fig. 4b) with 0.4% of the tracer dose in the thyroidal bed and lungs. She was given a treatment dose of 200 mCi of [131]I.

Perhaps the best article advocating withdrawal of T3 for two weeks is that of Goldman et al. [38]. The assets that they list in their article for this procedure is that the patient is more comfortable, there is less tumor growth (they supplied no references), there was a higher uptake at two weeks than at four weeks, and there are no new areas of uptake detected at four weeks.

The deficits that they listed in their article was that only one of their patients had distant metastases. The majority of their patients had a fairly sizable amount of normal thyroid tissue in the thyroidal bed. Seventeen had uptake in the thyroidal bed, five in cervical lymph nodes and one in lung metastases. The fact that the serum T4 increased in four patients and into the normal range in two is evidence for a sizable normal thyroid remnant. Further evidence is that in 2 of 29 patients, the uptake increased to greater than 50% at four weeks to as high as an 18% uptake.

They admitted that increased TSH might decrease the turnover time and therefore decrease the uptake at 48 hours. They used the 48 hour interval rather than our interval of 24 hours. They recalled that in persons with normal thyroids there is a rebound increased uptake after T3 in euthyroids. They also gave references in the literature to the fact that some patients with normal thyroids who had been on thyroid hormone did not have their pituitaries recover from thyroid hormone suppression for up to 35 days after cessation of thyroid therapy [39–40]. Basal serum TSH could not be used to differentiate euthyroid from hypothyroid patients for 35 days after withdrawal of thyroid therapy. The response to TRH does not improve this differentiation [39].

We commonly observe that patients treated for hyperthyroidism with radio-iodine may return at three months after ^{131}I treatment with sub-normal levels of serum T4 and T3 without any elevation of the serum TSH because their pituitaries have not recovered from the excess thyroid hormone.

9.4 *Why not use radioactive thallium-201* rather than ^{131}I and thus avoid taking the patient off thyroid hormone? It has been demonstrated that some patients may have their metastases detected with Thallium-201 that did not concentrate radio-iodine. It has also been demonstrated that some patients have their metastases detected with Thallium-201 equally well while they are on thyroid hormone as when they are off thyroid hormone [41]. Subsequent to these original Japanese observations, however, abundant evidence has appeared from our laboratory and others [42] that the use of Thallium is less reliable than [131]I. It may also image normal lymph nodes.

9.5 *Why not use serum thyroglobulin* (HTG) instead of the radioiodine uptake? There is abundant evidence that the serum HTG is increased in many thyroid diseases [43]. It is released from both benign and malignant tissue, particularly with increasing serum TSH. It detects non-functioning metastases. The serum HTG is higher with bone and lung metastases than with lymph node metastases.

Schneider et al. [44] found that 14 out of 15 patients had a serum HTG in the normal range (less than 10 milligram/milliliter) on T3. A high HTG did not distinguish residual tissue from metastases. The HTG was greater than normal in 18% of patients with negative scans. There were positive scans in 14 out of 32 patients (44%) where the HTG was less than 2 milligrams/milliter. A conclusion of this article was that the combination of radioiodine scans and HTG were better than the use of either alone. The work was substantiated by Echenique et al. from M.D. Anderson [45].

10. Why not give 29 millicuries of radioiodine ablating dose for thyroid remnant rather than 150 millicuries?

This question was addressed briefly in the first few pages of this chapter. The idea of giving less than 30 mCi of ^{131}I was initially advanced because the Atomic Energy Commission asked that all patients with 30 mCi or more of radioactivity in their bodies should be hospitalized so that their urine could go down a certified sewer.

We gradually moved up from an initial treatment dose of 5 millicuries to a more or less routine radioiodine uptake in the remnant ablating dose of 150 millicuries because of a high failure rate. The failure rate is best judged by a one to two year follow-up. We found that if we failed to ablate the uptake on a first dose that was small, we then had to give a larger second dose and actually increase the total

112

radiation dose to the patient. There is also increasing evidence that a sub-optimal radiation dose decreases the biologic half-life of subsequent radiation doses and therefore decreases the chance of curing the patient [46–47].

Figure 5a shows a good uptake in thyroid remnant and in one or two cervical nodes in a young man with carcinoma of the thyroid who had had a 'total' thyroidectomy and extensive lymph node plucking. He had a normal chest X-ray. There is such little uptake in lungs that it might be tempting to some to ablate the uptake in the remnant and in the cervical nodes first with 29 millicuries and then give a larger treatment dose for the lung metastases. Evidence that this is not necessary is shown by the striking uptake in the lungs after the therapy dose of 200 millicuries (Fig. 5b).

Figure 5c shows that one year later the patient has no evidence of uptake in the thyroidal remnant or cervical nodes or lung metastases.

11. Should you give a low iodine diet and/or diuretic therapy?

We do give a low iodine diet for the last week before the scan on radioiodine therapy to decrease the iodine pool and thus increase the specific activity of ^{131}I from a treatment dose. Milk is the principal source of iodine. This is found in cheese and pizzas. Iodine is also found in fish and X-ray contrast media.

12. Why not treat with X-ray therapy and/or chemotherapy instead of ^{131}I?

We do not use X-ray therapy before radioiodine because it will decrease the T 1/2b of ^{131}I in the thyroid cancer thus decreasing the radiation dose from ^{131}I [46, 47]. It is not effective in treating well-differentiated thyroid cancer [48]. It does not ablate the uptake of ^{131}I [49]. It increases the incidence of bone marrow

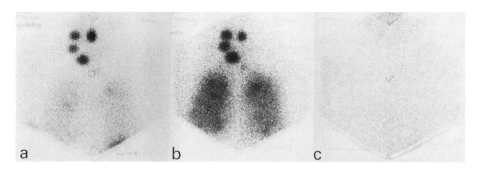

a   b   c

Figure 5. Good uptake of ^{131}I in thyroid remnant and in one or two cervical nodes in a young man who had had a 'total' thyroidectomy and extensive lymph node plucking (a). His chest roentgenogram was normal. When a 200 mCi treatment dose of ^{131}I was given, he was demonstrated to have lung metastases (b) and the uptake in both thyroidal remnant and lung metastases was ablated (c).

depression after ^{131}I treatment [50]. Mazzaferri found that X-ray therapy actually adversely affects the outcome [17]. Many people believe that it should be used only in the treatment of anaplastic carcinoma of the thyroid, adenocarcinomas refractory to ^{131}I therapy, lymphoma, and possibly in Hürthle cell and medullary thyroid carcinoma [51].

We have produced evidence that adequate surgery followed by radioiodine treatment is the most effective method of treating well-differentiated thyroid cancer today. We have referred above to the fact that whereas there is no recent evidence that radioiodine treatment of thyroid carcinoma increases the incidences of leukemia or second cancers, there is abundant evidence that there is a marked increased risk of acute leukemia after chemotherapy and second cancers after the combination of X-ray therapy and chemotherapy [30].

We have also produced evidence that radionuclide therapy can deliver orders of magnitude larger radiation doses than conventional X-ray therapy [30]. We have also produced evidence that radionuclide therapy is far less traumatic and invasive than X-ray therapy and chemotherapy. It should be pointed out that two authors produced most of the cases of leukemia in thyroid carcinoma with radioiodine [52, 53]. It is reassuring to note that these authors, like many of the first people using radioiodine therapy in thyroid carcinoma, gave fractionated doses at short intervals, as in conventional radiation therapy. Most of these cases of leukemia had also had X-ray therapy. This method of therapy resulted in deaths from intracerebral hemorrhage following thrombocytopenia at six to ten weeks after this fractionated therapy and resulting in bone marrow depression. It is reassuring that most of us have not observed a case of leukemia in 20 years [11]. We believe that this is because we now allow the bone marrow to recover for one year [11, 54, 55].

13. Should we use ^{131}I for the treatment of medullary thyroid carcinomas? (or anaplastic thyroid carcinoma?)

There have been four articles that suggest that radioiodine might be useful in the treatment of medullary carcinoma after total thyroidectomy with no known residual lymph node involvement, with demonstrated uptake in the thyroidal bed off T4 and T3 for six weeks, and stable elevated serum calcitonin levels for six months or more [56–59]. There is very recent evidence that C cells may be far more sensitive to the radiation from radioiodine than follicular cells [60].

Although almost no medullary thyroid carcinoma has been proved to concentrate ^{131}I, the initial rationale for treating thyroid carcinoma that did not concentrate ^{131}I was that uptake of ^{131}I in normal thyroid tissue in the thyroidal bed would kill the thyroid carcinoma not concentrating ^{131}I bij producing obliterative endarteritis or by cross irradiating with beta and/or gamma rays. None of our patients, however, with anaplastic carcinoma in the thyroidal bed have experienced an increased survival time from this treatment [26].

Medullary thyroid carcinoma may be a different case, however, because of the established increased sensitivity of cells to irradiation [60] and because papillary and follicular carcinomas that merely have some focal medullary changes do respond to ^{131}I therapy. At present, we believe it is justified to try it in patients without evidence of lymph node extension after adequate surgery, with significant ^{131}I uptake in thyroidal bed.

14. Why treat young healthy asymptomatic persons with lung metastases and cause pulmonary fibrosis?

Rall [61] answered this question in an article in 1957. He showed that when he achieved less than 100 millicuries uptake of radioiodine in the lungs there was no subsequent pulmonary fibrosis. He achieved that unfavorable result only when there was more than 100 millicuries of uptake in the lungs with patients with diffuse bilateral metastases. The highest percent uptake we have ever had in the lungs is 35% of the tracer at 24 hours. Since we never give over 200 millicuries in a dose, it has been impossible for us to achieve a 100 millicurie treatment dose in the lungs and we have never had a result of pulmonary fibrosis and deteriorating lung function.

15. Will ^{131}I therapy decrease the fertility or increase the incidence of birth abnormalities?

Dr. Sarkar and I published a follow-up on 40 children [62] that we treated for thyroid cancer, with a mean total dose of 196 millicuries and a maximum dose of 691 millicuries, followed for periods of up to 25 years. There was no decreased fertility or abnormal birth history.

16. Can radioiodine cause anaplastic transformation?

Mazzaaferi showed that only 1/2 of the reported patients with papillary and follicular thyroid carcinoma who developed anaplastic cancers had a documented history of previous irradiation [16].

17. Should we see the surgery and pathology reports and pathology slides before treating with [131]I?

Perhaps this warning should have been put first and last. We *never* treat or consult on treatment of a patient for thyroid carcinoma without seeing the surgery and pathology report and pathology slides.

17.1 *Wrong slides on wrong patient.* We have had patients referred to us for treatment of thyroid carcinoma who never had thyroid carcinoma. One patient had her slides mixed up with a patient who had had an operation in the same room immediately before her (who did have thyroid carcinoma). When we requested the slides on our patient, our pathologist reported that the slides showed osteomyelitis!

17.2 *Hürthle cells in Hashimoto's Struma.* One of these patients had Hashimoto's Struma. The Hürthle cells in Hashimoto's Struma may be confused with Hürthle cell carcinoma.

17.3 *Papillary carcinoma of the ovary* with calcospherite confused with papillary carcinoma of the thyroid gland with calcospherites. Another patient had a papillary carcinoma with calcospherites in cervical lymph nodes next to her thyroid gland. When our total thyroidectomy disclosed no carcinoma, we requested the slides from an oophorectomy performed at the referring hospital 8 years previously on the same patient. They revealed the identical pathology of a papillary carcinoma of the ovary with calcospherites.

17.4 *Focal areas of carcinoma* that falsely suggest that the patient is not a candidate for treatment with ^{131}I. In addition, some patients may have a small area of anaplastic change or medullary change or occult sclerosing carcinoma of the thyroid that may prove in more slides or blocks to be a papillary and follicular carcinoma of the thyroid that concentrates ^{131}I therapeutically.

17.5 *'Follicular adenoma' vs follicular carcinoma.* Some patients are said to have a follicular adenoma. Follicular carcinoma cannot be ruled out in such patients until all of the capsule has been examined for capsular or vascular invasion. We do not ablate thyroid remnants after surgery in patients with *proved* benign follicular adenomas.

17.6 *Hürthle cell carcinomas and ^{131}I therapy.* It is generally true that a pure Hürthle cell carcinoma does not concentrate ^{131}I or respond to ^{131}I therapy. We have referred to the fact that Hürthle cells are found in Hashimoto's Struma and Hashimoto's Struma may or may not co-exist with papillary and/or follicular carcinoma of the thyroid gland. Thus, we may ask for more slides and/or the blocks of tissue removed to decide this issue. Generally, Hürthle cell carcinoma is considered a variant of follicular carcinoma with a poorer prognosis.

17.7 *'Poorly differentiated'* thyroid carcinoma and ^{131}I therapy. It is a bad prognostic sign to have any pathologist read the frozen section as poorly differentiated thyroid carcinoma of unknown origin. Even on formaldehyde sections, a 'poorly' differentiated papillary or follicular carcinoma will rarely concentrate ^{131}I sufficiently to result in successful ^{131}I therapy.

17.8 *Invasion of surrounding tissues.* 'Invasion of the trachea' was always accompanied by a shortened survival time before the use of [131]I. When the thyroid carcinoma concentrates ^{131}I sufficiently, however, the prognosis is as good as in a patient without invasion of the trachea. If it concentrates ^{131}I poorly, all our patients referred to us with invasion of the trachea have died of their disease.

17.9 *'Anaplastic carcinoma'.* We have referred above to the fact that patients have been referred to us with 'anaplastic carcinoma' who have been treated satisfactorily with ^{131}I because the 'anaplastic' area was small and removable or because there were Hürthle cell change or focal medullary change or 'occult sclerosing' change in an otherwise predominantly papillary and follicular carcinoma that concentrated [131]I.

Small cell carcinomas in our experience should all be treated as lymphomas. Giant and Spindle cell sarcoma patients are almost always dead within one year regardless of the method of treatment. We have tried X-ray therapy, adriamycin and other chemotherapy routinely in such patients but all patients have died with little or no change in their clinical course.

18. Who will benefit and who will not benefit from medical treatment of thyroid carcinoma?

There is an intelligent effort today to quantitate % uptake of tracer or treatment dose in the thyroid carcinoma to be treated with eventual treatment response [63, 64]. Evans [65] was able to quantitate the spatial and temporal distribution of radium dial painters using the 'geometric mean' or conjugate view technique. We use this today with a 3 dimensional CAT scan to quantitate volume and allow calculation of rad dose delivered.

It is worthwhile to quantitate uptake before and one year after therapy to determine whether or not there is any relationship between degree of uptake and eventual 'cure'. It should be noted, however, that there is not sufficient data at present to make a decision to treat or not treat dependent upon a quantification of uptake to decide whether or not the dose will deliver a predetermined number of rads, for the following reasons:

1. Generally, the highest % uptake of ^{131}I in any well-differentiated thyroid carcinoma we see is in bone metastases. Generally the morphology of these metastases to bone show very well-differentiated thyroid carcinoma that may

even be read as 'normal thyroid gland'. This statement is also true for metastases to the brain. Rarely, if ever, however, are we successful in curing metastatic thyroid carcinoma to the brain or bone. These locations may offer immunologic sheltering. We have demonstrated [5] that it is easiest to free the patient of cervical and mediastinal metastases and to a lesser extent of lung metastases. These observations suggest that, in addition to radiation dose delivered to the carcinoma, the host defense mechanisms are at least equally important. Review of the sparse literature available does indicate that most 'cures' are associated with the delivery of 5000 rads or more [66].

2. Another mistake that is commonly made after a tracer dose is administered is to say that if the % uptake is below a certain figure (i.e., 0.5%) that treatment is not warranted. The fallacy in this reasoning is that to calculate rad dose, one must know the volume of the metastasis (usually determined by 2 or 3 dimensional CAT scanning) and the total amount of radioactivity in that lesion daily for a period of 5–8 days. Thus, a 0.5% dose in a 1mm^2 sized lesion may deliver a therapeutically effective dose, whereas it would be ineffective in a much larger lesion.

Most importantly, we have nothing better than ^{131}I after surgery for treatment. When everything fails, the patient is referred to us with the question: 'Are you positive that ^{131}I has nothing to offer this patient'? If you treat with [131] after surgery until you ablate uptake and the patient becomes worse, this question is easy to answer. [131]I should therefore be used first after surgery until there is no significant uptake or response.

Lastly, I have had occasional patients who had uptake only in the thyroidal bed, even 3 days after a therapy dose, who had very rapidly growing cervical nodes and obvious rapidly growing lung metastases who had all of their lesions disappear after merely ablating uptake in the thyroidal bed.

19. Recurrent lymph nodes after surgery and [131]I.

Occasionally, a young patient who has had adequate surgery and ^{131}I therapy returns with new palpable cervical lymph nodes. Some of these are 'benign lymphocytic hyperplasia' – an attempt of the lymphatic system to reinstitute itself after a cervical node dissection. This may occur years after the apparently successful surgical and ^{131}I therapy. Block et al. [67] have found that isolated enlargement of lymph node located to the posterior triangle of the neck after lateral cervical lymph node dissection is not the result of metastasis from thyroid carcinoma.

New supraclavicular metastases are usually recurrent thyroid carcinoma. If they do not show appreciable uptake of ^{131}I, I have had these patients apparently cured by surgical resection of these nodes.

118

20. Conclusion

We end then as we began. The young patient with well-differentiated thyroid carcinoma, even with distant metastases is almost always curable. If the physician does a 'conservative' nodulectomy or subtotal thyroidectomy and then waits 'conservatively' until recurrences in the thyroidal bed occur or distant metastases appear, there is a statistically increased likelyhood that the patient will be incurable. My closing prayer, therefore, is that physicians will treat patients aggressively as outlined above with surgery and ^{131}I when the patient is curable.

Acknowledgements

The author is indebted to all the physicians who call him daily to ask questions on how to treat their patients with thyroid carcinoma. The author is also grateful to numerous postgraduate course audiences that have taught him the main unanswered questions. I am particularly indebted to Drs. Sisson, Matovinovic and Shapiro in my Division of Nuclear Medicine today, and to many trainees in the past, for their suggestions and their requests to document my answers to their questions.

References

1. Third National Cancer Survey, N.C.I. Monograph 41, 1975.
2. Incidence, five leading cancer sites in young adult females (15–34) Ca-A. Cancer Journal for Clinicians 32: 39, Jan/Feb, 1982. (From Biometry Branch, National Cancer Institute)
3. Williams ED, Doniach MD, Bjorenson O, et al.: Thyroid cancer in an iodine rich area. Cancer 39: 215, 1977.
4. Thompson NW, Nishiyama RN, Harkness JK: Thyroid carcinoma: Current controversies. Curr Prob Surg 25: 1–17, 1978.
5. Beierwaltes WH, Nishiyama RN, Thompson NW, et al.: Survival time and 'cure' in papillary and follicular thyroid carcinoma with distant metastases: Statistics following University of Michigan therapy. J Nucl Med 23: 561, 1982.
6. Winship T and Rosvoll RW: Childhood thyroid carcinoma. Cancer 14: 734, 1961.
7. Rawson RW, Leeper RD: Chapter 27, Treatment of thyroid cancer with radioactive iodine. In: Nuclear Medicine, 2nd ed., Blahd WH. Blakiston: McGraw Hill Book Co., 1965, p 745.
8. Perzik SL: Total thyroidectomy in Graves' disease in children. J Pediatr Surg 11: 191, 1976.
9. Thompson NW, Dunn EL, Freitas JE, et al.: Surgical treatment of thyrotoxicosis in children and adolescents. J Pediatr Surg 12: 1009, 1977.
10. Leeper RD: The effect of ^{131}I therapy on survival of patients with metastatic papillary or follicular thyroid carcinoma. J Clin Endocrinol Metab 36: 1143, 1973.
11. Leeper RD: Controversies in the treatment of thyroid cancer: The New York Memorial Hospital approach. Thyroid Today, July/August, 1982.
12. Beierwaltes WH, Johnson PC: Thyroid carcinoma treated with radioactive iodine. An eight-year experience. J Mich State Med Soc 55: 410, 1956.
13. Beierwaltes WH: The treatment of thyroid carcinoma with radioactive iodine. Sem Nucl Med 8: 79–94, 1978.

14. Sawyer VL, Block MD, Bowman HE: Results of surgical management of carcinoma of the thyroid. J Mich State Med Soc 56: 468, 1957.
15. Block MD: Well differentiated carcinomas of the thyroid. In: Current Problems in Cancer. Vol 3, 1979, Year Book Med Publ Inc, 1979, pp 1–60.
16. Mazzaferri EL, Young RL, Oertel JE, et al.: Papillary thyroid carcinoma: The impact of therapy in 576 patients. Medicine 56: 171, 1977.
17. Mazzaferri EL: Papillary thyroid carcinoma: A 10 year follow-up report of the impact of therapy in 576 patients. Am J Med 70: 511, 1981.
18. Maheshuari YK, Hill CS, Jr., Haynie TP, et al.: [131]I therapy in differentiated thyroid carcinoma: M.D. Anderson Hospital experience. Cancer 47: 664, 1981.
19. Bestagno MF, Pagliaini R, Mavra G, Terzi A: The Use of radioiodine in the management of the differentiated thyroid cancer. Radioanalytical Chemistry 65: 239, 1981.
20. McCowen KD, Adler RA, Ehaed N, et al.: Low dose radioiodine thyroid ablation in post surgical patients with thyroid cancer. Am J Med 61: 52, 1976.
21. Kuni CC, Klingensmith WC: Failure of low doses of ^{131}I to ablate residual thyroid tissue following surgery for thyroid cancer. Radiol 137: 773, 1980.
22. Siddigarri AR, Edmanson J, Wellman HH, et al.: Feasibility of low doses of ^{131}I for thyroid ablation in post surgical patients with thyroid carcinoma. Clin Nucl Med 6: 158, 1981.
23. Chabner BA: Second neoplasm – A complication of cancer chemotherapy. N Engl J Med 297: 213, 1977.
24. Beierwaltes WH, Copp JE: Relationship of millicure dose of ^{131}I for ablation of thyroid remnants to results in patients with well-differentiated thyroid carcinoma. (In preparation).
25. Freedburg AS, Kurland GA, Blumgart HL: The pathologic effects of I-131 on the normal thyroid gland of man. J Clin Endocr 12: 1315, 1952.
26. Varma VM, Beierwaltes WH, Nofal MH, Nishiyama RH and Copp J: Treatment of thyroid cancer: Death rates after surgery, and after surgery followed by [131]I. JAMA 214: 1437–1442, 1970.
27. Benua RS, Cicale NR, Sonenberg M, et al.: The relation of radioiodine dosimetry to results and complications in the treatment of metastatic thyroid cancer. Am J Roentgen 87: 171, 1962.
28. Phillips AF: The gamma ray dose in carcinoma of the thyroid treated by radioiodine. Acta Radiol 41: 533, 1954.
29. Harness JK, Thompson NW, Sisson JC, et al.: Differentiated thyroid carcinomas: Treatment of distant metastases. Arch of Surg 108: 410, 1974.
30. Beierwaltes WH: New horizons for therapeutic Nuclear Medicine in 1981. J Nucl Med 22: 549, 1981.
31. Sisson JC, Beierwaltes WH: The effect of thyroidectomy with and without thyroxine replacement on transplantable thyroid tumors in rats. Endocrinology 74: 925–929, 1964.
32. Kumar MS, Chiang T, Deodhar SD: Enhancing effect of thyroxine on tumor growth and metastases in syngeneic mouse tumor systems. Cancer Res 39: 3515, 1979.
33. Vonderhaar BK, Greco AE: Effect of thyroid status on development of spontaneous mammary tumors in primiparous C3H mice. Cancer Res 42: 4553, 1982.
34. Krishnamurthy GT, Blobd WH: Human reactions to bovine TSH. J Nucl Med 18: 629, 1977. (abstract).
35. Hays MT, Solomon DH, Beall GN: Suppression of human thyroid function by antibodies to bovine thyrotropin. J Clin Endocrinol Metab 27: 1540, 1967.
36. Hershman JM, Edwards CL: Serum thyrotropin (TSH) levels after thyroid ablation compared with TSH levels after exogenous bovine TSH: Implications for ^{131}I treatment of thyroid carcinoma. J Clin Endocrinol Metab 34: 814, 1972.
37. Gershengorn MC, Weintraub BD, Robbins J: Response to oral thyrotropin releasing hormone in athyreotic patients with thyroid cancer. In: Proceedings of 7th International Thyroid Conference, Boston 1975, Robbins J, Braverman LE (eds). In: Excerpta Medica International Congress Series #378, 1975, p 575.

38. Goldman JM, Line BR, Aamodt RL, Robbins J: Influence of triiodothyronine withdrawal time on ^{131}I uptake postthyroidectomy for thyroid cancer. J Clin Endocrinol Metab 50: 734, 1980.
39. Singer PA, Nicoloff JF, Stein RB, Joravillo J: Transient TRH deficiency after prolonged thyroid hormone therapy. J Clin Endocrinol Metab 47: 512, 1978.
40. Krugman LG, Hershman JM, Chapra IV, et ai.: Patterns of recovery of the hypothalmic-pituitary thyroid axis in patients taken off chronic thyroid therapy. J Clin Endocrinol Metab 41: 70, 1975.
41. Fukuchi M, Tachibana K, Kuuata K, Nishikawa A, et al.: Thallium-201 imaging in thyroid carcinoma – appearance of a lymph node metastasis. J Nucl Med 19: 195–196, 1978.
42. Haroda T, Ito Y, Shimaoka K, Tanigachi T, Watsudo A, Senoo T: Clinical evaluation of 201 Thallium Chloride scan for thyroid nodule. Eur J Nucl Med 5: 125–130, 1980.
43. Pacini F, Pinchera A, Giani C, Grasso L, Doveri F, Baschieri: Serum thyroglobulin in thyroid carcinoma and other thyroid disorders. J Endocrinol Invest 3: 283, 1980.
44. Schneider AB, Line BR, Goldman JM, Robbins J: Sequential serum thyroglobulin determinations, ^{131}I scans, and ^{131}I uptakes after triiodothyronine withdrawal in patients with thyroid cancer. J Clin Endocrinol Metab 53: 1199, 1981.
45. Echenique RL, Kasi L, Haynie TP, Glenn HJ, Samaan NA, Hill CS: Critical evaluation of serum thyroglobulin levels and I-131 scans in post-therapy patients with differentiated thyroid carcinoma: Concise communication. J Nucl Med 23: 235, 1982.
46. Rawson RW, Rall JE, Peacock W: Limitations and indications in treatment of cancer of thyroid with radioactive iodine. J Clin Endocrinol 11: 1128, 1951.
47. Henk JM, Hirtsman S, Own CM: Whole body scanning and ^{131}I therapy in the management of thyroid carcinoma. Br J Radiol 45: 369, 1972.
48. Cady B: Risk factor analysis in differrentiated thyroid cancer. Ann Surg 18: 541, 1976.
49. Carr EA, Jr., Dingledine WS, Beierwaltes WH: Premature resort to X-ray therapy. A common error in treatment of carcinoma of the thyroid gland. Lancet 78: 478–483, 1958.
50. Haynie TP, Beierwaltes WH: Hematologic changes observed following I-131 therapy for thyroid carcinoma. J Nucl Med 4: 85–91, 1963.
51. Halron KE: The non-surgical treatment of thyroid cancer. Br J Surg 62: 769, 1975.
52. Pochin EE: The occurrence of leukemia following radioiodine therapy. In: Advances in Thyroid Research, Pitt-Dinen. New York: Pergammon Press, p 392.
53. Brinckner H, Hanren HR, Anderson AP: Induction of leukemia by ^{131}I treatment of thyroid carcinoma. Br J Cancer 28: 232, 1973.
54. Rubin P, Landman S, Mayer E: Bone marrow regeneration and extension after extended field irradiation in Hodgkin's disease. Cancer 32: 699, 1973.
55. Knorpe WH, Royudu LMS, Cartello M: Bone marrow scanning with 52 Iron ([52]Fe) regeneration and extension after ablative doses or radiotherapy. Cancer 37: 1432, 1976.
56. Hellman DE, Kartchner M, VanAntwerp JD, Salmon SE, Patton DD, O'Mara R: Radioiodine in the treatment of medullary carcinoma of the thyroid. J Clin Endocrinol Metab 48: 451, 1979.
57. Deftos LJ, Stein MF: Radioiodine as an adjunct to the surgical treatment of medullary thyroid carcinoma: J Clin Endocrinol Metab 50: 967, 1980.
58. Porthasarathy KL, Shimaoks K, Bokski SP, et al.: Radiotracer uptake in medullary carcinoma of the thyroid. Clin Nucl Med 5: 45, 1980.
59. Nusynowitz ML, Pollard E, Benedetto AR, Lecklitner ML, Ware RW: Treatment of medullary carcinoma of the thyroid with [131]I. J Nucl Med 23: 143, 1982.
60. Thereston V, Williams ED: The effect of radiation on thyroid C-cells. Acta Endocrinol 99: 72, 1982.
61. Rall JE, Alpers JB, LeWallen CG: Radiation pneumonitis and fibrosis: A complication of radioiodine treatment of pulmonary metastases from cancer of the thyroid. J Clin Endocrinol 17: 1263, 1967.
62. Sarker SD, Beierwaltes WH, Gill SP, et al.: Subsequent fertility and birth histories of children and adolescents treated with ^{131}I for thyroid cancer. J Nucl Med 17: 460–464, 1976.

63. Thomas SR, Maxon NR, Keriakes JG, et al.: Quantitative external counting techniques enabling improved diagnostic and therapeutic decisions in patients with well-differentiated thyroid cancer. Radiology 122: 731, 1977.
64. Koral KF, Adler RS, Carey JE, Kline RC, Beierwaltes WH: Two-orthogonal-view method for quantification of rad dose to neck lesions in thyroid-cancer-therapy patients. Medical Physics 9(4): 497–505, 1982.
65. Evans RC: Radium poisoning: II. The quantitative determination of the radium contect and radium elimination rate in living persons. Am J Roetgenol 32: 368, 1937.
66. Scott JS, Halran KE, Shimmins V, et al.: Measurement of dose to thyroid carcinoma metastases from radioiodine therapy. Br J Radiol 43: 256, 1970.
67. Block MA, Mitter JM, Horn RC, Jr.: Thyroid carcinoma with cervical lymph node metastasis. Effectiveness of total thyroidectomy and node dissection. Am J Surg 122: 458, 1971.

6. The impact of needle biopsy on the diagnosis of the thyroid nodule

JOEL I. HAMBURGER, J. MARTIN MILLER and SUDHA R. KINI

1. Introduction

Management of the patient with a thyroid nodule has been the subject of debate for many years. The essential question for any given nodule is whether the risk of cancer is great enough to justify the risk of surgical treatment. Granted the risks are very small when operations are performed by expert thyroid surgeons in first rate hospitals. Nevertheless, even these small risks must be justified when one is dealing with a problem which is as common as thryoid nodules, especially since most thyroid nodules are benign, most of those which are malignant are not very agressive, and the few highly lethal are almost always incurable by surgical methods.

For example, if as many as 5% of thyroid nodules are papillary carcinomas (the most common thyroid malignancy) a disease with about a 1% mortality rate [1], for any given nodule patient the risk of death from papillary carcinoma might be estimated to be about 0.05%. This approximates the usual mortality rate associated with thyroidectomy, even in very good institutions. Foster reports a mortality following thyroid operations for nontoxic nonmalignant goiters which increased with age from a low of 0.02% for patients less than 50 to 0.66% for those 70 years and older [2]. A somewhat higher mortality rate was observed for patients with malignant goiters.

Of course, the low death rate from papillary carcinoma applies to patients who were treated surgically. The risk of untreated papillary carcinoma is not known. Thus it is difficult to arrive at a mathematically precise assessment of the risks of thyroid nodules even though there is a vast body of published data. This may explain why some physicians (usually surgeons) still advise surgical treatment for all thyroid nodules [3], while others believe that there is no benefit to be obtained from the removal of any. These positions, of course, are the extremes. The majority of prudent and experienced thyroidologists recommend that thyroid nodules be evaluated individually for the findings which are associated with malignant or benign disease. Those nodules which seem to have a high risk of being malignant are excised, while the remainder are observed.

Selection of nodules for surgery has been employed for many years in many

Santen, R.J. and Manni, A. (eds.), Diagnosis and management of endocrine-related tumors. ISBN 0-89838-636-5.
© *1984, Martinus Nijhoff Publishers, Boston. Printed in the Netherlands.*

centers with more or less success. Medical history, physical examination and laboratory testing, including thyroid function tests, assays for antithyroid antibodies, thyroid imaging, and diagnostic ultrasound have been the tools employed in the selection process. Although reasonable accuracy may be achieved with this conventional clinical evaluation, there are many false positive diagnoses and some false negatives as well. For example, in most reported series of nodules selected for surgery the incidence of malignancy is about 20–30% [4–8]: i.e. the false positive diagnostic rate is 70–80%. Data upon the rate of false negative diagnoses is more difficult to acquire, because nodules considered benign are not ordinarily operated upon. The comparison of clinical with biopsy diagnoses in our patients suggested that the false negative rate by clinical evaluation might be about 9%.

The type of cancer for which operation might be delayed because of a false negative clinical diagnosis is not likely to prove rapidly lethal. More often followup examinations will make it evident that an error has been made while the lesion is still curable. Therefore we have been more concerned about the individual and public health implications of a 70–80% false positive diagnostic rate. The costs of the unnecessary surgery which these figures imply, both in terms of money and human suffering are staggering. In one of our clinics (JIH) about 500 patients with thyroid nodules are seen annually. When we were advising surgery on the basis of clinical evaluations about half the patients were operated upon and three-quarters of the operations were for benign disease, and thus in retrospect were unnecessary [9]. At an average cost of $3000 per patient [10], 180 unnecessary operations yearly means $540,000 wasted for patients from just one center. If these figures are representative of what happens in the hundreds of thyroid clinics in the United States one can appreciate the need for a more cost-effective approach to the diagnosis of the thyroid nodule.

Cost consideration aside, one must also reckon with the surgical risks to which these patients are subjected. One of us (JIH) has had four patients who died following thyroidectomy in the past 22 years. Three of these were operated upon for thyroid nodules, two of which were benign. If one adds to this toll the number of patients who are treated for hyperparathyroidism, suffer voice impairment and unsightly scars, and considers the implication of these numbers nationwide, one can begin to appreciate the scope of the human problem.

Unfortunately there is no perfect solution. Nevertheless our experience with needle biopsy procedures suggests that the diagnostic data provided by these techniques are substantially more precise than those obtainable by any combination of conventional clinical methods. However a high degree of diagnostic precision is achieved only after considerable experience. Experience is necessary to acquire the skills to permit one to obtain an adequate biopsy specimen, and to recognize from the gross appearance whether a specimen is likely to be adequate for diagnostic purposes. In addition the pathologist must learn to recognize the microscopic features which permit one to confirm or exclude the diagnosis of malignancy in the small biopsy specimens. The first, and one of the most important, judgements the pathologist must make is whether there is an adequate sampling to permit a diagnosis. For best results there must be close correlation between the physician performing the biopsy and the one who interprets the specimen.

It is of interest to note that needle biopsy diagnosis of thyroid nodules has been under investigation for more than 50 years [11]. However it has only been in the last few years that there has been widespread acceptance of the usefulness of these techiques [12–15]. Credit is due to the European, especially Scandanavian, workers for demonstrating the practicality of cytological evaluations of fine needle aspirates of thyroid nodules [16–23]. North Americans have been the principal pioneers in the use of larger needle biopsy procedures [24–26], designed to provide tissue cores or fragments for histological evaluation.

2. Needle biopsy techniques

There are three basically different methods of needle biopsy for thyroid nodules. These are:

Fine needle aspiration biopsy (FNAB), which provide specimens containing cellular clusters and small tissue fragments which are examined on the basis of cytological criteria. The usual needle employed is 25 gauge $1^1/_2$ inches long. Larger or small needles may be preferable in special situations.

Large needle aspiration biopsy (LNAB)which provide larger tissue fragments for examination on the basis of histological criteria. The usual needle employed is 18 or 16 gauge, $1^1/_2$ inches long.

Larger needle cutting biopsy (LNCB) which provides tissue cylinders for examination on the basis of histological criteria. The 14 gauge Silverman ($2^3/_8$ or $3^3/_8$ inches long) or the Tru-Cut (3 inches long) needles are used for these biopsies.

FNAB has advantages of greater simplicity and safety. Also it can be employed in nodules which are too small for the larger needles. LNAB is only slightly more difficult than FNAB. LNCB procedures are technically more difficult and potentially hazardous. They should not be attempted without a period of training.

FNAB specimens are adequate in most cases to make diagnoses of benign disease, Hurthle cell tumors, papillary carcinoma, anaplastic carcinoma, metastatic carcinoma to the thyroid and usually for medullary carcinoma. For most follicular tumors, and some medullary carcinomas, large needle biopsy specimens are preferred. Also, for the differential diagnosis of lymphoma of the thyroid from Hashimoto's thyroiditis (with which the most common lymphoma of the thyroid, histiocytic lymphoma, almost always coexists [27] large needle biopsy specimens are very helpful.

2.1 *FNAB method*

Patient preparation. Prior to beginning any needle biopsy procedure the patient should be prepared with liberal doses of reassurance, and a description of what will take place. To secure a satisfactory specimen patient cooperation is essential. An apprehensive patient may not remain still during the biopsy, and is very likely to contract the cervical musculature so that the necessary palpatory guidelines for the insertion of the needle are lost. The patient is placed in the recumbent position with a pillow under the shoulders to permit hyperextension of the neck. In the elderly the hyperextension must be limited to prevent occlusion of the vertebal arteries. The neck is cleansed with alcohol and the skin anesthetized. We advocate local anesthesia, using 0.5 ml of 1% Xylocaine, to minimize patient discomfort. Some workers consider this unnecessary when very fine needles are used [12]. However we routinely prepare six to eight grossly satisfactory smears. This may require 10 to 15 punctures. Patient comfort is necessary to maintain cooperation.

Needle selection. The needle we employ for FNAB in most cases is a 25 gauge, $1^1/_2$ inch disposable needle. Some physicians have advocated 27 gauge and even finer needles [28]. It is more difficult to aspirate though such fine needles, and more important, the needles are so flexible that one has more difficulty in maintaining control of the tips for the placement desired. Larger needles may produce too much disruption of the tissue so that bleeding will dilute the specimen to make it worthless.

The FNAB procedure. The needle is attached to a 10 ml disposable syringe, and inserted into the nodule in a direction perpendicular to the anterior surface of the skin. The nodule is held in a fixed position by the fingers of the opposite hand (Panel A of Fig. 1).

The initial aspiration is a test aspiration to assess the consistency of the nodular material and the appropriateness of the needle gauge and force of suction. The plunger of the syringe is withdrawn half way (Panel B, of Fig. 1) and then allowed to return to the initial position. No material should enter the barrel of the syringe. A small amount of fresh blood entering the barrel of the syringe is usually the result of excessive suction. The procedure should then be repeated with less suction, and success may be achieved. If one obtains the greenish-brown fluid suggestive of degeneration, placing the needle at the periphery of the nodule, rather than the center, may be more effective, because degeneration is usually most extensive centrally. Aspiration of old blood or clear straw-colored fluid may indicate that one is dealing with a cyst. In this case one should change to a 20 gauge needle and attempt to evacuate the cyst completely. Some cysts contain very thick, even gelatinous material. Only a small amount may enter the tip of the needle, but when this kind of material is expressed on a glass slide the operator should try to aspirate with a larger needle, e.g. 18, 16 or even 14 gauge. On rare occasions one may encounter the water clear to opalescent fluid characteristic of a parathyroid cyst. A high concentration of parathormone in the fluid confirms the diagnosis.

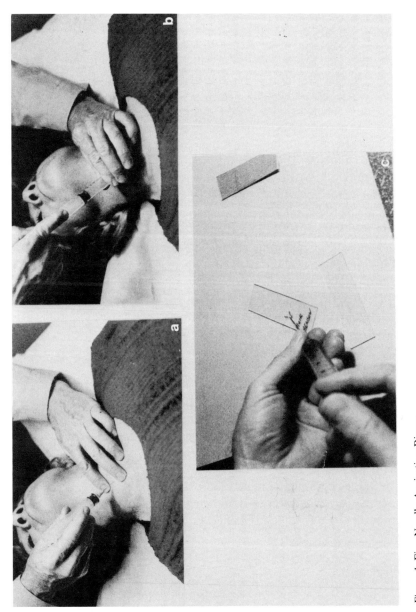

Figure 1. Fine Needle Aspiration Biopsy

A. Insertion of needle. Note that fingers of left hand fix the nodule in position.

B. Suction is applied.

C. The specimen is expressed on a glass slide.

When aspiration easily and repeatedly produces bloody to greenish-brown fluid in a noncystic nodule, regardless of needle placement, one may infer that there has been extensive degeneration. Since degenerated areas of nodules do not have much available epithelial elements to be aspirated, it may be impossible to obtain a satisfactory FNAB specimen. These nodules may be suitable for either LNAB or LNCB as will be discussed below.

In some instances very scanty material will be obtained with the 25 gauge needle. A 22 gauge or larger needle may then be employed. To obtain a satisfactory FNAB specimen from a hard, internally fixed papillary cancer may necessitate the use of an 18 gauge needle.

An alternative to larger needles is moving the needle in an in and out direction through a few millimeters distance to produce disruption of tissue so that a specimen can be obtained [29]. Suction must be maintained throughout this maneuver. One should stop just as bloody fluid enters the needle hub. The plastic hub of a disposable needle facilitates this visual check.

After aspiration has been completed, the needle is withdrawn from the nodule, detached from the syringe, a few ml of air taken into the syringe, the needle reattached, and the air forced through the needle to express the specimen onto a glass slide (Panel C of Fig.1). The material evacuated is then assessed for quantity and quality.

An ideal specimen will consist of one or two drops of orange red fluid. For each nodule we prepare four to six smears with aspirates obtained from different parts of the nodule. Bloody specimens or those consisting of greenish gray, cheesy white or thick oily degeneration fluid will contain too few epithelial cell for adequate evaluation.

A satisfactory specimen is smeared on the slide as if it were a routine blood smear. To prevent air drying the smear must be sprayed immediately with fixative (we use hair spray). In the case of relatively avascular nodules rather scanty relatively dry specimens may be obtained. For such material it may be advisable to place a drop of fixative on the slide, evacuate the specimen directly into the fixative, and then make the smear. The smear is stained with a modified Papanicolaou technique (30). The preparation is then examined microscopically considering the usual cytological criteria for benign or malignant lesions. Satisfactory FNAB specimens have been obtained on nodules as small as 0.5 cm in diameter.

2.2 LNAB method

Needle selection. For the LNAB method we have employed principally 1½ inch 16 gauge disposable needles. Initially we achieved some success with 18 gauge needles, and we still employ this size for smaller nodules. The patient position is the same as for FNAB.

Patient preparation. The skin overlying the nodule is cleansed with alcohol and infiltrated with 1% Xylocaine.

The LNAB procedure. The needle is attached to a 20 ml disposable syringe. To avoid clotting we draw up 1 ml of citrate solution (Heparin is just as effective and may be more readily available) into the syringe before beginning the aspiration. The needle is inserted into the nodule, usually in a direction perpendicular to the anterior surface of the neck. Skin incision is unnecessary with the LNAB since the 16 gauge needle is sharp enough and small enough to penetrate without much difficulty. A right-handed operator will hold the needle in his right hand while fixing the nodule with his left hand (Panel A of Fig. 2). With exercise of reasonable care by an experienced operator, the risks of inadvertent damage to adjacent structures are negligible. Having inserted the needle into the nodule the operator then rotates the barrel of the syringe through 360 degrees while suction is maintained [31]. This maneuver causes the sharp bevel of the needle to rotate through the tissue, cutting off small fragments which will be aspirated into the needle shank, or into the syringe itself. With suction maintained, the needle is withdrawn to the peripherry of the nodule and then reinserted for repeat aspiration in different directions three or four times. Two or three ml of bloody fluid are usually obtained. After the final aspiration, suction is maintained until the needle is withdrawn into a position just beneath the skin. Suction is then gently released. This minimizes the chances of fragmentation of any portion of the specimen within the needle which would otherwise be aspirated into the syringe as the needle is withdrawn through the skin.

Upon completion of the biopsy 10 ml of normal saline is aspirated into the syringe, the plunger withdrawn, and the diluted specimen poured out the proximal end of the barrel onto a paper towel or coffee filter. (This prevents the additional trauma to the specimen which might be produced if it were expelled through the needle). The residue is inspected and tissue fragments are readily visible (Panel C of Fig.2). Using this technique one can tell immediately whether tissue has been obtained. If there is no tissue the procedure may be repeated. The specimen is then placed in fixative (Bouin's solution followed by buffered formalin [32] and submitted for sectioning and histological examination.

LNAB has been employed for nodules as small as 1 cm in diameter. Hence this method makes it possible to have material for examination histologically as well as cytologically (FNAB) for these smaller nodules. This may be important since many of the suspicious palpable nodules are in the size range between 1 and 2 cm in diameter. FNAB must be done before LNAB because the tissue disruption of the latter precludes the former. LNAB is particularly suited to nodules which have undergone partial degeneration and have a low cell to amorphous material ratio.

Our initial success rate in obtaining a specimen adequate for diagnosis with LNAB was only about 50%. After greater experience we have been able to obtain useful specimens 60 to 70% of the time.

130

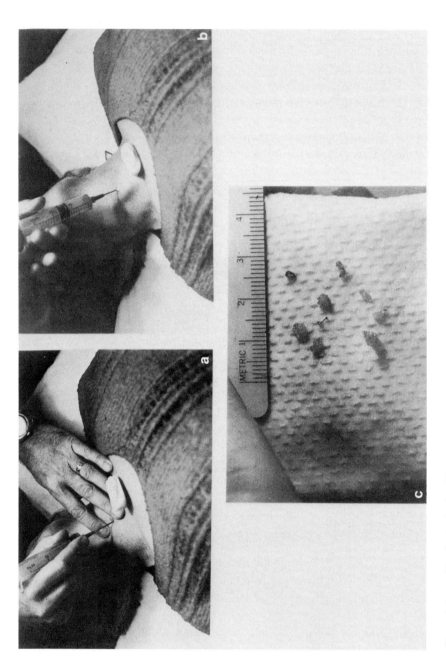

Figure 2. Large Needle Aspiration Biopsy

  A. Insertion of the needle. Note that fingers of left hand fix the nodule in position.

  B. During suction and rotation bloody fluid containing the tissue fragments enter the syringe.

  C. Tissue fragment residuals after filtration of the specimen on paper.

2.3 LNCB method

Needle selection. For LNCB a $2^3/_8$ inch or $3^3/_8$ inch 14 gauge Silverman needle or a 3 inch Tru-Cut needle is employed. The patient is positioned as described above for FNAB.

Patient preparation. The skin is prepared with iodine and alcohol and draped with a plastic drape. The area through which the needle is to be inserted is infiltrated with 1% Xylocaine. A fold of skin over the nodule is raised by pinching between thumb and forefinger, and with a number 11 Bard-Parker blade a nick large enouch to permit the insertion of the needle is made through the skin and subcutaneous tissue (Panel A of Fig. 3). The skin nick is usually made at the junction of the trachea and the upper medial pole of the nodule. This location may be adjusted to conform to the physical characteristics of the patient's neck, or to the location, size and shape of the nodule.

The LNCB procedure. The needle should be inserted in a direction parallel to the long axis of the neck to minimize the potential for damage to major vessels or nerves (Panel B of Fig. 3). The remainder of the biopsy proceeds in standard fashion. If blood appears when the obturator of the Silverman needle is removed, the needle should be withdrawn and may be repositioned in the nodule for another biopsy attempt. If the needle has provoked more extensive bleeding within the nodule, it may not be possible to obtain a satisfactory specimen. Actually this is the most common cause of biopsy failure with both the Silverman needle and the Tru-Cut needle. In the case of the Tru-Cut needle, blood fills the biopsy notch more readily than tissue.

Success can be expected with the Silverman needle for most firm nodules. Some very firm nodules can be penetrated with the needle, but the cutting element will not hold the specimen tightly enough to permits its extraction. These have usually been nodules consisting primarily of fibrous tissue. The Tru-Cut needle is especially useful in obtaining samples from softer nodules, particularly those with moderately extensive degeneration. The Tru-Cut needle seems to cut more efficiently than the Silverman needle for these nodules. The Silverman needle has a sharp point which may be improved and maintained by grinding on a stone. The Tru-Cut needle has a more nearly blunt tip which may be more difficult to insert into a thyroid nodule. If the cover of the biopsy notch is not flush with the needle shaft, the Tru-Cut needle may hang up at this point on the subcutaneous tissue or the capsule of the nodule. Also, if the Tru-Cut needle is inserted into a nodule and the cutting sheath retracted prior to the cutting stroke (the procedure recommended by the manufacturer), the sheath may catch on the capsule during the cutting stroke. In this case instead of the sheath severing a specimen within the notch, the needle shaft will be retracted to the capsule, and no specimen obtained. With experience the operator will appreciate that it is better to insert the needle just through the capsule; then, while holding the cutting sheath in a fixed position, to advance the pointed needle tip and its proximal shaft and notch. Care should be exercised not to penetrate through and

132

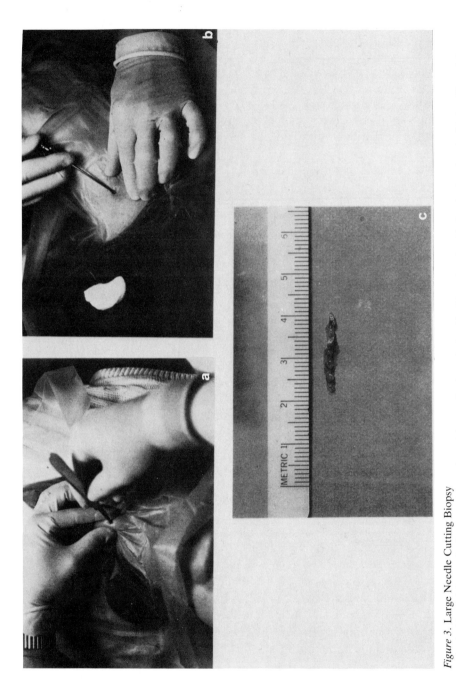

Figure 3. Large Needle Cutting Biopsy

A. A skin nick is required to permit insertion of the needle through the skin. Note that the skin is raised so that the blade will not injure underlying structures, and that the nick is made parallel with the skin lines.

B. Insertion of the needle in a direction parallel to the long axis of the neck and to the major vessels.

C. The specimen

beyond the opposite capsule. In this position the nodular tissue can prolapse in the open notch. Then, while the needle shaft is held in a fixed position, rapidly advance the outer cutting sheath over the notch severing the specimen. This technique is efficient for cutting and avoids the problem of inadvertent backup of the needle shaft and notch as the biopsy is being taken [33]. Although the Tru-Cut needle is intended to be a disposable item, it may be reutilized after gas sterilization. Since the Tru-Cut needle is not hollow (as in the Silverman needle) it is possible to penetrate a large vessel and be unware of it.

LNCB procedures are limited to nodules of size and location that permit the insertion of a 14-gauge needle. We prefer nodules at least 2.5 cm in largest diameter. Occasionally we have been successful with nodules as small as 1.5 cm, especially if they were not too deep in the neck.

It is best to obtain tissue samples from more than one portion of the nodule, especially in larger nodules, for there may be variations in histologic architecture for which multiple samples will provide a measure of assurance. Usually we try to obtain three satisfactory pieces of tissue, but sometimes we must settle for one or two if it proves more difficult to obtain tissue.

Figures 4–6 demonstrate representative needle biopsy specimens from various kinds of thyroid nodules.

3. Needle biopsy complications

The most common complication we have observed has been local bleeding. This has never been severe enough to require ligation of a bleeding vessel. Local pressure has been adequate. Occasionally bleeding will occur from a skin nick several hours after the procedure. Patients should be advised that local pressure for a few minutes will control it. One of our patients developed hoarseness from a transient nerve palsy. Within a few months both voice and vocal cord function were normal. We have had no instances of seeding of the needle track after biopsy of a malignant nodule. We must add that we have seen two patients who did not have needle biopsies, but still developed subcutaneous implants after thyroidectomy. Both of these were excised successfully under local anesthesia. One of these patients, a 73-year-old-woman, was described in a earlier publication in which one of us (JMM) was a co-author [34]. This patient had an attempt at aspiration of a nodule erroneously diagnosed as a cystic lesion by ultrasound. When no fluid was obtained surgery was performed. A papillary carcinoma was excised. Six months later a subcutaneous implant developed. The lesion was excised under local anesthesia as an outpatient. Unfortunately in an abstract of this report in the 1982 Year Book of Endocrinology, one of the editors (TBS) concluded that the implant had been in the needle track [35]. Actually it was in a location remote from the needle track, adjacent to the surgical scar.

Nevertheless there is a potential for damage to large vessels and nerves in the

134

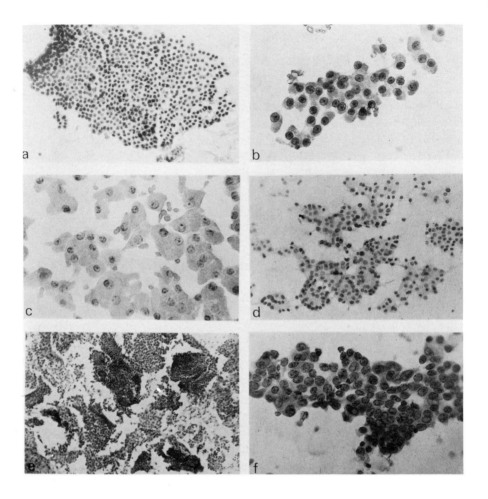

Figure 4. Microscopic Viewes of Fine Needle Aspiration Biopsy Specimens

A. Nodular goiter. A large monolayered sheet of follicular cells with a honeycomb pattern. Note uniform nuclei with finely granular chromatin.

B. Nodular goiter. Here the nuclei are enlarged, with prominent nucleoli. The cytoplasm is dense and abundant. These cells resemble the single cells seen in papillary carcinoma. However the latter have irregular muclei with clumped chromatin.

C. Hurthle cell tumor. Large polygonal cells, isolated and forming sheets with distinct cell borders and abundant dense granular cytoplasm. Nuclei are mostly eccentric with prominent macronucleoli.

D. Follicular adenoma. A very cellular aspirate containing multiple follicles formed by cells with crowded uniform nuclei. Overlapping and molding of nuclei is apparent. The chromatin is bland.

E. Papillary carcinoma. An extremely cellular specimen containing single cells, papillary fronds and monolayered sheets.

F. Papillary Carcinoma. A monolayered tissue fragment of carcinoma cells with enlarged hyperchromatic nuclei. Note loss of nuclear polarity and crowding of the cells. Cell borders are poorly defined. Note intranuclear cytoplasmic inclusions (clear zones within the nuclei).

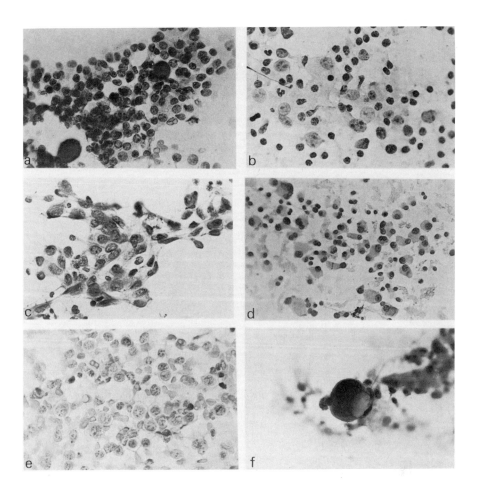

Figure 5. Microscopic Views of Fine Needle Aspiration Biopsy Specimens

A. Follicular carcinoma. Loosely grouped carcinoma cells, occasionally forming follicles containing colloid. The nuclei are enlarged, hyperchromatic with clumped chromatin and prominent nucleoli.

B. Hashimoto's thyroiditis. Atypical follicular cells obscured by lymphocytes, plasma cells and transforming lymphocytes.

C. Anaplastic carcinoma. Small groups of loosely coherent spindle shaped malignant cells. Nuclei are hyperchromatic and quite variable in size. There are multiple nucleoli. Cell boundries are ill-defined and the cytoplasm is variable in amount.

D. Medullary carcinoma. A very cellular specimen containing single cells of variable size. Most of them resemble plasma cells with eccentric nuclei. The chromatin is coarse and the nuclei are prominent.

E. Lymphoma of tne thyroid. A very cellular aspirate containing a monotonous population of large malignant cells with eccentric large nuclei, coarse chromatin and prominent nucleoli. The cytoplasm is variable. Note the absence of thyroid follicular cells or Hurtle cells.

F. Metastatic colon carcinoma to the thyroid. Note the single large carcinoma cell with a large secretory vacuole.

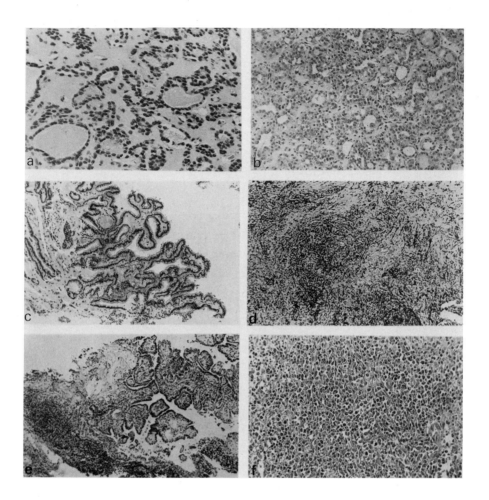

Figure 6. Large Needle Biopsy specimens

A. Follicular adenoma. Note the presence of variable size follicles, including many small ones, all contaning colloid.

B. Follicular carcinoma. Note the architectural disarray. The follicular cell nuclei are moderately pleomorphic.

C. Nodular goiter. Note the branching hyperplasatic papillae, superficially suggestive of papillary carcinoma. A higher power view showed more clearly the basal location of uniform nuclei with compact chromatin.

D. Hashimoto's thyroiditis, fibrous variant. Note the extensive fibrosis, diffuse lymphocytic infiltration and follicular atrophy

E. Hashimoto's thyroiditis with coexistent papillary carcinoma. Malignant papillation is seen in association with extensive lymphocytic infiltration.

F. Lymphoma of the thyroid. The specimen contains a proliferation of poorly differentiated neoplastic lymphocytes. Note the variation in size and shape of nuclei. Compare to fine needle aspirate, Figure 5, panel E.

neck with serious consequences, especially with LNCB.If the operator is not certain that the cutting portion of the needle is in the nodule, or at least within the thyroid, the biopsy should not be completed. Some such nodules are located at or beneath the suprasternal notch, an area where major vessels may be expected. Using the thyroid image as an anatomic guide we have been successful in obtaining specimens from a number of these nodules without any problems. However, this is not an area for the novice.

4. Impact of needle biopsy on diagnostic precision for the thyroid nodule

The worldwide experience with needle biopsy has served to establish these procedures in the first rank for the diagnosis of the thyroid nodule [36]. The physicians who still express doubt about the usefullness of needle biopsy diagnoses base their objections upon the indisputable fact that needle biopsy diagnoses are not always reliable. Both false positive and false negative errors are possible, even after considerable experience has been acquired. Although this statement is unassailable it is also irrelevant to the clinical setting, for implicit in the argument are two fundamental fallacies. The first is that for needle biopsy data to be useful they must be as accurate as surgical findings. Second is the assumption that surgical diagnoses are necessarily more accurate than needle biopsy diagnoses. We shall discuss the first of these fallacies now, and comment on the second later.

Obviously surgical specimens can only be studied after some portion of the nodule population has been selected for operation, or if all nodules were excised. Assuming that the reader has been persuaded to reject the advice that all thyroid nodules should be excised [3], then it is evident that accuracy of needle biopsy data in providing a basis for selecting nodules for operation cannot, in fairness, be compared to the accuracy of the diagnosis made on the surgical specimens, but rather comparison must be made with the accuracy of alternative clinial methods of preoperative diagnosis. In other words to be useful in the preoperative selection of nodules for surgery or observation, needle biopsy data do not have to be as accurate as diagnoses on surgical specimens, but only more accurate than other clinical methods of diagnosis.

For many years these authors evaluated thyroid nodules by means of the conventional clinical methods listed above [9]. On the basis of this kind of data nodules were classified into three groups: Probably Malignant, Possibly Malignant, and Probably Benign.

To study the relative accuracy of needle biopsy data consecutive patients were first classified on the basis of the conventional clinical evaluation, and then subjected to needle biopsy.

Needle biopsy procedures may yield one of four possible results:

1. *Specimen inadequate for diagnostic purposes.* This includes biopsies which

produced no specimens or specimens too scant to assure adequate sampling of the nodule. A fundamental and obvious limiting consideration for needle biopsy is the fact that one can only obtain the type of material which the nodule contains. For example, if the nodule has undergone extensive degeneration, and consists largely of a multiloculated structure containing a mixture of necrotic, bloody, calcific, fibrotic and amorphous matter it will not be possible to obtain useful material for diagnostic purposes. Similary, if the nodule is very small or located deep in the neck it may be very difficult to place the needle in the nodule. These are the two principle reasons for failing to obtain a satisfactory specimen by at least one of the needle biopsy techniques.

How much material is required before one can consider a needle biopsy specimen adequate for diagnosis depends upon the diagnosis one is attempting to establish. In this regard it is important to differentiate between the amount of biopsy material necessary to establish a diagnosis of a malignant nodule from what is needed to exclude a diagnosis of malignancy. Malignant cells or tissue can be obtained only from a malignant lesion. Benign cells or tissue can be obtained from benign nodules or benign tissue adjacent to a malignant lesion. With these facts in mind it should be evident that although a small amount of malignant tissue may be adequate to permit a reliable diagnosis of cancer, a few benign cells or a small fragment of benign tissue would not necessarily exclude a malignant nodule if there had been an error in needle placement. To minimize the potential for false negative sampling errors we require multiple clusters of benign cells on at least two of the six FNAB specimens before a diagnosis of a benign nodule is made. Similarly we prefer to have several benign tissue samples to make a benign large needle biopsy diagnosis.

An inadequate biopsy is of no diagnostic value, either positive or negative. Five of 37 patients who had unsatisfactory needle biopsies and were subsequently operated upon had cancer (all were papillary carcinomas).

An attempt at needle biopsy which identifies a cystic nodule for which aspiration produces complete regression of the lesion is no different than an unsatisfactory biopsy. No tissue has been obtained. In some instances aspiration of cyst fluid will make it possible to biopsy a solid residual component. Most cystic nodules are benign, but some are malignant. When repeated aspirations fail to eliminate a cystic nodule, and the aspiration is repeatedly bloody one should consider the possibility of a malignancy [37, 38].

2. *Malignant, either definitely or probably.* In most cases a specific type of malignancy can be identified.

3. *Inconclusive, i.e. malignancy can neither be confirmed nor excluded.* These are usually follicular neoplasms for which careful study of the entire tumor may be required to establish a diagnosis. Note that this diagnosis is different from that of 'inadequate'. This problem is not a lack of material. An abundant supply of tissue may have been obtained, however the microscopic features are such that one cannot exclude a malignancy.

One of the most important lessons which the pathologist must learn is to identify specimens which do not permit a diagnosis of cancer, but do suggest a neoplastic lesion which could be malignant, and to segregate these from specimens which are clearly from benign nodules (neoplastic or non-neoplastic).

4. *Benign.* In Table 1 clinical diagnoses are compared with the biopsy diagnoses for the first 2000 study patients for whom needle biopsy has produced specimens which were initially considered adequate for diagnostic purposes.

Only 37% of the nodules considered probably malignant by clinical evaluation had biopsy diagnoses of malignancy. More than half the biopsy diagnoses of malignancy were on nodules clinically diagnosed only possibly malignant or probably benign. Clinical diagnoses identified only 38% of the nodules as probably benign, whereas needle biopsy diagnosed 66% benign. If one has the objective of minimizing unnecessary surgery for thyroid nodule patients, perhaps the most important improvement in diagnostic accuracy provided by needle biopsy relates to patients for whom the clinical diagnosis was 'possibly malignant'. Given such a doubtful diagnosis a substantial proportion of patients will be advised to have surgery. Yet operation on these patients resulted in the excision of a malignant nodule only 7% of the time in an earlier series published by one of us (JIH) [9]. Therefore it would be helpful if one could substantially reduce the proportion of patients classified as possibly malignant. In this series of 2000 patients 43% were diagnosed clinically as possibly malignant. Only 18% were left with this inconclusive diagnosis after needle biopsy. Most of the nodules diagnosed 'possibly malignant' by clinical methods had benign biopsy diagnoses, thus greatly reducing the number of surgical candidates.

The data supplied to this point compared the findings of clinical and biopsy diagnoses. When we embarked upon our study of the usefulness of needle biopsy we wanted both to define the accuracy of diagnosis achieved with needle biopsy, while not exposing our patients to any increased risk of diagnostic error (especially false negative errors) than would have occurred in the absence of needle biopsy data. At the same time we could not, in good conscience, advise all patients whom we biopsied to have surgery simply to provide us with data upon which to assess the accuracy of needle biopsy diagnoses. After all, our primary

Table 1. Comparison of clinical diagnoses with needle biopsy diagnoses – 2000 consecutive thyroid nodule patients

Clinical diagnoses		Biopsy diagnoses		
		Malignant	Inconclusive	Benign
Probably malignant	394 (20%)	145 (37%)	79 (20%)	70 (43%)
Possibly malignant	850 (43%)	101 (12%)	171 (20%)	578 (68%)
Probably benign	756 (38%)	65 (9%)	104 (14%)	587 (77%)
Total	2000	311 (16%)	354 (18%)	1335 (66%)

objective in studying needle biopsy was to reduce the number of unnecessary thyroid operations. We were therefore unprepared to take a major step backward and advise all of our nodule patients to have surgery, even for a limited period of time. To achieve these objectives, as we commenced our study we established the following criteria upon which to advise operation:

1. All patients with clinical diagnoses of probable or possible malignancy, regardless of the biopsy findings.
2. All patients with biopsy findings of inconclusive or malignant, regardless of the clinical diagnosis.
3. Observation was advised only for patients with benign diagnoses by both clinical and biopsy methods.

Exceptions to these general rules were made for the following reasons:

1. Some patients for whom operations were advised refused the advice.

2. Some patients for whom surgery would have been advised were not operated upon because of overriding health considerations which made surgery unacceptably risky.

3. Some patients for whom needle biopsy findings of benign disease might have indicated observation were still advised to have operation because of continuing concern on the part of the patient, the attending physican or one use. An example is a 42 year old woman with a history of radiation therapy for acne as a teenager, and a hard 1 cm nodule for which the FNAB diagnosis was benign. Treatment with thyroid hormone for one year failed to alter the nodule. Diagnosis upon a repeat FNAB was again benign. Nevertheless operation was advised. The lesion was benign.

4. After studying the data from our initial 1000 satisfactory biopsies [39], we no longer advised operation for patients with benign biopsy diagnoses. Some of these patients still had surgery for reasons discussed above.

In assessing the accuracy of needle biopsy one must consider the false positive and false negative risks. If one defines a false positive biopsy diagnosis as any diagnosis for which operation would be recommended, but would produce a surgical specimen which could not be diagnosed malignant, then one must consider the results of surgery for nodules with biopsy diagnoses of 'inconclusive' as well as 'malignant'. After all, whether the biopsy diagnosis is malignancy or malignancy cannot be excluded (i.e. "inconclusive') makes no difference to the patient if an operation is performed in either case. There were 453 such patients operated upon and 204 (45%) did not have cancer. A similar analysis for a prebiopsy series published by one of us (JIH) revealed 76% false positive diagnoses (9). This is consistent with the 20–30% incidence of cancer in surgical reports of clinically selected thyroid nodules. Thus if a recommendation for surgery were based upon needle biopsy data the instance of malignancy in the nodules excised would increase from 24% to 55%; a substantial improvement in diagnostic precision. Translated in terms of the proportion of nodule patients operated upon, needle biopsy data could reduce this proportion by 50%; the proportion operated upon only to remove a benign nodule could be reduced by 75%. The economic and public health implications of these data are impressive when applied to the 2000 patients from our clinics, and would be staggering if applicable to the thyroid nodule population as large.

Important as a reduction in false positive diagnoses is, many physicians may be more concerned about the false negative risk of needle biopsy. How often will a benign needle biopsy diagnosis lead to the erroneous decision to observe a malignant nodule? We have already shown that 9% of the clinical diagnoses of benign nodules were reversed by biopsy diagnoses of malignancies. In fact of the 256 malignant nodules which were excised during this study 39 (15%) had been diagnosed benign clinically. Only 3 of 87 patients with benign biopsy findings had cancer. All of these errors were made early in our experience, and none contributed adversely to patient management as we shall see. One patient was an elderly woman with a large neck mass which seemed obviously malignant clinically. We suspected an anaplastic carcinoma and performed FNAB, expecting to make the diagnosis simply and easily. To our surprise the diagnosis was Hashimoto's thyroiditis (which she had). Although large needle biopsy was advised, the patient was hospitalized for open biopsy, which revealed a histiocytic lymphoma. This was the first lymphoma patient in our series. We quickly learned to do large needle biopsy whenever this diagnosis was a reasonable consideration.

The second patient had both FNAB and LNAB. The diagnosis on the former was inconclusive, that provided by LNAB was benign. In the case of discrepancies between fine and large needle biopsy findings we had decided to place primary reliance upon the latter, assuming that the diagnosis based upon the larger and more familiar histological specimens would be more dependable. The patient had a papillary carcinoma composed of 95% of well-differentiated follicular elements. In retrospect the size of the LNAB specimen should have been considered borderline in adequacy for diagnosis. Also, this specimen was fixed in formalin, rather than Bouin's solution. The latter produces a microscopic appearance more closely resembling that which is seen in sections of surgical specimens, and is preferred for fixation of large needle biopsy specimens [32]. Using Bouin's fixation routinely we have not had trouble diagnosing similar lesions correctly.

The third patient had a false negative FNAB diagnosis, corrected on routine review of FNAB specimens after one year's additional experience. The review diagnosis of suspected follicular carcinoma was confirmed at surgery

Hence we attribute these errors to inexperience. However, our data clearly show that the biopsy team made benign diagnoses on a much smaller proportion of cancers (3 of 256) by needle biopsy, than by conventional clinical methods (39 of 256). Nevertheless it is reasonable to assume that some of the nodules that we diagnosed benign and have not as yet been excised are actually malignant.

The improved diagnostic accuracy of FNAB for papillary carcinoma achieved with experience is indicated by finding that only 37 of the first 70 cases were diagnosed specifically as papillary carcinoma, and four were called benign. Of the last 105 cases 99 were diagnosed specifically as papillary carcinoma and none was called benign.

5. Comprison of usefulness of fine and large needle biopsies

FNAB is technically simpler and potentially less hazardous than the large needle procedures. For these reasons FNAB has gained wide acceptance in recent years. Our studies show that with experience one can achieve a considerable degree of diagnostic accuracy with FNAB alone. However there are important advantages to large needle biopsies which deserve increased attention.

On the first 1000 satisfactory FNAB specimens false negative diagnoses were made 11 timcs. Ten of these were corrected by large needle biopsies. Seven of the 11 errors were attributed to failure to recognize that the specimens were inadequate for diagnosis. Three other patients had lymphomas, diagnosis which in retrospect should have been suspected even on the FNAB specimens which were obtained. The final patient had an atypical adenoma (a lesion some might consider noninvasive follicular carcinoma) diagnosed nodular goiter by FNAB.

As we gained experience we have found that large needle procedures are most useful in the following situations:
1. When FNAB fails to produce a satisfactory specimen.
2. For nodules 3.5 cm or larger, to assure adequate sampling.
3. When FNAB suggest a follicular neoplasm.
4. In patients with Hashimoto's thyroiditis and a large discrete mass suspicious for malignancy (especially to confirm or exlude lymphoma).

6. Relative accuracy of needle biopsy and surgical diagnosis

Before closing this discussion it is necessary to consider the assumption that diagnoses on surgical specimens are more reliable than those on needle biopsy specimens. To address this point we must call attention to a sizable number of false negative diagnostic errors made on surgical specimens in community hospitals in our area, even though our biopsy team pathologist had made the diagnosis of cancer preoperatively. In one case the surgical pathologist made a diagnosis of benign disease, and provided us with the remainder of the gross surgical specimen for our review. Not only was the nodule a papillary carcinoma but the lesion was multifocal sparing hardly any of the thyroid and its adjacent lymph nodes. The point we are making is that difficulty of diagnosis relates not only to the microscopic features of the lesion, but also the experience level of the pathologist. Even experienced pathologists sometimes have problems differentiating benign from malignant follicular neoplams. On occasion this results from failure to take enough sections.

Thus, a comparison of the accuracy of needle biopsy diagnoses with diagnoses made on surgical specimens is not a simple matter. Needle biopsy diagnoses made by a very experienced thyroid pathologist might easily be more accurate than diagnoses on surgical specimens made by a pathologist without special interest or training in thyroid disease. Obviously this does not provide a fair comparison. Nevertheless, in actual practice, certainly in the area in which we practice, the experience level of our biopsy team pathologist is much higher than that of most of the pathologists who render diagnoses on the surgical specimens. We suspect that this is likely to be a common problem related to the development of skilled needle biopsy teams. Physicians should be aware of this fact.

7. Needle biopsy diagnosis of the follicular neoplasm

It is still widely held that segregation of benign from malignant follicular neoplasms by needle biopsy may be difficult, if not impossible in some instances [34, 40]. Diagnosis may present problems even when entire surgical specimen is available, even if the pathologist is very skilled. However it is a mistake to think that this is the rule for follicular neoplasms. Actually it is the exception. Most benign follicular nodules can be identified accurately and so can most malignant follicular lesions. Only a minority will have inconclusive needle biopsy findings. Nevertheless, follicular lesions do constitute the majority of the nodules with these inconclusive biopsy findings. As already noted when diagnostically adequate specimens are obtained, only about 15% will have inconclusive findings. This would not justify rejecting the benefits of needle biopsy for the remaining approximately 85%.

Recent investigations suggest that it is possible to classify follicular neoplasms in categories with decreasing probabilities of malignancy [41]. This information, if confirmed by further study, would be useful in management decisions for some patients, especially those with other health problems which adversely influence surgical risks.

8. Commonly asked questions about needle biopsy

Before closing it may be helpful to address a selection of the qestions we are asked most frequently when the issue of needle biopsy is under discussion. These questions deal with important practical considerations.

8.1 *Who should do biopsies?* It is probable that most needle biopsies currently are being done by internists, usually those with special interest in endocrinology or

144

thyroidology. However there is no reason why anyone who has a special interest in thyroid diseases, and is experienced in palpation of the thyoid gland, could not learn these procedures. We know of one pathologist who not only interprets the specimens but performs the biopsies as well.

More important than the type of specialty training is the number of patients needing biopsies available to the physician. The skills required to permit one to obtain adequate needle biopsy specimens with a high degree of consistency cannot be acquired and maintained unless the physician is performing these procedures on a regular basis, say ten to twenty times monthly. In any given community it is far better to pool the available cases so that a small number of physicians can achieve a high degree of technical proficiency. Pooling the specimens for study by pathologists with special interest and expertise in thyroid disease is equally or even more important. In our area with increasing frequency we are rebiopsying patients who have had unsuccessful procedures by inexperienced physicians.

8.2 *Should patients be hospitalized for needle biopsy?* All of the patients which we have biopsied had their procedures done as outpatients, excepting only a few who had biopsies while in the hospital for other reasons. We hold patients for observation for 20 to 30 minutes after larger needle procedures.

8.3 *Should all thyroid nodules be subjected to needle biopsy?* From the general tone and content of our presentation one might infer that our answer to this question would be affirmative. Actually there are several exceptions. Nodules which either function autonomously, or have developed on the basis of compensatory hyperplasia may, for practical purposes, be considered invariably benign. These diagnoses are easily established by appropriately sequenced tracer studies [42]. Although there have been isolated case reports of tiny foci of differentiated thyroid carcinoma within an otherwise benign autonomous nodule, one should not suspect that this is the probable cause of a zone of reduced imaging activity within an autonomously functioning nodule. These findings are common, and nearly always reflect areas of degeneration, most commonly central in location. We consider the risk of cancer in these nodules too small to justify needle biopsy.

Essentially all nodules which have reduced function on imaging should be considered for needle biopsy. The only exception might be patients for whom surgical treatment, even of a limited degree, is contraindicated by other health problems. For example, recently a patient with advanced inoperable breast cancer was referred for needle biopsy. The lesion was benign. In retrospect it is probable that regardless of the findings the data were too unlikely to influence future patient management to have justified the procedure.

The cystic thyroid nodule is another lesion that is hypofunctional on imaging, for which biopsy will not be done unless there happens to be a solid component to the lesion.

8.4 *If I am confident on the basis of my clinical evaluation that a nodule is malignant, is needle biopsy still necessary, or may the patient proceed directly to surgery?* We advised needle biopsy for two reasons. First the clinical diagnosis of malignancy may be right; and second, it may be wrong. Let us suppose that the lesion is malignant. All malignancies of the thyroid are not best treated surgically. For example, anaplastic carcinoma or lymphoma of the thyroid may be treated without operation (the former for paliation, the latter for cure). For metastatic carcinoma to the thyroid, thyroidectomy would seldom improve the patient's prognosis. For medullary carcinoma a preoperative diagnosis will permit screening for pheochromocytoma, and obtaining calcitonin levels for comparison with postoperative findings. True enough, these are unusual forms of thyroid cancer. Most of the time we will be dealing with papillary or follicular carcinoma. How will needle biopsy data help in these cases if the clinical picture is 'obvious'?

The data are helpful in a number of ways. In the first place if one tells a patient 'You need a thyroidectomy because I think you have thyroid cancer', he will obtain a certain measure of compliance. However, if one tells a patient 'You need a thyroidectomy because the needle biopsy findings show that you have thyroid cancer' he is likely to obtain a far better level of compliance. Also, knowing the diagnosis in advance of surgery permits the surgeon to explain the operation more precisely, and to plan for the appropriate operation in advance. He may find it suitable to dispence with frozen section, or where these procedures are routine, he may not be misled by false negative diagnosis (far more common with frozen sections than needle biopsies, once reasonable competence has been achieved by the pathologist member of the biopsy team). In this fashion we have virtually eliminated the previously common sequence of a diagnostic lobectomy, followed several days later by a second operation to complete the thyroidectomy because permanent sections reversed a false negative frozen section diagnosis.

On the other hand, having frequently made false positive clinical diagnoses of malignancy for thyroid nodules which proved to be benign, we are convinced that this is a risk even for very skilled clinicians. Needle biopsy can correct these clinical errors and eliminate unnecessary operations. Needle biopsy is now so wide-spread that a physician who fails to suggest it, to his discomfiture, may find himself upstaged by the second opinion physician.

8.5 *If I am confident on the basis of my clinical evaluation that a nodule is benign, is needle biopsy still necessary?* It should not be surprising if we answer this question in the affirmative, in this instance principly because the benign diagnosis might be wrong. We have already shown that 9% of the patients for whom we had made clinical diagnoses of benign disease had biopsy findings indicative of cancer. These were usually soft less discrete lesions in older people. One patient was particularly instructive. She was first seen at age 77 with a 3 cm nodule which was only moderately firm. We were not doing needle biopsies at that time, and advised observation. The patient returned annually with no discernible change.

At age 80 a needle biopsy revealed a medullary carcinoma which was successfully excised under local anesthesia. Screening of the family established the diagnosis in several additional members.

8.6 *If the patient has a history of prior head-neck radiation therapy, does this mean that surgery is necessary, or is needle biopsy still appropriate?* It is clear that prior radiation therapy increases the incidence of thyroid nodules. However it has not been proved that for any given nodule the chances of cancer are significantly increased. In fact our data are to the contrary [43]. This issue has recently been discussed in depth by a panel of authorities [43]. We conclude that a history of radiation therapy does not vitiate the usefullness of needle biopsy.

8.7 *Should needle biopsy be done if a nodule is discovered in a pregnant woman, or should one defer evaluation until after parturition?* We advise needle biopsy. If the lesion is benign there is no need to prolong the patient's anxiety. If the lesion is malignant, this information may permit her to plan more efficient management. For example, she may prefer to have the thyroidectomy in the third trimester or even while she is in the hospital for delivery, rather than having to leave her newborn in the care of someone else while she re-enters the hospital for thyroidectomy because the diagnosis was deferred until after delivery.

8.8 *Does the advent of needle biopsy render thyroid imaging obsolete?* This point is arguable. We prefer to have imaging data so that we can exclude from needle biopsy autonomously functioning and hyperplastic nodules. These imaging findings essentially exclude malignancy, needle biopsy specimens usually suggest cellular neoplasms for which malignancy cannot be excluded. Imaging thus would eliminate the necessity for needle biopsy for the 10–15% of nodules which are autonomous or hyperplastic. On the other hand, one could biopsy all nodules and image only those with 'inconclusive' or unsatisfactory biopsy findings. This would eliminate the necessitity for imaging for 50–60% of patients, at the expense of more biopsies. It is not clear that either approach is substantially more economical. Most physicians will probably continue to follow the path which minimizes the number of invasive procedures.

8.9 *Does the advent of needle biopsy render diagnostic ultrasound studies obsolete?* In our opinion the answer to this question is yes. Even if ultrasound studies were completely reliable in differentiating cystic from solid nodules (and they are not) we consider them a redundant expense. If the nodule is cystic one would want to do needle aspiration to evacuate the cyst, both to exclude a solid component, and in the hopes of eliminating the lesion. If the nodule is solid one would do a needle biopsy for diagnosis. Hence, regardless of ultrasound findings a needle will be inserted, and that needle alone would reliably permit the determination of whether the nodule were cystic or solid. Therefore we see no point to diagnostic ultrasound for thyroid nodule patients.

8.10 *What are the medical-legal implications of needle biopsy?* One could view this question from several perspectives: i.e.,

  a. The risk of false negative diagnoses.
  b. The risk of false positive diagnoses.
  c. The risk of complications.

If one were concerned about false negative or false positive needle biopsy diagnoses, he must appreciate that the risk of both types of errors are much greater when selection of nodules for surgery is based on conventional clinical methods. Only operation for all thyroid nodules will eliminate the risk of a false negative diagnosis. Of course the price would be a tremendous increase in the false positive diagnoses with an unavoidable attendant morbidity and mortality (ignoring practical considerations of cost, availability of hospital beds, surgeons and other personel), which make this alternative unacceptable. The legal implications of diagnostic error, in our judgement is an argument for needle biopsy, not against it.

With regard to the risks of complications we can only say to date the growing number of reports which deal with the subject do not reveal any serious problem. Our good record would seem to be readily duplicable as long as reasonable care is taken not to exceed the bounds of one's experience level. Once again the risk of complications must be viewed not in the absolute, but in the perspective of the risks of the alternatives- i.e. diagnostic errors of clinical selection, or morbidity and mortality of surgery for all thyroid nodules.

9. Conclusions

In considering what final words of encouragement to offer physicians who have yet to utilize needle biopsy in the diagnosis of the thyroid nodule we can do no better than quote directly from the comprehensive review of Ashcraft and VanHerle [36].

'How often has surgery been advocated because a thyroidal lesion is diagnosed as cold, solid, and solitary?' Just utter the words 'cold thyroid nodule' and watch how many colleagues react with furrowed brows and immediate decisions to perform a thyroidectomy. Yet the literature is filled with data and advice warning against the use of radioiodine scanning techniques as the criterion for surgery.

Primarily because of a single case report in 1952, the work of the previous 22 years and the following 28 years dealing with needle biopsy of the thyroid was largeley discarded by most American physicians. Instead, they turned to scanning techniques that offered a predictive value so poor that if introduced today, these techniques would not be accepted. Yet a technique of clearly demonstrated value is still rebuffed in lieu of these other modes. Why?

Needle biopsy is not new and has been practiced for 50 years. It is not perfect, but, as can be seen in Figs. 1 and 2, it clearly has the best predictive value of any technique currently available to differentiate benign from malignant thyroidal diasease. The medical community tends to be conservative – careful, cautious, and deliberate. Tumor implantation has led physicians to be especially wary; however, it has been shown that this caution is overstrated.

To continue to scorn the usefulness of fine needle aspiration must reflect either unwarranted conservatism or ignorance of the data. Indeed, based on the data presented in this review, it is possible to conclude (as several authors have already done) that fine needle aspiration should be the initial diagnostic test to the thyroid nodule.'

References

1. Mazzaferri EL, Young RL, Oertel JE, Kemmerer WT, Page CP: Papillary thyroid carcinoma: The impact of therapy in 576 patients. Medicine 56: 171–196, 1977.
2. Foster RS Jr: Morbidity and mortality after thyroidectomy. Surg Gynecol & Obset 146: 423–429, 1978.
3. Colcock BP: Evaluation of the thyroid nodule. Surg Clin N America 50: 541–544, 1970.
4. Shimaoka K, Badillo J, Sokal JE, Marchetta FC: Clinical differentiation between thyroid cancer and benign goiter. JAMA 181: 179–185, 1962.
5. Kendall LW, Condon RE: Prediction of malignancy in solitary thyroid nodules. Lancet I: 1071–1073, 1969.
6. Hoffman GL, Thompson NW, Heffron C: The solitary thyroid nodule. Arch Surg 105: 379–385, 1972.
7. Thomas CG Jr, Buckwalter JA, Staab EV, Kerr CY: Evaluation of dominant thyroid masses. Ann Surg 183: 463–469, 1976.
8. Liechty RD, Stoffel PT, Zimmerman DE, Silverberg SG, Solitary thyroid nodules. Arch Surg 112: 59–61, 1977.
9. Hamburger JI: Clinical Exercises in Internal Medicine, Vol 1, Thyroid Disease, Phila.: Saunders, 1978, pp 221–222.
10. Hamburger JI: Is long term antithyroid drug therapy for Graves' disease cost-effective. In: Controversies in Clinical Thyroidology, Hamburger JI, Miller JM (eds). New York: Springer-Verlag, 1981, pp 151–152.
11. Martin HE, Ellis EB: Biopsy by needle puncture and aspiration. Ann Surg 92: 169–181, 1930.
12. Walfish PG, Hazani E, Strawbridge HTG, Miskin M, Rosen IB: Combined ultrasound and needle aspiration cytology in the assesment and management of hypofunctioning thyroid nodule. Ann Intern Med 87: 270–274, 1977.
13. Gershengorn MC, McClung MR, Chu EW, Hanson TAS, Weintraub BD, Robbins J: Fine-needle aspiration cytology in the preoperative diagnosis of thyroid nodules. Ann Intern Med 87: 265–269, 1977.
14. Lopez Cardozo P: Le Cytodiagnostic immediat par la ponction thyreodienne. Arch Anat Pathol 12: 25–32, 1964.
15. Esselstyn CB, Grile G Jr: Needle aspiration and needle biopsy of the thyroid. World J Surg 2: 45–53, 1978.
16. Soderstrom N: Puncture of goiters for aspiration biopsy. A preliminary report. Acta Medica Scandinavica 144: 235–244, 1952.
17. Persson PS: Cytodiagnosis of thyroiditis: A comparative study of cytological, histological, immunological and clinical findings in thyroiditis, particularly in diffuse lymphoid thyroiditis. Acta Medica Scandinavica supplementum 483: 7–25, 1967.
18. Nilsson LR, Persson: Cytological aspiration biopsy in adolescent goitre. Acta Paediat 53: 333–338, 1964.

19. Ljunberg O: Cytologic diagnosis of medullary carcinoma of the thyroid gland with special regard to the demonstration of amyloid in smears of fine needle aspirates. Acta Cytol 16: 253–255, 1972.
20. Einhorn J, Franzen S: Thin-needle biopsy in the diagnosis of thyroid disease. Acta Radiol 58: 321–336, 1962.
21. Galvan G: Thin needle aspiration biopsy and cytological examination of hypofunctional 'cold' thyroid nodules in routine clinical work. Clin Nucl Med 2: 413–421, 1977.
22. Droese M, Kempken K: Die Feinnadelpunktion in der Schilddrüsendiagnostik. Med Klin 71: 229–234, 1976.
23. Löwhagen T, Sprenger E: Cytologic presentation of thyroid tumors in aspiration biopsy smear. Acta Cytol 18: 192–197, 1974.
24. Wang C, Vickery AL Jr, Maloof F: Needle biopsy of the thyroid. Surg Gynec Obstet 143: 365–368, 1976.
25. Crile G Jr, Hawk WA Jr: Aspiration biopsy of thyroid nodules. Surg Gynec Obstet 136: 241–245, 1973.
26. Martin H: Surgery of Head and Neck Tumors. New York: Hoeber-Harper, 1957, pp 29–33.
27. Miller JM, Kini SR, Rebuck J, Hamburger JI: Is lymphoma of the thyroid a disease which is increasing in frequency? In: Controversies in Clinical Thyroidology, Hamburger JI, Miller JM (eds). New York: Springer-Verrlag, 1981, pp 267–297.
28. Walfish PG, Miskin M, Rosen IB, Strawbridge H: Application of special diagnostic techniques in the management of nodular goitre. CMA J 115: 35–40, 1976.
29. Löwhagen T, Willems J-S, Lundell G, Sunblad R, Granberg, P-O: Aspiration biopsy cytology in diagnosis of the thyroid cancer. World J Surg 5: 61–73, 1981.
30. Hamburger JI, Miller JM, Kini SR: Clinical-Pathological Evaluation of Thyroid Nodules. Handbook and Atlas. Southfield: Private Publication 1979, p 13.
31. Rudowski W: Critical evaluation of aspiration biopsy in the diagnosis of tumors of the thyroid. Amer J Surg 95: 40–44, 1958.
32. Hamburger JI, Miller JM, Kini SR: Clinical-Pathological Evaluation of Thyroid Nodules. Handbook and Atlas. Southfield: Private Publication 1979, pp 16–17.
33. Hamburger JI, Miller JM, Kini SR: Clinical Pathological Evaluation of Thyroid Nodules. Handbook and Atlas. Southfield: Private Publication 1979, pp 14–15.
34. Block MA, Miller JM, Kini SR: The potential impact of needle biopsy on surgery for thyroid nodules. World J, Surg 4: 737–745, 1980.
35. Schwartz TB: Comment on Block MA, Miller JM and Kini SR: The potential impact of needle biopsy on surgery for thyroid nodules (abst). In: Year Book Endocrinology, Schwartz TB, Ryan WG (eds). Chicago: Year Book, 1982, p 138.
36. Ashcraft MW, Van Herle AJ: Management of thyroid nodules. II: Scanning techniques, thyroid suppressive therapy, and fine needle aspiration. Head and Neck Surg 3: 297–322, 1981.
37. Sykes D: The solitary thyroid nodule. Br J Surg 68: 510–512, 1981.
38. Miller JM, Hamburger JI, Taylor CI: Is needle aspiration of the cystic thyroid nodule effective and safe treatment? In: Controversies is Clinical Thyroidology, Hamburger JI, Miller JM (eds). Springer-Verlag, 1981, pp 209–236.
39. Hamburger JI, Miller JM, Kini SR: Clinical-Pathological Evaluation of Thyroid Nodules. Handbook and Atlas. Southfield: Private Publication, 1979, pp 74–86.
40. Goldfarb WB, Bigos TS, Eastman RC, Johnston H, Nishyama RH: Needle biopsy in the assessment and management of hypofunctioning thyroid nodules. Am J Surg 143–409–412, 1982.
41. Miller JM, Kini SR, Hamburger JI, Messner WA: Needle Biopsy of the Thyroid: Current Concepts. New York: Praeger (In press).
42. Miller JM, Hamburger JI: The thyroid scintigram. I. The hot nodule. Radiology 84: 66–74, 1965.
43. Hamburger JI, Miller JM Garcia M: Do all nodules appearing in patients subsequent to radiation therapy to the head and neck area require excision? In: Controversies in Clinical Thyroidology, Hamburger JI, Miller JM (eds). New York: Springer Verlag, 1981, pp 237–266.

7. Endocrine neoplasms: carcinomas of the thyroid

TIMOTHY S. HARRISON

1. Introduction

Confined to the thyroid, its carcinomas can be cured surgically. With extrathyroidal spread, surgical cure of thyroid cancer is uncertain. These two facts conspire to make risk prevention for developing the tumor, early detection of the thyroid cancer, and deeper understanding of the biology of the tumor's growth truly important for progress in successfully dealing with thyroid cancers. From this perspective we will discuss the four most common cancers of the thyroid, emphasizing shortcomings and limitations in our current therapy and goals for improved future management.

2. Differentiated thyroid cancers

2.1 Papillary adenocarcinoma

2.1.1 *Background and etiology.* The most common and least aggressive of thyroid cancers, papillary adenocarcinoma, occurs in children and in the elderly, and between those extremes is evenly spaced in patients of both sexes of any age and is slightly more frequent in women.

When present, prior exposure to ionizing or X-radiation to the neck and face unquestionably is an important etiologic force in the development of the tumor. Roughly 30 years ago, external X-radiation to the enlarged thymus, hypertrophic adenoids and tonsils, and to acneiform facial eruptions was all too common a practice. Duffy and Fitzgerald [1] first noted in 1950 an increase in thyroid nodules among those radiated patients, and a straightforward increased incidence of papillary adenocarcinoma in their thyroid nodules. A number of investigators, most particularly DeGroot and his colleagues, relentlessly pursued this lead, confirming not only the increased incidence of thyroid nodules and cancer but establishing as well an inordinately high incidence of multicentricity in the papillary adenocarcinoma of patients to whom antecedent X-radiation had once been delivered externally [2]. I discuss later the obvious therapeutic implications of post-radiation multicentricity of papillary thyroid cancer.

Santen, R.J. and Manni, A. (eds.), Diagnosis and management of endocrine-related tumors. ISBN 0-89838-636-5.
© 1984, Martinus Nijhoff Publishers, Boston. Printed in the Netherlands.

X-radiation exposure in adults carries with it a definite but lower incidence for radiation-induced cancer than that seen in radiated children [3]. Given an X-radiated population, Kaplan [4] studied five risk factors within a group of 95 patients with prior X-radiation to the neck: serum free thyroxine index, serum thyrotropin level, and palpable thyroid abnormalities, plus a history of lymphangiography, and finally X-radiation in excess of 3000 rads. Three patients had localized papillary carcinomas, 40 had elevated thyrotropin levels, and seven subnormal free thyroxine indices. Radiation in excess of 300 rads and/or lymphangiography increased the risk for elevated thyrotropin ($p<.01$), but duration of follow-up did not.

Concerted efforts to understand radiation injury to the thyroid indicate no increase in thyroid disease of any type in children exposed to fallout radiation from nuclear weapons testing in Nevada in the early 1940s [5]. Adult Marshall islanders exposed to fallout in 1954 had a high prevalence of hypothyroidism (14 of 86 subjects examined), and two were clinically hypothyroid. Most marked TSH increases were seen in children less than six years old when exposed. Most of this group subsequently had thyroid nodules. In 18 Marshall islanders with thyroid problems, there was one cancer and 15 patients with benign thyroid nodules. The Marshallees are far too mobile and inaccessible to complete evaluation, including surgery, to permit an accurate prevalence of thyroid cancer to be calculated for the risk of that fallout [6].

Other etiologic factors are difficult to implicate in human thyroid cancer. Experimentally, long-term iodide deficiency or exposure to goitrogens will ultimately result in thyroid cancer due in part, it is thought, to prolonged stimulation of the thyroid by endogenous thyroid-stimulating hormone. An overt correlation to human thyroid cancer is, however, lacking.

2.1.2 *Diagnosis*. The diagnosis of papillary adenocarcinoma is clinical. A palpable thyroid nodule picked up on a routine physical examination in a pregnant mother; visible metastases in cervical lymph nodes of an 11-year-old girl; suspicious enlargement of a longstanding goiter in a charming 82-year-old dowager – the need for early clinical diagnosis is easily apparent. An estimated 20% of patients with papillary adenocarcinoma of the thyroid have metastases at the time their tumor is first detected.

Currently there are two major efforts to enhance earlier detection of papillary adenocarcinoma. As yet, neither shows much prospect for success. Cytology of fine and coarse needle aspirates from the thyroid is in vogue and there is almost unbelievable preoccupation with it in most centers treating thyroid cancer today. While doubtless many patients can be spared surgical removal of benign thyroid nodules and cysts by aspiration cytology negative for malignant cells, falsely negative cytologies are possible and the more important goal of earlier detection of the tumor, when still pre-metastatic, is not changed by having aspiration cytology available.

A suitable serum tumor marker for papillary adenocarcinoma has long been sought, but to date none is dependable. Great hopes were raised and convictions expressed that serum thyroglobulin, or antibodies to thyroglobulin, would be a useful marker for papillary adenocarcinoma. Often one or both are elevated in papillary adenocarcinoma, but inconsistently so, preventing reliance on thyroglobulin or its antibodies as an important help in detecting thyroid cancers in populations at risk or in patients who unknowingly harbor occult thyroid cancer. In patients with known thyroid cancer, if thyroglobulin or its antibodies are elevated, this can signal early recurrences of the tumor before any other clinical clue exists. It is intriguing that serum thyroglobulin levels vary between normal and statistically significant elevations in rare thyroid cancer patients whose tumor size in unchanged from one observation time to the next.

Logically, more emphasis should be given in the future to discovering and evaluating by intensive computer analysis more risk factors contributing to papillary thyroid carcinoma in the way that X-radiation has been demonstrated so convincingly to influence the biological background from which papillary adenocarcinoma of the thyroid may develop.

2.1.3 *Treatment*. Immediately visible underneath the glass top of his desk, a prominent, well trained thyroid surgeon has a photograph of a mother and her 20-year-old daughter. Twenty-one years earlier the mother was three months pregnant and had a complete lobectomy for what was considered on frozen section a benign thyroid adenoma. Permanent section microscopy showed the invasiveness unmistakable as papillary adenocarcinoma. Then a chief surgical resident, the surgeon was advised by his chief to seek an opinion from a professor of surgery in another institution. 'Terminate the pregnancy and complete the thyroidectomy' was the 'expert's' advice. The resident refused to do either and now all three, mother, daughter and surgeon, are grateful that common sense prevailed.

The intensity of the conviction in a few centers that all differentiated thyroid carcinoma be treated by total thyroidectomy makes careful analysis of this point important. An estimated 80% of papillary adenocarcinoma is confined to one lobe of the thyroid when patients are first seen.

The most cogent analysis of lobectomy for thyroid cancer has come from the Mayo Clinic, where careful actuarial life table analysis was used to study survival of patients with all thyroid cancers including papillary adenocarcinoma [7]. A generous biopsy or subtotal lobectomy of the opposite lobe was also done in the Mayo Clinic patients. Compared to an age- and sex-matched population, the post-lobectomy patients's survival was identical with normal subjects without thyroid carcinoma. Admirably, the follow-up continued for at least 20 years and for some patients as long as 40 years (Fig. 1).

Of a number of studies reinforcing and amplifying the effectiveness of lobectomy, that of Tollefsen et al. from the Sloan-Kettering Memorial Center for

154

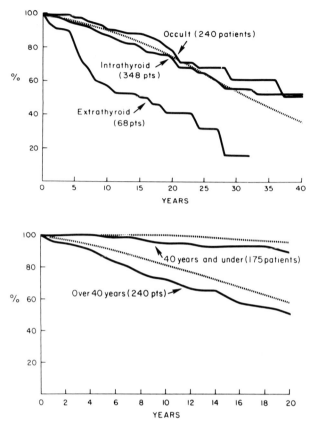

Figure 1. In the upper panel survival curves are shown for papillary adenocarcinoma of the thyroid at the Mayo Clinic for patients with occult, intra-thyroidal and extra-thyroidal tumor. Note that survival for occult and palpable intra-thyroidal tumors is the same as it is for an age and sex-matched control population shown with the cross hatched line.

In the lower panel the lower survival of older patients with papillary adenocarcinoma is apparent but in fact survival of age and sex matched controls decreases comparably. The curves therefore do not support the recently held contention that papillary adenocarcinoma is a more virulent disease in the elderly. Beahrs O, Pasternak B, *Current Problems in Surgery,* 1969.

Cancer is among the more persuasive [8]. In 216 patients with papillary adenocarcinoma followed for 18 years, treated only by total lobectomy, clinically palpable lesions developed in the opposite lobe in only two; in both of these patients the opposite lobe was uneventfully removed and the disease controlled. Five patients had a contralateral lobe removed for elective reasons. Five had the opposite lobe removed to control clinical recurrence or as part of a neck dissection for involved contralateral cervical nodes.

The incidence of multicentricity of papillary cancer is known to be low — the occurence of microscopic nests of papillary cells need not be viewed as multicentric tumor because such nests are a recognized postmortem occurence and it is uncertain that thyroid carcinoma would ever develop from them. Thus true, multicentric, clinically important papillary adenocarcinoma probably occurs in no more than 5% of those patients originally presenting with solitary nodules at the time of their initial treatment of papillary adenocarcinoma.

When the primary tumor involves both lobes, when there is a history of prior X-radiation to the neck, and when the papillary adenocarcinoma has metastasized to regional lymph nodes in either side of the neck or distantly to the lung or elsewhere, there is no question that total extracapsular thyroidectomy should be done.

Unfortunately, the control of extrathyroidal papillary adenocarcinoma is uncertain at best. The Mayo Clinic actuarial survival analysis shows 40% mortality in patients with extrathyroidal papillary adenocarcinoma 20 years after detection of their disease. Of the variety of available treatments, two offer some hope in treating metastatic thyroid of cancer: TSH suppression by exogenous thyroid hormone and [131]Iodine radiation.

Chronic TSH stimulation produces experimental thyroid cancer in many laboratory species. The use of thyroid suppression in managing clinically metastatic thyroid cancer is interesting. Mazzaferri and his colleagues studied metastatic papillary adenocarcinoma in depth by retrieving from the United States Air Force computer entry all patients with papillary thyroid cancer followed for 15 years [9]. The patients were Air Force personnel and their families; distinctly younger than a randomly sampled population with papillary adenocarcinoma. Surveillance for thyroid cancer is likely to be higher in the Air Force patients than in civilians. Studying 15-year cumulative recurrence rates, rather than actuarial survival rates, Mazzaferri ct al. found significant protection against recurrence in all patients with papillary thyroid cancer treated with exogenous thyroid; this includes patients with disease confined to one lobe and also those with metastatic thyroid cancer. A difficulty in Mazzaferri's data is that other centers have not analyzed and reported their follow-up data in the same way. Dilution of their patient pool with disproportionately many with surgically curable papillary adenocarcinoma confined to one lobe of the thyroid would, of course, favorably skew their results. The central question is not, does thyroid hormone influence a disease which is cured already, but rather does thyroid hormone protect against recurrence of, or mortality from, papillary thyroid cancer in those patients known to have extrathyroidal tumor? Until data such as that of Mazzaferri et al. are analyzed from this perspective, the potential significance of their findings on thyroid hormone suppression of papillary adenocarcinoma is interesting but unclear.

Recently at the Lahey Clinic, Cady has examined actuarially the influence of thyroid hormone treatment on survival from thyroid cancer[10]. The study is carefully done statistically and shows no survival benefit whatsoever from thyroid hormone therapy in papillary adenocarcinoma. Cady's analysis includes individual examination of high and low risk categories for death from papillary cancer, and in neither group is any protection seen (Fig. 2).

Therapeutic [131] Radio-iodine given to papillary adenocarcinoma patients with

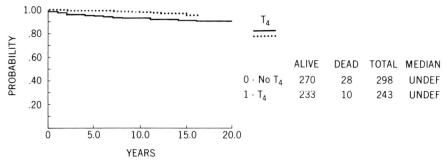

Figure 2. Shown are Survival curves for thyroid papillary adenocarcinoma patients with (————) and without (·······) Thyroid Hormone administration. There is no difference in survival between the two groups. In the same study high and low risk subgroups are analyzed independently for the effect of endogenous thyroid hormone on mortality from papillary adenocarcinoma of the thyroid and no protective effect is seen. Cady, B. et al. [10].

demonstrably metastatic disease has many ideal features. The treatment is simple and noninvasive. Serious sequelae to [131]Iodine have not appeared even on prolonged and careful observation. Concerted efforts with [131]Iodine achieve much anecdotal success. However, the lack of extended follow-up data on ^{131}I-treated metastatic papillary adenocarcinoma patients and, in particular, the total lack of actuarial life table follow-up mortality by those administering ^{131}I is serious. A recent noteworthy attempt to overcome this vacuum is that of Beierwaltes et al. [11]. They selected for extended actuarial follow-up patients with demonstrably extracervical differentiated thyroid cancer. They divided ^{131}I-treated metastatic papillary adenocarcinoma patients into two groups, those free from disease as judged by resolution of their extracervical ^{131}I uptake, and secondly, those with residual disease in spite of their ^{131}I treatment. Those patients free from disease were three times more likely to be alive at 15 years than those with residual disease after [131]I. The disease-free patients were also in closer conformity to Beierwaltes' stipulated criteria for successful treatment of thyroid cancer. Any study analyzing as a subgroup only those patients showing favorable response is bound to show a favorable influence. It is striking that there is still a large mortality from metastatic thyroid cancer in both the 'disease-free' subjects and others with disease persisting after radio-iodine treatment. It is interesting that the survival shown for disease-free patients is same as that for extrathyroidal papillary cancer in the Mayo Clinic series in which ^{131}I treatment did not figure prominently. The underlying virulence of papillary adenocarcinoma emerges as the single most telling determinant of mortality in metastatic thyroid papillary adenocarcinoma. Possibly both thyroid hormone and ^{131}I treatment of metastatic papillary thyroid cancer are ineffective. Ideally, there should be a prospective mortality study of extracervical papillary thyroid carcinoma patients analyzing those who have had ^{131}I treatment and those who have not.

For patients whose only metastasis from papillary adenocarcinoma is in the neck, long-term control and quite possibly cure of the papillary adenocarcinoma is possible with total thyroidectomy and removal of involved lymph nodes. Several operations years apart may be needed to remove palpably enlarged nodes. [131]I treatment is often given these patients, but if further tumor develops in the neck after ^{131}I treatment, surgical removal of the lymph nodes is still wise. In young patients, particularly, long-term control of the papillary adenocarcinoma is possible and likely with surgery. Radical dissection of cervical lymph nodes containing papillary thyroid cancer is advocated by Colin Thomas and his colleagues at the University of North Carolina [12]. In this operation, both sternocleidomastoid muscle and internal jugular vein are sacrificed and there is a noticeable cosmetic defect. Permanent hypoparathyroidism in 10% of their patients makes radical neck dissection unattractive treatment for papillary adenocarcinoma. Most surgeons remove sternocleidomastoid and jugular vein only if they are invaded by tumor – a rare occurrence. Thomas et al. carefully analyzed their long-term results actuarially with life table analysis for controlled and metastatic papillary adenocarcinoma, but the survival rates are no higher than those of the Mayo Clinic where a less destructive operation was used.

3. Follicular Adenocarcinoma

3.1. Background

Less common and noticeably more aggressive than papillary adenocarcinoma, follicular adenocarcinoma occurs in older patients. To the extent that it is understood, comparable etiologic factors are thought to be responsible for development of follicular carcinoma. Uncertainty is always raised by tumors which have a mixed papillary and follicular pattern. The tendency is to regard them in their more favorable light – that is, as papillary adenocarcinomas. This is a somewhat arbitrary solution to the problem of the mixed pattern, and a variety of other views have been offered, prominent among them that follicular and papillary cancers are, in fact, extremes of all differentiated thyroid tumors. Perhaps follicular carcinoma patients' being older accounts for its greater aggressiveness (Fig. 3), although papillary adenocarcinoma is considered a more aggressive tumor in older patients. New approaches such as carefull genetic analysis of both tumors are needed to examine more fully tumor heterogeneity in differentiated thyroid cancer.

3.1.1 *Treatment.* The opinion is prevalent, largely through Mazzaferri's study, that follicular adenocarcinoma is less suppressible by exogenous thyroid hormone than is papillary adenocarcinoma. However, follicular adenocarcinoma is thought to be more responsive to ^{131}I radiation than the papillary tumor. It is not difficult to find these convictions expressed, but it cannot be emphasized too

158

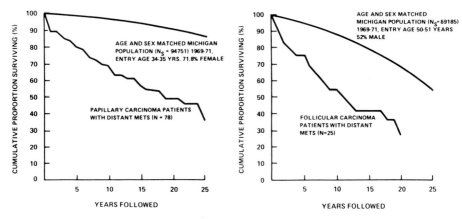

Figure 3. Survival for metastatic papillary adenocarcinoma with distant metastases is 45% at 20 years followup and about 28% for follicular carcinoma. This is strong evidence that follicular carcinoma is a more aggressive tumor than papillary adenocarcinoma of the thyroid. Beierwaltes, W.B. et al. [11].

strongly that actuarial life table mortality analysis is needed to assess these convictions adequately and such actuarial data are sparse.

In the Mayo Clinic actuarial analysis to which we referred previously follicular adenocarcinoma confined to one lobe of the thyroid is cured by lobectomy. Survival is identical to an age- and sex-matched population without thyroid cancer. However, 30% of follicular carcinoma is extrathyroidal at the time of diagnosis, and for these patients treated by total thyroidectomy and removal of extrathyroidal foci of tumor when feasible, survival is less possible than for patients with papillary adenocarcinoma, being only 22% 20 years after treatment. Radio-iodine treatment did not figure prominently in the Mayo Clinic series at the time of their study.

The innately greater aggressiveness of follicular cancer compared to papillary is reflected convincingly in the actuarial survival of patients with demonstrated extracervical disease studied by Beierwaltes et al. In 25 metastatic follicular carcinoma patients available for study, they found only 28% survival at 20 years compared to 45% for 78 patients with metastatic papillary adenocarcinoma (Fig. 3).

Follicular adenocarcinoma of the thyroid metastasizes to bone far more often than papillary adenocarcinoma. There can be brilliant resolution of bony metastases by ^{131}I treatment in follicular adenocarcinoma with complete destruction of ^{131}I uptake in a metastasis that originally took up ^{131}I avidly. Exciting as such results are, they are inherently anecdotal. The chief value of ^{131}I treatment, then, is pain relief and arrest or slowing of tumor growth followed objectively and sensitively by calculated ^{131}I uptake. It is hard to restrain enthusiasm for such progress when caring for follicular carcinoma patients with bony metastases. In fact, the long-term prognosis is poor and progression of the metastatic follicular adenocarcinoma elsewhere is most often inexorable and the patients often die of their tumor.

4. Medullary carcinoma of the thyroid

4.1 *Background*

'(There is) a multitude of histologic variants of thyroid cancer . . . (and) . . . the addition of a new diagnostic term should be recommended only upon established necessity'. Hazard 1955 [13].

In an appraisal of thyroid carcinoma several years ago, Hazard noticed a tumor which had not been recognized before, although it had special clinical and pathologic features.

In this setting, Hazard and his colleagues were the first to appreciate medullary thyroid cancer. Estimates vary from 2% to 10% for the incidence of medullary carcinoma in thyroid cancer patients. Whithout doubt, medullary carcinoma is common enough to require the educated interest of any physician caring for thyroid disease.

Neural crest derived parafollicular C-cells give rise to medullary cancer preceded, in the view of most, by C cell hyperplasia. Thyroid C-cells synthesize and release the peptide hormone calcitonin, and medullary carcinoma cells synthesize and release increased calcitonin. Calcitonin turns out to be a dependable marker for medullary carcinoma. Calcitonin as a medullary carcinoma marker is particularly important in screening kindreds at risk for medullary carcinoma in Sipple's Syndrome, MEN-II, in which an autosomal dominant trait transmits a high risk for medullary carcinoma. Using glucose 6 phosphate dehydrogenase Type A as a clonal marker, Baylin and his colleagues identified a mono-clonal cell line in MEN-II kindreds' medullary carcinomas and pheochromocytomas. [14] Subsequently, they recognized a mono-clonal origin for normal C-cells, C-cell hyperplasia, and finally medullary thyroid carcinoma itself in given MEN-II kindreds.

I subsequently comment in detail about calcitonin surveillance of MEN-II kindreds. For the moment, it is sufficient to realize significant improvement in mortality from medullary carcinoma in MEN-II is gained by aggressive calcitonin screening and total thyroidectomy in those patients with abnormally high serum calcitonins at rest or after appropriate stimulation. Other thyroid cancers lack as sensitive and specific a marker and do not occur in such clearly defined risk groups. Consequently, the treatment of other thyroid cancers is less likely to improve in the future than is that of medullary thyroid carcinoma.

5. Diagnosis of medullary (C-cell) thyroid carcinoma

5.1 *Sporadic and familial medullary thyroid cancer*

An estimated 80% of medullary cancer occurs with no familial predisposition for the disease. This is important because in roughly 40% of medullary carcinoma patients the tumor has metastasized to regional nodes by the time of clinical detection. The results of treating extrathyroidal medullary thyroid cancer are poor and have not yet improved with chemotherapy or external radiation even though these modalities are often fruitlessly tried.

It is in MEN-II kindreds at increased risk for medullary carcinoma that vigorous calcitonin screening is unquestionably effective. As soon as an elevated serum calcitonin is found either at rest or after stimulation with either calcium or pentagastrin or, most ideally, as pointed out by Wells [15], with both, total thyroidectomy should be done. The most sensitive calcitonin screening possible is with the inferior thyroid vein cannulated and inappropriately high calcitonins found far in excess of expected values but no tumor objectively demonstrated and normal peripheral calcitonins (Fig 4.) Wells and his colleagues have aggressively used this approach in surveying several MEN-II kindreds. The results are truly impressive, and there is no question that total thyroidectomy in those MEN-II patients with elevated calcitonins has, in fact, increased the percentage of medullary carcinoma patients presenting without metastatic disease. Although it is too

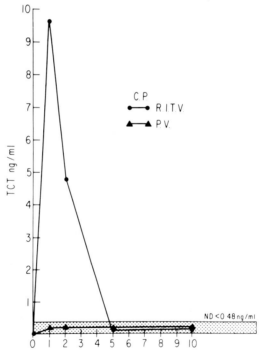

Figure 4. Following pentagastrin stimulation increased Calcitonin levels in the catheterized right inferior thyroid vein (RITV) contrast sharply to normal levels drawn simultaneously from a peripheral vein (PV). The patient, a 40 year old male is from a MEN-II kindred. Foci of C-cell hyperplasia were seen in his total thyroidectomy specimen.

I have never seen a stimulated Calcitonin level from a normal subject's inferior thyroid vein and this information while crucial may be difficult to obtain. Wells, S.A., Jr et al. [15].

soon for actuarial confirmation by life table analysis, this approach in MEN-II improves survival in those MEN-II subjects who, fortunately, were screened.

In sporadic MEN-II, A and B, a degree of increased surveillance is possible. Since MEN-II-A is a coincidence of pheochromocytoma, mild hyperparathyroidism and medullary thyroid carcinoma, it is important to measure resting and stimulated serum calcitonin in all pheochromocytoma and primary hyperparathyroidism patients. Only after consistent screening of large numbers of these patients will we know if the true incidence of sporadic MEN-II is high enough to justify this approach. The need for such study is an obvious and current concern.

5.1.1 *Treatment of medullary thyroid cancer.* Much has been made of total thyroidectomy and dissection of the cervical lymph nodes in the 'central compartment' of the neck as the surgical treatment of choice for medullary carcinoma. Of the wisdom of performing total thyroidectomy there can be no doubt. Medullary carcinoma is multicentric and the microscopic nests of 'hyperplastic' C-cells so often develop into cancer that one wonders if the term hyperplasia is really apt. This contrasts strikingly to papillary adenocarcinoma in which microscopic nests discovered at postmortem and in other circumstances are found which obviously hold little if any potential of becoming clinical carcinoma.

Central compartment dissection includes those lymph nodes lying between the medial edge of the sternocleidomastoid muscles. It is valuable to include these nodes with total thyroidectomy, not for any supposed therapeutic advantage because there is none, but because it is helpful to know if the lymph nodes are microscopically positive when staging the disease for intelligent discussion of the prognosis with patients and their families.

If palpable lymph nodes are present in the jugular chain, or elsewhere outside the central compartment of the neck, obviously it is wise to extend the dissection to include those nodes which are suspicious.

Although often resorted to, externally delivered X-radiation and chemotherapy, unfortunately, have no important effect on metastatic medullary thyroid carcinoma. Similarly, ^{131}I delivered to the thyroid is ineffective with medullary carcinoma because ^{131}I is not taken up by calcitonin-secreting C-cells and the effective radiation reaching the C-cells themselves is not large. Metastatic medullary carcinoma cannot be expected to take up ^{131}I at all.

In sporadic and familial MEN-II-B, a characteristic Marfanoid facies and habitus, occurrence of submucosal neuromas and pheochromocytoma, most often bilateral, all signal the disease. This physiognomy permits diagnosis at first glance. Not to obtain resting and stimulated serum calcitonin values in all sporadic and familial MEN-II-B patients is unthinkable, and if the calcitonins are initially normal screening these individuals who are at risk for the rest of their life. So far as we know, and the reported numbers are still small, sporadic MEN-II subjects are at an inordinately high risk for the eventual development of medullary thyroid carcinoma.

5.1.2 *Case reports*. An 11-year-old girl with two normal siblings and normal parents has a typical Marfanoid facies and body and bumps on her lips. In her lifetime she visited a pediatrician at least five times for routine childhood physical examination and illnesses. Along with a routine cold, the mother notices swellings in the neck, both in the thyroid and in the back of the neck. Two weeks later, the cold is gone but the swellings persist. The child has metastatic, incurable medullary carcinoma of the thyroid and dies four months later.

A 26-year-old schoolteacher and housewife is in the fifth month of her first pregnancy. Violent hypertension and pulmonary edema and massively increased urinary catecholamine excretion rates led to the diagnosis of pheochromocytoma. After appropriate alpha and beta adrenergic receptor blockade, her pregnancy is terminated and bilateral pheochromocytomas weighing a total of 980 grams are removed. Convalescence is smooth.

Postoperatively, resting calcitonin is elevated on two determinations. There is no scanning defect in the thyroid and no thyroid nodules are felt. Total thyroidectomy yields a multicentric medullary carcinoma. The patient is well 10 years postoperatively. Modest calcitonin elevations persist but may not be related to persistent medullary carcinoma since there have been no other stigmata of recurrent cancer in 10 years.

In MEN-II-B, the Marfanoid subtype previously mentioned, sustained postoperative calcitonin elevations may occur with no recurrent tumor for years. These patients may be cured and watchful waiting, repeated calcitonin measurements, and appreciation of the lack of continued increase in absolute calcitonin levels all may tip off the patients' cure. The submucosal neuromas of MEN-II-B contain calcitonin and possibly are responsible for the prolonged but definite serum calcitonin increases seen postoperatively in MEN-II-B patients evidently cured of their medullary carcinoma.

5.1.3 *Postoperative follow up*. Once operated upon, medullary carcinoma patients are conveniently followed by periodic serum calcitonin measurement. This should be done every year or so, and if a normal postoperative calcitonin level is followed by a persistently higher level, metastases should be suspected and probably searched for even though there is no definitive treatment for metastatic medullary carcinoma of the thyroid

6. Anaplastic undifferentiated carcinoma of the thyroid

6.1 *Background and pathology*

In elderly patients there is a devastating thyroid tumor from which survival is negligible after two years. Far more aggressive than either differentiated thyroid cancer or medullary (C-cell) carcinoma, anaplastic carcinoma kills patients by directly invading structures contiguous to it in the neck, particularly the trachea, carotid artery or jugular vein, with fatal consequences to the airway or blood vessels. Airway obstruction, bleeding into the trachea or uncontrollable bleeding often cause death in these unfortunate patients.

The tumor is diverse clinically and pathologically. It may be stony hard or soft. In addition to involving vital structures of the neck, it can metastasize into lymph nodes or disseminate into the blood stream and distantly throughout the body.

Microscopically, the predominant cell is usually small and round with sparse cytoplasm. Variations occur in which giant cells are prominent, and there is a suggestion by some that the giant cell variants be considered as a separate tumor, but to date there is no consistently clearcut therapeutic advantage in doing so. Spindle cell variants are seen and in a few patients, patterns of papillary and follicular carcinoma are present, suggesting that the tumor can arise from pre-existing follicular or papillary adenocarcinoma.

6.1.1 *Diagnosis of undifferentiated thyroid cancer.* The clinical presentation of a hard, large, ill-defined thyroid mass in the elderly will usually alert physicians to anaplastic carcinoma. Chronic thyroiditis may mimic the picture, and this can be resolved not only by measuring circulating levels of antimicrosomal thyroid antibodies but by adequate biopsy, either open or by adequate cutting needle biopsy of the mass in question. Anaplastic carcinoma must also be differentiated from thyroid lymphosarcoma since the latter can be treated by chemotherapy and radiation. Generous open biopsy of the thyroid is the best way to differentiate between lymphosarcoma and anaplastic thyroid carcinoma.

6.1.2 *Treatment of anaplastic thyroid carcinoma.* Very little is gained by attempting total surgical removal of anaplastic thyroid carcinoma. In the giant cell variant of anaplastic carcinoma, radical surgery of the neck with en bloc removal of the thyroid followed by X-radiation was encouraging and resulted in five-year survival of two patients treated at the M.D. Anderson Hospital in Houston [16]. Shrinkage of tumor followed aggressive chemotherapy in two of our anaplastic carcinoma patients. It is doubtful that appreciably longer life is given to anaplastic carcinoma patients by intensive chemotherapy, but the shrinkage in tumor size and improved appearance have been positive psychologic benefits to these patients and their families.

A common therapeutic dilemma in anaplastic carcinoma is posed by acute early airway obstruction from the tumor. Tracheostomy can be extremely difficult through the bed of anaplastic tumor and, again, longevity achieved by such heroics is apt not to be followed by significantly prolonged life.

Externally delivered X-radiation is almost invariably useless in reversing local complications in the neck or distant metastases of anaplastic thyroid carcinoma.

References

1. Duffy BJ Jr, Fitzgerald PJ: Cancer of the thyroid in children: A report of 28 cases. J Clin Endocrinol 10: 1296–1308, 1950.
2. DeGroot L, Frohman LA, Kaplan EL, et al. (eds): Proceedings of the Conference on Radiation-Induced Thyroid Cancer, September 30–October 1, 1976. New York: Grune and Stratton, Inc., 1977.
3. Maxon HR, Thomas SR, Saenger EL, et al.: Ionizing radiation and the induction of clinically significant disease in the human thyroid gland. Am J Med 63: 967–978, 1977.
4. Kaplan MM, Garnick MB, Gelber R, et al.: Risk factors for thyroid abnormalities after neck irradiation for childhood cancer. Am J Med 74: 272–280, 1983.
5. Refetoff S, Harrison T, Karafinski ET, et al.: Continuing occurrence of thyroid carcinoma after radiation to the neck in infancy and childhood. N Engl J Med 292: 171–175, 1975.
6. Larsen PR, Conard RA, Knudsen KD, et al.: Thyroid hypofunction after exposure to fallout from a hydrogen bomb explosion. JAMA 247: 1571–1575, 1982.
7. Woolner LB, Bzahas OH, Black BM, et al.: Thyroid carcinoma: General considerations and follow-up data on 1181 cases. In: Thyroid neoplasia, Young S, Inman DR (eds). London: Academic Press, 1968, p 51.
8. Tollefsen HR, Shah JP, Huvos AG: Papillary adenocarcinoma of the thyroid: Recurrence in the thyroid gland after initial surgical treatment. Am J surg 124: 468, 1972.
9. Mazzaferri EL, Young RL, Oertel JE, et al.: Papillary thyroid carcinoma: The impact of therapy in 576 patients. Medicine 56: 171–196, 1977.
10. Cady B, Cohn K, Rosse RL: The effect of thyroid hormone administration upon survival in patients with differentiated thyroid carcinoma. Surgery (in press).
11. Beierwaltes WB, Nishiyama RH, Thompson NW, et al.: Survival time and 'cure' in papillary and follicular thyroid carcinoma with distant metastases: Statistics following University of Michigan therapy. J Nucl Med 23: 561–568, 1982.
12. Buckwalter JA, Thomas CG Jr: Selection of surgical treatment of well differentiated thyroid carcinoma. Ann Surg 176: 565, 1972.
13. Hazard JB, Hawk WA, Crile G Jr: Medullary (solid) carcinoma of the thyroid: A clinicopathology entity. J Clin Endocrinol 19: 152, 1959.
14. Baylin SB, Gann DS, Hsu SH: Clonal origin of inherited medullary thyroid carcinoma and pheochromocytoma. Science 193: 321–323, 1976.
15. Wells S, Baylin SB, Linehan WM et al.: Provocative agents and the diagnosis of medullary carcinoma of the thyroid gland. Ann Surg 188: 139–141, 1978.
16. Rogers JD, Lindberg RD, Hill CS Jr: Spindle and giant cell carcinoma of the thyroid: A different therapeutic approach. Cancer 34: 1328–1332, 1974.

8. Primary hyperparathyroidism: pathophysiology, differential diagnosis and management

JUSTIN SILVER and LOUIS M. SHERWOOD

1. Introduction

The routine availability of serum calcium screening in both hospitals and the physician's office has produced a dramatic increase in the apparent prevalence of primary hyperparathyroidism [1, 2]. This growth in recognition has stimulated a number of additional questions concerning the pathogenesis, criteria for diagnosis and management of such patients, particularly those with asymptomatic disease [3]. The physiologic abnormalities that characterize primary hyperparathyroidism as well as other disorders in which hypercalcemia is found can best be understood in relation to the multiple advances in our knowledge of the biochemistry and physiology of bone and the calcium-regulating hormones in the past two decades. The introduction to this discussion of hyperparathyroidism will concentrate, therefore, on aspects of normal calcium homeostasis and the biochemistry and physiology of the hormones which will be helpful in understanding the clinical disorders.

Some of the problems of calcium homeostasis in man can best be appreciated from a brief review of comparative endocrinology, as follows:

Fish live in an environment rich in calcium and do not synthesize parathyroid hormone (PTH). They also do not have the ability to activate vitamin D to its most active metabolite, 1,25-dihydroxycholecalciferol, which is also a calmobilizing hormone. Calcitonin, which tends to inhibit calcium mobilization, is present in fish, and is produced by their ultimobranchial glands [4]. In salmon, the ultimobranchial glands undergo hyperplasia during migration and spawning. In the phylogenetic development of amphibians and terrestrial animals which live in a relatively calcium-poor environment, the ability to conserve calcium becomes more critical [5]. The parathyroid glands appear in amphibians, and PTH and 1,25-dihydroxycholecalciferol are synthesized and secreted [6, 7].

For birds with the added stress of egg-laying, the conservation of calcium is even more critical than for mammals, and they have an amplified calcium hormonal system. With the adjustment to terrestrial life, calcitonin becomes less important in normal calcium homeostasis.

In this review we shall discuss normal calcium metabolism and its homeostasis

Santen, R.J. and Manni, A. (eds.), Diagnosis and management of endocrine-related tumors. ISBN 0-89838-636-5.
© 1984, Martinus Nijhoff Publishers, Boston. Printed in the Netherlands.

by PTH and vitamin D. We shall then review primary hyperparathyroidism, its differential diagnosis and management.

2. Calcium balance: forms of calcium and functions.

Calcium in plasma is ionized, complexed to phosphates and citrates and bound to proteins, predominantly albumin [5]. It is the free ionized form (40–50%) which is functional, but its measurement requires an ion electrode which is not standard laboratory equipment. Total calcium is usually measured and is in the range of 8.8–10.5 mg/dl. A low serum albumin would therefore lead to a low total calcium, despite a normal ionized (and functional) calcium. Rarely, a serum calcium reading might be falsely high because of a calcium binding serum paraprotein while the ionized calcium is, in fact, normal [8].

The physiologic functions of calcium are multiple. It is critical to neuromuscular excitation, smooth muscle contraction, membrane potential, neurotransmitter and hormone secretion and in regulating enzyme function and the coagulation cascade. These functions are sensitive to small variations in extracellular calcium concentration which is maintained via the mobilization of calcium from calcium stores (mainly bone) and the controlling influences of the two major hormones, PTH and vitamin D.

The average American dietary content of calcium is 1000 mg, with 150–200 mg excreted in the urine and 800 mg in the feces, the latter representing calcium that is not absorbed as well as that secreted into the gut. The enteric circulation of calcium accounts for 400–500 mg of calcium per day and is normally all reabsorbed unless there is malabsorption or vitamin D deficiency. About 500 mg of calcium per day is deposited in bone and an equivalent amount resorbed. Bone contains 99% of the total body calcium (>1.0 kg) as calcium hydroxyapatite. The finely tuned mechanism carrying out the flux of calcium into and out of bone in relation to the serum calcium is carried out primarily by PTH [5, 9] and the physical chemical equilibrium of calcium and phosphate ions in the extracellular fluid and in the labile mineral bone pool.

3. Parathyroid glands and parathyroid hormone (PTH) (Fig. 1)

PTH is a polypeptide hormone secreted by the parathyroid glands which are derived from the third (lower parathyroids) and fourth (upper parathyroids) branchial pouches and in man are situated at the upper and lower poles of the thyroid gland. Their number and location may vary considerably, e.g. in the mediastinum, within the thyroid or behind the esophagus. A single human gland is approximately 5 × 5 × 3 mm, and the combined weight of all glands is about 120 mg. The glands are pinkish with a vascular stalk. The main epithelial cell is the

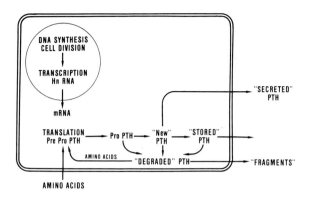

Figure 1. Potential control points in the biosynthesis, storage, degradation and secretion of PTH.

chief cell which has numerous granules containing PTH. Water clear cells and perhaps oxyphil cells are derived from chief cells and are present in smaller numbers. Fat cells separate the cords of parenchymal cells [10, 11], with the amount of fat increasing directly with age. This is a useful parameter in determining the presence of hyperplasia or adenoma in which fat diasappears.

3.1 *Chemisty [12]*. Human, like bovine and procine PTH, is a single peptide chain of 84 amino-acids (9,500 daltons). The amino-terminal region of 34 amino acids (1–34) has been synthesized and retains complete biological activity. The carboxyl-terminal region (35–84) is devoid of biologic activity but has a much longer half-life in the circulation. There are no disulfide bands in the hormone, and there is a single tyrosine residue which can be iodinated for use of the peptide in the radioimmunoassay.

3.2 *Biosynthetic precursors of PTH*. The initial product of the messenger RNA for PTH is a hormone precursor called pre-proPTH [12]. The pre-hormone extension of pre-proPTH consists of a 25 residue hydrophobic 'signal' peptide connected to the six amino acid highly basic pro region. The pre-protein includes the 'signal' peptide that permits the newly synthesized protein to enter the endoplasmic reticular membrane and to penetrate into the cisternal space. The pre-protein undergoes extremely rapid cleavage and exists in the cell only in minute quantities. Once the prohormone is formed, it is transported to the Golgi apparatus by an energy-requiring mechanism. PTH is then formed by rapid cleavage within the secretory granules by a trypsin-like enzyme. The hormone is then secreted, stored or degraded.

3.3 *Regulation of the secretion of PTH*. PTH secretion is exquisitely sensitive to ionic calcium concentration [5, 13]. The secretory response to hypocalcemia occurs within seconds, but it is as yet unknown whether calcium exerts its primary effect on the plasma membrane or in the cytoplasm. Studies of PTH secretion *in vitro* have shown that PTH secretion is regulated by ionic calcium and that most of the change in secretion occurs at concentrations equivalent to a total serum calcium of 7–10 mg/dl. At very high concentrations of calcium, the secretion of PTH is suppressed but not completely abolished [5].

Abe and Sherwood first showed that dibutyryl cAMP stimulated PTH secretion and that theophylline potentiated its action [14]. Other agents which raise intracellular cAMP (β-agonists such as epinephrine and iso-proterenol, prostaglandins, dopamine, etc.) also enhance secretion of PTH *in vitro* and *in vivo* [15]. However, the effects of calcium and agents that stimulate parathyroid cAMP appear to differ in the manner in which they affect PTH secretion. Calcium causes relatively small changes in intracellular cAMP and large changes in hormone secretion and may regulate secretion through a mechanism independent of cAMP. Furthermore, the agents which increase intracellular cAMP appear to have effects over a short period of time, whereas low calcium causes sustained release of hormone. Low calcium stimulates release of both stored and newly synthesized hormone, while the other agents may only release stored hormone [13, 16].

Magnesium, like calcium, has a suppressive effect on PTH release at high concentrations. At very low concentrations, however, PTH release is blunted both *in vitro* and *in vivo* [17]. This may result in a clinical syndrome in which hypomagnesemia causes hypocalcemia due to inadequate PTH secretion and perhaps impairment of its action. Examples include the short bowel syndrome, prolonged intravenous infusion and acute alcoholism. Lithium has recently been shown to increase PTH secretion and may be a cause of biochemical hyperparathyroidism in some manic-depressive patients on chronic therapy [18].

It is unclear whether vitamin D or its metabolites affect parathyroid secretion. There are conflicting reports of the effect of 1,25-dihydroxycholecalciferol on the release of PTH from incubated parathyroid tissue [19-21], some of which suggest that it decreases secretion and others showing no effect. On the other hand, 1,25-dihydroxycholecalciferol localizes in the chick parathyroid gland [22], and a specific receptor for the metabolite is present in both chick and human glands [23]. Its biological function remains to be elucidated.

3.4 Parathyroid secretory protein. Parathyroid secretory protein is a high molecular weight glycoprotein of unknown function that is secreted by the parathyroid gland [24]. It accounts for more of the synthesized protein in the parathyroid cell than does PTH, and it coexists in the same secretory granule as PTH. Its secretion is inversely proportional to extracellular calcium concentration [13, 25]. Although its function is as yet unknown, it has recently been shown to be phosphorylated [26], and a similar protein is apparently present in many secretory cells.

3.5 Peripheral metabolism of PTH [27] (Fig. 2). The bulk of circulating PTH consists of carboxyl-terminal fragment(s). Some of these may be derived from the

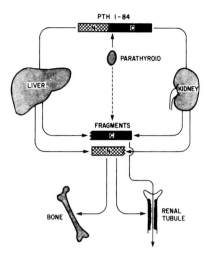

Figure 2. Peripheral metabolism of parathyroid hormone – this figure emphasizes the important role of the liver in cleaving 1-84 PTH and releasing fragments back into the circulation as well as the important role of the kidney in both cleaving and clearing PTH. As yet controversial is the issue of whether amino-terminal PTH is the primary peptide active in bone.

gland during secretion, but most are produced after secretion from the intact hormone which is rapidly cleaved into fragments, principally by the liver and kidney [12]. There appears to be a receptor on the surface of the hepatic Kupfer (reticuloendothelial) cell which binds PTH, effects a cleavage and then releases amino and carboxyl fragments back into the circulation. Some investigators believe that the amino terminal fragment is the biologically active moiety in bone. Intact and amino-terminal PTH have a relatively short half-life (5–10 minutes or less) whereas that of carboxyl-terminal PTH is of the order of several hours. In patients with chronic renal failure, the carboxyl fragments, which are normally cleared by the kidney, accumulate to very high levels [27]. An amino-terminal radioimmunoassay is therefore more useful in such patients in getting a truer indication of the level of circulating biologically-active hormone.

3.6 *PTH radioimmunoassay.* Most antisera are raised against bovine PTH and recognize predominantly the inactive carboxy-terminal fragment. The use of this assay in differentiating hyperparathyroid patients from normal is aided by relating the PTH levels to the serum calcium (see Fig. 3), because a high serum calcium should normally result in marked suppression of PTH activity. For the routine diagnosis of primary hyperparathyroidism, the carboxyl-terminal assay is perfectly satisfactory, particularly when the value is interpreted in relation to the serum calcium. It should be understood, however, that the carboxyl-terminal assay actually measures a metabolite of the hormone (e.g. analagous to measuring urinary 17-OH corticoids instead of plasma cortisol in assessing adrenal function.) Recently, highly sensitive amino-terminal assays have also been de-

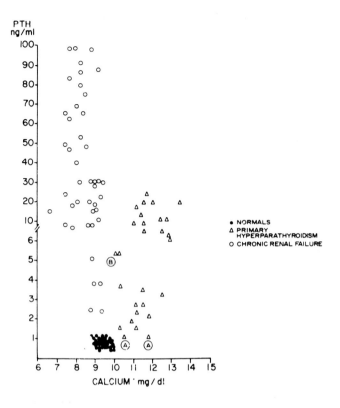

Figure 3. Radioimmunoassay results in author's laboratory using a highly sensitive carboxyl-terminal assay which can detect PTH in the serum of all normal subjects. The assay used differentiates clearly between 35 normal subjects and patients with primary hyperparathyroidism, particularly when PTH in relation to calcium is considered. Two patients (A) with high normal levels of PTH were franklly hypercalcemic. Two patients (B) with high normal calcium had markedly increased PTH. In patients of the A or B type, more careful analysis to rule out familial hypocalciuric hypercalcemia should be undertaken. Patients with secondary hyperparathyroidism have much higher levels of PTH.

veloped, and they are particularly useful in chronic renal failure and in assessing acute physiologic changes in hormone secretion. The levels of circulating hormone measured by amino-terminal assays are significantly lower than those of carboxyl-terminal assays.

3.7 *Actions of parathyroid hormone.* PTH elevates the serum calcium and lowers serum phosphorous, through its actions on bone and kidney, thus maintaining the level of serum calcium [10–12]. In bone it appears to stimulate osteocytic osteolysis and has a slower effect in increasing the size of the osteoclast pool. PTH exerts its effect upon bone cells by an increase in cAMP concentration as well as an increase in the uptake of calcium into the cell, but how these lead to increased osteoclastic activity is not clear (since the principal receptor for PTH is actually on the osteoblast). Whether factors are released by the osteoblast that increase osteoclast activity or stimulate their recruitment from the monocyte-macrophage pool is at present unclear. However the net result is a release of bone matrix calcium into the extracellular fluid and an elevation in the serum calcium [28].

Of prime importance to calcium homeostasis is the effect of PTH on the kidney where its net effect is to retain calcium and excrete phosphorus [10–12]. Within minutes of PTH infusion into a renal artery there is activation of adenylate cyclase and increased conversion of ATP to cAMP which results in an increased urinary excretion of cAMP. This is followed by phosphaturia. Micropuncture studies have shown that in the proximal tubule PTH blocks the reabsorption of sodium, calcium, phosphorus and bicarbonate while in the distal tubule it enhances the tubular reabsorption of calcium. The effect of PTH on bicarbonate excretion results in a mild renal tubular acidosis in patients with primary hyperpara-thyroidism.

PTH exerts its action on the renal cell by stimulating adenylate cyclase and enhancing the uptake of calcium into the cell. The former action increases cellular cAMP which activates protein kinase and phosphorylation of proteins. Cytosolic calcium concentration also acts as a messenger in PTH action. Increased renal cell cytosolic cAMP affects ion transport. Adenylate cyclase is present in the con-traluminal (basal-lateral membrane) fractions of the renal tubular cells but not in the luminal (brush border microvilli) fractions.

4. Vitamin D

The other hormone essential to calcium homeostasis is vitamin D [29, 30]. Vitamin D_3 or cholecalciferol is a secosteroid synthesized in the skin from 7-dehydrocholesterol under the influence of ultraviolet light. Some vitamin D is also absorbed from the diet in the form of chylomicrons. This dietary vitamin D might also be vitamin D_2 (ergocalciferol), the plant sterol which has been a supplement in milk or other products, but vitamin D_2 and D_3 are metabolized identically in man, so they are considered as one. Vitamin D is rapidly transferred to a specific vitamin D binding globulin and then either transferred to tissue stores (muscle, fat) or metabolized further by the liver [29, 30]. A hepatic microsomal mixed-function hydroxlyase metabolizes vitamin D_3 to 25-hydroxycholecalciferol (25-OH-D_3) which reappears in the circulation bound to the vitamin D binding globulin. Some 25-OH-D_3 is metabolized further in the kidney by mitochondrial enzymes of the proximal tubules to 1α,25-dihydroxycholecalciferol (1,25-$(OH)_2D_3$) and 24R, 25-dihydroxycholecalciferol (24,25$(OH)_2D_3$). The former is the most active biological metabolite of vitamin D_3, and its production is finely controlled. The metabolite 24,25$(OH)_2D_3$ may have a role in bone mineralization or it may be an inactive metabolic product; its production is determined by the amount of 25-OH-D_3 substrate available, with its serum level being about 10% that of 25-OH-D_3.

The production of $1,25(OH)_2D_3$ is responsive to a low serum calcium, since its synthesis is enhanced by PTH as well as hypophosphatemia [29, 30]. Thus PTH not only mobilizes calcium from bone and retains it by renal tubular reabsorption, but it also stimulates the production of $1,25(OH)_2D_3$ which increases the intestinal absorption of both calcium and phosphorus. Hence, the action of PTH on the intestine is through the active metabolite of vitamin D. The action of PTH on renal $25\text{-}OH\text{-}D_3\text{-}1\alpha$-hydroxylase is cAMP-mediated.

The active metabolite of vitamin D acts like a steroid hormone. In the small intestinal cell, it is transported by a specific cytoplasmic receptor to the nucleus and activates a specific gene locus responsible for coding mRNA for the synthesis of calcium-binding protein. The latter in some way is related to transcellular calcium transport, although the mechanism is unclear [29, 30]. Alternatively, $1,25(OH)_2D_3$ might act on the brush border of the intestinal cell.

Vitamin D deficiency leads to poorly mineralized bone matrix or osteoid (rickets and osteomalacia), which is corrected rapidly by vitamin D therapy. Therefore, vitamin D is necessary for normal bone mineralization, but it is not clear which metabolites of vitamin D perform this action. In organ culture, $1,25(OH)_2D_3$ actively resorbs bone.

5. Calcitonin

Calcitonin (CT) is produced by the C-cells (parafollicular cells) of the thyroid [4]. These cells, which are derived from the ultimobranchial body, are of ectodermal origin, being cells derived from the neural crest. They are related, therefore, to the agentaffin cells of the adrenal medulla. Clinically, these embryologic origins are of interest in the association of medullary thyroid carcinoma (a calcitonin producing tumour), bilateral pheochromocytomas, and hyperparathyroidism (multiple endocrine neoplasia Type 2; Sipple's Syndrome).

Calcitonin is a small peptide of 32 amino acids with a disulfide loop at the amino terminal end. It is synthesized as part of a larger precursor molecule which is processed to calcitonin and other peptides whose function has not yet been clarified. Calcitonin inhibits osteoclastic bone resorption and pharmacologically is useful in the treatment of Paget's disease of bone and in some patients with hypercalcemia. However, it does not appear to be of major physiologic importance to calcium homeostasis [31]. Total thyroidectomy does not affect calcium homeostasis, and in medullary carcinoma of the thyroid, calcium levels are usually normal despite the very high levels of calcitonin. Although calcitonin's actions are opposite to those of PTH and vitamin D, the peptide is of little physiologic significance in normal calcium homeostasis.

6. Pathogenesis of hypercalcemia (Fig. 4)

The actions of both PTH and $1,25(OH)_2D_3$ are to increase the serum calcium via their effects on bone, kidney and the intestine. The two hormones work in concert to mobilize calcium from bone. When the serum calcium is increased, their secretion or production is decreased, and with a normal calcium and phosphorus concentration in the extracellular fluid, bone is mineralized. In hyperparathyroidism this finely-regulated calcium homeostasis is disrupted.

Hypercalcemia occurs when there is excessive mobilization of calcium, a process which may be mediated by the unmodulated activity of PTH or vitamin D, or diseases in which there is abnormal mobilization of calcium from bone [5].

Hypercalcemic disorders. The presence of persistent hypercalcemia (i.e. not a laboratory error) requires that its cause be determined. We shall consider the differential diagnosis of hypercalcemia based on the physiology and biochemistry of normal calcium homeostasis.

7. Primary hyperparathyroidism

The classical hypercalcemic disorder is primary hyperparathyroidism, a condition due to abnormal proliferation of parathyroid tissue. Usually there is a single benign adenoma consisting of solid masses of chief cells. In various series between 5 and 20% of patients have hyperplasia of more than one gland [32]. Very large tumours are more likely to be associated with skeletal rather than other manifestations of the disease. These patients present with higher serum calcium and PTH concentrations [33] than those with smaller tumors. Currently, however, large tumors are uncommon. Occasionally a patient may have multiple adenomas, which may be familial, and rarely a carcinoma of the parathyroid

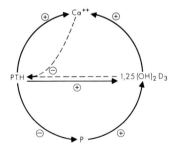

Figure 4. Interactions of PTH and $1,25(OH)_2D_3$ in regulating calcium and phosphorous metabolism. This figure emphasizes the effects of PTH on increasing serum calcium, stimulating production of $1,25(OH)_2D_3$ and decreasing serum phosphorus and the inhibitory effects of calcium and possibly $1,25(OH)_2D_3$ on PTH production. It also emphasizes the role of $1,25(OH)_2D_3$ in raising the plasma calcium and the impact of a low serum phosphorous on stimulating $1,25(OH)_2D_3$ production.

which is usually functional. Primary hyperplasia of all four parathyroid glands presents a more difficult therapeutic problem and may be an expression of an autosomal dominant trait or a sporadic disorder.

7.1 *Pathogenesis and pathophysiology.* The pathogenesis of hyperparathyroidism remains obscure, although a variety of factors have been considered [3]. Genetic factors are involved in patients with multiple endocrine neoplasia, with the histologic abnormality being hyperplasia of all the glands. No humoral or other factors responsible for the hyperplasia have been identified and it is presumably on a genetic basis. Patients who have received irradiation to the head and neck in childhood are at increased risk not only for thyroid carcinoma but also for parathyroid adenomas [34, 35]. Analysis of the two variants of glucose-6-phosphate dehydrogenase in parathyroid adenomas from women suggests that these tumors are of polycellular rather than monocellular origin [3, 36]. If so, it is unclear what hormonal factors might cause multicellular hyperplasia.

An abnormality in hormone secretion has been well-documented which accounts for the pathogenesis of hypercalcemia [3, 37, 38]. Oversecretion of hormone in this disorder can result from an increase in the set point for individual parathyroid cells (calcium level at which 50% suppression of hormone release occurs) and/or an increased mass of normally responsive cells (which cannot be suppressed completely).

Increased PTH secretion leads to osteocytic osteolysis, osteoclastic bone resorption, increased distal tubular calcium retention, and increased production of $1,25(OH)_2D_3$, which in turn increases intestinal calcium absorption. These all result in an elevated serum calcium. In the kidney, PTH also increases phosphate and bicarbonate clearance, causing hypophosphatemia and a mild hyperchloremic acidosis.

7.2 *Clinical features.* With the widespread use of the autoanalyzer to analyze serum calcium, the incidental finding of hypercalcemia is now the most common presentation of hyperparathyroidism. This represents a development of the last 15 years or so when such routine screening has been practiced widely in the United States. Two recent studies suggest a prevalence greater than earlier figures of 1 per 800–1000 patients and show an annual case finding index of up to 7.8/100,000, with the incidence in women over age 60 going as high as 188/100,000 [1, 2].

Primary hyperparathyroidism has now been noted with increasing frequency in the elderly, and in a recent series, 1.5% of a geriatric population of 1129 individuals was found to have primary hyperparathyroidism [39]. In a retrospective 10 year study of 158 geriatric patients treated surgically, 10% were asymptomatic, 80% had neuromuscular symptoms, 16% renal insufficiency and kidney stones and 30% anorexia and/or constipation. Symptomatology attributable to hyperparathyroidism may affect multiple organ systems and be quite variable [9, 32].

Patients may be entirely asymptomatic, or complaints may vary from non-specific lethargy or constipation to mental disturbances such as irritability, depression and frank psychosis or more specific problems involving the gastrointestinal system, kidneys, bone or cardiovascular system. One must differentiate between symptoms attributable to hypercalcemia of any cause and specific organ system problems related to hyperparathyroidism [5, 9]. The latter includes duodenal ulcers which are more prevalent in primary hyperparathyroidism, possibly as a result of calcium-stimulated gastrin release. A decrease in lower esophogeal sphincter pressure in these patients has also been described [40]. Pancreatitis is also more likely in hyperparathyroidism although the etiology is uncertain [41, 42]. Bone pain may suggest osteitis fibrosa cystica, but it is only rarely of clinical significance in patients with primary hyperparathyroidism and much more prominent in secondary hyperparathyroidism. Radiologically the bones are usually normal, but they may show evidence of generalized decalcification including a loss of density in all bones, a loss of the lamina dura surrounding the teeth or the characteristic subperiosteal bone resorption in the phalanges. Rarely, a so-called 'brown tumor' or giant cell tumor is present. Single or dual beam absorption densitometry in many patients reveals a decrease in bone mass not detectable by routine radiographs and is required in following asymptomatic patients in whom a decision not to undertake surgery is made. Bone biopsy commonly reveals osteitis fibrosa cystica with increased formation and resorption (osteoclastic) [3].

The most characteristic complication of primary hyperparathyroidism is renal colic due to nephrolithiasis, but even this is much less common in recent studies [1, 43]. The polyuria and polydipsia found in many patients reflects the inhibition of vasopressin action by hypercalcemia. An impairment in renal concentrating ability which may not be reversible is present in some patients with primary hyperparathyroidism. Hypertension is frequently found in primary hyperparathyroidism as are both gout and pseudogout. The increased prevalence of these associations is unexplained. A recent report [44] suggests that patients with hypertension and hyperparathyroidism have a lower serum phosphorus.

7.3 *Laboratory diagnosis*. In a patient suspected of having hyperparathyroidism, at least three serum calcium determinations should be performed by a reliable laboratory. Venesection should be performed without venous stasis which may falsely elevate the serum calcium, and the samples should be obtained in the fasting state. Once hypercalcemia is established, its cause must be determined. This involves a careful clinical evaluation to exclude other common causes of hypercalcemia (vidé infra) and their specific tests. Before this evaluation is started, it must be determined whether the patient is taking a thiazide-containing diuretic. The latter may raise serum calcium but usually only in patients with underlying primary hyperparathyroidism or occasional patients receiving vitamin D [45]. The initial laboratory evaluation includes several serum calcium determinations and a radioimmunoassay for PTH. Documented fasting hypercalcemia together with an increased immunoreactive PTH is generally sufficient to document the diagnosis of primary hyperparathyroidism. Hypophosphatemia, hyperchloremic acidosis, marked phosphaturia (tubular reabsorption of phosphorus (TRP) less than 80%), and mild to moderate hypercalciuria are all compatible with hyperparathyroidism but are not required to establish the diagnosis. An elevated urinary cAMP or nephrogenous cAMP was thought to be specific for hyperparathyroidism, but it is apparent now that renal cAMP is increased in some patients with humoral hypercalcemia of malignancy [46, 47]. Ancillary tests which have very limited applicability in diagnosing primary hyperparathyroidism include lack of steroid suppressibility of the serum calcium and the inability to increase the TRP to more than 95% after phosphate deprivation. Protein electrophoresis and X-ray of the chest should be performed to exclude multiple myeloma and sarcoidosis where they are suspected. In some patients it is necessary to do repeated measurements to document clearly the calcium abnormality. In such patients it is also important to measure 24 hour urinary calcium excretion to rule out a rare but confusing disorder, familial hypocalciuric hypercalcemia (vidé infra) [48]. Hypercalcemia and an immunoreactive PTH greater than 1.25 times the upper limit of normal (when performed by a reliable laboratory) definitively establish the diagnosis of primary hyperparathyroidism if renal function is normal. Some patients with primary hyperparathyroidism, however, have only slightly elevated PTH or even high normal PTH values in the face of hypercalcemia (Fig. 3).

A definitive diagnosis of primary hyperparathyroidism unfortunately does not rule out coexisting disorders which also cause hypercalcemia. Because primary hyperparathyroidism has a prevalence of greater than one per thousand people and may coexist with other common causes of hypercalcemia such as metastatic tumors of the breast, lung and other organs, differential diagnosis is sometimes confusing. Surgery for hyperparathyroidism is warranted if the prognosis of the malignancy is satisfactory.

Following a diagnosis of hyperparathyroidism, it is almost always determined at surgery whether the patient has an isolated parathyroid adenoma or hyperplasia of one or more glands. The latter may be suspected if there is a family history of renal stones or any clinical evidence of multiple endocrine neoplasia, types I or II.

Once the disorder is diagnosed, there has been up to now very limited value in preoperative localization of an adenoma by cineesophogram, ultrasound or computerized tomography and even less value in selective various sampling for PTH before a first neck exploration. In a patient with previous unsuccessful surgery, there is value in doing selective venous catheterization with radioimmunoassay and selective angiography prior to a repeat neck exploration [49]. Noninvasive techniques have been useful primarily in suggesting the location of fairly large tumors which are readily identified by the surgeon, but with radiologic technology advancing rapidly, this perspective may change [50–52]. Very recent studies from the Mayo Clinic suggest a marked increase in preoperative localization of parathyroid adenomas using high resolution ultrasonography, and these promising results must be pursued further [52].

7.4 *Primary hyperparathyroidism and vitamin D deficiency.* A relatively rare combination of hyperparathyroidism and vitamin D deficiency may mask the hypercalcemia and hence provide diagnostic difficulties in a symptomatic patient [53]. Vitamin D deficiency itself, whether it be nutritional or due to malabsorption or renal disease, leads to a low serum calcium and secondary hyperparathyroidism; correction of the vitamin D deficiency with a small dose of vitamin D further increases the serum calcium. Primary hyperparathyroidism itself increases the metabolism of vitamin D to $1,25(OH)_2D_3$, and when vitamin D stores are marginal, vitamin D deficiency might be precipitated. The condition is important because it is likely to be present in elderly patients who are symptomatic, with both osteomalacia and osteitis fibrosa cystica. Serum 25-OH-D_3 levels would be low, reflecting the vitamin D deficiency. Therapy involves careful management of both disorders.

7.5 *Hyperparathyroidism after renal transplantation for chronic renal failure.* Virtually all patients with chronic renal failure have secondary hyperparathyroidism. Patients on chronic intermittent hemodialysis occasionally require subtotal parathyroidectomy because of the skeletal complications of the hyperparathyroidism (osteitis fibrosa cystica), vascular calcification due to calcium mobilization together with a high serum phosphorus or hypercalcemia which may be associated with intractable pruritus and subcutaneous calcification [54].

After renal transplantation, there is very slow involution of the hyperplastic parathyroid glands, which may take several years [55]. These allografted patients now have secondary hyperparathyroidism in the presence of a normal-functioning kidney responsive to PTH action. Many experience hypercalcemia, and some require parathyroidectomy.

7.6 *Severe primary hyperparathyroidism of the neonate.* There have been isolated cases of neonates presenting with severe hypercalcemia due to primary hyperparathyroidism involving hyperplasia of the parathyroids [48]. This may occur in mothers with hypoparathyroidism. Marx et al. [56] have recently presented evidence that it may also be a neonatal expression of the parathyroid hyperplasia of familial hypocalciuric hypercalcemia (FHH).

7.7 *Hyperparathyroidism and pregnancy.* This uncommon condition is associated with a high calcium concentration in the amniotic fluid and fetal plasma, which falls shortly after birth and may result in neonatal tetany. Maternal PTH does not cross the placenta but the maternal hypercalcemia may cause transient hypoparathyroidism in the newborn.

7.8 Hyperparathyroidism in Multiple Endocrine Neoplasia (MEN). In MEN Type I, primary hyperparathyroidism is associated with one or more of the following: the Zollinger-Ellison syndrome (gastrin producing pancreatic islet cell tumors) producing severe gastric and duodenal ulcers; other islet tumors producing hypoglycemia and other syndromes, and functioning or nonfunctioning tumors of the anterior pituitary. MEN Type II includes adrenal pheochromocytoma (often bilateral), medullary carcinoma of the thyroid, and primary hyperparathyroidism. Hyperparathyroidism in these conditions is due to hyperplasia of all four parathyroids [57], and it presumably occurs on a genetic basis.

7.9 Asymptomatic hyperparathyroidism. Considerable controversy exists regarding the treatment of asymptomatic patients with primary hyperparathyroidism. First of all, many patients with 'asymptomatic' disease actually have vague symptoms of malaise or weakness, which only become apparent in retrospect following successful surgery. In order to define a patient as truly asymptomatic, one must rule out insidious bone loss (as with absorption densitometry) and subtle renal disease. There is unfortunately as yet no well-controlled study in which this issue has been studied. The Mayo Clinic followed a group of 140 patients with very mild hypercalcemia and no complications [58–59]. Approximately 25 needed surgery within two years, and many of the others were difficult to follow because of anxiety on the part of the patient and the physician. In the 10 years following, it was impossible for them to predict from clinical or laboratory criteria which patients would get into trouble [58]. At present, many investigators, including the authors, recommend surgery (unless it is contraindicated) when the diagnosis is firmly established. Others choose to follow patients with asymptomatic disease clinically.

7.10 Medical treatment for hyperparathyroidism. There is no ideal medical treatment for hyperparathyroidism [60]. Patients who cannot have surgery should remain well hydrated and take oral furosemide if necessary. Propranolol and cimetidine are of no value [61, 62]. Oral phosphorus is useful if renal function is good and serum phosphorus is normal or low. Although chronic phosphorus therapy may lower $1,25(OH)_2D_3$ and calcium excretion, it may also cause an increase in immunoreactive PTH and nephrogenous cAMP excretion [63]. Intermittent mithramycin has been used in some patients with chronic severe hypercalcemia (e.g. parathyroid carcinoma) or humoral hypercalcemia of malignancy [64].

7.11 Treatment by an experienced surgeon. Parathyroidectomy is the established therapy for primary hyperparathyroidism although in an asymptomatic mildly hypercalcemic patient the indications for surgery are not clear-cut. All parathyroid glands should be identified and single or multiple adenomas removed in toto. If there is hyperplasia of all four glands as determined by frozen section, the surgeon should remove three and a half glands leaving about 30–50 mg of the fourth gland [65, 66]. An alternative form of surgery which is successful is total parathyroidectomy followed by autotransplantation [67, 68]. The risk of biopsying normal glands or of doing subtotal parathyroidectomy in these patients is small [69]. About 10% of the tumors are in aberrant positions (e.g. intrathyroidal, retroesophageal, mediastinal) and might require extensive cervical exploration. Mediastinal exploration should generally not be performed at the time of initial neck exploration. Post-operatively, in patients with overt osteitis fibrosa cystica, there may be accelerated deposition of calcium in bone ('hungry bone syndrome'), and tetany requiring therapy with intravenous calcium and then oral calcium plus $1,25(OH)_2D_3$ therapy for several weeks or longer. In the usual successfully operated patient, there is a transient drop in calcium for several days postoperatively, and there are usually no symptoms. Intravenous or oral calcium therapy is rarely needed in the usual postoperative period. There is a small but definite risk of permanent hyperparathyroidism, but this is almost always in patients who have needed repeat explorations. Limited studies using transcatheter infarction of parathyroid adenomas suggests that in selected patients who might not be candidates for surgery this approach might be useful [70].

7.12 Differential diagnosis of hyperparathyroidism

1. *Familial Hypocalciuric Hypercalcemia (FHH).* Familial hypercalciuric hypercalcemia (familial benign hypercalcemia, FHH), represents a rare but important autosomal dominant disorder in which hypercalcemia presents before the age of 10 years [48]. Usually family members are asymptomatic although chondrocalcinosis and pancreatitis have been reported. Mild hypercalcemia and a ratio of clearance of calcium to creatinine of less than 0.01 are supportive of the diagnosis. Mild hyperplasia of the parathyroids may be present but there is no place for parathyroidectomy in this condition. Occasionally, severe primary hyperparathyroidism occurs among neonates in FHH kindreds, and parathyroidectomy is indicated [56]. The underlying biochemical defect is at present unknown.

2. *Idiopathic hypercalciuria.* Patients with idiopathic hypercalciuria present with renal stones associated with an increased urinary calcium excretion and a *normal* serum calcium [71]. Some have a low serum phosphorus and exaggerated phosphaturia with $1,25(OH)_2D_3$ levels being reportedly high. Moreover, circulating PTH and nephrogenous cAMP may be elevated in a subgroup of these patients with increased renal calcium loss [71]. These features may also be characteristic of the patient with hyperparathyroidism, but the cardinal feature differentiating them is a well-documented increase in serum calcium in hyperparathyroidism. Patients with idiopathic hypercalciuria also have a greater degree of hypercalciuria than patients with primary hyperparathyroidism (in whom the primary effect of PTH is stimulating renal tubular calcium-reabsorption).

3. *Sarcoidosis.* Less than 5% of patients with sarcoidosis have hypercalcemia, and it almost always responds to steroid therapy [5]. Hypercalciuria is more

common in the disease. The hypercalcemia is related to high $1,25(OH)_2D_3$ levels which also decrease when steroids are given. How this granulomatous disease increases $1,25(OH)_2D_3$ is not known, although it has recently been suggested that mononuclear cells in the granuloma have 25-hydroxyvitamin D_3-1α-hydroxylase [72]. Hypercalcemia has also been reported in patients with sarcoidosis after bilateral nephrectomy. Other granulomatous diseases such as tuberculosis and coccidiomycosis may also rarely be associated with hypercalcemia [73–75].

4. *Vitamin D toxicity.* Chronic excess intake of vitamin D results in toxicity. The body has defenses against vitamin D toxicity in the form of storage in fat and in the specific serum α globulin which binds vitamin D and its metabolites and is normally less than 5% saturated. However, with chronic vitamin D excess the binding globulin becomes saturated with vitamin D and significant amounts appear in lipoproteins. When in lipoproteins, the metabolism of vitamin D is not regulated and it, or its metabolites, might produce toxicity [76]. Clinically, vitamin D toxicity is manifested by hypercalcemia, a normal or high serum phosphorus, the usual complications of hypercalcemia (e.g. polyuria leading to dehydration, nephrocalcinosis and renal failure) and a high serum 25-hydroxy-vitamin D_3 concentration. More recently, with its market availability, toxicity with $1,25(OH)_2D_3$ has been reported. However, the half-life of this metabolite is short, so with close monitoring of serum calcium, its toxicity is more readily controllable.

5. *Malignant hypercalcemia* [9,47]. Hypercalcemia is a frequent complication of malignancy, where it may be produced both by local or humoral mechanisms [47]. Local factors include bone metastases (lung, breast, kidney, thyroid, etc.) or bone involvement by the primary disease e.g., multiple myeloma, lymphomas and rarely leukemias. The mechanism of bone destruction by myeloma and possibly some lymphomas involves the production of osteoclast activating factor (OAF) [9]. Production of factors locally such as prostaglandins, epidermal growth factor or others may be, in fact, responsible for the hypercalcemia in patients with metastatic disease. Another large group of hypercalcemic cancer patients has a humorally-mediated increase in serum calcium due to a circulating factor. This involves the synthesis of an as yet unidentified hormone with actions similar to PTH [46]. These patients have a high serum calcium with a low serum phosphorus and phosphaturia, and low levels of immunoreactive PTH, but very high levels of cAMP excretion. The hypercalcemia, phosphaturia and high cAMP excretion are compatible with a PTH effect; however, these patients have a low immunoreactive PTH, low serum $1,25(OH)_2D_3$ concentrations and higher fasting calcium excretions than hyperparathyroid patients. The tumor hormone is therefore not the same as PTH. Recent studies suggest that this protein binds the PTH receptor in the kidney, but it is significantly higher in molecular weight and is not one of the known precursors in PTH synthesis [77].

6. *Hyperthyroidism.* Patients with hyperthyroidism often have hypercalciuria because of thyroxine-stimulated bone resorption, and in about 8–10% of patients

very mild hypercalcemia [78]. Serum PTH would be expected to be low.

7. *Adrenal insufficiency.* Hypercalcemia has been reported in patients with adrenal insufficiency. The mechanism is not known, but the hypercalcemia responds rapidly to steroid replacement [79].

8. *Milk-alkali syndrome.* In the past, patients who ingested large amounts of milk and soluble absorbable alkali developed hypercalcemia and renal failure [5]. The differential diagnosis must include hyperparathyroidism where duodenal ulcers are common. This condition should not occur very frequently now with the use of non-absorbable antacids and histamine receptor blockers.

9. *Thiazide administration.* Chronic thiazide therapy in a PTH-dependent action increases renal calcium reabsorption [80]. In patients who already have hyperparathyroidism or have a high bone turnover this may result in increased hypercalcemia.

10. *Immobilization.* Prolonged immobolization may cause hypercalcemia in a patient with a high rate of bone turnover (e.g., underlying Paget's disease or hyperparathyroidism) and in growing children or teenagers with sudden paralysis [81]. Coexisting hyperparathyroidism should first be excluded, particularly in elderly patients who become hypercalcemic after immobilization.

11. *Vitamin A toxicity.* Chronic excessive vitamin A ingestion increases osteoclastic bone resorption and therefore may cause hypercalcemia and bone pain [82]. A high serum vitamin A concentration will be present.

12. *Acute renal failure.* Occasionally patients with acute renal failure have hypercalcemia due to a failure to excrete calcium [83]. Moreover, patients with acute rhabdomyolysis causing renal failure may sequestrate calcium in necrotic muscle [84]. Together with the elevated extracellular phosphorus of renal failure, this sequestration leads to a low serum calcium. With recovery from the acute renal failure, the calcium is mobilized from the muscle tissue, occasionally resulting in hypercalcemia.

7.13 *Approach to the hypercalemic patient* First, a technical error in measurement should be excluded as in all clinical disorders. The approach is at first historical. Has the patient taken medications which contain thiazides, vitamin D or A? Is there a family history? Is there any sign of systemic disease or complications of known hypercalcemic disorders such as hyperparathyroidism? The next question is the clinical effects of the hypercalcemia, such as polyuria, polydipsia etc.? Finally the diagnostic workup for hyperparathyroidism and its differential diagnosis should be initiated.

Management involves therapy of the underlying disorder, but an elevated serum calcium of more than 12 mg/dl itself warrants treatment, with saline hydration, with furosemide, steroids, phosphorus, mithramycin or calcitonin, or, if necessary, with peritoneal or hemodialysis [9, 59].* (Table 1). Dichloromethylene disphosphonate has also been found to be effective in some patients but is not now clinically available because of side effects [85]. There are occa-

Table 1. Treatment of acute hypercalcemia

Form of therapy	Dosage	Route of administration	Effects on urinary calcium	Mechanism of action	Potential complications	Limitations to use
Sodium chloride infusion	2–3 liters of 0.9% sodium chloride over 6 h. (1.45% saline may also be used)	Intravenous	Increased	Increased urinary excretion of calcium associated with natriuresis	Sodium overload; hypernatremia; hypokalemia; hypomagnesemia	Hypertension: congestive heart failure, renal insufficiency
Furosemide	40–80 mg/h 40–160 mg/day	Intravenous Oral	Increased	Increased urinary excretion of calcium	Hypokalemia; volume depletion; hypomagnesemia; calcium depletion	Renal failure with oliguria not responsive to furosemide and saline
Sodium sulfate infusion	3 liters of isotonic sodium sulfate over 9 h.	Intravenous	Increased	Increased urinary excretion of calcium	Sodium overload; hypernatremia; hypokalemia; hypomagnesemia	Hypertension; congestive heart failure; renal insufficiency
Phosphate	1–3 g P per day	Oral	Decreased	Bony or extraskeletal deposition of calcium phosphate; prevention of bone resorption; increased bone formation; binding of calcium in gastrointestinal tract	Hyperphosphatemia; hypotension and shock; extraskeletal calcification	Renal insufficiency; high normal or elevated serum phosphorus
Phosphate	50 mmol over 6–8 h.	Intravenous	Decreased	As above, except for gastrointestinal binding	As above	As above, use only when all other methods are inadequate
Corticosteroids	30 mg prednisone (or equivalent) or more per day	Oral or parenteral	Variable	Antagonism to vitamin D effects on intestine; inhibition of bone mobilization of calcium (anti-OAF?)	Hypercorticism or acute steroid complications	Delayed effect; generally not effective in hyperparathyroidism
Mithramycin	25 μg/kg of body weight	Intravenous	Not increased	?Antagonism to calcium mobilization from bone (interference with parathyroid hormone and/or vitamin D effect and physicochemical equilibrium)? anti-tumor	Bleeding disorder; hepatic dysfunction; renal insufficiency	Bone marrow or liver failure

sional patients with clinically elevated calcium levels in the range of 13–15 mg/dl who are asymptomatic, and it may not be necessary to be aggressive therapeutically in such patients while diagnostic workup is proceeding. Hypercalcemia is a relatively common disorder which requires appropriate clinical and laboratory evaluation and then therapy.

References

1. Heath H III, Hodgson SF, Kennedy MA: Primary hyperparathyroidism. Incidence, morbidity and potential economic impact in a community. N Engl J Med 302: 189–193, 1980.
2. Mundy GR., Cove DH, Fisken R: Primary hyperparathyroidism: changes in the pattern of clinical presentation. Lancet 1: 1317–1320, 1980.
3. Frame B, Potts JT Jr. (eds): Clinical Disorders of Bone and Mineral Metabolism. Amsterdam: Excerpta Medica, 1983, pp 129–168.
4. Copp DH: Comparative endocrinology of calcitonin. In: Handbook of Physiology, Sect. 7, Aurbach GD (ed). American Physiological Society, Washington, D.C. 7: 431, 1976.
5. Schneider AB, Sherwood LM: Calcium homeostasis, and the pathogenesis and management of hypercalcemic disorders. Metabolism 23: 975–1007, 1974.
6. De Luca HF, Schnoes HK: Metabolism and action of vitamin D. Annu Rev Biochem 45: 631–636, 1976.
7. De Luca H, Schnoes HK: Vitamin D: Recent Advances. Annu Rev Biochem 52: 411–440, 1983.
8. Lindgärd F, Zettervall O: Characterization of a calcium-binding IgC myeloma protein. Scand J Immunol 3: 277–285, 1974.
9. Rodman JS, Sherwood LM: Disorders of mineral metabolism in malignancy. In: Metabolic Bone Disease Vol. II, Avioli LV, Krane SM (eds). New York: Academic Press, 1978, p 555–631.
10. Phang JM, Weiss IW: Maintenance of calcium homeostasis in human beings. In: Handbook of Physiology, sect. 7, Aurbach GD (ed). American Physiological Society, Washington, D.C., 7:157, 1976.
11. Talmage RV, Meyer RA Jr: Physiological role of parathyroid hormone. In: Handbook of Physiology, sect. 7, Aurbach GD (ed). American Physiological Society, Washington, D.C. 7:343, 1976.
12. Potts JT Jr, Kronenberg HM, Rosenblatt M: Parathyroid hormone: chemistry, biosynthesis and mode of action. Adv Protein Chem 35: 323–396, 1982.
13. Cohn DV, MacGregor RR: The biosynthesis, intracellular processing, and secretion of parathormone. Endocr Rev 2: 1–26, 1981.
14. Abe M, Sherwood LM: Regulation of parathyroid hormone secretion by adenyl cyclase. Biochem Biophys Res Commun 48: 396, 1972.
15. Brown EM, Gardner DG, Windeck RA, Aurbach GD: Relationship of intracellular cAMP accumulation to parathyroid hormone release from dispersed bovine parathyroid cells. Endocrinology 103: 2323–2333, 1978.
16. Hanley DA, Takatsuki K, Birnbaumer M, Schneider AB, Sherwood LM: In vitro perifusion for the study of parathyroid hormone secretion. Calcif Tissue Int 32: 19–27, 1980.
17. Takatsuki K, Hanley DA, Schneider AB, Sherwood LM: The effects of magnesium ion on parathyroid hormone secretion in vitro. Calcif Tissue Int 32: 201–206, 1980.
18. Davis BM, Pfefferbaum A, Krutzik S, Davis K: Lithium effect on parathyroid hormone. Am J Psychiat 138: 489–492, 1981.
19. Canterbury JM, Lerman S, Claflin AJ, Henry H, Norman AW, Reiss E: Inhibition of parathyroid hormone secretion by 25-hydroxycholecalciferol and 24,25-dihydroxycholecalciferol in the dog. J Clin Invest 61: 1375, 1978.

184

20. Chertow BS, Baker GR, Henry HL, Norman AW: Effects of vitamin D metabolites on bovine parathyroid hormone release in vitro. Am J Physiol 238: 384, 1980.
21. Golden P, Greenwalt A, Martin K, Bellorin-Font E, Mazey R, Klahr S, Slatopolsky E: Lack of a direct effect of 1,25-dihydroxycholecalciferol on parathyroid hormone secretion by normal bovine parathyroid glands. Endocrinology 107: 602, 1980
22. Wecksler WR, Henry HL, Norman AW: Studies on the mode of action of calciferol subcellular localization of 1,25-dihydroxy-vitamin D_3 in chicken parathyroid glands. Arch Biochem Biophys 183:168, 1977.
23. Wecksler WR, Ross FP, Mason RS, Posen S, Norman AW: Biochemical properties of the $1\alpha,25$-dihydroxyvitamin D_3 cytoplasmic receptor from human and chick parathyroid glands. Arch Biochem Biophys 201:95, 1980.
24. Kemper B, Habener JF, Rich A, Potts JT, Jr: Parathyroid secretory protein: Discovery of a major calcium-dependent protein. Science 184: 167–168, 1974.
25. Sherwood LM, Takatsuki K, Porat A, Shin KY, Jackimek A: Parathyroid secretory protein: Intracellular concentration and release by calcium. Clin Res 29: 579A, 1981.
26. Bhargava G, Russell J, Sherwood LM: Phosphorylation of parathyroid secretory protein. Proc Natl Acad Sci USA 80: 878–881, 1983,
27. Martin KJ, Hruska KA, Freitag JJ, Klahr S, Slatopolsky E: The peripheral metabolism of parathyroid hormone. N Engl J Med 301: 1092–1098, 1979.
28. Raisz LG, Kream BE: Regulation of bone formation. N Engl J Med 309: 29–35, 1983.
29. DeLuca HF: The vitamin D system in the regulation of calcium and phosphorus metabolism. Nutr Rev 37: 161–193, 1979.
30. Norman AW, Roth J, Orci L: The vitamin D endocrine system: steroid metabolism, hormone receptors, and biological response (calcium binding proteins). Endocr Rev 3: 331–366, 1982.
31. Sherwood LM: The relative importance of parathyroid hormone and calcitonin in calcium homeostasis. N Engl J Med 278: 663–669, 1968.
32. Mallette LE, Bilezikian JP, Heath DA, Aurbach GD: Primary hyperparathyroidism: clinical and biochemical features. Medicine (Baltimore) 53: 127–146, 1974.
33. Lloyd HM: Primary hyperparathyroidism: an analysis of the role of the parathyroid tumors. Medicine (Baltimore) 47: 53–71, 1968.
34. Rao SD, Frame B, Miller MJ, Kleerekoper M, Block MA, Parfitt AM: Hyperparathyroidism following head and neck irradiation. Arch Intern Med 140: 205–207, 1980.
35. Katz A, Braunstein GD: Clinical, biochemical and pathologic features of radiation-associated hyperparathyroidism. Arch Intern Med 143: 79–82, 1983.
36. Fialkow PJ, Jackson CE, Block MA, Greenwald KA: Multicellular origin of parathyroid adenomas. N Engl J Med 297: 696–698, 1977.
37. Brown EM, Brennan MF, Hurwitz S, Windek R, Marx SJ, Spiegel AM, Koehler JO, Gardner DG, Aurbach GD: Dispersed cells prepared from human parathyroid glands: Distinct calcium sensitivity of adenomas vs primary hyperplasia. J Clin Endocrinol Metab 46: 267–276, 1978.
38. Birnbaumer ME, Schneider AB, Palmer D, Hanley DA, Sherwood LM: Secretion of parathyroid hormone by abnormal human parathyroid glands in vitro. J Clin Endocrinol Metab 45: 105–113, 1977.
39. Tibblins S, Palsson N, Rydberg J: Hyperparathyroidism in the elderly. Ann Surg 197: 135–138, 1983.
40. Mowschenson PM, Rosenbergs S, Pallotta J, Silen W: Effect of hyperparathyroidism and hypercalcemia on lower esophageal sphincter pressure. Am J Surg 153: 36–39, 1982.
41. Paloyan D, Simowowitz D, Paloyan E, Snyder TJ: Pancreatitis associated with primary hyperparathyroidism. Ann Surg 48: 366–368, 1982.
42. Gardner EC, Jr, Hersh T: Primary hyperparathyroidism and the gastrointestinal tract. South Med J 74: 197–199, 1981.
43. Parks J, Coe F, Favus M: Hyperparathyroidism and nephrolithiasis. Arch Intern Med 140: 1479–1481, 1980.

44. Daniels J, Goodman AD: Hypertension and hyperparathyroidism Relation of serum phosphate level and blood pressure. Am J Med 75: 17–23, 1983.
45. Klimiuk PS, Davies M, Adams PH: Primary hyperparathyroidism and thiazide diuretics. Postgrad Med J 57: 80–83, 1981.
46. Stewart AF, Horst R, Deftos LJ, Cadman EE, Lang R, Broadus AE: Biochemical evaluation of patients with cancer-associated hypercalcemia: Evidence for humoral and non-humoral groups. N Engl J Med 303: 1377–1382, 1980.
47. Sherwood LM: The multiple causes of hypercalcemia in malignancy. N Engl J Med 303: 1412–1413, 1980.
48. Marx SJ, Spiegel AM, Levine MA, Rizzoli RE, Lasker RD, Santara AC, Downs RW Jr, Aurbach GD: Familial hypocalciuric hypercalcemia. The relation to primary parathyroid hyperplasia. N Engl J Med 307: 416–426, 1982.
49. Eisenberg H, Pallotta J, Sherwood LM: Selective arteriography, venography and venous hormone assay in diagnosis and localization of parathyroid lesions. Am J Med 56: 810–817, 1974.
50. Sommer B, Walter HF, Spelsberg F, Scherer U, Lissner J: Computed tomography for localizing enlarged parathyroid glands in primary hyperparathyroidism. J Comput Assist Tomog 6: 521–526, 1982.
51. Stark DD, Moss AA, Gooding GA, Clark H: Parathyroid scanning by computed tomography. Radiology 148: 297–299, 1983.
52. Reading CC, Charboneau JW, James EM, Karsell PR, Purnell DC, Grant CS, Van Heerden JA: High resolution parathyroid sonography. Am J Radiol 139: 539–546, 1982.
53. Stanbury WE: Vitamin D and hyperparathyroidism: Lumleian Lecture 1981. J R Coll Phys (London) 15: 205–217, 1981.
54. Slatopolsky E, Rutherford WE, Hoffsten FH, Elkan IO, Butcher HR, Bricker NS: Nonsuppressible secondary hyperparathyroidism in chronic progressive renal disease. Kidney Int 1: 38, 1972.
55 David DS, Sakai S, Brenne BL, Riggio RA, Cheigh J, Stenzel KH, Rubin AL, Sherwood LM: Hypercalcemia after renal transplantation: Long-term follow-up data. N Engl J Med 289: 398, 1973.
56. Marx SJ, Attie MF, Spiegel AM, Levine MA, Lasker RD, Fox M: An association between neonatal severe primary hyperparathyroidism and familial hypocalciuric hypercalcemia in three kindreds. N Engl J Med 306: 257–264, 1982.
57. Marx SJ, Spiegel AM, Brown EM, Aurbach GD: Family studies in patients with primary parathyroid hyperplasia. Am J Med 62: 698–706, 1977.
58. Scholz DA, Purnell DC: Asymptomatic primary hyperparathyroidism. Ten year prospective study. Mayo Clinic Proc 56: 473–478, 1981.
60. Bilezikian JP: The medical management of primary hyperparathyroidism. Ann Intern Med 96: 198–202, 1982.
59. Russell CF, Edis AJ: Surgery for primary hyperparthyroidism: experience with 500 consecutive cases and evaluation of the role of surgery in the asymptomatic patient. Br J Surg 69: 244–247, 1982.
62. LJunghal S, Akerström G, Rudberg C, Selking O, Johansson H, Wide L.: Treatment with cimetidine in patients with primary hyperparathyroidism. Acta Endocrinol 99: 546–550, 1982.`
61. LJunghal S, Rudberg C, Akerström G, Wide L: Effects of beta adrenergic blockade on serum parathyroid hormone in normal subjects and patients with primary hyperparathyroidism. Acta Med Scand 211: 27–30, 1982.
63. Broadus AE, Magee JS, Mallette LE, Horst RL, Lang R, Jensen PS, Gertner JM, Baron R: A detailed evaluation of oral phosphate therapy in selected patients with primary hyperparathyroidism. J Clin Endocrinol Metab 56: 953–961, 1983.
64. Mundy GR, Wilkinsen R, Heath DA: Comparative study of available medical therapy for hypercalcemia of malignancy. Am J Med 74: 421–432, 1983.

65. Wang CA, Castleman B, Cope O: Surgical management of hyperparathyroidism due to primary hyperplasia. Ann Surg 195: 384–392, 1982.
66. Brennan MF, Marx SJ, Doppman J, Costa J, Saxe A, Spiegel A, Krudy A, Aurbach G: Results of reoperation for persistent and recurrent hyperparathyroidism. Ann Surg 194: 671–676, 1981.
67. Wells SA Jr, Ellis GJ, Gunnels JC, Schneider AB, Sherwood LM: Parathyroid autotransplantation in primary parathyroid hyperplasia. N Engl J Med 295: 57–63, 1976.
68. Saxe AW, Brennan MF: Reoperative parathyroid surgery for primary hyperparathyroidism caused by multiple gland disease: total parathyroidectomy and autotransplantation with cryopreserved tissue. Surgery 91: 616–621, 1982.
69. Anderberg B, Gillquist J, Larsson L, Lundstrom B: Complications to subtotal parathyroidectomy. Acta Chir Scand 147: 109–13, 1981.
70. Doppman JL: The treatment of hyperparthyoidism by transcatheter techniques. Cardiovasc Intervent Radiol 3: 268–276, 1980.
71. Sherwood LM: Idopathic hypercalciuria: A 'mixed bag' of stones. J Lab Clin Med 90: 951–952, 1977.
72. Bell NH, Stern PH, Pantzer E, Sinha TK, DeLuca HF: Evidence that increased circulating $1\alpha,25$ dihydroxyvitamin D is the probable cause for abnormal calcium metabolism in sarcoidosis. J Clin Invest 64: 218–225, 1979.
73. Shai F, Baker RK, Addrizzo JR, Wallach S: Hypercalcemia in mycobacterial infection. J Clin Endocrinol 34: 251–256, 1972.
74. Braman SS, Goldman AL, Scharz MI: Steroid-responsive hypercalcemia in disseminated boned tuberculosis. Arch Intern Med 132: 269–271, 1973.
75. Lee JC, Catanzaro A, Parthemore JG, Roach B, Deftos LJ: Hypercalcemia in disseminated coccidioidomycosis. N Engl J Med 297: 431–433, 1977.
76. Silver J, Shvil Y, Fainavu M: Vitamin D transport in an infant with vitamin D toxicity. Br Med J 2: 93–94, 1978.
77. Strewler GJ, Williams RD, Nissenson RH: Human renal carcinoma cells produce hypercalcemia in the nude mouse and a novel protein recognized by parathyroid hormone receptors. J Clin Invest 71: 769–774, 1983.
78. Parfitt AM, Dent CE: Hyperthyroidism and hypercalcaemia. Q J Med 39: 171–187, 1970.
79. Walser M, Robinson BHB, Duckett JW: The hypercalcemia of adrenal insufficiency. J Clin Invest 42: 456–465, 1963.
80. Popovtzer MM, Subryan VL, Alfrey AC, Reeve EB, Schrier RW: The acute effect of chlorothiazide on serum-ionized calcium: Evidence for a parathyroid hormone-dependent mechanism. J Clin Invest 55: 1295–1302, 1975.
81. Lerman S, Canterbury JM, Reiss E: Parathyroid hormone and the hypercalcemia of immobilization. J Clin Endocrinol Metab 45: 425–428, 1977.
82. Frame B, Jackson CE, Reynolds WA, Ymphrey JE: Hypercalcemia and skeletal effects in chronic hypervitaminosis A. Ann Intern Med 80: 44–48, 1974.
83. de Torrente A, Berl T, Cohn PD, Kawamoto E, Hertz P, Schrier RW: Hypercalcemia of acute renal failure. Am J Med 61: 119–123, 1976.
84. Koffer A, Friedler RM, Massry SG: Acute renal failure due to nontraumatic rhabdomyolysis. Ann Intern Med 85: 23–28, 1976.
85. Shane E, Baquiran DC, Bilezikian JP: Effects of dichloromethylene diphosphonate on serum and urinary calcium in primary hyperparathyroidism. Ann Intern Med 95: 23–27, 1981.

9. Surgery of the parathyroid glands

EDWIN L. KAPLAN and ALLAN FREDLAND

Surgery of the parathyroid glands

To be successful, a parathyroid surgeon must have a working knowledge of the anatomy of the neck region, an understanding of the pathophysiology of the parathyroid glands and a clear concept of the potential postoperative complications that might occur, along with their treatment.

The first operation for hyperparathyroidism was performed by Dr. Felix Mandl of Vienna in 1925 [1]. His patient Albert, a Viennese railway driver, had severe osteitis fibrosa cystica, the classical bone disease of hyperparathyroidism. After unsuccessful treatment of his condition with parathyroid pills and a parathyroid graft, Albert was operated upon. At neck exploration, a large parathyroid gland was removed and his bone disease improved temporarily, only to later recur.

In the United States the first diagnosis of hyperparathyroidism was based more on physiologic parameters. Collip [2] and Hanson [3] had each independently extracted parathyroid extract in 1925. When injected into dogs [2], parathyroid extract resulted in hypercalcemia, hypophosphatemia and an increase of urinary calcium output, as well. Aub [4], at the Massachusetts General Hospital was using this new preparation to mobilize lead from the bones of children with chronic lead poisoning. These youngsters were found to manifest similar chemical changes in the blood and urine after injection of parathyroid extract. Charles Martell, a merchant marine captain with a severe bone disease of unknown etiology, was also found to have hypercalcemia and hypophosphatemia. Hence, Dr. Eugene DuBois, Professor of Medicine at Cornell sent him to Aub's unit in Boston for further study. An overfunction of the parathyroid glands was postulated and Charles Martell was operated upon in May, 1926 [5]. The surgeons were unaware of the experience in Vienna, which had not yet been reported. Unfortunately, the abnormal gland was not found at this operation or several subsequent neck and chest explorations. Finally, during his *seventh* operation in 1932, a parathyroid adenoma was successfully removed from Captain Martell's mediastinum. Now, hypocalcemic and certainly hypoparathyroid, he died in

Santen, R.J. and Manni, A. (eds.), Diagnosis and management of endocrine-related tumors. ISBN 0-89838-636-5.
© 1984, Martinus Nijhoff Publishers, Boston. Printed in the Netherlands.

tetany following another operation six weeks later to remove a calculus which had blocked his ureter [6].

Such a tragic demise for the first patient operated upon in this country for primary hyperparathyroidism! However, if one understands all of the problems associated with his medical and surgical care, one knows a great deal about parathyroid surgery as it is practiced today.

Embryology [7]

The upper parathyroid glands arise embryologically from the fourth branchial pouch along with the lateral lobes of the thyroid (Fig. 1). They descend only slightly during embryologic life along with the thyroid and continue to remain in close association with the upper portion of the lateral thyroid lobes. Because of

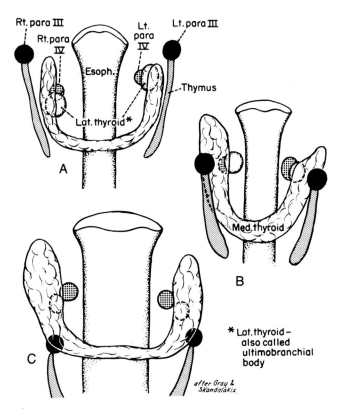

Figure 1. Schematic representation of the embryologic shifts in location of the thyroid, parafollicular, and parathyroid tissues. C. Approximates the adult position. From Sedgwick and Cady [7].

their relatively circumscribed migration, their position in adult life remains quite constant.

The lower parathyroids arise from the third branchial pouch along with the thymus and descend with the thymus. Because they travel so far in embryologic life, they have a very wide range of distribution in the adult. They may be found all the way from just beneath the mandible to the pericardium. When the lower parathyroid descends into the mediastinum, it is almost always anterior and is usually supplied by the inferior thyroid artery.

Anatomy

Normal parathyroid glands. Gilmour [9], in an extensive autopsy study, found that roughly 80 percent of individuals had four glands, 6 percent had five, and 13 percent had three. Two glands or six glands were present very rarely. In nearly 75 percent of the cases the upper gland lay on the posterior portion of the middle third of the thyroid, usually toward the superior part of this area, either in a groove on the thyroid or on a projecting nodule (Fig. 2a and 2b). It usually was found cephalad to the inferior thyroid artery and close to the recurrent laryngeal nerve.

The inferior parathyroid glands were more variable. In somewhat more that 50 percent of the cases the lower parathyroid was found on the lateral or posterior surface of the lower pole of the thyroid gland, or not more than 0.5 cm below the lower pole. The next most common location, in 12.8 percent, was 1 cm below the lower pole of the thyroid. In most of the remaining individuals, the lower parathyroid gland was found within the tongue of the thymus (also called the thyrothymic ligament). The tongue of the thymus usually is present just below the lower pole of the thyroid gland on each side, adjacent to the inferior thyroid veins. Less frequently, the inferior parathyroids can be located in the superior mediastinum within the thymus, and rarely they are found high in the neck, the so-called undescended parathyroid glands.

Gilmour [9] found that the parathyroids were occasionally included within the thyroid capsule or lay beneath it and that they were sometimes carried partially into the substance of the thyroid by the thyroid vessels. Sometimes, however, a parathyroid was completely covered by the thyroid. These intrathyroidal lesions usually involved the inferior parathyroid glands.

The average weight of a normal parathyroid gland is about 35 mg [10] but some authors think that normal glands may be heavier if they contain a great deal of fat. The total weight of four normal parathyroids is about 120 to 140 mg.

The usual positions for the superior and inferior thyroid arteries, the recurrent laryngeal nerve, and the parathyroids are shown in Fig. 3. The superior para- thyroid gland is usually supplied primarily by the superior thyroid artery; while the inferior gland is almost always supplied by the inferior thyroid artery. How-

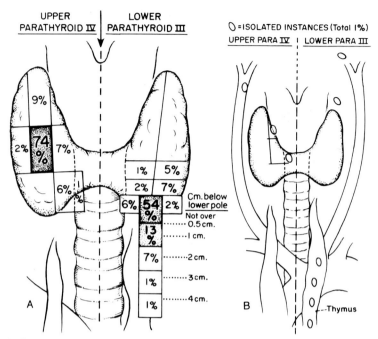

Figure 2a. A. Frontal view of anatomic location of upper and lower parathyroid glands as dissected by Gilmour [9]. B. Location of uncommon aberrant upper (left) and lower (right) parathyroid glands. From Sedgwick and Cady [8].

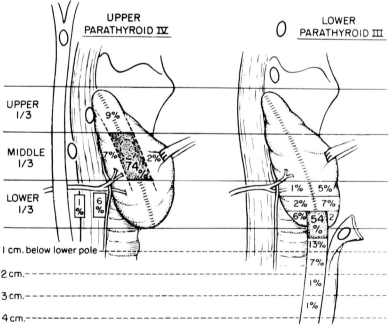

Figure 2b. Lateral view of anatomic location of upper and lower parathyroid glands as dissected by Gilmour [9]. From Sedgwick and Cady [8].

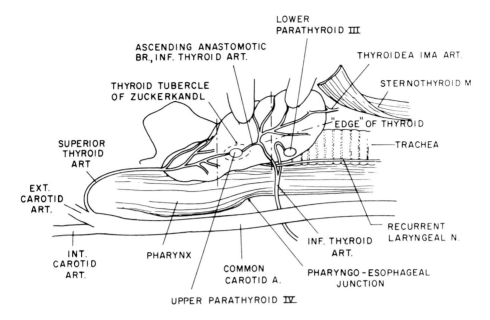

LOWER
PARATHYROID Ⅲ

ASCENDING ANASTOMOTIC
BR., INF. THYROID ART.

THYROIDEA IMA ART.

THYROID TUBERCLE
OF ZUCKERKANDL

STERNOTHYROID M

"EDGE" OF THYROID

SUPERIOR
THYROID
ART

TRACHEA

EXT.
CAROTID
ART.

RECURRENT
LARYNGEAL N.

INF. THYROID
ART.

INT.
CAROTID
ART.

PHARYNX

COMMON
CAROTID A.

PHARYNGO-ESOPHAGEAL
JUNCTION

UPPER PARATHYROID Ⅳ

Figure 3. Lateral view with the thyroid retracted anteriorly and medially to show the surgical landmarks for locating the parathyroids. From Kaplan [11].

ever, in many instances, these two arterial systems join and intercommunicate. The inferior gland which descends into the mediastinum because of the development of an adenoma is always supplied by the inferior thyroid artery, while an adenoma which develops in a gland that has come to be located in the mediastinum embryologically may be supplied by branches from the internal mammary or thymic vessels, or rarely from the aorta.

Abnormal parathyroid glands. When parathyroid glands enlarge and become adenomatous or hyperplastic their position can change. Large upper parathyroid glands frequently fall back, posterior to the recurrent laryngeal nerve and the inferior thyroid artery and are found along the esophagus down into the posterior-superior mediastinum. Lower parathyroid glands are displaced into the anterior-superior mediastinum, either separately or along with the thymus gland. Usually they remain anterior to the recurrent laryngeal nerves.

While 80 to 85% of parathyroid adenomas will be found adjacent to the thyroid gland in their normal locations, fifteen to twenty percent will be ectopically located in the anterior-superior mediastinum, along the esophagus into the posterior-superior mediastinum, or less commonly, within the carotid sheath or high up in the neck. Finally, up to 3 percent of all parathyroid adenomas can be intrathyroidal, usually within the lower pole of the thyroid gland. Fortunately, most of these can be felt as a mass within the thyroid lobe, but in other instances they are found only after thyroid excision or thyroidotomy.

Pathology of primary hyperparathyroidism

Primary hyperparathyroidism may be due to a parathyroid adenoma, hyperplasia of the parathyroid glands, carcinoma, or a nonparathyroid tumor which produces a parathyroid-like substance. The symptoms are similar whatever the actual cause of the primary hyperparathyroidism. It is also possible for a patient with secondary hyperparathyroidism due to renal or bowel disease to develop hypercalcemia. This condition is commonly referred to as *tertiary hyperparathyroidism*, but perhaps a better name is severe secondary hyperparathyroidism.

The relative frequency of entities producing primary hyperparathyroidism is shown in Table 1. Several points are important to note. Primary chief cell hyperplasia was described by Cope in 1958 [13]. Hence studies which include data prior to 1958 can be misleading for, at that time, multiple enlarged glands were called multiple adenomas instead of hyperplasia. It is apparent that the incidence of primary chief cell hyperplasia differs markedly as diagnosed in different institutions. While some authors believe that the increased incidence of primary hyperplasia is due to the fact that primary hyperparathyroidism is being diagnosed and operated upon earlier, most likely these discrepancies are the result of nonuniformity of diagnostic criteria among different pathologists. Furthermore, it has been shown by Edis [14] that when more glands are removed by the surgeon

Table 1. Relative frequency of parathyroid adenoma, hyperplasia, and carcinoma in reported series

Author and year	No. of patients	Adenoma %	Primary hyperplasia %	Carcinoma %
Goldman et al., 1971	300	96	3	1
Krementz et al., 1971	100	96	3	1
Hoehn et al., 1969	788	93	6	1
Davies, 1974	350	90	7	3
Palmer et al., 1975	250	90	9	<1
Satava et al., 1975	307	90	10	–
Myers, 1974	185	82	11	1
Werner et al., 1974	129	84	14	1
Wang, 1976	431	82	14	4
Romanus et al., 1973	274	81	19	–
Block et al., 1974	121	80	20	–
Bruining, 1971	242	60	40	–
Haff and Armstrong, 1974	35	57	43	–
Esselstyn et al., 1974	100	51	49	–
Haff and Ballinger, 1971	74	50	50	–
Paloyan et al., 1973	84	33	65	2

Source: A.J. Edis: Surgial anatomy and technique of neck exploration for primary hyperparathyroidism. Surg Clin North Am 57: 495, 1977 [12].

at operation, the pathologist is more likely to diagnose hyperplasia. In those series in which a high incidence of primary chief cell hyperplasia is found, the surgeon usually practices subtotal parathyroidectomy as a routine procedure. On the other hand, when a single enlarged gland is removed by the surgeon, it will be most likely called an adenoma.

Classically, an adenoma was defined as an enlarged gland with a rim of normal tissue. However, Roth [15] and other pathologists now state that this appearance can be found in cases of hyperplasia as well, and that it is not possible to tell the difference between hyperplasia and adenoma from looking at only one gland; other glands must be examined.

The greatest differences of opinion relate to what constitutes *mild* hyperplasia and whether or not mildly hyperplastic glands are of physiologic importance. Some pathologists consider that normal-sized or mildly enlarged glands are hyperplastic if they do not contain enough *extracellular* fat. Others [16] do not feel that these glands are necessarily abnormal and feel that the amount of *intracellular* fat is the most important criterion in this differentiation.

The major problem at the time of operation is to differentiate an adenoma from chief cell hyperplasia, or single gland disease from multiglandular disease of the parathyroids. In general, most experienced surgeons feel that by evaluating the size, shape and color of the parathyroid glands at operation, they can differentiate normal glands from enlarged ones. If one gland is enlarged and the others are perfectly normal visually and by biopsy with frozen section, this is an adenoma. If all four glands are enlarged this is hyperplasia (or multiglandular disease). Occasionally two glands are enlarged and the others are normal; this has been called a double adenoma by some, although it probably represents a form of multiglandular disease or hyperplasia.

Today, in most series, primary hyperparathyroidism is found to be caused by an adenoma in the majority of cases. Chief cell hyperplasia is found in 15 to 30% of non-familial cases, but this entity is present in virtually all of the instances of familial hyperparathyroidism or of the multiple endocrine neoplasia (MEN 1 or 2) syndromes. Carcinoma of the parathyroids is uncommon.

The treatment of each of these entities and the results obtained by operation will be discussed later in this chapter. Undoubtedly, the ultimate proof that a lesion was correctly diagnosed and treated is the lack of persistence or recurrence of hypercalcemia in later years.

Carcinoma of the parathyroid. Carcinoma of the parathyroid is rare and probably represents less than one percent of cases in non-selected series of primary hyperparathyroidism (Table 1). Many lesions which originally were thought to represent carcinoma have been discarded on review, since benign adenomas can sometimes have cells with bizarre nuclear patterns.

Eighty-five percent of all patients with parathyroid cancer presented with hypercalcemia [17, 18]. In fact, 75% of these patients had serum calcium concentrations of greater than 14 mg/dl while only 9% of adenomas have calcium values over this level. Bone disease was present in 73 percent, a palpable neck mass in 52 percent, and renal disease in 32 percent. Thus, hypercalcemia and a palpable neck mass should alert one to the possibility of parathyroid carcinoma. Cervical metastases were found in 32 percent and distant metastases (liver, lung, bone, pancreas, and adrenal) in 21 percent. Local neck recurrences following surgery occurred in 65 percent of patients. Typically hypercalcemia recurred several months after surgery in many instances and was the first sign of recurrent tumor.

Often a diagnosis of malignant disease cannot be made by the microscopic features of the tumor, a situation which also pertains to other endocrine neoplasms. Very wild-looking tumors histologically may persue a completely benign course; the reverse is also true. Occasionally the original tumor was diagnosed as an adenoma but the tumor recurred after operation. Capsular infiltration is a particularly inadequate sign of malignancy, since this is sometimes seen in benign adenomas. The only completely acceptable criteria for malignancy are recurrence of the tumor following its removal, distant metastases, or invasion of adjacent structures. Some carcinomas can be identified grossly because they are attached to adjacent tissues by a thick fibrous capsule which gives the gland a whitish hue. Fifty percent of reported cases were adherent to or invading into adjacent structures at the time of surgery. If suspicious lesions of this type are recognized at operation, they should be widely excised. A thyroid lobectomy should be performed. Special care should be exercised not to enter the capsule to prevent seeding of the neck with tumor. Appropriate lymph node dissections should be performed if nodes are involved.

Though some individuals die because of tumor growth and spread, more commonly morbidity and mortality are related to the complications related to persistent and progressive hypercalcemia, which is very difficult to control chronically. Because of this, several authors [19] recommend aggressive reoperation to try to totally excise or to debulk metastatic lesions in order to lessen the serum calcium level.

Indications for operation

Patients with primary hyperparathyroidism in whom the diagnosis has been established with relative certainty should definitely be subjected to parathyroid surgical treatment if they have either bony or renal manifestations of the disease, since these will almost inevitably become worse with time [20]. The urgency is greater the higher the calcium level, the most impelling example being the patient with hypercalcemic crisis. Treatment is also indicated if peptic ulcer or pancreatitis is secondary to the hyperparathyroidism. Hypertension may or may not be benefited by parathyroidectomy, depending upon its relation to permanent renal damage which has been incurred by long-standing hypercalcemia.

As newer methods for establishing the diagnosis of hyperparathyroidism have developed, more and more cases are operated upon at an earlier stage. We have found that mild symptoms such as decreased appetite, arthritis, tiredness and depression are common, especially in elderly patients, and that they are frequently helped by parathyroidectomy. The mortality and morbidity for this operation are so low that unless the patient presents an unusually poor risk, operation should be undertaken when any of the indications listed above present themselves.

Some completely asymptomatic paients with minimal hypercalcemia (serum Ca, 11 mg/dl) have been followed without surgery at the Mayo Clinic even though the diagnosis of primary hyperparathyroidism was definitively made [21]. At the end of a 10-year study period, over 20 percent of these individuals required operation because of complications attributable to the disease or a rise in serum calcium levels to above 11.0 mg/dl. Another 20 percent were dropped from the study because of lack of cooperation in the follow-up program. Other patients requested the operation because of the uncertainty of being followed for this disease. No criteria are evident that would permit identification of those patients who will ultimately require a parathyroid operation. The Mayo group have concluded that surgical treatment is correct in this asymptomatic group in most cases. We follow this same recommendation.

Preoperative management of hypercalcemia

Hypercalcemia is a serious and potentially lethal complication of many diseases. When it is severe, the approach to therapy must be tempered by an appreciation of the underlying disease state and whether or not emergency reduction of serum calcium is required. Individual tolerance to hypercalcemia is variable and may reflect the rapidity with which the concentration of serum calcium has risen. It is not uncommon, for example, to observe nearly asymptomatic patients with hyperparathyroidism with a serum calcium of 13 to 15 mg/dl, yet virtually moribund patients with rapidly progressive cancer have a similar serum calcium.

Since patients with hypercalcemia often have had anorexia, nausea, vomiting and polyuria for some time prior to seeking medical assistance, severe dehydration is a common presenting feature. Thus perhaps the most important initial treatment is restoration of the extra-cellular fluid volume with 0.9% sodium chloride. Hypokalemia is frequently present and may require replacement of large amounts of potassium for correction.

Calcium and digitalis are synergistic in their effect on the myocardium and conducting system. Hence the fully digitalized patient may manifest digitalis toxicity if he becomes hypercalcemic. Thus it may be necessary to reduce or stop digitalis. Similarly, if digitalization is necessary in a hypercalcemic patient, a lower dose is generally required.

Treatment of hypercalcemic crisis. While most patients with hyperparathyroidism require little or no preparation before operation, those who have severe hypercalcemia often present with many symptoms and signs (Table 2) and surely are severe medical and surgical risks. Many treatment regimens are available to lower the serum calcium concentration, depending upon the underlying cause of this metabolic abnormality (Table 3). The mainstay of preoperative management when the hypercalcemia is due to hyperparathyroidism is saline infusion and diuresis with furosemide (Lasix). No longer is parathyroidectomy necessary as an absolute emergency procedure. However, once the diagnosis is made and the patient's condition is stabilized, results are far better if a parathyroidectomy is performed without unnecessary delay.

Strategy of the initial parathyroid exploration

The role of the surgeon in the first parathyroid exploration is to remove the parathyroid adenoma or hyperplastic glands appropriately and thus to cure the hyperparathyroid state. While Wang [24] and Tibblin [25] recommend unilateral neck exploration if one large gland (an adenoma) and a normal gland are found on the first side, and Paloyan [26] has recommended subtotal parathyroidectomy for all patients, I think that a middle-ground approach is appropriate. Both sides of the neck should be carefully explored in all cases and the number of glands removed should fit the disease process.

Table 2. Symptoms and signs in 42 patients with hypercalcemic crisis due to hyperparathyroidism

Symptoms	Percent of cases	Signs	Percent of cases
Muscular weakness	80	Hypotonia	44
Nausea and vomiting	80	Neck mass	42
Weight loss	65	Hypertension	35
Fatigue	65	Dehydration	31
Lethargy and drowsiness	65	Tachycardia	26
Confusion	57	Fever	22
Bone pain	55	Abdominal tenderness and distension	15
Abdominal pain	48	Band keratopathy	9
Polyuria	40	Tracheal deviation	4
Constipation	37		
Coma	26		
Polydipsia	24		
Renal colic	22		
Neck swelling	9		
Dysphagia and neck pain	4		

Source: From Lemann and Donatelli, 1964 [22].

Table 3. Usual doses of hypocalcemic agents

Drug	Route	Dosage	Reported complications	Contraindications
Sodium chloride solution (isotonic)	Intravenous	1 liter every 3–4 h	Pulmonary edema	Congestive heart failure, renal insufficiency, hypertension
Furosemide	Intravenous	100 mg/h	Volume depletion, hypokalemia	Renal insufficiency
EDTA	Intravenous	50 mg/kg body weight over 4–6 h	Renal failure, hypotension	Renal insufficiency
Cortisone	Oral or parenteral	150 mg/day	Hypercorticism	Emergency reduction of serum calcium required
Mithramycin	Intravenous	25 μg/kg body weight	Hemorrhage, thrombo-cytopenia, nausea, vomiting	Bleeding disorder, renal insufficiency, liver impairment
Phosphate	Oral	1–2 mM*/kg body weight daily	Diarrhea	–
Calcitonin	Parenteral	1–5 MRC units/kg body weight/day	Nausea, vomiting	Thrombotic disorders

* 1 mM of phosphate is equivalent to 31 mg of phosphorus.
Source: Modified from W.N. Suki, J.J. Yium, M. Von Minden et al.: Acute treatment of hypercalcemia with furosemide. N Engl J Med 283: 836–840, 1970 [23].

In general, parathyroid surgery requires an unrushed, meticulous dissection with a bloodless field. Hence, try to keep the operative field as dry as possible. Neither methylene blue nor toluidine blue are used by most parathyroid surgeons in either primary or secondary neck explorations. Undoubtedly, the more thyroid or parathyroid operations that one performs, the more readily he will be able to recognize the parathyroid glands. Abnormal parathyroid glands are enlarged, more spherical and often have a darker color that can range from tan to reddish-brown. Normal parathyroid glands are usually more yellowish in color, they bleed more than fat when a small biopsy is taken, and sometimes they can be recognized by the small hematoma that often occurs within their substance following manipulation.

At neck exploration the surgeon must be a diagnostician as well as a therapist. In most cases, at the time of operation, it is up to him to recognize the pathologic process that is present. If one gland is enlarged and the others are normal, this is an adenoma. The adenoma should be removed and one or two normal glands should be biopsied. We no longer biopsy the fourth normal gland, because in our experience this practice leads to a greater degree of transient postoperative hypocalcemia.

If four glands are found to be enlarged, this is hyperplasia. In such cases a subtotal parathyroidectomy is necessary. Three glands and part of the fourth are excised, leaving a well-vascularized remnant of 50 to 80mg of tissue. Each thymic tongue is also excised to be certain that more parathyroid tissue is not present, therein. The partial resection of one parathyroid gland should always be performed first, so that one can see that the remnant remains well-vascularized before removing the other three glands. In cases of familial hyperparathyroidism or of the MEA-1 syndrome one might consider doing a total parathyroidectomy with an autotransplant to the arm, as recommended by Wells [27].

When two parathyroid glands are enlarged and the others appear normal, this is probably a variant of hyperplasia (or multi-glandular disease); others call this a double adenoma. In such cases, we have found that resection of the two enlarged glands and biopsy of the two normal glands has been curative. Always mark the remaining parathyroid remnant (or remnants) with a hemoclip or a nonabsorbable suture so that, if necessary, it can be found more readily in the future.

Operative technique

Under general endotracheal anesthesia with the neck hyperextended, a transverse incision is made in the lower neck (Fig. 4). The platysma muscle is elevated with the skin flap, and the superior flap is dissected to the hyoid superiorly, the lower flap to the upper border of the sternum inferiorly. The skin flaps may be held apart by a self-retaining retractor or by sutures, and the deep cervical fascia is divided longitudinally in the midline from the hyoid bone to the suprasternal

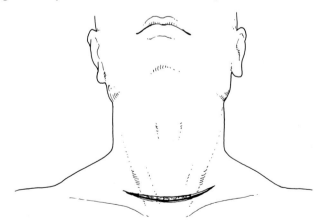

Figure 4. Technique of parathyroidectomy. With the neck extended, a transverse collar incision is made in the lower neck.

notch. Others prefer to divide the sternohyoid and sternothyroid muscles transversely at the junction of the upper and middle third to facilitate exposure; however, we usually do not find this necessary. The thyroid gland is mobilized by dividing the middle thyroid veins and rolling the lobe of the thyroid medially (Fig. 5). The recurrent laryngeal nerve is then identified, usually in the groove between the trachea and esophagus. The recurrent nerve may also be identified at the inferior cornu of the thyroid cartilage, and followed inferiorly. Parathyroid adenomas are frequently found down under the lateral lobe of the thyroid in a space alongside the esophagus lying just slightly posterior to the groove between the esophagus and the trachea or thyroid cartilage (Fig. 6). Tracing the branches of the inferior thyroid artery may sometimes be helpful in locating the hyperfunctioning parathyroid gland, since this vessel usually supplies the parathyroid adenoma with blood. After a preliminary search in this area the inferior parathyroid will often be found just below the point at which the recurrent laryngeal nerve intersects the inferior thyroid artery or within the thymic tongue inferior to the thyroid. The superior parathyroid will often be found within 1 or 2 cm above this point, usually on a little prominence of the posterior surface of the thyroid.

An adenoma, particularly one of the lower gland, can be tucked well behind the thyroid or between the trachea and esophagus, so that it is not readily apparent until the thyroid has been rotated forward and the fatty tissue in this area has been gently teased away. The adenoma is not usually bound down to the

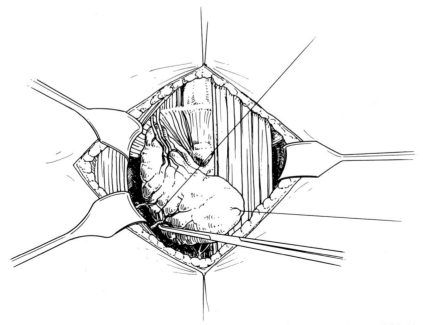

Figure 5. After upper and lower subplatysmal flaps are developed, the strap muscles are divided in the midline, the thyroid lobe is mobilized anteriorly and medially and, as shown here, the middle thyroid vein is ligated to facilitate exposure of the parathyroid glands.

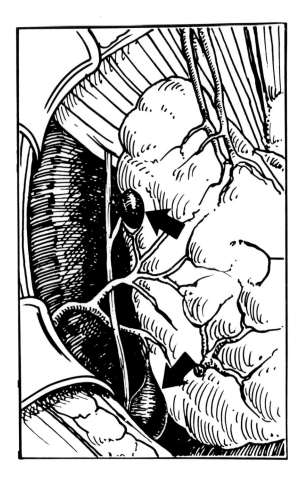

Figure 6. By blunt dissection, the recurrent laryngeal nerve is identified and both parathyroid glands are visualized. A large right lower parathyroid gland (lower arrow) and a normal-appearing right upper parathyroid gland (upper arrow) are seen. The left side of the neck should then be explored. If normal parathyroid glands are found there, the parathyroid adenoma is then removed and one or two other glands are carefully biopsied.

surrounding tissues and can be popped out of its hiding place. It is generally red-brown, or yellow-brown, smooth, and with a surface which is vascular and bleeds easily when rubbed or cut. On rare occasions, particularly when it lies beneath the capsule of the thyroid, it may look extremely similar to thyroid tissue itself.

Once the provisional location of the normal or abnormal glands has been established, the procedure is repeated on the other side. We make it a policy to examine both sides of the neck and to evaluate all of the parathyroid glands that can be found before removing any of them. This is to protect against the possibility of removing three enlarged parathyroids glands as they are encountered, only to find that the patient has no fourth gland. When all the parathyroids cannot be found adjacent to the thyroid gland, further search is facilitated by dividing the superior pole vessels of the thyroid on the side of a missing upper gland and performing the manuevers described below.

When the operation is to be completed, the strap muscles are loosely opposed with several sutures. A small suction catheter is inserted. The dermis is approximated with interrupted subcuticular sutures and the epidermis with sterile skin tapes (Fig.7).

The search for ectopic parathyroid glands. About 80 percent of all parathyroid adenomas are found near the thyroid. However, the others are located in ectopic sites. If an adenoma cannot be found in the usual locations at exploration the following procedures should be performed. Each normal parathyroid gland should be biopsied, and after positive identification as parathyroid tissue on frozen section, a diagram should be made of its location for later reference; each gland should be marked with a hemoclip. Do *not* remove normal parathyroid glands; this complicates the situation when the adenoma is ultimately found.

If three normal parathyroid glands are found and the fourth cannot be located, the surgeon should try to assess whether an upper or a lower parathyroid gland on that side is missing. If it is the lower parathyroid gland, as much of the thymus as possible should be pulled up into the neck and resected. Often the inferior adenoma will be found within the thymus.

Very frequently, it is an adenoma of the upper parathyroid gland which is overlooked. These fall down along the esophagus into the posterior-superior mediastinum. The mistake in this case is that the dissection was not carried out deep enough back to the prevertebral fascia of the neck. When this is done near the upper pole of the thyroid, a finger can be safely inserted behind the inferior thyroid artery and posterior to the recurrent laryngeal nerve. Not infrequently an

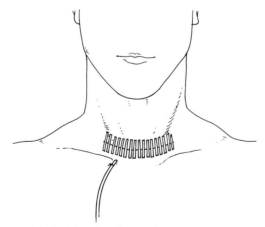

Figure 7. The appearance of the incision after closure of the dermis with fine interrupted subcuticular sutures and approximation of the epithelial layer with sterile skin tapes. The suction catheter is almost always removed on the following morning.

adenoma will be palpable beside or behind the esophagus and this gland can be pulled up and easily removed.

If the parathyroid gland still cannot be found after these manuevers, the dissection should be carried up in a cephalad direction to the hyoid bone where occasionally an 'undescended' adenoma will be found. Next, the thyroid lobe on the side of the missing gland should be carefully palpated. Any lump within the thyroid should be excised for this might represent an intrathyroidal parathyroid adenoma. It is also important to remember that many patients, particularly those that have been exposed to low-dose external radiation in the past, have benign or malignant lesions of the thyroid gland that require proper surgical resection, along with parathyroidectomy [33]. Even if no lump is present, a 'blind' subtotal excision of the thyroid lobe on the side of the missing gland should be performed. Sometimes a nonpalpable parathyroid adenoma will emerge. Others use a thyroidotomy and incise the lower pole of the thyroid rather than resecting it. Finally, the carotid sheath should be opened from the level of the clavicle upwards. Occasionally, a parathyroid adenoma which cannot be palpated because it is flattened out like a pancake, will be found.

Even if four normal glands are found in the neck, the surgeon should search all of these ectopic sites for a fifth gland that is adenomatous. Similarly, if four hyperplastic glands cannot be found, these same sites should be explored.

Should a sternotomy be performed at this time? Only rarely should a sternotomy and formal mediastinal dissection be done as part of the first exploration. This procedure is probably indicated only if the patient is extremely ill from hypercalcemia which cannot be adequately managed medically. The reasons for this approach are several: First of all, sometimes the diagnosis is in error. Secondly, occasionally hypercalcemia regresses or is eliminated by this first neck exploration despite the fact that no abnormal parathyroid tissue has been removed. This probably occurs when an adenoma is infarcted by accidental ligation of its arterial supply. Finally, it is well-known that in most cases of persistent hyperparathyroidism, the offending gland or glands can later be removed through a neck incision, particularly if the first surgeon is not very experienced in this area (Fig. 8). This fact is clearly demonstrated in the Mayo Clinic series [28] in which, until 1970, 1,000 parathyroid explorations were performed and only twelve required a sternotomy, an incidence of 1.2 percent. At the Massachusetts General Hospital [29] 21% of cases of primary hyperparathyroidism involved ectopically placed parathyroid adenomas. However, almost all of these could be removed through a neck incision, and only 5 percent required a sternotomy. At the University of Chicago Hospitals, in a personal series of over two hundred cases, about two percent of cases required a sternotomy and in each instance this operation was curative. Thus, *do not rush to do a sternotomy* as part of the first operation.

Management of persistent or recurrent hyperparathyroidism

Persistent disease means that hypercalcemia remains after operation. This occurs when the diagnosis of hyperparathyroidism is incorrect, or when the hyperfunctioning gland or glands have not been adequately removed. In the hands of experienced neck surgeons, this should occur only infrequently, probably 5 percent of the time or less for initial neck explorations. Recurrent disease means that the calcium returns to normal postoperatively but that months to years later, hypercalcemia due to hyperparathyroidism returns. This condition is relatively uncommon except in familial hyperparathyroidism or MEA, type 1 syndromes [30] (Table 4), and is most often seen if primary chief cell hyperplasia is not recognized and one or two enlarged glands are removed because they are diagnosed as adenomas. When recurrent hyperparathyroidism does occur, the parathyroid disease should be treated as hyperplasia with subtotal parathyroidectomy or a total resection of all glands with autotransplantation. A lesser procedure will be once more doomed to failure. Hypercalcemia recurring several months after an apparently successful parathyroidectomy should alert the physician to the possibility of a parathyroid carcinoma, although inadequately treated hyperplasia is more likely. It is necessary to follow patients for many years following parathyroidectomy if the results of therapy are to be truly assessed.

Before reoperation for a missed parathyroid adenoma, it is important to consider the following factors.

Confirmation of the diagnosis. It is imperative hat the surgeon and endocrinologist reassess the diagnosis. Does the patient truly have primary hyperparathyroidism or is there a different etiology for the hypercalcemia? The differential diagnosis of hypercalcemia is long and the correct analysis at times can be very difficult. Consider the following clinical situation: A 75-year-old woman was recently referred to us for sternotomy after having been explored elsewhere for primary hyperparathyroidism; four normal parathyroid glands were confirmed to be in the neck. Her serum calcium levels were elevated, the phosphorus values were low, the alkaline phosphatase was elevated and the circulating parathyroid hormone (PTH) concentration was borderline high. The chloride level was elevated but she had been receiving intravenous fluids for a prolonged period. The chloride/phosphorus ratio was greater than 40. Her appetite was poor and she had lost 20 to 30 pounds over several months. At the University of Chicago Hospitals her serum values were similar, except that the high alkaline phosphatase was found to be hepatic in origin, and by using a different assay, the parathyroid hormone concentration was within the normal range. A liver-spleen scan demonstrated multiple filling defects and a percutaneous liver biopsy confirmed the presence of a primary hepatoma, a known cause of ectopic PTH secretion.

While carcinoma elsewhere and a parathyroid adenoma can occur together in

Table 4. Incidence of recurrent hyperparathyroidism and severe hypoparathyroidism following operation for primary hyperparathyroidism

Author and year	Total no. of patients	Multiple gland involvement, %	Recurrent hyperpara-thyroidism, %	Severe hypo-para-thyroidism, %	Follow-up
Paloyan et al. (1969)	I 27	18	15	19	7 mo–3 yr
	II* 26	58	0	8	–
Haff and Ballinger (1971)	38	50	3	5	18 mo or longer
Bruining (1971)	I 267	45	0	1.2	3^1/$_2$ yr (average)
	II* 11	–	0	27	–
Clark and Taylor (1971)	99	15	1	2	–
Johanssen et al. (1972)	203	18	0	3.8	
Paloyan et al. (1973)	98	65	1	2	–
Romanus et al. (1973)	274	20	1	7	4 yr average
Hines and Suker (1973)	51	10	0	–	To 15 yr
Wang (1973)	256	–	0.8	–	10 mo–15 yr
Davies (1974)	350	10	3	5	mo–38 yr
Myers (1974)	82	13	1	–	1–65 yr
Purnell et al. (1974)	475	13	0.6	0.2	–
Block et al. (1974)	121	20	1	4	4^1/$_2$ yr (average)
Muller et al. (1975)	352	50	1	–	–
Palmer et al. (1975)	250	15	0.5	2	15 yr
Farr (1976)	100	5	2	4	–
Block (1976)	182	20	0	0	–
Clark et al. (1976)	263	12	2.7	4	6 mo–40 yr
MEA or FHP[a]	21	71	33	24[b]	–
Without MEA or FHP	242	6	0.4	2.6	–

* Subtotal parathyroidectomy.
Source: Adapted from O.H. Clark, L.H. Wang, and T.K. Hunt. Ann Surg 184: 391, 1976 [30].
[a] MEA, multiple endocrine adenomatosis; FHP, familial hyperparathyroidism.
[b] None permanent.

the same patient, this seems unlikely in this individual, for with chemotherapy and better nutrition, her serum calcium and phosphorus values returned to normal.

Evaluation of the severity of disease. It is important that the severity of the parathyroid disease be reassessed and be considered sufficient to justify the increased risk of reexploration with possible sternotomy. One might argue that 'minimal hyperparathyroidism' in an asymptomatic patient does not warrant this risk, particularly in an individual who is elderly and has other medical complications. In such cases, oral phosphate might be tried, although one should be cognizant that renal deterioration has been reported to occur in some instances. On the other hand, the mortality of a neck reexploration even with sternotomy is low even in the elderly, and sometimes one gets into greater difficulty by waiting. This is a matter of clinical judgement.

Familial hypocalciuric hypercalcemia (F.H.H.) [31]. Nine percent of recent patients referred for reexploration to the National Institutes of Health have been shown to have familial hypocalciuric hypercalcemia [32]. This familial disease is probably a benign variant of hyperparathyroidism. Despite hypercalcemia and elevated parathyroid concentrations in most instances, these patients suffer few complications of their disease. The diagnosis is made by demonstrating a low urinary calcium output despite hypercalcemia and a calcium to creatinine clearance ratio of less than 0.01. Such patients will not benefit from parathyroidectomy since less than a total parathyroidectomy will not correct the hypercalcemia. Thus, if the correct diagnosis is made, a reoperation should not be contemplated.

Careful documentation of the findings of the previous operation. Before reoperation, the operative note and the pathology report or slides should be carefully examined in order to find documentation of the *number* and *location* of normal or abnormal parathyroid glands that had been removed or biopsied. The location of each gland found at the initial operation and whether to expect an adenoma or hyperplasia are very helpful factors. Unfortunately, at times, it is very difficult to gain this information from the notes which are available.

To localize or not to localize? A number of preoperative tests are now available which can sometimes localize the site of enlarged parathyroid glands preoperatively with greater or lesser certainty. *Palpation* of the neck is occasionally helpful. However, 54% of our patients were found to have gross thyroid abnormalities as well as parathyroid disease [33] making a palpatory finding less meaningful. A reliable *isotope scan* would be very important; thallium scanning with ^{99m}Tc subtraction of thyroid uptake shows promise. *Ultrasonography* using a high resolution, high-frequency, real-time, small parts scanner has been reported to be quite efficacious in some series [34]. However, many hospitals have neither the proper equipment nor an experienced physician to make this technique useful. This technique can be combined with fine needle aspiration with cytologic evaluation to confirm the diagnosis and differentiate the lesion from a thyroid mass. *Computed tomography* (CT scanning) with or without contrast material can sometimes be of help, particularly when larger glands are present [35]. Approximately half of the parathyroid adenomas found substernally within the thymus were identified preoperatively by this technique.

Among the invasive tests, *arteriography* can be useful in up to half of the cases [32] but is not without risk. Occasional cases of quadraplegia, hemiparesis and other neurologic deficits have occurred, presumably from high concentrations of dye going to the spinal cord by way of small vessels of the thyrocervical trunk. While rare, these complications are devastating to both the patient and the physician. For this reason highly selective injections into the inferior thyroid artery should probably not be performed. Rather, dye injections into the subclavian and the internal mammary arteries can be done with far less risk. In our experience, four mediastinal parathyroid adenomas have been visualized successfully by this technique. Finally, *selective catheterization* of the neck veins with sampling of blood for parathyroid hormone analysis [36] has also been used effectively in about half of our patients. However, this technique is laborious, time-consuming and expensive and never pinpoints the site of disease as well as arteriography.

Presently we do not perform invasive localization tests on any patient whom we are exploring for the first time. However, we might utilize ultrasonography or CT scanning on all patients if these techniques were shown to be reliable in our hospital. We reserve invasive localization studies for the patient who has had a prior exploration by an experienced neck surgeon, for these patients are very likely to have ectopically placed glands. There are differences of opinion concerning the value and appropriateness of invasive localizing studies when the patient has been explored by someone without much experience in this field. While it is recognized that in most of these patients the gland will be found in the neck; on the other hand, it is easier and less time consuming during operation if its site is known beforehand. The risk-benefit value of localization should be weighted for each patient.

Strategy and technique of reoperation [37]

Reoperations of the neck are more difficult because of the scarring, changes in anatomy and loss of tissue planes which occur as a result of the first exploration, whether it was for a thyroid or parathyroid disorder. Frequently, for example, the strap muscles will be densely adherent to the anterior surface of the thyroid lobes making entry into the usual anatomical planes more difficult. Furthermore, the recurrent laryngeal nerve is in greater jeopardy, first of all because it may be encased in scar tissue, but especially because it might lie immediately beneath the strap muscles if the thyroid lobe was previously removed. Finally, since one's knowledge of how many parathyroid glands remain in the neck after the first exploration is often limited, the chance of creating permanent hypoparathyroidism after removal of one or more abnormal parathyroid gands found at reexploration is increased. Usually there is not a rush to reoperate and it is better to allow some time to pass in order to permit the wound to heal, to reevaluate the diagnosis, and to assess the findings of the previous operation.

When reoperating, we always explore the neck again first unless an adenoma is localized to the mediastinum or an experienced parathyroid surgeon did the initial operation and was 'certain' that the lesion was not in the neck. Only under these circumstances would a sternotomy be performed initially.

The prior transverse neck incision is used and subplatysmal flaps are elevated. The strap muscles are often adherent to the thyroid lobes; hence, instead of separating them in the midline, it is often easier to dissect the vertical plane between each sternocleidomastoid muscle and the strap muscles (Fig. 9). Not infrequently this plane is totally unscarred and by retracting the carotid sheath laterally and the thyroid gland medially, a 'fresh' area containing the recurrent laryngeal nerve and parathyroid glands will be entered. If this area is scarred, the dissection should be started as low in the neck as possible since this region is often untouched. Once the recurrent nerve is identified, it can be safely followed in a cephalad direction. If the adenoma was not localized beforehand, a bilateral neck exploration is usually necessary. In the case of either positive localization, or retrospective determination of the side of the neck of the missing gland, the cervical dissection might be started there initially.

One of the most rewarding manuevers that should be done early is to dissect the upper thyroid area posteriorly to the prevertebral fascia and to introduce one's finger downward behind the inferior thyroid artery along the esophagus into the posterior mediastinum as far as one can reach [38]. Often the missing adenoma will be palpated here before it can be seen. This is the area in which many missing adenomas will be found because the initial dissection was not carried out deep enough.

If this is unsuccessful, all of the sites described above under the heading 'The search for ectopic parathyroid glands' should be explored. This involves pulling up and dissecting the thymus on each side into the neck and removing all of the tissue down to the innominate artery, dissecting as high in the neck as the hyoid bone, removing a part of one or both thyroid lobes, and finally opening and exploring the carotid sheath areas. A careful neck reexploration in this manner will almost always yield the missing adenoma or the elusive hyperplastic gland or glands that remain.

Before operation, consent for a possible sternotomy should be obtained, if that is your operative plan. Another approach used by many surgeons, however, is to plan to only reexplore the neck as carefully as possible, and to postpone the sternotomy for another time, especially if no localization studies were performed before the neck reexploration.

Either a partial sternotomy to the third intercostal space or a complete sternotomy can be performed. First the thymus and surrounding fat pads should be palpated. Several times we could feel a mass, which proved to be the missing adenoma and only a partial thymectomy was necessary. Otherwise, the entire thymus should be removed. If the parathyroid gland is not found therein, a posterior dissection should then be performed. Lesions have been found along

208

the esophagus, between the aorta and pulmonary artery and even very rarely in an intrapericardial location. Needless to say, these dissections can be very long and tedious.

When an adenoma is found in the neck or chest it should be totally removed. If one additional normal gland was left after the first operation, the patient will have normal postoperative parathyroid function (thus, stressing the importance of *not* removing normal parathyroid glands during an unsuccessful initial operation). If hyperplastic glands are identified at reoperation, either a subtotal parathyroidectomy be can performed, or others prefer a total parathyroidectomy, arguing that if recurrence were to occur in a remnant that is left, this would necessitate a third neck operation. If total parathyroidectomy is used, or following removal of an adenoma when one thinks that no other parathyroid tissue remains, one has the option of either immediately autotransplanting some of the abnormal parathyroid to the arm [39] or else cryopreserving the tissue and awaiting to see whether or not hypocalcemia occurs postoperatively [32]. If hypoparathyroidism

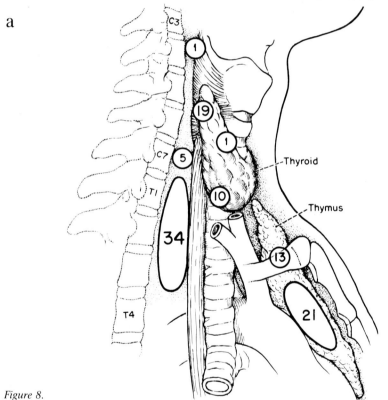

a

Figure 8.

a. Location of all parathyroid adenomas found at reoperation after failure to cure hyperparathyroidism initially, as described by Wang [45]. Note that most of these glands could be removed through a neck incision.

b. Location of 21 parathyroid adenomas that required a median sternotomy for resection. Open circles represent glands enclosed in thymus; closed circles indicate those behind thymus.

occurs, a subsequent autotransplant to the arm could be employed, especially if the preserved tissue were shown to be suppressible.

Each of these approaches has advantages and disadvantages. In our hands, cryopreservation has not been developed to the extent described by Wells [40] and Brennan [32] and, hence, we would be more likely to utilize immediate autotransplantation if it were thought necessary, but only if we felt strongly that *all* other parathyroid tissue had been removed from the patient. The frequency of recurrent hyperparathyroidism when part of an adenoma or of a hyperplastic gland is used as an autotransplant to the arm remains a fruitful area for study.

Postoperative complications of parathyroidectomy

The surgeon, house officers, and nurses must be cognizant of the possible complications that may occur following parathyroid operations. All complica-

b

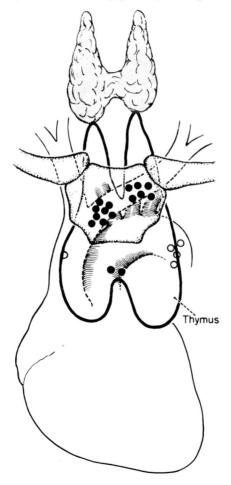

Thymus

210

tions should be anticipated and treated expeditiously and effectively if they occur. As with all operative procedures, nausea, vomiting, headache, and some minor chest problems are common occurrences immediately after operation. Wound infections are rare, however, following these procedures.

Hemorrhage and hematoma. Bleeding can occur from an artery or vein in the thyroid or neck region that has not been effectively ligated. We routinely drain these wounds with a small suction catheter. In most cases, this is removed on the morning after operation. If significant bleeding occurs, however, the drain is often ineffective and a hematoma can still form deep to the strap muscles. To prevent this, the scrap muscles are only loosely approximated at the end of the procedure. The greatest danger in such cases is compression of the trachea, respiratory comprimise, and possible death.

If respiratory compromise from a hematoma is diagnosed, the wound should be opened without delay, even at the bedside, and the hematoma should be evacuated. This may be a life-saving procedure. Later the patient can be taken to the operating room if necessary for a more leisurely exploration. It is our practice to keep a sterile tracheostomy pack at the bedside of each patient who has recently undergone parathyroidectomy so that proper instruments will be available if necessary. Respiratory compromise is a very rare complication, but it is a very serious one.

Recurrent laryngeal nerve injury. Damage to the recurrent laryngeal nerve is a dangerous but uncommon complication. If this nerve is injured during operation, the ipsilateral vocal cord becomes paralyzed and can no longer abduct. The voice

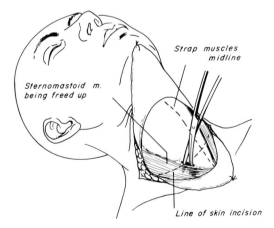

Figure 9. During reoperative parathyroid operations, the strap muscles are often fixed to the surface of the thyroid lobes making their usual mobilization difficult. Hence, rather than dissecting the midline, it is often easier to enter the plane between the strap muscles and the sternocleidomastoid muscle, an area that is often unscarred and allows easy access to the recurrent laryngeal nerve and to the parathyroid glands. Adapted from Kaplan [11].

usually becomes husky and hoarse since, in most cases, the cords no longer approximate one another. Occasionally the cord can be fixed in a midline position, in which case the speaking voice will not be greatly impaired. In other instances, with time, the opposite cord may spontaneously compensate and move across the midline to approximate the paralyzed cord. In this case, a husky voice might become much better in quality.

A recurrent nerve injury may occur because of trauma or rough dissection during operation. In these instances, the vocal cord paralysis is usually *transient*, and function may spontaneously return after several months. But if a recurrent nerve is divided at operation or severely damaged, *permanent* vocal cord paralysis will occur. If division of the nerve is recognized at the time of operation, the two ends should be approximated carefully by microsurgical technique. Return of function may occur after several months or longer. If no return of function occurs following a period of six months to one year after nerve injury, Teflon injection into the paralyzed vocal cord may greatly improve the quality of the patient's speaking voice, since this usually leads to better vocal cord approximation.

Bilateral recurrent nerve injury with bilateral vocal cord paralysis represents a very serious situation but is extremely rare following parathyroid surgery. The patient is susceptible to aspiration when swallowing and cannot cough effectively. Furthermore, if the cords are approximated near the midline, the airway may be inadequate and the patient may be dyspneic at rest or with mild activity. Even if the cords are fixed in the paramedian position, there is a danger that they may move toward the midline with time. Thus, many of the patients require a tracheostomy immediately postoperatively or later. An alternative treatment, if no vocal cord function returns, is to move one vocal cord laterally in order to insure an adequate airway. Other reinnervation operations are also being tried.

Superior laryngeal nerve injury. Damage to the external branch of the superior laryngeal nerve during operation may occur when the superior thyroid vessels are ligated in order to mobilize the upper pole of the thyroid gland (Fig. 10). This nerve innervates the cricothyroid muscle, which is a general tensor of the vocal cords. Following this injury, the patient cannot sing as well as before and cannot shout or project the voice effectively. Fortunately, in most people there is great improvement of these functions within several months.

Hypoparathyroidisim

Following parathyroid surgery, hypoparathyroidism may occur [41] (Table 4). The symptoms of this disease are primarily due to a significant fall in concentration of the serum calcium ion, the physiologically active form of circulating calcium.

When severe hypocalcemia is present, the patient often becomes tense and anxious. Not uncommonly he or she states that the fingers and toes tingle or 'feel

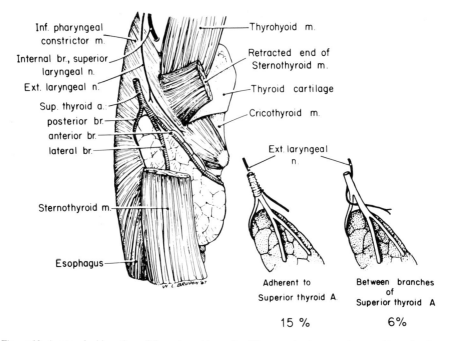

Inf. pharyngeal constrictor m.

Internal br., superior laryngeal n.

Ext. laryngeal n.

Sup. thyroid a.
posterior br.
anterior br.
lateral br.

Sternothyroid m.

Esophagus

Thyrohyoid m.

Retracted end of Sternothyroid m.

Thyroid cartilage

Cricothyroid m.

Ext. laryngeal n.

Adherent to Superior thyroid A.

15 %

Between branches of Superior thyroid A

6%

Figure 10. Anatomical location of the external branch of the superior laryngeal nerve. Note that in at least 21 percent of cases this nerve is intimately associated with the branches of the superior thyroid artery. Thus, it is easily damaged during mobilization of the upper pole of the thyroid if care is not exercised. From Thompson NW, Olsen WR and Hoffman GL [38].

asleep', and the area around the mouth is numb. Physical examination reveals that the deep tendon reflexes are usually hyperactive. If the area in front of the patient's ear over the facial nerve is tapped, twitching and contraction of the facial muscles will occur (Chvostek's sign). Initially the response is very subtle, and only a slight, almost imperceptible movement of the upper lateral lip area is seen. As the serum calcium concentration decreases further, this reaction is more readily observable. The presence of significant hypocalcemia may also be clinically determined by the Trousseau sign. A blood pressure cuff applied to the patient's upper arm is inflated to just above systolic pressure for several minutes. A positive test is indicated by carpal spasm; the affected wrist and metacarpophalangeal joints become flexed, while the interphalangeal joints are extended. The hand cannot be voluntarily opened to a normal position because of the spasm. When hypocalcemia is full-blown, carpopedal spasm or tetany often occur spontaneously; both hands and feet may be held involuntarily in a spastic state. Abdominal cramps, urinary frequency, and even intestinal ileus may also occur with severe hypocalcemia.

The greatest risks of hypocalcemia result from two other complications, each of which may be life-threatening. With severe hypocalcemia, *convulsions* may occur, especially in children. Secondly, *laryngeal spasm* may occur, and it results in stridor and inability to breathe effectively. Respiratory death may result if treatment is not instituted immediately.

Hypoparathyroidism is characterized by a decrease in serum calcium and an increase in serum phosphorus concentrations. The urinary calcium output also decreases as the serum calcium level falls. The urinary phosphorus output also decreases in hypoparathyroidism as the phosphaturic effect of parathyroid hormone on the renal tubule is diminished. When hypocalcemia exists a prolongation of the Q-T interval is often seen on the electrocardiogram.

While patients differ somewhat in their individual responses to a fall in serum calcium concentration, most develop mild symptoms by the time the serum calcium level reaches 8.0 mg/dl or less. Severe symptoms usually represent a circulating calcium level of 7.5 mg/dl or less in most patients. Some individuals develop symptoms of hypocalcemia at higher levels of serum calcium, which suggests that the *change* in serum calcium concentration rather than the absolute level is most important.

During parathyroidectomy, all parathyroid tissue might be inadvertently removed, irrevocably damaged, or devascularized; each leads to *permanent hypoparathyroidism*. Fortunately, however, most hypoparathyroidism that occurs following parathyroidectomy is *transient* and is spontaneously reversed in less than one week.

Transient hypoparathyroidism can be noted after removal of a parathyroid adenoma or a resection of most of the tissue in parathyroid hyperplasia. This is made worse when the patient has renal disease or when the patient has serious bone disease. Postoperatively the calcium tends to be deposited in the bone, thus producing hypocalcemia. This process is referred to as 'bone hunger' and should be expected when the patient has a high alkaline phosphatase concentration preoperatively due to severe bone disease. The biopsy of three normal glands after removal of an adenoma also results in a greater degree of postoperative hypocalcemia in our experience [33]; hence we leave the fourth gland untouched.

For the first few postoperative days, it is impossible to determine by laboratory tests whether the hypocalcemia is transient or permanent. However, in transient hypoparathyroidism, the lowest serum calcium level usually occurs between 24 and 72 hours postoperative and then begins to rise spontaneously. Usually, the lowest serum calcium concentration is 7.5 mg/dl or greater in these cases. In permanent hypoparathyroidism, on the other hand, the serum calcium concentration falls at the same rate shortly after the operative procedure but remains low thereafter, often decreasing to 7 mg/dl or below if no treatment is instituted.

Treatment of postoperative hypocalcemia. Since hypocalcemia following parathyroidectomy is usually transient, a period of careful observation will suffice for most patients until the serum calcium level returns toward normal. However, during this period, it is imperative that no harmful effects of hypocalcemia occur in the patient. The serum calcium concentration should be determined on the evening following operation and every 12 hours thereafter for several days then daily until the patient is discharged. Serum phosphorus concentration is measured if hypocalcemia persists.

When mild hypocalcemia occurs, no treatment is needed. However, if the patient becomes symptomatic secondary to the lowered calcium level, 1 gm of calcium gluconate can be given by intravenous injection. Then 1 or 2 g of calcium gluconate are added to the intravenous fluid regimen and given continuously over each eight hour period. This is the amount of choice since it generally relieves all symptoms without greatly raising the serum calcium concentration. Within several days, all calcium therapy can usually be stopped. It must be remembered that calcium chloride and calcium gluconate are not interchangeable ampule for ampule, for each gram of calcium chloride contains about twice as much calcium ion as does calcium gluconate.

For more persistent hypocalcemia, oral calcium is begun at a dose of 1.5 to 2.0 g of calcium ion per day. In order to provide 1 g of elemental calcium daily, 4 g of calcium acetate, 5.5 g of hydrated calcium chloride, 8 g of calcium lactate, or 11 g of calcium gluconate must be administered [42]. Calcium gluconate is palatable and can be given in a liquid form. It is well tolerated by the patient; unfortunately, diarrhea is a major side effect of all of these calcium preparations. Once started, the oral calcium can be tapered and discontinued after several weeks in most patients. It is preferable not to add vitamin D to this regimen early unless it is necessary to raise the serum calcium concentration still further or unless one strongly suspects that permanent hypoparathyroidism has occurred. The addition of vitamin D makes follow-up more difficult, since the effects of these preparations may last for weeks or even several months after they are discontinued (Table 5). In most patients who are given about 20 g of calcium gluconate orally daily, the serum calcium level rises sufficiently after several days without the administration of vitamin D.

If *permanent hypoparathyroidism* is suspected, in addition to the oral calcium therapy, the patient should be started on a vitamin D preparation (Table 5). Vitamin D3 50.000 to 100,000 units per day (1.25 to 2.5 mg per day) is commonly

Table 5. Clinical comparison of substances with vitamin D action

Characteristic	D_2 or D_3	DHT*	$1,25(OH)_2$-D_3
Daily dose in hypoparathyroidism (mg)	0.75–3.0	0.25–1.0	0.5–2 μg
Relative potency	1	3	1500
Time to restore normocalcaemia (weeks)[a]	2–4	1–2	3–6 days
Time to reach maximum effect (weeks) [a]	4–12	2–4	3–6 days
Persistence after cessation (weeks)	6–18[b]	1–3	3–6 days

* DHT = dihydrotachysterol.
[a] For constant daily dose; shorter if a loading dose is given.
[b] Up to 18 months after severe intoxication[41].

used. Others prefer dihydrotachysterol, 0.125 to 1.0 mg per day or 1,25 dihydroxy D, 1 to 2 μg daily. Several days usually pass before the serum calcium begins to rise after vitamin D3 therapy is begun; however, the rise of this ion is faster after the use of the other preparations (Fig. 11). The serum calcium concentration must be measured frequently, since some patients are insensitive to these preparations and require larger doses, while others develop vitamin D intoxication with severe hypercalcemia while receiving relatively small doses. Good control means that the serum calcium level remains within the normal physiologic range.

Serum PTH concentrations should be measured at regular intervals in patients being treated for permanent postoperative hypoparathyroidism. Several patients whom we have seen have been treated unnecessarily with vitamin D therapy for many years because postoperative tetany occurred. If serum PTH levels are in the normal range, vitamin D therapy should be tapered and finally terminated, if possible.

Other nonspecific factors may tend to influence the treatment of hypocalcemia [42]. A diet high in phosphate or oxalate content should be avoided, since it may impair calcium absorption. Concomitant ingestion of anticonvulsants and tranquilizers may lower intestinal absorption of calcium both directly and by interfering with vitamin D metabolism. Estrogen and oral contraceptive therapy lower the serum calcium level by suppressing bone resorption. Diuretics, such as furosemide, result in increased calcium excretion in the urine. On the other hand, a low sodium diet with chlorthalidone has been reported to raise the serum calcium concentration [44]. Finally, hypomagnesemia should be avoided since this leads to resistance to vitamin D therapy.

Prevention of permanent hypoparathyroidism. To avoid permanent hypoparathyroidism, the surgeon should not remove normal parathyroid glands when an adenoma cannot be found; rather carefully biopsy them with a fine scissors. The inferior thyroid artery should not be ligated laterally, since this might completely

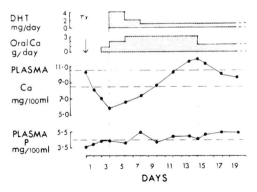

Figure 11. Following total thyroidectomy and parathyroidectomy for medullary carcinoma of the thyroid (Tx), severe hypocalcaemia was treated with dihydrotachysterol (DHT) and oral calcium. Note the rapid response achieved by this therapy. From Parfitt [43].

devascularize the parathyroid glands, especially when the superior thyroid vessels are also ligated. Finally, the use of autotransplantation of parathyroid tissue, either during operation [39] or later following cryopreservation [40] in a 'parathyroid bank' is a powerful tool that can prevent the need for a lifetime of treatment for hypoparathyroidism when it is used appropriately.

Acknowledgements

This work was supported by a generous grant from The Nathan and Frances Goldblatt Society for Cancer Research. The assistance of Ms. Joey Czerwonka in preparing this manuscript is greatly appreciated.

References

1. Mandl F: Therapeutischer Versuch bei Ostitis fibrosa generalisata mittels Exstirpation lines Epithelkorperchentumors. Wein klin Wchnschr 50: 1343, 1925.
2. Collip JB: Extraction of parathyroid hormone which will prevent or control parathyroid tetany and which regulates level of blood calcium. J Biol Chem 63: 395–438, 1924.
3. Hanson AM: Hydrochloric X Sicca: parathyroid preparation for intramuscular injection. Mil Surgeon 54: 218, 1924.
4. Hunter D, Aub JC: Lead studies XV. Effect of parathyroid hormone on excretion of lead and of calcium in patients suffering from lead poisoning. Quart J Med 20: 123–140, 1927.
5. Richardson EP, Aub JC, Bauer W: Parathyroidectomy in osteomalacia. Ann Surg 90: 730–741, 1929.
6. Bauer W, Federman DD: Hyperparathyroidism epitomized: case of Captain Charles E. Martell. Metabolism 11: 21–29, 1962.
7. Sedgwick CE, Cady B: Embryology and developmental abnormalities, Chapter 2. In: Surgery of the Thyroid and Parathyroid Glands, Sedgwick and Cady (eds). Philadelphia: WB Saunders Co., 1980, pp 6–18.
8. Sedgwick CE and Cady B: Surgical Anatomy, Chapter 3. In: Surgery of the Thyroid and Parathyroid Glands, Sedgwick and Cady (eds). Philadelphia: WB Saunders Co., 1980, pp 19–38.
9. Gilmour JR: The embryology of the parathyroid glands, the thymus and certain associated rudiments. J Pathol 45: 507, 1937.
10. Gilmour R: The weight of the parathyroid glands. J Pathol Bacteriol.44: 431, 1937.
11. Kaplan EL: Thyroid and parathyroid, Chapter 38. In: Principles of Surgery, Schwartz SI, Shires GT, Spencer FC, Storer EH (eds). New York: McGraw-Hill Book Co., 1983, pp 1545–1635.
12. Edis AF: Surgical anatomy and technique of neck exploration for primary hyperparathyroidism. Surg Clin N Am 57: 495, 1977.
13. Cope O, Keynes WM, Roth SI, Castelman B: Primary chief-cell hyperplasia of the parathyroid glands: A new entity in the surgery of hyperparathyroidism. Ann Surg 148: 375, 1958.
14. Edis AJ, Beahrs OH, van Heerden JA, Akwari OE: 'Conservative' versus 'Liberal' approach to parathyroid neck exploration. Surgery 82: 466, 1977.
15. Roth SI: Pathology of the parathyroids in hyperparathyroidism: Discussion of recent advances in the anatomy and pathology of the parathyroid glands. Arch Path (Chicago) 73: 495, 1962.
16. Roth SI, Gallagher MJ: The rapid identification of 'normal' parathyroid glands by the presence of intracellular fat. Amer Path 84: 521–528, 1976.

17. Holmes EC, Morton DL, Ketcham AS: Parathyroid carcinoma: A collective review. Ann Surg 169: 631, 1969.

18. Schantz A, Castleman B: Parathyroid carcinoma: A study of 70 cases. Cancer 31: 600, 1973.

19. Flye MW, Brennan M: Surgical resection of metastatic parathyroid carcinoma. Ann Surg 193: 425, 1981.

20. Clark OH, Arnaud CD: Hyperparathyroidism: incidence, diagnosis and problems. In: Surgery of the Thyroid and Parathyroids. Clinical Surgery International V6, Kapla EL (ed). Edinburgh: Churchill Livingstone, 1983, pp 144–157.

21. Purnell DC, and Heath III H: The dilemma of asymptomatic hypercalcemia. In: Surgery of the Thyroid and Parathyroids. Clinical Surgery International V6, Kaplan EL (ed). Edinburgh: Churchill Livingstone, 1983, pp 211–223.

22. Lemann JL Jr, Donatelli AA: Calcium intoxidation due to primary hyperparathyroidism. A medical and surgical emergency. Ann Intern Med 60: 447, 1964

23. Suki WN, Yium JJ,VonMinden M, et al.: Acute treatment of hypercalcemia with furosemide. N Engl J Med 283: 836, 1970

24. Wang CA, Potts JT Jr, Neer RM: Controversy of parathyroid surgery. In: Calcium Regulating Hormones, RV Tamage (ed). Amsterdam: Excerpta Medica, 1975, p 82.

25. Tibblin S, Bondeson AG, Ljunberg O: Unilateral parathyroidectomy in hyperparathyroidism due to single adenoma. Ann Surg 195: 245–252, 1982.

26. Paloyan D, Pickleman JR: Hyperparathyroidism Today. Surg Clin North Am 53: 211, 1973.

27. Wells SA Jr, Ellis GJ, Gunnells JC, et al.: Parathyroid autotransplantation in primary parathyroid hyperplasia. N Engl J Med 295: 57, 1976.

28. Scholz DA, Purnell DC: Asymptomatic Primary Hyperparathyroidism 10-year Prospective Study. Mayo Clin Proc 56: 73, 1981.

29. Nathaniels EK, Nathaniels AM, Wang C-A: Mediastinal parathyroid tumors: A clinical and pathological study of 84 cases. Ann Surg 171: 165, 1970.

30. Clark OR, Way L, Hunt TK: Recurrent hyperparathyroidism. Ann Surg 184: 391, 1076.

31. Marx SJ, Attie MF, Levine MA, Spiegel AM, Downs RW Jr, Lasker RD: The hypocalciuric of benign variant of hypercalcemia: Clinical and biochemical features in fifteen kindreds. Medicine 60: 397, 1981.

32. Brennan MF: Reoperation for suspected hyperparathyroidism. In: Surgery of the Thyroid and Parathyroids. Clinical Surgery International V6, Kaplan EL (ed). Edinburgh: Churchill Livingstone. 1983, pp 168–176.

33. Lever EG, Refetoff S, Straus II FH, Nguyen M, Kaplan EL: Coexisting thyroid and parathyroid disease – Are they related? Surgery 94: 893–900, 1983.

34. Edis AJ, Evans TC: High resolution real-time ultrasonography in the preoperative localization of parathyroid tumors. N Engl J Med 301: 532, 1979.

35. Doppman JL, Brennan MF, Koehler JQ, Marx SJ: Computed tomography for parathyroid localization. J Comput Assist Tomogr 1: 30, 1977.

36. Brennan MF, Doppman JL, Krudy AG, Marx SJ, Spiegel AM, Aurbach GD: Assessment of techniques for reoperative parathyroid gland localization in patients undergoing reoperation for hyperparathyroidism. Surgery 91: 6–11, 1982.

37. Saxe AW, Brennan MF: Strategy and technique of reopertive parathyroid surgery. Surgery 89: 417–423, 1981.

38. Thompson NW, Olsen WR, Hoffman GL: The continuing development of the technique of thyroidectomy. Surgery 73: 913–927, 1973.

39. Edis AJ, Linos DA, Kao PC: Parathyroid autotransplantation at the time of reoperation for persistent hyperparathyroidism. Surgery 88: 588, 1980.

40. Wells SA Jr, Gunnells CJ, Gutman RA, Shelburne JD, Schneider AB, Sherwood LM: The successful transplantation of frozen tissue in man. Surgery 81: 86, 1977.

41. Kaplan EL, Sugimoto J, Yang H, Fredland A: Postoperative hypoparathyroidism: diagnosis and

management. In: Surgery of the Thyroid and Parathyroids. Clinical Surgery International V6, Kaplan EL (ed). Edinburgh: Churchill Livingstone, 1983, pp 262–274.

42. Alvioli LV: The therapeutic approach to hypoparathyroidism Am J Med 57: 34, 1974.

43. Parfitt AM: Surgical, idiopathic and other varieties of parathyroid hormone-deficient hypoparathyroidism. In: Endocrinology, DeGroot LJ (ed). New York: Grune and Stratton, pp 755–768.

44. Porter RH, Cox BG, Heaney D, Hostetter TH, Stinebaugh BJ,Suki WN: Treatment of hypoparathyroid patients with chlorthalidone. N Engl J Med 298: 577–581, 1978.

45. Wang C-A: Parathyroid re-exploration: A clinical and pathological study of 112 cases. Ann Surg 186: 140–145, 1977.

10. Adrenocortical tumors

O. PETER SCHUMACHER

Adrenocortical nodules more than a centimeter in diameter are found in approximately 1.5–8.7% of unselected postmortem examinations [1, 2] and are more frequent in older people and those with high blood pressure. Benign nonfunctional adrenocortical tumors [3] are only rarely diagnosed during life but may be diagnosed more with the increasing use of CT scans [4, 5], particularly sector CT scans and abdominal ultrasound studies. Malignant nonfunctional tumors are also very infrequent, comprising only about 0.2% of all reported carcinomas [6].

Most adrenal tumors are described as benign or malignant or functional as opposed to nonfunctional. From an endocrinologist's point of view, patients with tumors that function are more likely to come to his attention than those that are nonfunctional simply because of the clinical expression. Patients who are more virilized are more likely to have carcinomas than patients who have evidence of excess cortisol production.

Functional tumors may cause hypertension, excess aldosterone production, excess catecholamines, Cushing's syndrome (excess cortisol production), and very rarely excess estrogen or hypoglycemia.

The excellent study by Bertagna and Orth [7] is a review of one of the larger clinical series in recent literature. This study emphasized that adrenal tumors occur throughout life, having a peak in the first decade and then another peak at 35 years for adenoma and 50 years for carcinoma. In their group there were no nonfunctional tumors occurring in children and most occurred in the 30–70 year age group. Relatively few of their patients were men; 4 out of 26 adenomas and 2 of the carcinomas occurred in men, but 7 of the 10 patients with nonfunctional carcinomas were men.

Most of their patients with functional tumors (as in other series) presented with Cushing's syndrome often associated with virilization. As mentioned early in their series, women with carcinomas might present with virilization alone. Two patients apparently had hypertension as the only possible endocrine manifestation.

Of the 36 patients who presented with Curshing's syndrome, 22 had an adenoma and 14 had a carcinoma. During that same time they had 136 patients with pituitary Cushing's syndrome and 23 with ectopic ACTH syndrome. The dura-

Santen, R.J. and Manni, A. (eds.), Diagnosis and management of endocrine-related tumors. ISBN 0-89838-636-5.
© 1984, Martinus Nijhoff Publishers, Boston. Printed in the Netherlands.

tion of symptoms before diagnosis was quite long (29 months) in patients with an adenoma and 14 months for a patient with a carcinoma.

The 30 patients with tumors who underwent high dose dexamethasone suppression (2 mg every 6 hours for 2 days) did not demonstrate suppression with dexamethasone. In reviewing the information obtained with such a test, one has to be aware of the fact that the secretion of steroids from an adrenal tumor may fluctuate a great deal from day to day and one must be certain to obtain at least a number of baseline assays in order to be certain of the baseline levels and the variations that would occur spontaneously. Most of our patients with adrenocortical tumors with Cushing's syndrome have had suppressed ACTH but at least one has had a normal ACTH level (132 pg/ml plasma) at 8:00 a.m. on repeated occasions.

None of the 23 patients with an adenoma or carcinoma reported by Bertagna and Orth [7] had an increase in urinary hydroxycorticoid levels on the day following metopirone. In the Bertagna study, ten patients with an adenoma responsed normally to an eight hour infusion of ACTH and none with carcinoma. In nine other patients with adenoma and ten with carcinoma, the 17 hydroxycorticoids increased by less than 50% after ACTH. They felt that approximately half the patients would respond to ACTH.

There was no difference in the plasma cortisol levels between the two groups and there was a lack of normal diurnal rhythm. Plasma cortisol was also not suppressed by low or high dose dexamethasone.

In their series, only one patient with adrenal carcinoma is still living, almost 17 years after surgery. Metastases or recurrence was found in the others 4 months to 11.7 years after surgery. In two patients treated with o,p'DDD clinically detectable tumor disappeared for 1–2½ years but in nine others treated there was only slight imporvement if any. Patients died in intervals from immediately to 16 years after surgery.

Tests of assessment of adrenocortical function

Plasma ACTH values [8] can be very helpful in assessing whether a patient has primarily a pituitary or ectopic source of ACTH or an adrenal source of the primary cause of excess cortisol production. We have had one case with a normal ACTH level (132 pg/ml), previously mentioned, in the presence of Cushing's syndrome secondary to an adrenal tumor. The explanation of this is not totally clear but it certainly represents something to consider clinically. It is assumed that the patients with ectopic ACTH syndrome [9] have much higher levels of ACTH than those with the ACTH coming from pituitary origin. There seems to be a number of patients with ectopic sources of ACTH, carcinoid, etc., who have relatively normal levels of ACTH and yet have an ectopic source. There is hope that it may be possible in the future to distinguish the ectopic ACTH as having a different protein structure than pituitary ACTH, but at the present time the clinical immunoassays are not able to detect these differences.

Cortisol can be measured by many different methods. Initially they were estimated by a measurement of 17 ketogenic steroids [10] and 17 hydroxycorticoids using the Porter-Silber reaction [11]. At the present time, however, it would seem best to measure cortisol production by the measurement of urinary free cortisol. One must be careful, however, that the fluorometric methods [12] may be distorted by a number of drugs, particularly aldactone and dyazide (spironolactone, triamterene, and hydrochlorothiazide). If a patient is essentially normal appearing who has urinary free cortisols 10–50 times the normal level, one has to be very suspicious that the assay was done by a fluormetric technique and the patient is taking a drug that interferes with the assay. Immunoassay, however, by Ruder *et al.* [13] certainly has been very helpful clinically to us and we have essentially stopped using any other method for both plasma and urinary free cortisols.

Urinary hydroxycorticoids steroids (17-OHCS) [10] have been used for a long period of time but are gradually becoming less useful. One advantage of it is that it does not deteriorate very rapidly in a receptacle without preservation. It also measures a number of other products in addition to that related to the breakdown of cortisol. It is particularly useful in a metopirone test where it also measures 11-dexoxycortisol production which is the precursor of cortisol. This increased production of 11-dexoxycortisol is due to the feedback mechanism of the pituitary stimulated by the decrease in cortisol production secondary to the metopirone block. We usually measure creatinine with 17 hydroxycorticoids in order to judge the adequacy of collection. Also the 17 hydroxycorticoids/creatinine ratio helps compensate for increased 17 hydroxycorticoids secondary to obesity.

Aldosterone is also best measured by immunassay method [14]. One must be very careful, however, in assessing the values of urinary aldosterone at the same time one measures the level of the amount of sodium in the urine and with consideration of the previous sodium in the diet of the patient.

17-ketosteroids. The oldest chemical method for measuring steroids was developed by Calahoe in 1940 employing the Zimmerman reaction [10]. Many hospitalization programs are no longer willing to pay for 17-ketosteroids because it is felt by many that it is no longer a useful test. We, however, have still felt that in certain stituations it may be useful, particularly in patients with adrenocortical carcinoma where these values may be unusually high. The 17-ketogenic steroid is one that is used very little any more but does have the advantage of measuring pregnantriol in addition to hydroxycorticoids.

Plasma cortisol levels. It may be very helpful to measure plasma cortisol levels [13] both in the morning and in the afternoon because most patients with adrenocortisol dysfunction do not have the normal diurnal variation. One must be careful, however, that patients with tumors may have great fluctuations in their steroid levels and this may be misinterpreted as a diurnal variation or suppression by dexamethasone when in actual fact it may be a normal spontaneous fluctuation of the tumor.

Dehydroepiandrosterone sulfate (DHEAS) [15] may be very useful in measuring adrenal androgen production because of its long plasma half life. Often this can be helpful in considering patients with what is called adrenal hirsutism and the stimulation to the hirsutism is mild adrenal hyperfunction. Measurements of DHEAS may be slightly elevated in patients with hirsutism whereas patients with adrenocortical tumor and particularly with carcinoma will be quite high.

Plasma 17 hydroxyprogesterone. In early detection of congenital adrenal hyperplasia, the measurement of the plasma 17 hydroxyprogesterone [16] can be most helpful and this is probably the best single test for this.

Tests of pituitary adrenal axis function

The most commonly used tests in our institution to assess adrenocortical reserve is the use of synthetic ACTH or Cortrosyn (Table 1). The test is typically done by obtaining a baseline plasma cortisol, giving cortrosyn 0.25 mg. intramuscularly and measuring the plasma cortisol at one half hour and again at one hour. If the patient is presumed to be normal, measurement of the level at an hour often is sufficient with a response above $30\,\mu g/24$ h after cortrosyn representing a normal response. A more careful assessment of adrenocortical reserve can be done by giving 40 units of ACTH every 12 h in continuous I.V. for two days. We collect a baseline urinary free cortisol or hydroxycorticoid and urine each 24 h of the ACTH infusion. In addition, we measure the plasma cortisol in the morning the infusion begins, at 8 hours, 24 hours, and 48 hours [17]. Typically, in a patient with normal pituitary adrenal function, the plasma cortisol will rise to above $60\,\mu g/ml$ and the urinary hydroxycorticoid will be greater than 20/mg/ 24 h. We usually place the patient on Florinef 0.1 mg a day and Decadron 0.5 mg twice a day during the baseline urine and during the days of the ACTH infusion. We have felt that it is very important to place the ACTH in 5% glucose and normal saline rather than just 5% glucose [18] because we have had a number of patients with Addison's disease who have developed marked hyponatremia when only given 5% glucose or 5% glucose and $^1/_4$ normal saline.

Patients with hypothyroidism or partially suppressed adrenal function, such as patients following removal of an adrenal tumor with cortisol production, will

Table 1. Cushing's syndrome diagnostic flow chart

In favor		Against
Urinary free cortisol elevated		Urinary free cortisol normal
Urinary hydroxicorticoids (OHS) elevated		Urinary hydroxcorticoids normal Hydroxycorticoid/creatinine ration normal
	Dexamethasone suppression 1.0 mgm at midnight	
Greater than 6.0 μgm%		Less than 2.0 μgm%
	0.5 mgm every six hours × 2 days	
Greater than 4.0 mgm/24 h		Less than 2.0 mgm/24 h
	Suppression with 2.0 mgm Dexamethasone every six hours for two days/urine/ 24 h	
Cushing's		Adrenal tumor vs ectopic
Greater than 50% suppression of urinary hydroxicorticoids		No suppression of urinary hydroxycorticoids
Normal ACTH		Low ACTH High ACTH
	Metopirone 750 mgm every four hours for two days	
Double urinary OHS/24 h		No response No response

have a partial response to such aggressive testing but often will not have a normal response for at least six months to a year.

Pituitary ACTH reserve. There are a number of tests that can be used to measure pituitary function. To measure pituitary ACTH reserve we have usually used the metopirone test. This test inhibits the enzyme that controls the final step between Compound S (11 Deoxycortisol) and Compound F (11-betahydroxylase). Giving metopirone produces a decrease in cortisol production which results, in a normal person, with an increase in ACTH which stimulates steroid biosynthesis. Because of the increase in ACTH, the adrenal is stimulated to make more 11-hydroxy-steroids (cortisol precursors) in an attempt to produce normal cortisol secretion. Since the 11-hydroxycorticoids are measured in the urine as hydroxycorticoids, the value goes up. One also can see an increase in 11-dexoxycortisol in the blood at the same time and many use this test instead of the urine.

The test is usually done by administering metopirone in oral dosage 750 mg every four hours for two days [19], collecting the baseline urine and the urine during the two days on metopirone. One modification of this test is to give 3 GMs of metopirone at midnight and measure the plasma 11-dexoxycortisol [20] in the morning. In most normal patients there is a marked rise in 11-dexoxycorticoid steroid when this is done [19]. Some authors feel that one should demonstrate a drop in plasma cortisol at the same time in order to confirm that there is sufficient stimulus to increase the plasma Compound S. We have not routinely done this except in patients on Dilantin or other drugs. It is not appropriate to place the patient on steroids while doing the metopirone test despite the fact that if a patient has borderline pituitary adrenal reserve it is possible that the patient will become ill from hypocortisolism during the test. The patient, therefore, should be carefully monitored if this is a clinical possibility and the test should be stopped with the administration of aggressive steroid therapy if this occurs.

Dexamethasone suppression tests (Table 1). There have been a number of suppression tests proposed over the years but most use the one originally described by Liddle [21]. This standard test is to give a low dose (0.5 mg every six hours for two days) and collect a urinary hydroxycorticoid and/or free cortisol on the second day. In a normal person the urinary hydroxycorticoids decrease to less than 2.5 mg per day on the second day of the study. Most patients with Cushing's syndrome will not suppress completely on the low dose of dexamethasone. When a high dose of dexamethasone is given (2 mg every six hours for eight doses), however, patients with pituitary Cushing's syndrome will have a definite suppression of their urinary assays secondary to this whereas patients with adrenal tumors do not. The screening tests for Cushing's syndrome that have been recently popularized employ a single 1 mg dose of dexamethasone at midnight with a plasma cortisol being drawn in the morning. The plasma cortisol is generally said to stay above $5 \mu g$. if the patient has Cushing's from whatever cause. We have had patients with Cushing's syndrome who have clearly suppressed below this level.

Adrenocortical tumors. There is little difference clinically between patients with adrenocortical tumors as compared with those with Cushing's disease. Patients with adrenal tumors, however, tend to have clinical evidence of excess cortisol production but also have, in addition- some other feature such as virilization or excess aldosterone production more frequently than in patients with Cushing's disease on a pituitary basis. It is usually to be anticipated that when Cushing's syndrome is present in children, their growth would be suppressed. The fact that most patients with adrenocortical tumors have some androgen production along with the cortisol tends to accelerate the bone age in most children with adrenal tumors even though they may have clinical Cushing's syndrome [22].

Virilization, however, may be very subtle particularly because mild hirsutism is a common problem. We have had two patients who have received steroid therapy for 'adrenal hirsutism' who have turned out to have adrenocortical tumors and one with carcinoma. In view of this, one must be careful to exclude adrenocortical tumors before considering therapy with steroids for hirsutism.

Typically, however, patients with adrenocortical tumors have some virilization in addition to simple hirsutism. They have voice change, temporal balding, increased clitoral size, increased muscular mass, etc. At times, however, this excess androgen will only express itself in increased libido, in its early stages. The distinction between hirsutism and virilism is a most important clinical one and can be very useful in deciding whether the patient has a serious illness or not.

Drugs with potential use in the care of patients with adrenal tumors. A number of drugs have been shown to have an affect in controlling the production of adrenal steroids. Metopirone, as mentioned earlier, definitely decreases the production of Compound F. The effect of this drug is very short lived (a few hours) and if given continuously as therapy for adrenocortical hyperfunction, the adrenal may override it under the stimulation of increased ACTH. In view of this the long-term affect of metopirone by itself often does not control adrenal hyperfunction.

At the present time this drug is often used in conjunction with aminoglute-thimide. The dose we often use is metopirone 500 mg four times a day along with aminoglutethimide 250 mg four times a day. These two drugs together seem to be effective therapy. In recent times, we have prepared some of our patients with adrenocortical hyperfunction with this drug therapy in order to decrease post-operative morbidity and, we hope, mortality. In patients with adrenocortical tumors, however, when often the clinical symptoms are mild and there is more virilization, we have not delayed surgery. We have been particularly concerned about our inability to always detect whether the tumor represented an adenoma or a carcinoma preoperatively.

The third drug which is often used in patients with adrenocortical tumors, particularly carcinoma, is o,p'DDD (Mitotane or Lysodin). This drug was orig-inally demonstrated as the cause of adrenal necrosis in dogs [23]. A number of our patients have experienced permanent adrenocortical dysfunction with o,p'DDD even after it is stopped. Others have found that there can be recovery of adrenal function after cessation of o,p'DDD. It has been thought in the past that o,p'DDD affected the fasciculata and not the glomerulosa. In our patients who have been on this drug for a long period of time, there seems to be definite clinical and laboratory evidence of aldosterone insufficiency.

Spironolactone. Aldosterone antagonism with spironolactone can be used in some patients with hyperaldosteronism.

Evaluation of patients. The diagnosis of Cushing's syndrome is managed pri-marily by the clinical suspicion: the moon face with relatively little weight gain, thin skin, muscular weakness, osteoporosis, etc. Frequently patients have had a marked change in their personality, restlessness, manic behavior which can often be illicited from the patient's family after careful questioning. Since patients with adrenocortical tumors often excrete some excess androgen in addition to the excess cortisol, the muscular weakness may not be as severe as it is with pituitary or ectopic sources of Cushing's syndrome.

Once the suspicion of Cushing's syndrome is present, we often measure urinary free cortisol correlating this with urinary creatinine in order to ascertain the accuracy of collection. We usually do this collection as an outpatient because of the problems which multiple shifts in hospital and delay of laboratory reporting. Depending upon our suspicion, we move to small and/or large dose Decadron suppression followed occasionally by a metopirone study. We often correlate the plasma cortisol suppression with the urinary assay data. We rarely use an ACTH stimulation test. In the present state of the radiologic technology, most adrenocortical tumors can be found by the present CT scans. Pituitary tumors, however, are frequently not seen in patients with pituitary origin of the excess ACTH and CT scans frequently are interpreted as showing tumor when none are present [24, 25].

Adrenalectomy. If it is ascertained that an adrenal tumor is the primary problem, our adrenal surgeons use either the anterior or posterior approach once they have assessed the presence of a tumor with a CT scan. We have gradually come to favor the flank incision because of the decreased morbidity. We usually give the patient 200 mg of cortisone acetate intramuscularly 24–36 hours before surgery and another 200 mg of cortisone acetate intramuscularly 12 hours before surgery and another dose the morning of surgery. We have elected to plan the first injection far ahead of the surgery because of the delay in absorption. Postoperatively we then give another 100 mg of cortisone intramuscularly the day following surgery with 100 mg a day for a number of days until the patient is able to retain fludis and take medication orally. We then change to oral cortisone, perhaps 25 mg every 8 hours along with the addition of Florinef 0.1 mg a day as we taper the steroid dosage. We often send the patient home from the hospital on what is presumably an excess of cortisone because of the steroid withdrawal symptoms that are frequently a problem at this point. In a few weeks we gradually taper the dose of steroids getting closer to a total of $37\frac{1}{2}$ mg of cortisone acetate a day. We tend to use cortisone acetate rather than prednisone but other authors have used other steroids. As mentioned, in the immediate postoperative period the major problem is steroid withdrawal from the marked steroid excess. The greater the severity of the Cushing's syndrome preoperatively, the slower one must be in withdrawing the steroids because of the symptomatic difficulty with steroid withdrawal even though the patient does not have measureable andrenocortical insufficiency. Most of these patients get quite depressed during this time and need to be supported both emotionally and physically during this time. We frequently tell patients they will not feel 'normal' for at least a year.

Isotopes and adrenal gland imaging. Beierwaltes and his group have done extensive work with the scanning of the adrenal gland, both in cortisol producing tumors and in pheochromocytoma. Dr. Beierwaltes has successfully used 6-beta[131] I-iodomethyl-19-nor cholesterol for adrenocortical imaging [26, 27, 28,

29]. He has found that when there is a functioning adrenal tumor on one side, there is suppression of the function as measured by this technique on the other side. He has found this very helpful in distinguishing between bilateral hyperplasia from Cushing's Disease as opposed to adrenocortical tumors causing Cushing' Syndrome [30].

In the area of pheochromocytoma, he has been able to localize the tumors and also ectopic locations [31, 32].

It is also my understanding that Dr. Beierwaltes has successfully treated malignant pheochromocytoma with the use of the labelled material (pers. commun.).

Others have not found this as useful but according to Dr. Beierwaltes, there are 130 centers now using his material for adrenal schanning so that this may become more popular in the future.

Adrenocortical suppression postoperatively. It has been clearly shown that patients with Cushing's syndrome due to adrenal tumors have marked adrenal suppression for a considerable period of time postoperatively. We have not felt that giving small doses of ACTH intermittently in order to prime the adrenal was worthwhile and have not done so, simply tapering the dose of steroids gradually to a reasonable level and allowing the patient's clinical symptoms of Cushing's to disappear. We then cut the steroids even further depending on this response.

The patient should always receive increased doses of steroids during any major medical or surgical stress. Others [33] recommend that steroid therapy should be given in a single daily dose in order to minimize the possibility of further suppression. We, however, have simply followed the patient and if they don't have symptomatic adrenocartical insufficiency, we gradually withdraw the dose of steroids.

Adrenal hyperplasia. Although in most instances the differential diagnosis between adrenal tumor and congenital hyperplasia is rather clearcut, some patient's diagnosis can be difficult. Usually the onset of the clinical syndrome is at birth even if the patient is discovered at age 5 or 6. Most of the children that have a delay in diagnosis have had a marked increase in growth which goes all the way back to birth. Some patients with adrenocortical hyperplasia do not suppress initially with steroids. We have had one patient who had adrenal hyperplasia, first treated at age 12, who required large doses of steroids equivalent to greater than 100 mg of cortisone a day for more than a week before the steroid levels fell to a reasonably acceptable level. The patient clearly had congenital adrenal hyperplasia. Unfortunately, occasionally patients with congenital adrenal hyperplasia will develop an adrenocortical carcinoma in later life.

One problem that we have had from a clinical point of view has been the patients with what is sometimes called familial hirsutism or adrenal hirsutism. As mentioned earlier, these patients have been placed on steroids and then have been seen later with mild clinical Cushing's syndrome. It has been difficult in those patients to sort out clinically whether this syndrome is on the basis of the steroids used in treatment or whether the patient has an adrenocortical cause of hypercortisolism. In view of this we have felt that careful follow-up of patients that are presumed to have mild adrenal overactivity causing hirsutism is most important. We have also felt that a modified dexamethasone suppression test would be wise initially to be certain that one is not dealing with an unsuspected problem.

The use of o,p'DDD in adrenal cancer. o,p'DDD was originally observed by Nelson and Woodard [23] to cause necrosis and atrophy of the adrenal cortex when DDT was administered to dogs. Subsequent studies by Cueto and Brown [34] showed the effective constituent to be the o,p'DDD isomer, commercial name Lysodin or adopted name Mitotane. The drug has been useful in prolonging the survival time in a considerable number of patients as reported by Becker, Bergenstal, Downing, Hoffman, etc. [35–40]. Our experience was much like that of others in the sense that it would often produce a marked decrease in steroid production, but rarely a marked decrease in tumor size. There is evidence that o,p'DDD actually may interfere with the assay of the steroids themselves rather than just a decrease in steroid production. It also seemed quite clear that once a patient had definite metastases one could rarely hope for a cure from this very aggressive form of therapy [41, 42].

The life history of untreated inoperable adrenocortical carcinoma was reported by McFarland [43] to be short nearly without exception, being on the average 2.9 months from the time of diagnosis. It was 2.2. months in the hormonal group compared to 3.8 in the nonhormonal type. The mean survival of 107 of 115 inoperable adrenocortical carcinoma patients reported by Lubitz [44] was 8.4 months using o,p'DDD. There were no cures. By experience, it often seemed to slow down the markedly rapid rate of progression in adrenocortical metastases but did not really have a marked effect on the disease. The doses that were usually required to have some effect were quite large and produced significant side effects such as nausea, vomiting, psychosis, depression, or weakness.

Discussion

It is generally accepted practice to prescribe o,p'DDD for patients not surgically curable or with evidence of clinicially advancing disease. We suggest that earlier treatment is desirable and the use of o,p'DDD be considered postoperatively if there is uncertainty about residual disease and seeding especially if the tumor has clearly extended into the vena cava or the periadrenal tissue. Our results are markedly better than those described in earlier reports. Variations in growth rate of adrenal cancer makes it difficult to determine worthwhile survival statistics. In our series, in the five of eleven patients (Table 2) without recurrent tumor postoperatively treated with o,p'DDD the average time of follow-up is greater than 91 months. In patients where metastasis did occur postoperatively, the mean survival time is 27 months. There are two probable cures, Case 1 and 2. One of the patients has survived $15^1/_{12}$ years and the other $12^3/_4$ years. Two patients, Cases 3 and 4, have survived longer than 4 years without a recurrence to date. The patient, Case 5, died as a result of an auto accident without recurrence demonstrable postmortum 3 months after initiation of therapy. Case 6 died at $3^3/_4$ years with a lymph node and pulmonary metastases that were hormonally functioning, that occurred after the o,p'DDD had been stopped. This patient had been on o,p'DDD for $2^1/_2$ years without measureable recurrence. Case 7 had known adrenocortical carcinoma recurrence at the time the o,p'DDD was stopped and the patient died shortly thereafter. Patient 8 died of progressive metastases once the o,p'DDD was stopped because of gastro-intestinal toxicity. This patient died of widespread metastases involving the lungs, liver, and vagina 13 months after initiation of therapy. She received intermittent 5-fluorouracil once the DDD was stopped. Case 9 had rapidly advancing adrenocortical carcinoma and died with 7 months of cerebral metastatases. Case 10 died of liver metastatases at 8 months and this patient had received concomitant Cytoxan and Adriamycin. Case 11 had o,p'DDD stopped at 11 months because of psychosis and paranoia which cleared after cessation of o,p'DDD. At the time there was no measureable evidence of a recurrence. She died a little more than three years later of liver metastases.

In reviewing our cases, once there was evidence of advancing disease, increasing the dose of o,p'DDD did not seem to have any measureable affect on the tumor.

For protection from adrenal insufficiency, all patients received cortisone acetate and Florinef except during the study periods when dexamethasone was used. Clinically Florinef was used because of evidence of adrenocorticoid insufficiency as manifested by rising potassium. Two patients were studied with the results found in Table 3. Both cases showed a subnormal response of aldosterone to corticotropin on a normal salt diet.

Pheochromocytoma is a rare cause of secondary hypertension but the diagnosis is important. Undetected it is almost always fatal whereas hypertension is usually cureable by resection of the tumor. About 1,000 cases are found annually in the United States.

Pharmacologic tests. In the presence of typical signs and symptoms of pheochromocytoma, the diagnosis can be confirmed by either biochemical or pharmacologic means, or both. According to the recent work of Bravo [45], the demonstration of increased levels of plasma catecholamines should suffice to confirm the diagnosis. A major problem is that the patient needs to be off all drugs for a considerable period of time since some of the drugs will raise the test

Table 2. Clinical and laboratory data from eleven cases of adrenocortical carcinoma treated with o,p'DDD at the Cleveland Clinic

Case no.	Sex	Age (yrs.)	Endocrine status	Disease duration	Meas-urable	Findings at surgery Extent of metastasis	o,p'DDD How long	Why stopped	Survival Start of o,p'DDD
1	M	69	None	1 week	0	Ruptured adrenal CA with metastasis all over periadrenal fatty tissue	$6^1/_6$ yrs.	No recurrence	$15^1/_2$ yrs
2	M	$3^1/_3$	Virilism	2 mos.	+	Thought not curative with disease adherence to liver and venous invasion (C.C.)	$2^1/_2$ yrs.	No recurrence	$12^3/_4$ yrs
3	F	48	None	0	0	Left adrenal CA invading periadrenal fat	1 yr.	No recurrence	$5^1/_2$ yrs
4	F	23	Cushing's Syndrome	2 yrs.	+	Large 2,780 Cm left adrenal CA with marked vascular invasion and tumor nodule, either extention or lymph node metastasis	4 yrs.	4 yrs. Stopped because of cerebellar toxicity	4 yrs.
5	F	52	None	2 weeks	0	Right adrenal CA with periadrenal fat invasion	3 mo.	Accidental Death	3 ml. No Mets.
6	F	30	Cushing's Syndrome	3 yrs.	0	Left adrenal CA extended to fat and approx. line of resection	$2^1/_6$ yrs.	No recurrence Recurrence 10/78 Recurrence 4/79	$3^3/_4$ yrs. Abdominal Mets.
7	F	44	None	6 mo.	+	Large right suprarenal mass invaded IVC, right hemidiaphragm and liver	$4^1/_6$ yrs.	Stopped because extent of disease and refusal of further therapy	$4^1/_4$ yrs (died) Abdominal Mets.
8	F	71	Cushing's Syndrome	8 mo.	+	Left adrenal CA and multiple pulmonary nodules	5 mo.	GI intolerance	13 ml. (died) Pulmonary mets.
9	F	27	Cushing's Syndrome	3 mo.	+	Huge right kidney and adrenal with angio invesion	7 mo.	Died	7 mo. Cerebral mets.
10	F	53	Virilism	18 yrs.	+	Right adrenal CA metastatic liver	3 mo.	Died	8 mo. Liver mets.
11	F	45	Cushing's	3 mo.	+	Right adrenal CA with liver metastasis	11 mo.	Psychosis paranoia	$3^1/_6$ yrs (died) Liver mets.

Table 3. Effect of ACTH infusion on aldosterone in two cases

	Date	Plasma Adosterone ng/100 ml		Urinary Aldosterone μg/100 ml	
		Before ACTH	On ACTH for one hour	Before ACTH	On ACTH for one hour
CASE 3	2/7/79	10.1	8.1	1.4	2.1
	11/8/79	4.1	4.1	–	–
CASE 7	4/19/78	7.8	11.3	–	–
	10/14/78	9.3	10.9	–	–

results and some will lower them. Nevertheless, in the recent work by Bravo the morning resting plasma catecholamines is almost always clearly above the normal range in patients with pheochromocytoma and essentially always in the normal range in patients with essential hypertension.

The best test to suppress borderline plasma norepinephrine levels is the use of clonidine. The clonidine test is described in the Bravo paper [46]. The other tests that may be useful but have been used much less in the recent past are the various stimulation tests. The test that is primarily used now is the glucogon stimulation test. Provocative tests, however, should not be performed when the diastolic blood pressure is equal or greater than 110 mm of mercury or the patient has concommitant vascular problems.

The localization of pheochromocytoma. In the past many different studies were considered and used to determine the anatomic location of the pheochromocytoma once the diagnosis was made. Some authors have recommended venous catheterization particularly of the vena cava. In one of our patients [47] the tumor was found at the bifurcation of the carotid and the tumor was localized by venous sampling in the jugular vein. Now, however, the use of CT scanning should essentially eliminate most of the arteriographic and other studies necessary. Most of the CT scans can find tumors that are 1 cm or greater even though they are in an atypical location. The use of ^{131}I iodobenzylguanidine, a radioactive compound selectively taken up by adrenergic cells, has been used by some authors to find small tumors [30].

Management of pheochromocytoma. The only real cure of pheochromocytoma is surgical removal of the tumor. Since about 10% of the tumors are multiple, careful examination of the abdomen during surgery is most important. Preoperative preparation requires adrenergic blockade and volume repletion. Phenoxybenzamine, in doses of 20–60 mg per day was recommended by Bravo to successfully control the blood pressure. Bravo feels that beta adrenergic blocking agents should be withheld unless tachycardia and/or arrhythmia are present. Lidocaine and other antiarrhythimic drugs can be used to control arrhythmia.

During the operation, intra-arterial pressure should be monitored through a catheter and a large artery. The blood pressure rises can be managed with infusion of sodium nitroprusside.

Postoperatively the most common problem is hypotension which can be the result of either bleeding or decreased blood volume. It is important to consider the possibility of associated diseases such as Von Hippel-Lindau disease, Von Recklinghausen's neurofibromatosis, Sipple's syndrome (MEN Type IIa), muco-cutaneous neuromata (MEN Type IIb). We have also had patients with pheochromocytoma that produced ACTH causing Cushing's syndrome.

Primary aldosteronism. The author recommends review of the paper by Bravo et al. [14] reviewing a prospective study of 80 patients with primary aldosteronism for a true assessment of the clinical syndrome.

In the study, the demonstration of excessive aldosterone production after three days of salt loading provide the best sensitivity (96%) and best specificity (93%) in identifying patients with primary aldosterone. As they reported, severe persistent hypokalemia, increased 18-hydroxycorticosterone values, and an anomalous postural decrease in the plasma aldosterone concentration, when present, provided the best indicators of the presence of an adenoma. The best localization procedure was the measurement of adrenal venous plasma aldosterone concentration when this was possible. The presumptive diagnosis of primary aldosteronism was suspected in 32 cases because of spontaneous hypokalemia and in 43 because of moderately severe hypokalemia (less than 3 mcq/l produced by conventional doses of potassium wasting diuretic agents. Five, however, had no previous history of hypokalemia.

Localization procedures. All patients in the Bravo series [46] had adrenal venous sampling for plasma aldosterone and cortisol followed by adrenal venography. Catheterization of the adrenal vein on the left side was successful but failed on the right in 30 patients (38%). Adrenal computer tomography and bilateral adrenal vein sampling with venography were successfully performed in 26 patients. Results in these patients form the basis for comparison in their series. Adrenal venography and adrenal computer tomographic scan identified the site of the lesion in 73 and 83% of the cases. The smallest tumor visualized by adrenal venography measured 1.5 cm while the computed tomographic scan identified tumors as small as 0.8 cm. Adrenal venous sampling for plasma aldosterone concentration accurately localized the site of the lesion in all patients studied. The practical problem from the standpoint of adrenal venography is the inability frequently to get into the right adrenal vein because of the variation in anatomy.

References

1. Symington T: Functional Pathology of the Human Adrenal Gland. Baltimore: Williams & Wilkins, 1969, p 151.
2. Hedeland H, Ostberg G, Hokfelt B: On the prevalence of adrenocritical adenomas in an autopsy material in relation to hypertension and diabetes. Acta Med Scand 184: 211, 1968.
3. Shamma AH, Goddard JW, Sommers SC: A study of the adrenal status in hypertension. J Chronic Dis 8: 587, 1958.
4. Prinz RA, Brooks MH, Churchill R, et al.: Incidental asymptomatic adrenal masses detected by computed tomographic scanning: Is operation required? JAMA 248: 701, 1982.
5. Siekavizza JL, Bernardino ME, Sammaan NA; Suprarenal mass and its differential diagnosis. Urology 18: 625, 1981.
6. Lipsett MB, Hertz R, Ross GT: Clinical and pathophysiologic aspects of adrenocortical carcinoma. Am J Med 35:374, 1963.
7. Bertagna C, Orth DN: Clinical and laboratory findings and results of therapy in 58 patients with adrenocortical tumors admitted to a singly medical center (1951 to 1978). Amer J Med 71: 855, 1981.
8. Yalow RS, Glick SM, Roth J, Berson SA: Radioimmunoassay of plasma ACTH. J Clin Endo Metab 24: 1219, 1964.
9. Liddle GW, Nicholson WE, et al.: Clinical and laboratory studies of ectopic humoral syndromes. Recent Progr Horm Res 25: 238, 1969.
10. Appleby JI, Gibson G, Norymberski JK, Stubbs RD: Indirect analysis of corticosteroids. Biochem J 60: 453, 1955.
11. Porter CC, Silber RH: A quantitative color reaction for cortisone and related 17, 21 dihydroxy-20 ketosteroids. J Biol Chem 185: 201, 1950.
12. Mattingly D: A simple fluorimetric method for the estimation of free 11-hydroxycorticoids in human plasma. J Clin Path 15: 374, 1962.
13. Ruder HJ, Guy RL, Lipsett MB: A radioimmunoassay for cortisol in plasma and urine. J Clin Endo Metab 35: 219, 1972.
14. Bravo EL, Tarazi RC, Dustan HP, et al.: The changing clinical spectrum of primary aldosteronism. Amer J Med 74:641, 1983.
15. Buster JE, Abraham CE: Radioimmunoassay of plasma dehydroepiandrosterone sulphate. Analytical letters 5: 543, 1972.
16. Youssefnejadian E, Florensa E, Collins WP, Sommerville IF: Radioimmunoassay of 17-hydroxy-progesterone. Steroids 20: 773, 1972.
17. Rose LI, William GH, Jagger PI, Lauler DP: The 48-hour adrenocorticotropin infusion test for adrenocortical insufficiency. Ann Int Med 73: 49, 1970.
18. Sheeler LR, Schumacher OP: Letter to the Editor: Hyponatremia during ACTH infusions. Ann Int Med 90: 709, 1979.
19. Liddle GW, Estep HL, et al.: Clinical application of a new test of pituitary reserve. J Clin Endo 19: 875, 1969.
20. Newsome HH, Clements AS, Borum EH: The simultaneous assay of cortisol, corticosterone, 11-Deoxycortisol, and cortisone in human plasma. J Clin Endo Metab 34: 743, 1972.
21. Liddle GW: Test of pituitary-adrenal suppressibility in the diagnosis of Cushing's syndrome. J Clin Endo 20: 1539, 1960.
22. Hayles AB, Hahn HB, Sprague RG, et al.: Hormone-secreting tumors of the adrenal cortex in children. Pediatrics 37: 19, 1966.
23. Nelson AA, Woodard G: Severe adrenal cortical atrophy (cytotoxic) and hepatic damage produced in dogs by feeding 2, 2-bis (parachlorophenyl 1-1, 1-dichloroethane (DDP or TDE). Arch Pathol 48: 387, 1949.
24. Chambers EF, Turski PA, LaMasters D, Newton TH: Regions of low density in the contrast-

enhanced pituitary gland: normal and pathologic processes. Radiology 144: 109, 1982.

25. Swartz JD, Russell KB, Basile BA, et al.: High resolution computed tomographic appearance of the intrasellar contents in women of childbearing age. Radiology 147: 115, 1983.

26. Beierwaltes WH, Lieberman LM, Ansari AN, Nishiyama H: Visualization of human adrenal glands in vivo by scintillation scanning. JAMA 216: 275, 1971.

27. Lieberman LM, Beierwaltes WH, Conn JW, et al.: Diagnosis of adrenal disease by visualization of human adrenal glands with $_{131}$I-19 iodocholesterol. N Engl J Med 285, 1387, 1971.

28. Morita R, Lieberman LM, Beierwaltes WH, et al.: Percent uptake of $_{131}$I-radioactivity in the adrenal from radioiodinated cholester. J Clin Endo Metab 37: 36, 1972.

29. Sarkar SD, Beierwaltes WH, Ice RD, et al.: A new and superior adrenal scanning agent, NP-59. J Nuc Med 16: 1038, 1975.

30. Schteingart DE, Seabold JE, Gross MD, Swanson DP: Iodocholesterol adrenal tissue uptake and imaging in adrenal neoplasms. J Clin Endo Metab 52: 1156, 1981.

31. Wieland DM, Brown LE, Tobes MX, et al.: Imaging the primate adrenal medullae with [123$_1$] and [131$_1$] meta-iodobenzylguanidine; concise communication. J Nuc Med 22: 358, 1981.

32. Wieland DM, Wu JI, Brown LE, et al.: Radiolabeled adrenergic neuronblocking agents; adrenomedullary imaging with [131$_1$] iodobenzylguanidine. J Nuc Med 21: 349, 1980.

33. Liddle GW: The Adrenals. Textbook of Endocrinology, Sixth Edition, Robert H. Williams. Philadelphia: WB Saunders Co., pp 249–292.

34. Cueto C, Brown JHU: Biological studies of an adrenocorticolytic agent and the isolation of the active components. Arch Int Med 138: 301, 1978.

35. Becker D, Schumacher OP: o,p'DDD therapy in invasive adrenocortical carcinoma. Ann Int Med 82: 677, 1975.

36. Bergenstal DM, Hertz R, Lipsett MS, Moy RH: Chemotherapy of adrenocortical cancer with o,p'DDD. Ann Int Med 53: 672, 1960.

37. Downing V, Eule J, Juseby RA: Regression of an adrenal cortical carcinoma and its neovascular bed following Mitotane therapy: A case report. Cancer: 34: 1882, 1974.

38. Hoffman DL, Mattox VR: Treatment of adrenocortical carcinoma with o,p'DDD. Med Clin N A 56: 999, 1972.

39. Hutter AM, Kayhole DE: Adrenocortical carcinoma – results of treatment with o,p'DDD in 138 patients. Am J Med 41: 581, 1966.

40. Newton MA, Laragh JH: Effect of corticotropin on aldosterone excretion and plasma renin in normal subjects in essential hypertension and in primary aldosteronism. J Clin Endo 28: 1006, 1968.

41. Halmi KA, Lascari AD: Conversion of virilization to feminization in a young girl with adrenal carcinoma. Cancer 27: 931, 1971.

42. Ostruni JA, Roginsky MS: Metastatic adrenal carcinoma – documented cure with combined chemotherapy. Arch Int Med 135: 1257, 1975.

43. MacFarlane DA: Cancer of the adrenal cortex – the natural history, prognosis and treatment in a study of fifty-five cases. Ann Royal Coll of Surg of Engl 23: 155, 1958.

44. Lubitz JA, Freeman L, Okun R: Mitotane use in inoperable adrenal cortical carcinoma. JAMA 223: 1109, 1973.

45. Bravo EL: The clinical values of plasma catecholamine measurement. Lab Mgmt, 1982.

46. Bravo EL: Pheochromocytoma: current concepts in diagnosis, localization, and management. Primary Care 10: 75, 1983.

11. Diagnosis and treatment of 'insulinoma'*

STEFAN S. FAJANS and AARON I. VINIK

1. Introduction

Insulin-secreting pancreatic islet cell tumors and other forms of organic hyperinsulinism causing fasting and postprandial hypoglycemia are not common disorders that afflict a large portion of any physician's practice. The fact of the matter is that they are rare disorders. However, endocrinologists continue to see patients by referral in whom the proper diagnosis had been delayed because of a mistaken diagnosis of functional hypoglycemia or other disorders followed by inappropriate therapy for years. The advent of more precise definitions of pancreatic islet cell physiology and of expanded techniques for the study in man, have facilitated a more dependable, simpler and sometimes earlier diagnosis of 'insulinoma' and other forms of organic hyperinsulinism. Further, advances have been made in the pre-operative localization of insulin-producing islet cell tumors and in the preoperative differentiation of islet cell tumors from other forms of organic hyperinsulinism. In this contribution we will omit a discussion of the spontaneous hypoglycemias which occur in infancy and childhood.

2. Characteristics of symptom complex of spontaneous hypoglycemia

The symptom complex of spontaneous hypoglycemia has four general characteristics. First there is periodicity of symptoms, spells or attacks at very specific times of the day, but they may occur at irregular intervals. Symptoms occur either in the fasting state (after an overnight fast or more than 5–6 hours after the last meal), or postprandially two to four hours after meals. In many patients with organic hyperinsulinism, symptoms may occur both in the fasting and postprandial states. The patient who has symptoms of a chronic unremitting nature or has symptoms within minutes to one hour after ingestion of food or a carbohyratecontaining drink is unlikely to be symptomatic due to hypoglycemia. The second characteristic of the symptom complex of spontaneous hypoglycemia is the

* Supported in part by U.S. Public Health Service Grant AM-00888; NIH-5 M01 RR-42 General Clinical Research Centers; and Michigan Diabetes Research and Training Center Grant 5-P60-AM20572.

Santen, R.J. and Manni, A. (eds.), Diagnosis and management of endocrine-related tumors. ISBN 0-89838-636-5.
© *1984, Martinus Nijhoff Publishers, Boston. Printed in the Netherlands.*

repetitive nature of complaints. The constellation of symptoms is usually similar in any given patient, but the type of symptoms may differ from patient to patient. The third characteristic of the symptom complex is the ease of confirmation of a low plasma concentration of glucose if symptoms are indeed due to hypoglycemia, particularly in patients with organic or fasting hypoglycemia. However the relationship between the degree of hypoglycemia and onset of symptoms is not always consistent. In an occasional patient with postabsorptive hypoglycemia it may be difficult to document a relationship between symptoms and low blood glucose concentration because of the transient nature of hypoglycemia. A fourth characteristic of the symptom complex is the fact that administration of readily absorbed carbohydrate or injected glucose will usually relieve syptoms due to hypoglycemia promptly or prevent symptoms from progressing. Patients who have symptoms that are relieved by the ingestion of foods containing protein and fat only (cheese, meat, nuts) or have very slow improvement after a sugar-containing drink, are unlikely to have a hypoglycemic disorder.

3. Symptoms of hypoglycemia

Symptoms of hypoglycemia that occur in any given patient vary with the rate of decline of plasma glucose levels, the degree of hypoglycemia, the duration of hypoglycemia and with the variable susceptibility of the patient's sympathetic and central nervous systems. Symptoms may be due to activation of the autonomic nervous system including the release of epinephrine or they may be due to central nervous system glucopenia or due to involvement of both branches of the nervous systems. Symptoms due to adrenergic stimulation are usually associated with a rapid decline in plasma glucose to levels below fasting. These symptoms consist of sweating, flushing, pallor, shaking, tremulousness, tachycardia, palpitations, anxiety, nervousness, restlessness, weakness, fatigue, hunger, nausea and vomiting. Symptoms due to hyperepinephrinemia are not specific for hypoglycemia. Any condition and state which may be associated with the release of epinephrine may produce similar symptomatology. Symptoms of central nervous system glucopenia result from decreased uptake of glucose and decreased utilization of oxygen by the brain. They may occur when the decline in plasma glucose levels is gradual and slow, or when hypoglycemia is severe or prolonged, or under both circumstances. There is a gradient of sensitivity of the nervous system to glucopenia, which parallels the hierarchial levels of central nervous system function. Cerebral cortex and cerebellum are generally affected first, followed by basal ganglia, thalamus and hypothalamus, proceeding through midbrain, brain stem, spinal cord, and ganglia to peripheral nerves. Symptoms due to neuroglucopenia include headache, disturbances of vision as blurring of vision or diplopia, lethargy, yawning, faintness, lassitude, dizzy spells, restlessness, irritability, difficulty with speech and thinking, and inability to concentrate. This phase of dimished cerebral function may be subtle. Patients may not recognize these symptoms or misinterpret them as fatigue, particularly if they are not preceded or accompanied by symptoms secondary to autonomic nervous system activation. Other symptoms may be agitation, confusion, amnesia, somnolence, syncope, stupor, prolonged sleep, loss of consciousness, and coma. There may be twitching, convulsions, 'epilepsy' and bizarre neurological signs, motor as well as sensory in nature. Transient hemiplegia has occurred. Personality changes characterized by irrational behavior, aggressive behavior, outbursts of temper or bizarre and psychotic behavior have been seen. Repeated severe and prolonged hypoglycemic episodes may lead to a decrease in intellectual ability, although permanent central nervous system damage is rare in the adult. An infrequent manifestation of neuroglucopenia is hypothermia; hyperthermia and pyrexia have been reported as well. If the decline in plasma concentrations of glucose is rapid, profound and prolonged, the symptoms may be those due to both activation of the sympathetic nervous system as well as due to decreased cerebral glucose utilization. In elderly patients, with underlying cerebrovascular insufficiency, hypoglycemia may produce focal neurologic signs, simulating cerebrovascular accidents or cerebral metastases. Focal signs also occur in young patients without known cerebrovascular insufficiency.

Thus, the symptoms of hypoglycemia are varied and not specific. However, the demonstration of a low plasma concentration during the occurrence of symptoms compatible with hypoglycemia, and prompt relief of symptoms by correction of biochemical hypoglycemia, i.e., Whipple's Triad, constitute good evidence that the symptoms are indeed caused by hypoglycemia. (For definition of biochemical hypoglycemia see 8.1.1.1.) Not only in patients with postabsorptive (reactive) but occasionally also in patients with fasting hypoglycemia due to organic hyperinsulinism, symptoms of hypoglycemia subside without carbohydrate administration because of a spontaneous rise in blood glucose concentration. This may be due to fluctuation in insulin secretion by the tumor with corresponding fluctuations in hyperinsulinism and/or due to activation of counterregulatory mechanism.

A few patients with recurrent and protracted periods of severe hypoglycemia due to hyperinsulinemia caused by insulinomas, develop a syndrome which consists of the development of motor and sensory symptoms of neuropathy [1]. Characteristic findings are those of a predominantly or entirely motor peripheral neuropathy, which is distal and symmetrical. Upper limb involvement is more frequent and more severe than lower limb involvement. There is weakness associated with prominent distal muscle wasting but fasciculations are observed in only one-quarter of the patients. Motor nerve conduction velocities may be decreased. Painful or disagreeable distal paresthesias are common without being accompanied by objective signs of sensory disturbance. Among the more than 1000 patients reported with insulinomas, only 28 such patients have been reported [1]. The patients have a history of frequent and severe hypoglycemia manifested by disturbances in cerebral function, although permanent cerebral dysfunction is usually minimal or absent.

Electromyographic and nerve conduction studies performed are indicative of axonal peripheral nerve damage. Detailed analysis of nerve histology in one patient showed features indicative of axonal neuropathy. Damage to anterior horn cells and dorsal ganglia cells has not been ruled out. Jaspan et al. [1] have designated this syndrome as a 'hypoglycemia neuropathy' since they believe that it is hypoglycemia rather than hyperinsulinemia which leads to nerve damage.

4. Metabolic control of glucose homeostasis

4.1 Factors controlling blood glucose homeostasis in the fasting state

A 70 kg person generally requires about 2000 kilo calories (kcal) per day. Approximately 30% of that requirement must be in the form of glucose because the central nervous system, kidneys and adrenal medula and the formed elements of the blood have an absolute dependence upon glucose for metabolism. Table 1 indicates the energy reserves of a normal man weighing 70 kg and Table 2 the phases of starvation and the metabolic response [2, 3]. The minimum requirement of glucose in the circulation is no more than 3–5 g or 12–20 kcal and would be a sufficient source of glucose for a very short period of time. During fasting, the amount of glucose available from liver glycogen is generally 100 grams, little more than half that needed over a 24-hour period. Thus glycogenolysis insures adequate glucose for brain function only during the initial phases of food deprivation. As hepatic glycogen is depleted after 18–24 hours a third glucose source must come into play, namely, neoglucogenesis. Neoglucogenesis occurs in the liver,

Table 1. Energy reserves of normal man*

Fat	Adipose tissue	12–16	kg	100,000–150,000 Cal
Protein	Muscle	6	kg	25,000 Cal
Carbohydrate	Muscle glycogen	0.5	kg	2,000 Cal
	Liver glycogen	0.1	kg	400 Cal
	Free glucose	0.02	kg	80 Cal

* Normal man – 70 kg (154 lbs)

Table 2. Phases of starvation

1.	1–8 hours	Gastrointestinal absorption
2.	1–2 days	Glycogenolysis
3.	2–7 days	Gluconeogenesis
4.	2 days start; plateau at 7 days	Ketosis
5.	7 days onward	Diminished gluconeogenesis and increased cerebral ketone consumption

the substrates being lactate, glycerol, and most important, amino acids, particularly alanine, derived from muscle protein (Table 3). Lactate is the dominant neoglucogenic precursor accounting for 54%, glycerol 13%, amino acids 29%, half of which is due to alanine, and pyruvate 4%. The capacity of the liver to generate new glucose by neoglucogenesis is tremendous, about 200–300 g/day, and the process is essential to maintain glucose homeostasis if fasting is prolonged for longer than 24 hours. Early in the fast, blood glucose concentrations gradually decrease as consumption of glucose by the central nervous system and other organs continue. As the concentration of glucose declines, pancreatic beta cells decrease secretion of insulin and the catabolic hormones, glucagon and catecholamines, are released. This constitutes a new hormonal set of decreasing anabolism and increasing catabolism in response to the deprivation of glucose. In the midphase of the fast, i.e., between 18 and 24 hours when liver glycogen is depleted, gluconeogenesis becomes the essential process [4]. In the late phases of the fast but commencing within 48 hours, lipolysis ensues and the liver converts incoming free fatty acids to ketone bodies which serve as substrates for brain metabolism. Thus the obligatory demand for glucose decreases to 73–90 g/day with a reduction in the requirements of neoglucogenic substrate, especially of alanine, which may be explained teleologically as a compensatory mechanism to minimize protein breakdown for survival.

4.1.1 *The role of insulin.* When healthy subjects fast, the ensuing decrease in plasma glucose concentration is accompanied by a decrease in insulin secretion which results in a decrease in glucose utilization and an increase in hepatic glucose production. Insulin is the dominant glucose lowering hormone. It suppresses endogenous glucose production and stimulates glucose utilization, thereby lowering the plasma glucose concentration. Insulin has important actions on the liver as well as on peripheral tissues [5]. It inhibits hepatic glycogenolysis and gluconeogenesis, and, in the presence of hyperglycemia and a reduction in counter regulatory hormones, converts the liver into an organ of net glucose uptake and storage in the form of glycogen. Insulin also stimulates glucose uptake, storage and utilization by other insulin-sensitive tissues, such as muscle and fat. Suppression of endogeneous hepatic glucose production is more sensitive to changes in plasma insulin concentrations than is stimulation of glucose utilization [6]. An

Table 3. Substrates for glucose production

Prescursor	Total glucose production (%)	Gluconeogenesis
Lactate	13	54
Glycerol	4	13
Amino acids	7	29
(Alanine)	(4)	(15)
Pyruvate	1	4

increase of 15–20 μU/ml decreases glucose production 50% and completely inhibits it at a concentration of 50–60 μU/ml. Half maximal insulin stimulation of glucose utilization requires an increase of 50–60 μU/ml and maximal effects are only observed at around 200–500 μU/ml. Thus, mild to moderate hyperinsulinemia causes hypoglycemia primarily by inhibiting hepatic glucose production rather than by stimulation of glucose utilization. This is supported by the observation that patients with insulin-producing islet cell tumors have decreased rates of glucose production rather than increased rates of glucose utilization during the development of hypoglycemia at relatively low insulin concentrations [7]. Inhibition of neoglucogenesis requires greater plasma insulin concentration than does the inhibition of glycogenolysis [8]. Approximately 100 μU/ml are required to produce an 80% decrease in neoglucogenesis, whereas 500 μU/ml are required for total suppression [9].

Adipose tissue is far more sensitive to the effects of insulin in terms of lipolysis, and only 1/10 of the concentration required for stimulation of glucose utilization inhibits lipolysis [10].

Insulin, like other polypeptide hormones, initiates its biologic effect by binding to specific receptors on its target tissues [11]. Insulin receptors may, however, be occupied not only by insulin but by another class of compounds referred to collectively as the insulin-like growth factors (IGF) [11]. This class of compounds possesses insulin-like activities and there is considerable homology in the structure of certain IGF fractions and that of insulin. Although the IGFs, including the somatomedins, may bind weakly to the insulin receptor, i.e., with low affinity, when present in sufficient quantity, they can mimic the biological action of insulin [12]. Increased concentrations of IGF have been reported in some patients with extrapancreatic tumor hypoglycemia [13, 14, 15]. Other substances have also been found to bind to the insulin receptor and include autoantibodies to the receptor which may both inhibit the action of insulin or mimic the action of insulin [16, 17]. The clinical presentation of these patients with antibodies to the receptor varies from intractable hypoglycemia to severe insulin resistance and diabetes, depending upon whether the antibodies function primarily as insulin agonists or antagonists [18, 19]. After the binding event the insulin-insulin receptor complex is formed and one or more signals of insulin action are generated. The signal or second messenger may involve the generation of a chemical mediator, a conformational change within the plasma membrane, alterations in flux or other information transfer [20]. Studies of the nature of insulin action at the receptor and post-receptor levels have been carried out both in vivo and in vitro. Of all the in vivo methods currently available to evaluate insulin action at receptor and post-receptor levels, that which provides the greatest information is the euglycemic hyperinsulinemic clamp, as devised by DeFronzo, Andres and colleagues [21]. Utilizing this technique combined with isotopic measurement of glucose flux, Rizza et al. [7] showed that hypoglycemia in insulinoma patients was due to suppression of hepatic glucose output, without evidence of a change in receptor status. While these observations may generally be true there is need for simultaneous in vivo and in vitro measurements to determine overall receptor and post-receptor status.

4.1.2 *Regulation of insulin receptor*. It has been shown that the number of insulin receptors on the cell surface is regulated by the ambient insulin concentration. Gavin et al. [22] were the first to demonstrate that in vitro exposure of cultured lymphocytes to insulin caused a decrease in the number of insulin receptors. This observation has been substantiated in other in vitro systems.

In vivo, an inverse relationship has been found between the fasting plasma insulin concentration and insulin binding to monocytes, red blood cells and adipocytes in healthy control subjects [23, 24] and in a variety of pathological conditions [25, 26]. This strongly suggests that insulin is an important factor in the regulation of its own receptor number.

Changes in receptor binding may partially compensate for changes in the plasma insulin concentration. Hyperinsulinemia produced by insulin-secreting pancreatic tumors [27] or by infusion of insulin [28] decreases insulin binding. A reduction in the number and/or affinity of insulin receptors observed in patients with insulinoma [27] may constitute a protective mechanism against hyperinsulinemia and excessive hypoglycemia. On the other hand, the presence of a normal or low insulin concentration does not necessarily rule out hypoglycemia due to activation of the insulin receptor complex. These observations may explain why, in many instances, there is not a direct correlation between the actual insulin concentrations measured in plasma and the degree of hypoglycemia in a patient with an insulin-secreting tumor.

4.1.3 *Potentially important glucose counterregulatory factors to maintain euglycemia*

4.1.3.1 *Hormones*. Glucagon secreted from the A cell of the pancreas stimulates hepatic glycogenolysis and neoglucogenesis. Within minutes of its administration glucagon increases hepatic glucose production [29] which normally is transient and returns to approximately baseline levels within 90 minutes, despite sustained hyperglucagonemia. Basal glucagon secretion appears to account for a large proportion of glucose production during overnight fasting by glycogenolysis and to a lesser extent, by neoglucogenesis [30]. Glucagon is critical to acute phase hypoglycemic counterregulation [31, 32]. Like glucagon, epinephrine stimulates both glycogenolysis and gluconeogenesis and transiently increases hepatic glucose production within minutes. It promotes ketone formation by enhancing lipolysis. However, epinephrine also limits glucose utilization. The alpha-adrenergic activity of epinephrine inhibits endogenous insulin secretion and promotes a sustained prolonged inhibition of glucose assimilation [33]. This effect of epinephrine is mediated by inhibition of insulin-stimulated glucose uptake in peripheral tissues [33] and splanchnic glucose uptake [34]. Sustained hyperepinephrinemia results in sustained hyperglycemia, a result of both direct and indirect actions [35]. The direct actions appear to be mediated by a beta-adrenergic receptor mechanism, which includes the stimulation of hepatic glucose production and limitation of glucose utilization.

Growth hormone limits glucose transport into tissues and chronic growth hormone excess causes insulin resistance. This effect requires, however, several hours [36, 37]. Indeed, during the first two hours after plasma levels are increased growth hormone exerts a plasma glucose-lowering effect, or insulin-like effect, and levels of plasma glucose do not increase above control values for at least two hours thereafter. Cortisol limits glucose transport into tissues, promotes lipolysis and stimulates neoglucogenesis. Its hyperglycemic effects require several hours to become evident.

Infusions of cortisol for prolonged periods in humans causes no increase in hepatic glucose production [38] and a small increase in the plasma glucose concentration that occurs only after 2–1/2 or 3 hours of continous elevation of plasma levels which is due to a decrease in glucose utilization. Thus, it appears that neither growth hormone nor cortisol are likely to be important short-term glucose counterregulatory hormones, although they may serve a function in the long term. Certain neural mechanisms appear to be important in counterregulation as well. Stimulation of hepatic sympathetic nerves results in a rapid increase in hepatic glucose release and hyperglycemia [39]. Direct periarterial hepatic nerve stimulation also causes an increase in the plasma glucose concentration [40]. It seems that these effects may be mediated by local norepinepherine release from the axon terminals or the sympathetic postganglionic neurons.

4.1.3.2 *Auto regulation.* In the absence of hormonal responses to hypoglycemia there is considerable evidence that glucose per se affects hepatic glucose production [41]. The concept of auto regulation, i.e., that hepatic glucose production is an inverse function of the ambient plasma glucose concentration independent of hormonal and neural factors has received support from studies both in animals and in man [42]. Thus a decrease in the plasma glucose concentration per se is potentially an important glucose counterregulatory factor.

4.1.4 *Glucose counterregulation during hypoglycemia.* Studies of counterregulation during hypoglycemia have been carried out using insulin-induced hypoglycemia and emphasize the role of the counterregulatory hormones in restoring the blood glucose concentration to normal. Isotopically determined kinetic patterns of glucose recovery from insulin-induced hypoglycemia consists of: (1) a return of insulin-stimulated glucose utilization to baseline levels; (2) a rebound of insulin-suppressed glucose production above baseline levels. The temporal relationships between these changes in glucose kinetics and activation of glucose counterregulatory systems was first defined by Garber et al. [43]. Hypoglycemia stimulates the prompt release of glucagon, epinephrine and norepinephrine and slighly later, growth hormone and cortisol (see Fig. 1). There appear to be important synergistic actions between the counter regulatory hormones. In normal humans the combined infusion of epinephrine, glucagon and cortisol produces a greater than additive hyperglycemic response [38]. The relative roles of these various hormones in hypoglycemic glucose counterreglation have been extensively studied (Fig. 2) [44–47]. Recovery from hypoglycemia was impaired by approximately 40% during infusion of somatostatin which inhibits the secretion of many hormones, including glucagon and growth hormone. Growth hormone was shown to be unimportant in the recovery since replacement thereof did not correct the hypoglycemic unresponsiveness. Glucagon appeared to play an important and essential role in hypoglycemic counterregulation. However, substantial glucose recovery occurred, approximately 60% of normal, even in the absence of glucagon secretion. Recovery from insulin-induced hypoglycemia was little affected, if at all, by pharmacologial adrenergic blockade [45, 48] or by the

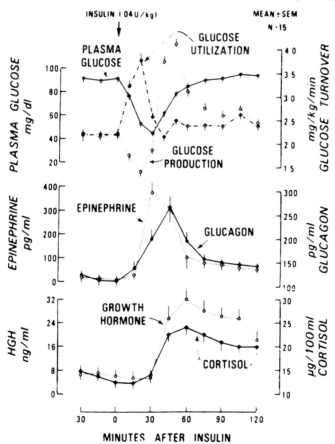

Figure 1. Counterregulatory hormone responses to insulin-induced hypoglycemia in normal persons. From Gerich et al. (Metabolism 29: 1164–1175, 1980). Reproduced with permission. HGH = human growth hormone.

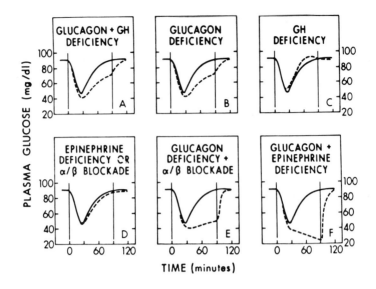

Figure 2. The role of glucagon, growth hormone (GH) and the autonomic nervous system in the recovery from insulin-induced hypoglycemia. From Cryer *et al.* Diabetes 30: 261–264, 1981. Reproduced with permission. Note that a deficiency of GH, adrenergic function or glucagon alone does not impair recovery but that the combination of adrenergic blockade or epinephrine deficiency with glucagon deficiency caused marked impairment of glucose counterregulation.

epinephrine-deficient state in bilaterally adrenalectomized persons [46]. However, when adrenergic blockade was combined with inhibition of glucagon secretion recovery from hypoglycemia was markedly impaired (see Fig. 2). Furthermore, when deficient glucagon and epinephrine secretion were combined glucose recovery failed to occur. The data were thought to be consistent with the fact that neither the secretion of growth hormone nor that of cortisol is critical to recovery from insulin induced hypoglycemia and that neither sympathetic neural epinephrine release nor glucose autoregulation is sufficiently potent to promote recovery from hypoglycemia in the absence of the key glucose counterregulatory hormones, glucagon and epinephrine [49].

While these hormonal responses to induced hypoglycemia and changes in blood glucose concentration within the normal range are well established, the counterregulatory responses to more sustained hypoglycemia as occurs in patients with insulin secreting tumors, or to chronic repeated episodes of hypoglycemia have not been thoroughly evaluated. Sustained fasting hypoglycemia as seen in patients with insulinomas is not associated with elevated plasma levels of growth hormone [50] or glucagon [51].

4.1.5 Hormonal and metabolic effects of associated exercise. It is well known that in certain patients with organic hyperinsulinism the demonstration of hypoglycemia may not occur even after prolonged fasting but that superimposition of a short period of exercise will produce an increase in glucose utilization above basal levels, followed by hypoglycemia. In healthy subjects, with the onset of exercise plasma insulin concentration usually declines [52, 53] and levels of glucagon [54, 55, 56] and catecholamines [55, 57] usually rise. These changes in general favor the stimulation of both glycogenolysis and neoglucogenesis. Exercise also causes a variable increase in the levels of plasma cortisol [58] and growth hormone [59]. Two factors appear to be primarily responsible for the increase in glucose utilization by exercising muscle. The first is the large increase in capillary surface area that results from vasodilatation and opening of previously closed capillary beds [60]. The second is a primary stimulation of glucose transport [61]. It should be noted, however, that the latter effect on glucose transport is dependent on the presence of circulating insulin and does not occur in the total absence of insulin [62, 63]. When exercise is performed in conjunction with hyperinsulinemia, the resultant increase in glucose utilization is greater than the effects of either exercise alone or the hyperinsulinemia alone [53], i.e., a true synergistic effect was observed between the exercise-induced increase in glucose metabolism and that induced by hyperinsulinemia. Patients with organic hyperinsulinism and autonomous insulin secretion do not lower plasma concentrations of insulin during exercise as occurs in healthy subjects. Other effects of exercise may be related to the associated increase in the number and affinity of insulin receptors.

4.2 Factors controlling blood glucose homeostasis in the fed state

In normal human beings plasma glucose concentrations are maintained in a narrow range between 70 and 140 mg/dl. This stability is remarkable in view of the widely varying composition of food ingested, the episodic nature of our eating habits, and the interspersed periods of fasting. In the fed state, i.e., immediately upon eating and for four hours thereafer, carbohydrate, protein and fat are absorbed from the gastrointestinal system and contribute to the circulating glucose level. Thus there is a refined system for disposal of ingested glucose to maintain the blood glucose concentration within these narrow limits. An important mechanism is carbohydrate storage which is primarily mediated by the secretion of insulin. Carbohydrate may be stored as glycogen in the liver and muscle and as triglycerides in the fat cells. Amino acids are converted into protein in muscle, and fat is stored as triglycerides in peripheral fat cells. The metabolic milieu after a meal is maximally anabolic with an increase in the circulating concentration of insulin, the primary anabolic hormone, and suppression of the catabolic hormones, glucagon and catecholamines. As an anabolic hormone, insulin enhances the uptake of amino acids, especially the branched chain amino acids, by the muscle cell and the liver for the synthesis of protein. Insulin stimulates the uptake of glucose by the liver, muscle and fat cell, oxidation of glucose and the synthesis of glycogen. It increases the synthesis of triglycerides in adipose tissue. While most of these actions of insulin are opposed by the counter-regulatory hormones, glucagon, epinephrine and to some extent, cortisol and growth hormone, the dominant action in the immediate postprandial state relates to the overall anabolic effects of insulin.

5. Factors which determine the insulin secretory response

Insulin is synthesized in the pancreatic B-cell from its precursor, proinsulin, which contains the insulin molecule and a connecting peptide linking the A and B chains of insulin. In the basal state after an 8–14 h fast, the circulating immunoreactive insulin (IRI) in non-obese humans ranges between 5–15 μU/ml with a mean of 10 μU/ml. Plasma concentrations of IRI are increased (to 45 μU/ml) in obese but otherwise healthy subjects. Of this, 5–20% is proinsulin. When the B-cell is stimulated, insulin is cleaved from proinsulin, and is released in equimolar quantities with C-peptide and 5–6% proinsulin. The insulin secretory responses are best considered as those related to glucose, which is the primary nutrient stimulus, and those related to nonglucose stimuli.

5.1 Glucose-stimulated insulin secretion

In normal man, glucose stimulation of the B-cell results directly in insulin secretion. In both man and animals a multiphasic insulin secretory response has been demonstrated [64, 65, 66]. In humans the first phase begins within one to two minutes after intravenous injection of glucose, reaches a maximum within 3–5 minutes, which is 8–10 times the basal concentration and is generally over within 10 minutes and is not dependent upon the prevailing glucose level. If the plasma glucose concentration remains elevated, a second phase of insulin secretion occurs subsequently and continues as long as hyperglycemia persists. The first phase is dependent upon immediate release of newly formed insulin, whereas the second phase depends upon insulin stores and is contingent upon protein synthesis [64, 65, 66]. This second phase of insulin secretion is dependent upon the steady state plasma glucose concentration. In other words, the higher the prestimulus glucose concentration the greater the magnitude of the second phase, and the lower the plasma glucose the smaller the increment in plasma insulin in response to induced hyperglycemia. Glucose probably interacts with islet cells in three separate ways – recognition as a molecule, metabolism specifically as glucose and generation of energy. As the glucose concentration is raised progressively by intravenously administered glucose, a progressive increment in insulin secretion occurs to maximal levels at blood glucose concentrations of around 240 mg/dl [67].

Below a blood glucose concentration of 50 mg/dl, insulin secretion reaches basal or near basal levels but does not disappear, an important factor in the prevention of ketoacidosis. When blood glucose levels reach the hypoglycemic level of about 30 mg/dl, peripheral insulin concentrations fall to 0–1 μU/ml. This threshold for insulin secretion may be important in the diagnosis of insulinomas, as will become apparent later.

Of the other nutrients ingested, protein and fat, their break-down products, i.e., amino acids and to a minor degree, fatty acids are also capable of stimulating insulin secretion [68]. Fatty acids and ketones, which may be effective in some species, have inconsistent effects on insulin secretion in man [65].

5.2 Amino acid stimulation of insulin secretion

Most amino acids stimulate the release of insulin [69, 70, 71]. Leucine was the first amino acid to be shown to stimulate insulin release [72, 73, 74]. Leucine can stimulate the release of insulin in vitro in the absence of glucose while arginine cannot. The action of leucine but not of arginine may be exaggerated in patients with B cell hyperplasia, islet cell tumors, and sulfonylurea-induced islet cell stimulation, even in the presence of hypoglycemia [75]. Leucine stimulates the release of insulin by a mechanism which is different from the mechanism by which arginine stimulates the release of insulin [71, 75]. The insulin secretory response to leucine has been used as a diagnostic test in states of pathological hyperinsulinism [75, 76, 77]. The nonmetabolizable amino acid analogs of leucine and arginine stimulate insulin secretion, thus these amino acids do not have to be metabolized to exert their insulin-stimulating action [78, 79]. The insulin secretory response to amino acids is multiphasic and is potentiated by glucose [80]. Thus, ingestion of mixed meals results in higher insulin levels, presumably due to the potentiating interaction between amino acids and glucose [80].

5.3 Gastrointestinal hormones and other factors influencing insulin secretion

Ingestion of an amount of glucose which produces a rise in circulating glucose equivalent to that found with its intravenous administration, elicits a greater insulin secretory response than the intravenous stimulus. This has led to the concept that the gut produces an 'incretin' which facilitates glucose stimulated insulin release [81]. A number of hormones in the gut have been considered as potential candidates for the role of this incretin, namely secretin [82], gastrin [81], cholecystokinin, and vaso-active intestinal polypeptide [83], but the major candidate appears to be glucose-dependent insulin releasing peptide or GIP [84, 85]. During meals these gut hormones are released in significant quantities and duplication of the circulating levels enhances the insulin secretory response to glucose stimulation [86]. Oral fat ingestion also causes the release of GIP [84].

Intraislet hormones may also be important modulators for insulin secretion [87]. Based upon studies by Samols and Weir [88, 89, 90], Bonner-Weir and Orci [91] and Unger [87] proposed that the pancreatic islet functions not as in individual cell, but as an organ in which the blood supply first reaches the B-cell and the effluent from the cell via an intraislet portal system impinges upon the A- and D-cells secreting glucagon and somatostatin. Pancreatic glucagon has been demonstrated to stimulate insulin secretion [88]. The intraislet hormone, somatostatin, has an inhibitory effect on insulin secretion [92], and the changes in secretion of somatostatin and glucagon may directly affect insulin secretion from the B-cell [93, 94]. Other substances, including serotonin and prostaglandin E, have been found in the pancreas and may have an inhibitory role on insulin secretion [95], but data in this regard are conflicting. Neural factors are clearly important in regulating insulin secretion; parasympathetic stimulation [96] appears to be a weak stimulus. Whereas sympathetic stimulation may cause an increase in insulin secretion by a beta-receptor mechanism [97], the predominant effect of catecholamines is alpha-receptor-mediated inhibition [98]. In the pancreatic islet alpha-adrenergic receptor activity predominates over the beta receptor [64] during hypoglycemia and the stimulation of release of catecholamines. This inhibitory role of alpha-adrenergic receptor activation appears to be an important mechanism whereby insulin secretion ceases. The action of the autonomic nervous system and a number of hormones, such as growth hormone and cortisol on insulin secretion, may be indirectly mediated since these have effects on the secretion of both somatostatin [90, 99] and glucagon [94, 100, 101].

Thus, as has been proposed by Unger [87], the pancreatic islet organ acts as an integrator. Meal-related nutrient concentrations interact with glucose as the primary stimulus subject to neural and hormonal signals to regulate the secretion of insulin. Insulin is the primary anabolic hormone which governs the distribution of the various fuels into their storage sites.

5.4 Sulfonylureas and insulin secretion

Intravenous administration of tolbutamide (1 g) stimulates a brisk rise in insulin secretion. In normal individuals, the peak level of insulin usually occurs within 5 minutes and returns to basal levels within 90–120 minutes. In contrast, profound and protracted hypersecretion of insulin may occur in patients with hyperfunctioning B-cells.

5.5 Relative potencies of secretagogues

The normal B-cell usually responds to secretogogues in the following order: glucose, tolbutamide, glucagon, leucine. The neoplastic B-cell may hyperrespond to these stimuli in the following sequence: tolbutamide, leucine, glucagon, and glucose. This transposition of the order forms the basis of certain provocative tests for insulinomas [76, 77].

6. Classification of spontaneous hypoglycemia (differential diagnosis of 'insulinoma')

The diagnosis or differential diagnosis of insulinoma is facilitated if the physician is familiar with an overall classification of spontaneous hypoglycemia. Table 4 presents a classification of spontaneous hypoglycemia divided into the fasting hypoglycemias and the postprandial or postabsorptive (reactive) hypoglycemias. In patients with one of the many types of fasting hypoglycemia, the presenting symptoms may occur in the fasting state and/or biochemical and symptomatic hypoglycemia can be precipitated by prolonging the overnight fast. In contrast, in patients with postprandial hypoglycemia, the symptoms of hypoglycemia or biochemical hypoglycemia occur only after ingestion of nutrients, and pathological hypoglycemia does not occur on prolongation of an overnight fast.

6.1 Fasting hypoglycemia

The various types of fasting hypoglycemia can be subdivided into 1) organic hypoglycemia associated with a recognizable anatomic lesion, 2) hypoglycemias due to a specific hepatic enzyme defect, rarely seen in adult patients, 3) the functional hypoglycemias without a recognizable or persistent anatomic lesion, uncommon in the adult, and 4) hypoglycemias induced by exogenous agents.

6.1.1 Organic hypoglyemia: recognizable anatomic lesion
6.1.1.1 Pancreatic islet B-cell disease with hyperinsulinism. Among adults with pancreatic islet cell disease and hyperinsulinism, a number of pathological entities involving islet tissues can be recognized (Table 5). Most adult patients with hyperinsulinism due to pancreatic islet cell disease have macroscopic pancreatic B-cell tumors. Approximately 75% to 80% of patients with organic hyperinsulinism have a single benign adenoma.

Functioning benign islet cell tumors have been found from birth to old age, with most occurring between 20 and 60 years of age. Table 6 gives the sex and age distribution of 69 patients with organic hyperinsulinism seen at the University of Michigan since 1960. Single benign islet cell adenomas in our series have varied in size from 0.15 to 5 cm in diameter, with 75% between 0.5 and 2 cm in diameter. Their weight varied from 0.35 to 12.3 g, with the majority weighing less than 2 g. The majority of multiple adenomas were less than 1 cm in diameter. Adenomas are usually encapsulated, firmer than the normal pancreas, highly vascular,

Table 4. Classification of spontaneous hypoglycemia

A. *Fasting Hypoglycemia*
 1. Organic hypoglycemia: recognizable anatomic lesion
    a. Pancreatic islet beta-cell disease with hyperinsulinism[a] *in the adult:*
       (1) adenoma, single or multiple
       (2) microadenomatosis, with or without macroscopic islet cell adenomas
       (3) carcinoma with metastases
       (4) adenoma(s) or carcinoma, associated with adenomas or hyperplasia of other endocrine glands (familial multiple endocrine adenomatosis or neoplasia, Type I)
       (5) nesidioblastosis
       (6) hyperplasia
       in infancy and childhood:
       (1) hyperplasia (leucine-sensitive[b] or -insensitive)
       (2) nesidioblastosis
       (3) adenoma
    b. Nonpancreatic tumors associated with hypoglycemia
    c. Anterior pituitary hypofunction (more frequently in infancy and childhood)
    d. Adrenocortical hypofunction (more frequently in infancy and childhood)
    e. Acquired diffuse hepatic disease
    f. Severe congestive heart failure
    g. Severe renal insufficiency in non-insulin dependent diabetic patients
 2. Hypoglycemia due to specific hepatic enzyme deficiency *(infancy and childhood)*
    a. Glycogen storage diseases
    b. Glycogen synthase deficiency
    c. Fructose 1, 6-diphosphatase deficiency
    d. Glutaric aciduria, Type II
 3. Functional hypoglycemia: no recognizable or no persistent anatomic lesion
    a. Deficiency of glucagon[b]
    b. Severe inanition
    c. Insulin autoimmune syndrome[c]
    d. Autoantibodies to insulin receptor
    e. ketotic hypoglycemia *(childhood)*
    f. Transient hypoglycemia in the *newborn* of low birth weight
    g. Transient hyperinsulinism of the *newborn* (hyperplasia of pancreatic islet cells reported)
 4. Hypoglycemia induced by exogenous agents
    a. Ethanol (and poor nutrition)
    b. Insulin administration ⎫
    c. Sulfonylurea administration ⎬ iatrogenic or factitious
    d. Ingestion of ackee fruit (hypoglycin)
    e. Miscellaneous drugs
B. *Postprandial (Reactive) Hypoglycemia*
 1. Functional hypoglycemia: no recognizable anatomic lesion
    a. Alimentary hyperinsulinism (usually previous G-I surgery)
    b. Reactive secondary to mild diabetes
    c. Reactive functional – idiopathic (may be heterogenenous)
 2. Hypoglycemia due to specific hepatic enzyme deficiency
    a. Hereditary fructose intolerance (fructose 1-phosphate aldolase deficiency) – *infancy and childhood*
    b. Galactosemia – *infancy and childhood*
    c. Familial fructose and galactose intolerance (two patients described)

[a] May manifest also as postabsorptive (reactive) hypoglycemia – glucose or leucine-induced.
[b] May manifest also as postabsorptive (reactive) hypoglycemia – protein (amino acid)-induced.
[c] May manifest also as postabsorptive (reactive) hypoglycemia – glucose-induced.

Table 5. Summary of types of islet cell pathology found in 69 patients with organic hyperinsulinism

Number of patients	Without MEN-Type I (%)	With MEN-Type I	Total (%)
1. Solitary adenoma	51* (81%)	1	52 (75%)
2. Adenomatosis	5 (8%)	4	9 (13%)
a. macroadenomas only	1	2	
b. macroadenomas + microadenomatosis	1	1	
c. macroadenomas + hyperplasia	3	1	
3. Nesidioblastosis	3 (5%)	–	3 (4%)
4. Hyperplasia	1 (1.6%)	–	1 (1%)
5. Carcinoma	3 (5%)	1	4 (6%)
Totals	63	6	69

MEN – Multiple endocrine neoplasia

* One patient had peritumor microadenomatosis, not of functional significance as patient has had normal glucose and insulin levels during 72-hour fasts with follow-up of 10 years

Table 6. Distribution of 69 patients with organic hyperinsulinism

Sex	Male: 32 (46%)		Female: 37 (54%)					
Age, Years	2–9	10–19	20–29	30–39	40–49	50–59	60–69	70–79
Total numbers	2	8	14	12	16	11	2	2
%	3	12	21	18	24	16	3	3
Single adenoma	1	5	12	10	11	8	1	2
Adenomatosis	0	2	1	1	4	2	0	0
Nesidioblastosis	1[a]	1[b]	0	0	1	0	0	0
Hyperplasia	0	0	0	1	0	0	0	0
Carcinoma	0	0	1	0	1	1	1	0
MEN-Type I	0	2	1	0	2	1	0	0

[a] Onset of symptoms age 2 years – first documentation of hypoglycemia age 17 years, first documentation of hyperinsulinism age 20 years.

[b] Onset of symptoms age 9 years – first documentation of hyperinsulinism age 11 years.

purplish or occasionally whitish-yellow, and may present a smooth or irregular surface. They are almost equally distributed among the head, body, and tail of the pancreas. Benign adenomas of islet cell tissue rarely occur outside the pancreas. A working classification of insulinomas based on the quantitative evaluation of ultrastructural features of tumor cells has been proposed [102] which is simpler than earlier classifications [103]. Group A tumors are characterized by abundant well-granulated typical B-cells, trabecular arrangement of cells, and uniform insulin immunofluorescence; functionally these tumors show a mean concentration of circulating proinsulin-like material which is within limits of normal or slightly elevated, and there is almost complete suppressibility of insulin secretion by somatostatin and diazoxide. Tumors in Group B are characterized by few typical well-granulated beta cells, and medullary-type histological structure, irregular insulin immunofluorescence, and functionally these patients show a mean concentration of proinsulin-like material which is more than twice the upper limit of normal, and there is marked resistance to the inhibitory effects of both somatostatin and diazoxide on insulin secretion.

Adenomatosis consisting of multiple macroadenomas or one or more macroadenomas together with microadenomatosis interspersed between normal islets occur in approximately 5–15% of patients with hyperinsulinism, though it is rarely discussed in the literature [105, 106]. Islet cell carcinoma (approximately 5% of patients with organic hyperinsulinism) can be diagnosed only with certainty when regional or distant metastases are present.

Nesidioblastosis (diffuse and disseminated neoproliferation of insulin-producing cells from pancreatic ductules) is the leading cause of hyperinsulinemia in the newborn and infants and has been recognized only at that age in the past [107]. This condition has recently been recognized in adolescents and adults as well [106, 108, 109], and it occurs in approximately 5% of patients with hyperinsulinism. Nesidioblastosis may be diffuse or focal and limited primarily to one part of the pancreas, such as the head. Diffuse islet cell hyperplasia (excessive and diffuse proliferation of beta cells in the islets of Langerhans) has been reported in adults. Stefanini et al. [110, 111] reported that of a total of 1,137 cases of organic hyperinsulinism, 1,067 (93.8%) were caused by insulinomas and 70 (6.2%) by diffuse islet cell disease. In 7 cases (0.6%) there was a combination of the two diseases. Some patients reported in the literature as having hyperplasia may today be classified more properly as nesidioblastosis if the appropriate immunofluorescent staining techniques are applied. We have seen one adult patient in whom hyperplasia was the only functional lesion. In four other patients, hyperplasia coexisted with adenomatosis. Other reports have appeared describing pancreatic islet cell adenomas with islet cell hyperplasia and nesidioblastosis in the adult [112]. Nesidioblastosis, islet hypertrophy, islet hyperplasia, focal hyperplastic adenomatosis and adenoma could be the expression of one and the same basic defect, termed 'islet cell dismaturation syndrome' by Gabbay [113], and 'endocrine cell dysplasia' by Jaffe et al. [114]. The recognition of microadenomatosis, nesidioblastosis or hyperplasia is important therapeutically since removal of a large portion of the pancreas is necessary for the relief of hyperinsulinism and hypoglycemia. In some patients, a 70–85% pancreatectomy will achieve a cure, but in others medical therapy or additional removal of pancreatic islet tissue is essential.

In patients with multiple endocrine neoplasia (MEN) Type I, and organic hyperinsulinism, single adenomas, multiple adenomas with and without adenomatosis or hyperplasia, islet cell carcinoma with regional metastases, microadenomatosis and nesidioblastosis and hyperplasia have been recognized [115]. Islet cell lesions in patients with MEN-Type I are found associated with adenomas or hyperplasia of the parathyroid and other endocrine glands and with peptic ulceration (ulcerogenic, Zollinger-Ellison Syndrome). Malignant or benign islet cell tumors found in this syndrome, as well as sporadic ones, have the capacity to secrete other polypeptide hormones as well, such as glucagon, gastrin, human pancreatic polypeptide, somatostatin, adrenocorticotrophin (ACTH), and melanophore-stimulating hormone (MSH). Some tumors, including heterotopic pancreatic islet cell tumors, may produce 5-hydroxytryptophan or serotonin, or both, and are associated with a carcinoid syndrome. Subcutaneous lipomas may be found in these patients.

A family history of diabetes has been found in 25–30% of patients with functioning islet cell tumors (22% in our series).

Table 5 summarizes the lesions encountered in our series of 69 patients with organic hyperinsulinism seen since 1960.

6.1.1.2 *Nonpancreatic tumors associated with hypoglycemia*. Severe hypoglycemia has been reported in more than 250 patients harboring nonpancreatic tumors of mesothelial, epithelial, or endothelial origin [116]. Most of these tumors are mesothelial and are classified as fibromas, sacromas, fibrosarcomas, mesotheliomas or hemangiopericytomas. They are usually situated in the thorax, the retroperitoneal space, or the pelvis. They may be attached to the diaphragm or found within the liver. Other cases of nonpancreatic tumors associated with severe hypoglycemia include patients with primary hepatic carcinoma, patients with carcinoma of the adrenal cortex, occasionally patients with pheochromocytoma, gastrointestinal carcinomas, pseudomyxoma peritonei, two patients with bronchogenic carcinomas, and one with a bronchial carcinoid tumor. The common clinical characteristics of these tumors, particularly of the fibrosarcomas, are their slow growth and their massive size. Hypoglycemia disappears after resection or, occasionally, after irradiation of the tumor. Various theories have been advanced to explain how these tumors cause hypoglycemia, but none are applicable to all patients. It has been postulated that the excessive secretion of insulin or an insulin-like substance may block hepatic glucose output and enhance peripheral glucose utilization [117]; in others there may be excessive glucose consumption by tumor tissue having a high rate of anaerobic glycolysis and weighing up to 10 kg or more. In the majority of patients, insulin-like activity in serum or in extracts of tumor tissues has been normal or subnormal. High levels of serum 'immunoreactive insulin' have been reported in only two patients, one of whom had a large fibrosarcoma and in another who had a bronchial carcinoid tumor with metastases. An insulin-like biological activity demonstrable in plasma of some patients and in extracts of some of these tumors may be the effect of a polypeptide (or polypeptides), synthesized by the tumor, which is not recognized immunologically as insulin. Plasma NSILA-s (non-suppressible insulin-like activity soluble in acid alcohol) or insulin-like growth factors, (IGF-like material), measured by radioreceptor assay, has been found to be elevated in 35–40% of patients with non-islet cell tumors and hypoglyemia [13, 14, 15, 118]. This finding is still controversial [119, 120].

6.1.1.3 *Anterior pituitary hypofunction.* See below.

6.1.1.4 *Adrenal cortical hypofunction.* Anterior pituitary hypofunction or adrenal cortical hypofunction or a combination of both may also induce fasting hypoglycemia. In adults, hypoglycemia is more likely in such patients if there is concomitant malnutrition. Growth hormone and cortisol deficiency interfere with glucose homeotasis at several steps in hepatic metabolism (decreased gluconeogenesis and glycogenolysis) and in peripheral tissues (increased glucose uptake). (See 4.1.3.1)

6.1.1.5 *Acquired diffuse hepatic disease.* Acquired diffuse and severe liver disease such as viral hepatitis or toxic necrosis can lead to fasting hypoglycemia by compromising hepatocellular components involved in gluconeogenesis and glycogenolysis. Fasting hypoglycemia without recognizable symptoms attributable to hypoglycemia, was found in 50% of severely cirrhotic patients with superimposed septicemia, particularly in those patients with circulatory failure and shock [121].

6.1.1.6 *Severe congestive heart failure.* Fasting hypoglycemia has been reported in patients with severe congestive heart failure. In this circumstance reduced hepatic blood flow and reduced delivery of gluconeogenetic substrate to the liver can be implicated, as can hepatic dysfunction.

6.1.1.7 *Severe renal insufficiency in non-insulin dependent diabetic patients.* Fasting hypoglycemia has also been observed in diabetic (and nondiabetic) patients who have severe renal insufficiency concomitant with a disappearance of need for insulin or oral hypoglycemic agents [122]. Inadequate delivery of gluconeogenic substrates (hypoalaninemia) to the liver [123], decreased glycogenolysis due to poor glycogen stores, decreased inactivation of insulin by the kidney, and, to some extent, decreased renal gluconeogenesis and decreased caloric intake and starvation may contribute to the development of hypoglycemia. This is a rare occurrence despite the frequency of renal failure in diabetes. Ingestion of certain drugs may precipitate hypoglycemia in these patients (see exogenous causes).

6.1.2 *Hypoglycemia due to specific hepatic enzyme deficiency.* Hypoglycemia due to specific hepatic enzyme deficiency (Table 4) such as glycogen storage diseases, glycogen synthase deficiency, or fructose 1, 6-diphosphate deficiency, seen primarily in infancy and childhood, will not be discussed here.

6.1.2.1 *Glutaric aciduria Type II.* Glutaric aciduria Type II, previously described only in a neonate, has now also been described in the adult [124]. A 19-year-old woman had several episodes of life-threatening hypoglycemia, nausea and vomiting, all precipitated by intercurrent infections. Hepatomegaly, jaundice, elevated serum transaminase, fatty infiltration of the liver, and a proximal lipid storage myopathy were associated features. There was a family history of similar attacks in two sisters. The entity is characterized by metabolic acidosis with a lack of ketosis, and elevated serum levels of free fatty acids consistent with the inhibition of oxidation of butyrate and isovalerate. The abnormality is similar to that seen in Jamaican vomiting stickness due to the ingestion of unripe ackee fruit (see below). The patient improved after the institution of frequent high carbohydrate meals.

6.1.3 *Functional hypoglycemia.* No recognizable or no persistent anatomic lesion.

6.1.3.1 *Deficiency of glucagon.* A deficiency of glucagon could be expected to lead to fasting hypoglycemia by interfering with gluconeogenesis and glycogenolysis. Hypoglycemia associated with decreased secretion of glucagon has not been well documented. In one patient hypoglycemia was induced either by a 28-hour fast, a diet high in protein and low in carbohydrate, or an arginine infusion. Plasma levels of glucagon were below the lower limits of normal and could not be elevated by fasting, hypoglycemia, or arginine infusion, potent stimuli of glucagon secretion [125].

6.1.3.2 *Severe inanition.* The severe fasting hypoglycemia seen occasionally in patients with extreme inanition reflects a limitation of gluconeogenesis. Probably, this condition is in part due to an insufficient supply of substrate – i.e., depletion of peripheral fat stores with decreased mobilization from them of the substrate glycerol and free fatty acids, and depletion of muscle proteins, with decreased mobilization of amino acids. Decreased mobilization of free fatty acids from depleted fat stores makes less free fatty acid available for energy and oxidative needs in the process of hepatic gluconeogenesis. A decrease in synthesis or activation of gluconeogenetic enzymes may also be involved in the hypoglycemia of inanition. The infusion of alanine, a substrate for gluconeogenesis, did elicit a rise in blood glucose in one cachectic patient studied by us and in a similar patient described by others.

Some patients with starvation-related hypoglycemia are not responsive to the infusion of glucose [126]. It was postulated that cells normally impermeable to glucose, when serum insulin levels are low, become permeable in some severely starved patients for unknown reasons.

6.1.3.3 *Insulin autoimmune syndrome.* Some patients have severe fasting or postprandial hypoglycemia due to the presence of insulin binding antibodies, although never having received exogenous insulin [127–133]. In addition to glucose intolerance, some of these patients also have evidence of other immunological disorders such as Graves' disease, particularly when treated with Methimazole. These patients have greatly elevated levels of 'total immunoreactive insulin' (up to 40,000 μU/ml), an artifact of the standard immunoassay procedure related to the high insulin binding capacity of these patients' plasma. In the absence of hypoglycemia, levels of 'free-insulin' are normal. During hypoglycemia, free insulin is elevated. The antibodies in patients with autoimmune hypoglycemia exhibit both high affinity and low affinity binding sites. Hypoglycemia develops when the free insulin is released from these sites, especially the low affinity sites, if the pool of antibody-bound insulin is large enough. Substantial quantities of free insulin are released by dissociation from antibody-bound insulin. Hypoglycemia occurs either when saturation of insulin binding capacity is approached but release of insulin from the B-cells continues, such as after a meal, or whenever excessive insulin becomes dissociated from the antigen-antibody complex. These autoantibodies resemble the antibodies recovered from patients treated with exogenous insulin. Insulin antibodies were found in the IgG globulin fraction, with kappa-type globulins predominating, as opposed to insulin-treated patients in whom lambda globulins coexist with kappa [131]. In an effort to ascertain that such patients have not been exposed to exogenous insulin, circulating antibodies to bovine or porcine proinsulin have been looked for and found to be absent, whereas they have been present in almost all diabetics who have been treated with insulin which is not highly purified and contains variable amounts of bovine and porcine proinsulin [134]. Other antibodies to contaminants in insulin preparations, such as antibodies to hPP, have not been found in patients with autoimmune insulin hypoglycemia.

Since its first description in 1970, Hirata has reported 85 such patients from Japan [133] while 5 such patients were reported in one publication from the USA [134].

It may also be possible to distinguish the insulin autoimmune syndrome from factitious hypoglycemia due to surreptitious administration of insulin by measuring the concentration of connecting peptide in plasma. Following stimuli, an increase in free C-peptide immunoreactivity has been demonstrated and indicates that the patient's beta cells are responsive rather than suppressed as by exogenous insulin taken surreptitiously. Markedly increased total C-peptide immunoreactivity is due to the fact that significant amounts of proinsulin (containing the C-peptide within its structure) may bind to insulin antibody [135].

6.1.3.4 *Hypoglyemia due to autoantibodies to the insulin receptor.* Studies of insulin resistance in patients with acanthosis nigricans and glucose intolerance or diabetes have defined a subgroup of patients with antibodies against the insulin receptor. These patients also have a high incidence of autoimmune disease. Of 13 patients with antireceptor antibodies, symptomatic hypoglycemia has developed in 5 at sometime during their clinical course [136]. Three of the five patients have died, and in two, hypoglycemia seemed to be the cause of death. Recently a patient has been described in deatil in whom hypoglycemia was the sole manifestation of antireceptor antibodies [137]. Fasting hypoglycemia results from the insulinomimetic effect of autoantibodies directed against the insulin receptor. At times when the patient demonstrated fasting hypoglycemia, levels of plasma insulin were elevated and averaged 11 μU/ml, with a range of 7 to 19 μU/ml. Proinsulin concentration was 5% of total insulin immunoreactivity. Anti-insulin antibodies were undetectable. Positive tests for antibodies were found to extractable nuclear antigen, antinuclear antibodies, rheumatoid factor and antimicrosomal thyroid antibodies. Hypoglycemia after subtotal pancreatectomy was refractory to diazoxide therapy. Postoperatively the patient had hemolytic anemia, thrombocytopenia and fever. Circulating autoantibodies to the insulin receptor were present in a titer of 1:20. The patient was treated with large doses of steroids, which restored euglycemia presumably because it antagonized the insulin-like bioactivity of antireceptor antibodies since there was no detectable change in the titer of antireceptor antibodies. After 10 weeks of therapy, the titer of antireceptor antibodies had fallen approximately 100-fold and prednisone could be discontinued without recurrence of hypoglycemia. In patients with fasting hypoglycemia and other manifestations of autoimmunity, antireceptor antibodies must be considered in the differential diagnosis of hypoglycemia.

A similar patient with hypoglycemia resulting from autoantibodies to the insulin receptor has been described in abstract form [138].

The entities listed in Table 4 as A.3.e.f.g. will not be discussed as these are seen in childhood only.

6.1.4 *Hypoglyemia induced by exogenous agents*

6.1.4.1 *Ethanol* (and poor nutrition). Ethanol ingestion, if superimposed upon an inadequate diet, can precipitate acute hypoglycemia [139]. Inhibition of gluconeogenesis due to a decrease in substrate oxidation, in conjunction with depletion of liver glycogen stores, is primarily responsible for the hypoglycemia. During alcohol oxidation, the ratio of co-factors $NADH_2/NAD$ inceases, reversing the equilibrium lactate $\rightleftarrows$ pyruvate, resulting in a decrease in the rate by which substrate (e.g., pyruvate produced by the oxidation of alanine) is available for gluconeogenesis. Alcohol precipitates hypoglycemia in healthy subjects after they have fasted for 48–72 hours. In some patients with decreased gluconeogenetic reserve (e.g., those with cortisol deficiency, thyrotoxicosis) alcohol may precipitate hypoglycemia after a short period of fasting.

6.1.4.2 *Factitious hyperinsulinism due to insulin administration* (see below.)

6.1.4.3 *Factitious hyperinsulinism due to sulfonylurea ingestion.* The possibility of factitious hyperinsulinism due to surreptitious administration of insulin or sulfonylurea drugs [140] should always be considered, particularly in paramedical personnel, diabetic patients and relatives of diabetic patients. Some such patients have had partial pancreatectomies in search of islet cell tumors. If self-administration of insulin is suspected, insulin antibodies may, and suppressed levels of C-peptide will be found [141, 142, 143]. Plasma and urinary concentration of sulfonylurea drugs should be determined to rule out ingestion of these agents.

6.1.4.4 Ingestion of ackee fruit (hypoglycin). In Jamaica, profound hypoglycemia has occurred in persons who have ingested the unripened ackee fruit containing the toxic amino acid, hypoglycin. Hypoglycin interferes with the oxidation of long-chained fatty acid by inhibiting several acyl co A dehydrogenases, thus limiting energy for gluconeogenesis [144].

6.1.4.5 Miscellaneous drugs. Fasting hypoglycemia secondary to the ingestion of a variety of drugs has been reported [145]. In three patients the antiarrhythmic drug, disopyramide phosphate (Norpace) resulted in fasting hypoglycemia [146, 147]. All patients were elderly and were not well-nourished.

The ingestion of certain sulfonamide drugs prescribed for the treatment of urinary tract infections has precipitated fasting hypoglycemia. Severe hypoglycemia with an inappropriately elevated insulin level occurred in a patient with chronic renal failure who was taking two tablets of sulfamethoxazole and trimethoprim twice a day [148]. The hypoglycemic episode was related to hyperinsulinemia, probably induced by the sulfonamide, in addition to other factors already listed, prevailing in patients with chronic renal disease and congestive heart failure.

Symptomatic and biochemical hypoglycemia may occur as a complication of pentamadine therapy [149]. Pentamidine, an aromatic diamidine, is used in the treatment of patients with acquired immunodeficiency syndrome who develop pneumocystis carinii infections. A patient reported recently to develop hypoglycemia while being treated with pentamidine also received trimethoprim and sulfamethoxazole [150].

Salicylate-induced hypoglycemia with metabolic acidosis is well described in the pediatric literature. In adults it has been reported primarily in diabetic patients concomitant with the use of other hypoglycemic agents. A case of clinical hypoglycemia, ketosis, and metabolic acidosis attributable to salicylate has been reported recently in a nondiabetic adult [151].

6.2 Postprandial (reactive) hypoglycemia

6.2.1 Functional hypoglycemia: no recognizable anatomic lesion. There are three major types of postprandial or reactive hypoglycemia (Table 4, Fig. 3): a) Reactive hypoglycemia secondary to excessive absorption of food stuffs containing carbohydrates, the so-called alimentary hypoglycemia or alimentary hyperinsulinism; b) Reactive hypoglyemia associated with mild diabetes mellitus; and c) Idiopathic reactive functional hypoglycemia.

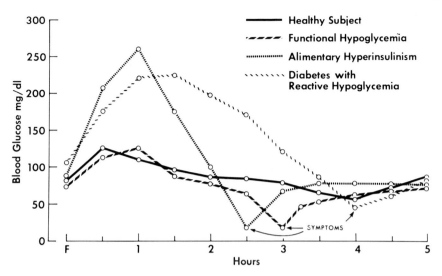

Figure 3. Glucose tolerance tests in healthy subject and in patients with three types of reactive hypoglycemia: reactive functional hypoglycemia, alimentary hyperinsulinism, and diabetes with reactive hypoglycemia. (Note: Biological fluid sampled is blood. Glucose concentration is 15% lower in blood than in plasma).

6.2.1.1 *Alimentary hyperinsulinism.* Alimentary hypoglycemia may occur in patients who have had a history of gastrointestinal surgery, such as subtotal gastrectomy or gastroenterostomy, or who have the functional equivalent because of a patulous pylorus. After a high carbohydrate meal, particularly one containing refined carbohydrate, there is rapid progression of carbohydrate into the upper small bowel with rapid absorption of the carbohydrate. Because of the rapid absorption, plasma glucose rises to a level higher than normal, frequently up to 250 mg/dl or more. This hyperglycemia stimulates excessive insulin release as compared to insulin release following the physiological rise of plasma glucose after meals, and the resultant hyperinsulinemia causes a rapid fall in plasma glucose. In addition there may be excessive stimulation of release of gastrointestinal hormones such as GIP, or glucose-dependent insulin-releasing polypeptide, also causing hyperinsulinism. Plasma glucose falls to hypoglycemic levels two to three hours after the beginning of a meal. The glucose tolerance test shows a normal fasting level of plasma glucose, a very high level of plasma glucose at one hour, a plasma glucose level in the normal or near normal range at two hours, and hypoglycemia by three hours (as low as 20–25 mg/dl). Usually symptoms of hyperepinephrinemia predominate. Since plasma glucose may fall to very low levels, symptoms of neuroglycopenia may occur. Since there is a rapid rebound from hypoglycemia to euglycemia, symptoms do not persist for long.

6.2.1.2 *Reactive hypoglyemia secondary to mild diabetes.* In patients with mild diabetes, characterized by normal or only slightly elevated fasting plasma glucose levels (usually below 130 mg/dl), reactive hypoglycemia may occur [152]. During the glucose tolerance test plasma glucose rises above 200 mg/dl at one hour and it is above this level at two hours, or in the case of the patient with 'impaired glucose tolerance', the plasma glucose may be between 140 and 200 mg/dl at two hours. Similar levels pertain after the ingestion of a meal high in refined carbohydrates. At 3–4-1/2 hours after ingestion of the meal or glucose load, plasma glucose levels will fall to levels below 50 mg/dl and the patients may have transient symptoms of hypoglycemia. It has been postulated that patients with reactive hypoglycemia secondary to mild diabetes mellitus have delayed insulin release in response to a rising blood glucose level. However, eventually, increases in plasma insulin exceed normal increases precipitating a secondary hypoglycemia.

6.2.1.3 *Idiopathic reactive or functional hypoglycemia.* Patients with this type of reactive hypoglycemia have neither mild diabetes mellitus nor an alimentary lesion. On a glucose tolerance test there will be a normal fasting concentration of plasma glucose, a normal rise in plasma glucose, a normal fall in plasma glucose thereafter, reaching hypoglycemic levels (<50 mg/dl or <45 mg/dl of plasma glucose). The majority of these patients do not have glucose-induced hyperinsulinism nor a detectable deficiency in counterregulatory hormones such as glucagon, epinephrine, hydrocortisone, or growth hormone. There may be some defect in the finer modulation of counterregulation by the autonomic nervous system. After hypoglycemic levels have been reached there is a rebound in plasma glucose toward or to normal levels between three and five hours (when there is no rebound one should suspect organic hyperinsulinism even though the patient does not have symptoms of fasting hypoglycemia). The patient with idiopathic reactive hypoglycemia has symptoms due to hyperepinephrinemia usually two to four hours after meals.

Demonstration of hypoglycemia during a glucose tolerance test does not justify a diagnosis of functional hypoglycemia. Up to 25% of normal young college students will have plasma glucose levels between 50–60 mg/dl and 3% may have levels below 50 mg/dl. Among a group of 400 subjects without diseases affecting carbohydrate metabolism the median nadir during the glucose tolerance test was 63 mg/dl, the 10th percentile 48 mg/dl and the 2.5th percentile 41 mg/dl [153]. Although some individuals may have symptoms following the nadir of plasma glucose during the glucose tolerance test they have no symptoms spontaneously after eating normal meals. Thus, they do not classify as having reactive hypoglycemia, nor does the patient who has symptoms of hyperepinephrinemia any time of the day or shortly after meals, but has a low plasma glucose on the glucose tolerance test.

The diagnosis of functional or reactive hypoglycemia should be considered only if three elements pertain: 1) spontaneous symptoms compatible with hypoglycemia at definite intervals after meals, such as 2–4 hours after eating, 2) demonstrable biochemical hypoglycemia (plasma glucose of less than 50 mg/dl) during the glucose tolerance tests, 3) reproduction of spontaneous symptoms at the time or following demonstration of biochemical hypoglycemia [154].

Reactive functional hypoglycemia occurs almost uniformly in tense, driving individuals with some emotional problems. The usual symptoms produced by reactive hypoglycemia are transitory and often subside spontaneously in 15 to 30 minutes. Weakness, hunger, inward trembling, sweating, palpitation and tachycardia are the most common symptoms in these patients. Severity of symptoms is not progressive. Attacks are more frequent when emotional stress and anxiety are greater. A family history of diabetes mellitus is usually absent. Recent publicity in the popular press and in books by some medical authors have led the public and some segments of the medical profession to believe that spontaneous hypoglycemia is a widespread and unrecognized cause of many physical and psychic ills. Promoting such a notion is a mistake. Persistent symptoms such as chronic fatigue, depression, lethargy, loss of vitality or anxiety that affect many people are not due to hypoglycemia ('nonhypoglycemia'). Because of the over-diagnosis of reactive hypoglycemia there has been scepticism that an entity such as reactive hypoglycemia exists. We believe that alimentary hypoglycemia and hypoglycemia secondary to diabetes are real entities and that idiopathic reactive hypoglycemia exists as well in a few patients.

It has been reported that hyperepinephrinemia may occur when the plasma glucose level falls from 90 to 60 mg/dl [155]. Thus, symptoms of hypoglycemia may occur at higher levels of plasma glucose than at a nadir below 50 mg/dl.

6.2.2 Hypoglycemia due to specific hepatic enzyme deficiency. These entities will not be discussed as they are seen in infancy and childhood only.

7. Evaluation of the patient with suspected hypoglycemia – history, physical examination, clinical course

The diagnosis of hypoglycemia, whether due to inappropriate hyperinsulinism due to pancreatic islet B-cell disease or to other etiological causes, should be suspected when symptoms, attacks, or spells occur as described under 3. Symptoms of Hypoglycemia. A careful history should be elicited differentiating between symptoms due to hyperepinephrinemia and symptoms due to neuroglucopenia. Important to ascertain are the type and severity of symptoms; relationship to meals, i.e., effect of fasting, delayed or skipped meals, temporal relationship of onset of symptoms to last meal; relief by carbohydrate-containing foods; effect of exercise; intervals between attacks; and progression or lack of progression of symptomatology in severity with time. Thus, a carefully obtained history should try to ascertain whether symptoms, potentially due to hypoglycemia, are more compatible with a postprandial (post-absorptive) cause of hypoglycemia or due to one of the fasting hypoglycemias. The presence of other diseases, such as hepatic, pituitary, adrenal disease, autoimmune disease; presence of a family history of multiple endocrine neoplasia Type I; possible access to or use of hypoglycemic agents; history of ethanol ingestion, and the nutritional status of the patient should also be ascertained.

Occasionally biochemical hypoglycemia will be found in the work-up of a patient not suspected to have hypoglycemia; if it occurs in the fasting state or if it is severe, it has to be pursued vigorously. On the other hand artifactual hypoglycemia may occur in patients with leukemia and polycythemia [156]. The spurious hypoglycemia is caused by accelerated in vitro metabolism of glucose by abnormal circulating cells.

Symptoms of hypoglycemia due to pancreatic B-cell disease may develop insidiously or rapidly and quite dramatically, with periodic attacks becoming more frequent and more severe. In contradistinction, symptoms due to the functional hypoglycemias are not progressive in terms of frequency and severity of symptoms. With organic hyperinsulinism, symptoms due to neuroglucopenia usually predominate over symptoms secondary to hyperpinephremia, although a combination of these two symptomatologies may occur. Table 7 lists the frequency of individual symptoms in 65 of our 69 patients with organic hyperinsulinism. The time of day of occurrence of initial symptoms is given in Table 8. Thirty-seven or 57% had symptoms with fasting or a missed meal, and 40 or 62% had postprandial symptoms. Classification of symptoms into neuroglucopenic and adrenergic symptoms at time of first attack are given in Table 9 with indication of the nature of their progression.

The majority of patients (36 of 65 or 55%) had both symptoms of neuroglucopenia and adrenergic symptoms with their first attack. Until diagnosis all patients continued with both types of symptoms. Twenty-one or 32% of patients had only neuroglucopenic symptoms during their first attack. Thus, 87% of the patients had symptoms of neuroglucopenia. Of the 21 patients who had symptoms of neuroglucopenia only with the initial attack, 14 had mixed symptoms during the following months, 7 within six months, 3 between 6–12 months, 3 between 12–24 months, and 1 between 24–36 months. Adrenergic symptoms only were seen with the first attack in 7 patients. All had experienced autonomic and neuroglucopenic symptoms in the following months, 3 within 6 months, 1 in 6 to 7 months, 2 in 12 to 24 months, and 1 in 24 to 48 months. One patient with multiple endocrine neoplasia type I had not experienced any symptoms, and another one only minor symptoms of hypoglycemia at the time the diagnosis of organic hyperinsulinism was made.

In 64 of the 65 patients in whom detailed information is available there was a progression in frequency and severity of symptoms. This occurred from within months after the first symptoms to within up to 5–7 years after the first symptoms were experienced.

The interval between onset of symptoms and recognition of their being due to hypoglycemia may be months to many years. In our patients with islet cell disease

Table 7. Frequency of symptoms in 65 patients with organic hyperinsulinism

		Adrenergic	Symptoms Adrenergic plus central nervous system	Central nervous system
1.	Sweating	54%		
2.	Confusion			48%
3.	Visual disturbance/diplopia			43%
4.	Clouding of consciousness			40%
5.	Weakness			35%
6.	Transient motor deficit			31%
7.	Fatigue		31%	
8.	Dizziness			29%
9.	Syncope			25%
10.	Inappropriate behavior			23%
11.	Headache			23%
12.	Seizures			23%
13.	Inability to concentrate			22%
14.	Shakiness, trembling, jitteriness	22%		
15.	Numbness and tingling			20%
16.	Speech difficulty			20%
17.	Memory failure			17%
18.	Circumoral paresthesia			15%
19.	Anxiety, nervousness	13%		
20.	Hunger, nausea	12%		
21.	Irritability		12%	
22.	Stupor			12%
23.	Amnesia for episode			11%
24.	Tachhycardia, palpitations	9%		
25.	Lethargy, lassitude			9%
26.	Twitching			6%
27.	Difficulty in arising in AM			6%
28.	Sleepiness during day			6%

Table 8. Periodicity of initial symptoms in 65 patients with organic hyperinsulinism

	Number of patients	% of total
1. Symptoms after overnight fast only	13	20
2. Fasting and postprandial symptoms	20	31
3. Symptoms after missed meal only	4	6
4. Postprandial symptoms only	20	31
5. Uncertain about timing of symptoms	7	11
6. No symptoms experienced	1	1
Totals	65	100
Symptoms exacerbated by exercise	23	35

Table 9. Classification of symptoms of first attack into neuroglucopenic and adrenergic and their progression among 65 patients with organic hyperinsulinism

First attack:	Number of patients	%
A. Neuroglucopenic and adrenergic symptoms Follow up – all patients continued with both types of symptoms	36	55
B. Neuroglucopenic symptoms only Follow up – 14 of 21 had mixed symptoms in following months, half within 6 months	21	32
C. Adrenergic symptoms only Follow up – all had mixed symptoms in following months, 4 within 12 months	7	11
D. No symptoms (patient with MEN-Type I)	1	1

Neuroglucopenic symptoms noted without adrenergic symptoms at same time: Peripheral and circumoral paresthesia, diplopia, dizziness, inability to concentrate, memory failure, speech difficulty, seizures, peristent neurological deficit, inappropriate behavior, syncope, clouding of consciousness.

the interval between the onset of symptoms and documentation of hypoglycemia was up to 17 years. In two patients biochemical hypoglycemia was noted before the first symptom, and in nine it was documented at the time of the first symptomatic episode. For the majority of patients the interval between the first symptom and documentation of hyperinsulinism or exploration of an insulinoma was fairly evenly distributed between a few months and 10 years. Symptoms, attacks, or spells may occur after an overnight fast when the patient has been fasting the longest, particularly when breakfast has been omitted or delayed because of an intercurrent illness of for religious reasons. In other patients only more prolonged fasting and exercise may precipitate attacks. When hyperinsulinism is severe, or in instances when the islet cell tumor secretes in response to food intake, symptoms may also occur two to four hours after meals. When symptoms occurring postprandially include severe symptoms of neuroglucopenia, organic hyperinsulinism in contradistinction to the more benign functional hypoglycemia should be considered. Thirty-one of 65 (48%) patients were admitted to a hospital emergency room because of severe CNS symptoms of hypoglycemia (Table 10). In 11 of these patients (35%) admission to the emergency room occurred for the first episode of symptoms. In the other 20 patients the time interval from first symptoms to visit to the emergency room ranged from one month to seven years, with the mean and median time span being two years.

In nine patients seen in an emergency room the initial diagnosis was a neurological or psychiatric one, including convulsive disorder or psyhomotor seizures while conversion hysteria was the diagnosis for the initial two episodes in a patient who had had multiple sclerosis for 15 years (Table 10). Plasma glucose was not measured during the first visit to the emergency room in seven patients.

Some patients learn to avoid symptoms by taking frequent feedings, including

Table 10. Admission to hospital emergency rooms because of symptoms of hypoglycemia in 65 of 69 patients with organic hyperinsulinism in whom information is available

31 (48%)	*Total number admitted to ER due to symptoms*
11 of 31 (35%)	For first symptomatic episode
20 of 31 (65%)	One month to seven years (median and mean time span two years) after first symptom.
Diagnoses at first ER visit	
15 (48%)	Hypoglycemia – 4 admitted immediately to rule out hyperinsulinism.
7 (23%)	Plasma glucose not measured – no diagnosis made.
9 (29%)	Psychiatric or neurological diagnosis
3	Convulsive disorder
1	Hysterical seizure vs. cerebral thrombosis
1	Conversion hysteria
1	Increase in frequency of psychomotor seizures of 34 yrs. duration
2	Possible CVA
1	Post automobile accident trauma (1 day previously)

feedings during the night. Obesity may thereby result, but it is not seen in the majority of our patients. Of 69 patients 41 or 63% were not obese (i.e., 121% or more of ideal body weight) at diagnosis.

In patients with insulinomas misdiagnosed as having functional hypoglycemia (6 patients), the institution of a low carbohydrate, high protein diet may aggravate symptoms of hypoglycemia or precipitate symptoms of neuroglucopenia (2 patients). If during a glucose tolerance test, performed because of suspected postprandial or functional hypoglycemia, postprandial hypoglycemia occurs but is not followed by a rebound of plasma glucose to normal levels, organic hypoglycemia should be suspected. Spontaneous remissions of symptoms from months to years have occurred. Symptoms are usually rapidly progressive in patients with malignant metastatic tumors (except for patient with multiple endocrine neoplasia – Type I).

In the absence of symptoms of hypoglycemia the physical examination is usually normal in patients with islet cell disease. Nonpancreatic tumors associated with hypoglycemia are usually large in size, are located in the chest, abdomen and pelvis, and may be found by a physical examination (or by appropriate radiological studies). When fasting hypoglycemia is secondary to hepatic, pituitary or adrenal disease the diagnosis of the underlying cause for hypoglycemia usually does not present diagnostic difficulties as physical findings of hepatic, pituitary or adrenal disease are obvious.

8. Evaluation of the patient with suspected hyperinsulinism – laboratory tests and procedures

8.1 Tests for suspected organic islet B-cell disease and hyperinsulinism

8.1.1 Essential diagnostic tests. The diagnosis of inappropriate hyperinsulinism due to pancreatic islet B-cell disease can be made by determination of fasting plasma levels of glucose and of immunoreactive insulin (IRI) from blood samples obtained after an overnight fast or during prolongation of the overnight fast. Characteristically, even though the patients major symptoms may occur post-prandially, hypoglycemia will occur on fasting, and the diagnosis can be con-firmed by the demonstration of an inappropriately raised plasma level of IRI.

8.1.1.1 Fasting plasma levels of glucose. In healthy males and females concentra-tions of plasma glucose after an overnight fast are rarely below 70 mg/dl. In healthy males, plasma glucose levels do not decline below 60 mg/dl during a 24-hour fast. During a 70–72 hour fast, they usually decline further but not below 55 mg/dl [157, 158]. Fasting results in greater decreases in blood glucose in healthy premenopausal females than in healthy males [157]. Merimee and Tyson [157] reported that in approximately 40% of lean women, blood glucose levels de-creased to less than 45 mg/dl during the 72-hour fast. Of these women, one-third had levels as low as 30–35 mg/dl, with occasional levels between 22 and 30 mg/dl. These authors suggest that after one day of fasting, a feasible lower limit of normal in women would be approximately 35 mg/dl for plasma glucose, and that after 36-hour fasting it is impossible to differentiate physiologic hypoglycemia from that secondary to hyperinsulinism. None of these subjects had symptoms unequivocally due to hypoglycemia. We confirmed [158] as did Haymond et al. [159] that there is a sex difference in plasma glucose levels during 72 hours of fasting (Fig. 4). However, in *none* of our 51 females fasted for 72 hours was plasma glucose *below 61 mg/dl* at *23 hours of fasting*. During the 72-hour fast, the lowest level in our females was 36 mg/dl, as compared to 42 mg/dl [160] and 47 mg/dl [161], respectively, in two other reports, and to 23 mg/dl in the group of females referred to above [157]. In many healthy females in whom plasma glucose falls below 50 mg/dl in the course of a 72-hour fast, the level will rise spontaneously again as the fast proceeds, presumably due to accelerated gluconeogenesis [158]. In all the females in our study, plasma glucose was 55 mg/dl or above after exercise between 70 and 72 hours of the fast (Fig. 4). The rise in plasma glucose during exercise can be attributed to hepatic conversion of lactate, derived from muscle glycogen, to glucose. During fasting, men have higher plasma levels of alanine and glutamine than do women [159]. Since men have a greater muscle mass than do women, both the increased plasma alanine and glutamine could be the result of increased release of these potential gluconeogenic amino acids. Increased availability of potential gluconeogenic substrates during fasting may be

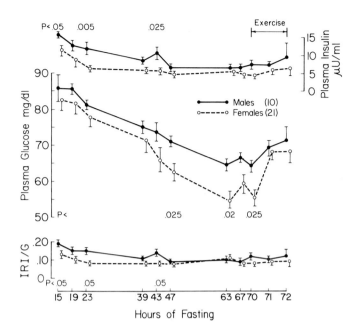

Figure 4. Levels of plasma insulin, plasma glucose, and IRI/G (immunoreactive insulin/glucose ratio) during 72-hour fast in 10 healthy, nonobese male and 21 female subjects (Mean ±S.E.M.). (Reprinted from Fajans, S.S. and J.C. Floyd, Jr., N. Engl. J. Med. 294: 776, 1976.)

partially responsible for the higher plasma glucose concentrations observed in men when compared to women. The differences between males and females in their plasma glucose responses to fasting are not due to differing concentrations of insulin [158] or counterregulatory hormones [159].

In many patients with pancreatic islet cell disease and hyperinsulinism, the level of plasma glucose after an overnight fast (10 hours) is below 60 mg/dl or even below 50 mg/dl. However, in only 53% of our patients with proven islet cell disease was the overnight fasting plasma glucose level below 60 mg/dl and in only 30% below 50 mg/dl on the first day of the study. When daily fasting plasma glucose levels were obtained for 6 or more days, 84% and 71% had at least one level below 60 mg/dl or 50 mg/dl, respectively. Thus, fasting plasma glucose may fluctuate from normal to subnormal levels from day to day. A more convenient and more reliable way to demonstrate fasting hypoglycemia in patients with organic hyperinsulinism is to prolong the overnight fast for four hours or more. This procedure usually will reduce plasma glucose to below 50 mg/dl. When the fast is lengthened to 20–24 hours, more severe fasting hypoglycemia (plasma glucose below 45 mg/dl, frequently below 40 mg/dl) will develop in the majority of patients. In men, this is clearly diagnostic of fasting hypoglycemia. According to Merimee and Tyson [157], such levels are nondiagnostic in females. In our experience, healthy females do not have concentrations of plasma glucose below 61 mg/dl during the first 23 hours of fasting. Thus, the differentiation between normal decreases in plasma glucose and pathological fasting hypoglycemia is usually made within the first 24 hours of fasting. If plasma glucose falls below 61 mg/dl during the first 24 hours of fasting in females, differentiation between normal and abnormal can usually be resolved by simultaneous measurements of plasma insulin and determination of the insulin to glucose ratio which stays normal in individuals without hyperinsulinism (see below). If after 24 hours of fasting, hypoglycemia is not induced in a patient with suspected fasting hypoglycemia or in whom fasting hypoglycemia needs to be excluded by more rigorous criteria, the fast should be continued for up to 72 hours. If symptomatic or biochemical hypoglycemia has not developed, the patient should be exercised vigorously for two hours at that time. In patients with insulinoma (and very low grade insulin secretion), or in patients with other types of fasting hypoglycemia, exercise will produce a further fall in blood glucose levels, but in healthy subjects and in patients with functional hypoglycemia it usually raises blood glucose. Exercise at any time during the fast can precipitate or aggravate hypoglycemia in patients with organic hyperinsulinism. The frequency of blood sampling during a fast depends on how well the patient tolerates deprivation of food. If the overnight fast or a short prolongation of the overnight fast results in levels of plasma glucose in the hypoglycemic range (below 40 mg/dl), further prolongation of the fast is unnecessary.

The time of onset of symptoms in hours after the last meal and after the beginning of a fast in 69 patients with organic hyperinsulinism is shown in Table 11. Thirty-eight patients or 55% had symptoms within 14 hours and 53 or 77% within 18 hours. Fifty-nine patients or 86% had their first symptoms within 24 hours. In another seven, the first symptom did not occur until between 28–48 hours of the fast. In all these patients the fast was terminated either immediately or several hours after the beginning of symptoms because of severe central nervous system symptomatology. Three patients were able to tolerate the fast for 72 hours. One patient had only mild intermittent diplopia. This patient was a member of a family with MEN-Type I. At operation he was found to have a multicentric islet cell carcinoma with regional lymph node involvement. He had an en bloc distal hemipancreatectomy which included involved lymph nodes and a focus of tumor toward the tail of the pancreas. An additional tumor was removed from the pancreatic head. It is now 15 years since the surgery and he continues to do well clinically. The other two patients had no symptoms whatsoever during the 72-hour fast. These patients had biochemical evidence of hypoglycemia for the last 48 hours of the fast with plasma glucose levels as low as 36 mg/dl. In general, many patients had biochemical hypoglycemia for many hours before the development of symptoms. When fasting is repeated in the same patient on different occasions, symptoms of hypoglycemia may occur many hours apart in these separate fasts even though they had similar decreases in plasma glucose.

Table 11. Time of onset of symptoms in hours after last meal and beginning of fast in patients with organic hyperinsulinism

Hours	Number of patients	
≤ 8	12	8 Single adenomas, 1 adenomatosis, 3 carcinomas
≤ 10	6	5 Single adenomas, 1 adenomatosis
≤ 12	11	10 Single adenomas, 1 adenomatosis
≤ 14	9	5 Single adenomas, 1 adenomatosis, 1 hyperplasia, 2 nesidioblastosis
≤ 16	11	10 Single adenomas, 1 adenomatosis
≤ 18	4	3 Single adenomas, 1 nesidioblastosis
≤ 20	3	3 Single adenomas
≤ 24	3	3 Single adenomas
≤ 28	1	1 Single adenoma
≤ 34	1	1 Single adenoma
≤ 40	1	1 Single adenoma
≤ 43	1	1 Single adenoma
≤ 48	3	2 Single adenomas, 1 adenomatosis
72	3 (no significant symptoms)	1 Single adenoma, 1 adenomatosis, 1 Ca-MEN-I (No symptoms in 2, transient diplopia in 1)
Total	69	

8.1.1.2 *Immunoreactive insulin after overnight or more prolonged fasting.* Determination of the concentration of plasma insulin after an overnight fast is essential to establish the presence of hyperinsulinism due to pancreatic islet cell disease. When fasting insulin levels are measured on several days, elevated levels of insulin in peripheral venous plasma can be found frequently in at least one specimen. Absolutely elevated levels are not found in all patients with functioning islet cell disease, owing in part to removal by the liver of some of the secreted insulin before it appears in peripheral blood and due to sporadic secretion of insulin from the tumor or other abnormal insulin secreting tissue. Insulinomas may secrete insulin in short bursts. This may provide wide fluctuations in plasma insulin concentrations. Thus, frequent measurements may be necessary to demonstrate inappropriately high levels of insulin in peripheral venous blood during fasting. Over a period of four hours during the prolongation of an overnight fast in one patient from 8:00 a.m. to 12:00 noon we have seen an extreme fluctuation of plasma insulin from $106 \mu U/ml$ to $4 \mu U/ml$. The patient was asymptomatic but had a constant concentration of plasma glucose of $32 mg/dl$ over this period of time. C-peptide, with its longer plasma half-life is less likely to show such marked changes in plasma concentration and should be a valuable adjunct in ascertaining the status of insulin secretion in patients with suspected insulinoma. Thus, although a diagnosis of insulinoma is confirmed by an elevated fasting insulin level, a 'normal' level does not rule out this diagnosis. In our laboratory, the normal upper limit of concentration of insulin (mean + 2SD) in peripheral blood of fasting nonobese healthy subjects was reported to be 24 μU/ml (10 + 14 μU/ml) [77]. More recently, in a larger group of healthy subjects we determined that the mean plus two standard deviations of fasting plasma IRI was 20 μU/ml [162]. Of the 67 patients with organic hyperinsulinism in whom plasma levels of immunoreactive insulin are available, after the first overnight fast only 52% of patients had an insulin concentration above 20 μU/ml and only 45% above 24 μU/ml. In many of these patients there were spontaneous fluctuations of insulin concentrations well above 20 μU/ml on other occasions. Of these patients, 88% had at least one elevated plasma level of insulin greater than 20 μU/ml and 74% greater than 24 μU/ml when six or more daily determinations were available (Table 12).

Among 51 patients with solitary benign insulinomas plasma levels of immunoreactive insulin (IRI) after on overnight fast ranged from 11 to 179 μU/ml. The six highest levels were 179, 116, 86, 70, 59 and 51μU/ml, respectively. The six lowest levels were 11, 11, 11, 12, 13, and 14 μU/ml, respectively. Examples of the range of daily fluctuation are from 10–40 μU/ml, 17–38 μU/ml, 28–64 μU/ml and 35–67 μU/ml, respectively. The patients with adenomatosis had fasting IRI levels which ranged from 15 to 115 μU/ml. The patient with the highest IRI level also had the extreme fluctuation, from 106 to 4 μU/ml within a 4-hour period, as mentioned above. Patients in whom organic hyperinsulinism was part of the syndrome of MEN-Type I had fasting IRI levels which ranged from 12–114 μU/ml. The three patients with sporadic metastatic insulinomas had insulin levels of 59, 64, and 1260 μU/ml, respectively. Thus, among the various groups of patients with organic hyperinsulinism, only the highest level of 1260 μU/ml in one patient with islet cell carcinoma was indicative of the type of disease present. However, by the time these patients were seen by us, hepatic metastases were obvious in all three patients with sporadic islet cell carcinoma. The patient with MEN-Type I in whom multicentric islet cell carcinoma and regional lymph node involvement was found at operation, had a fasting plasma IRI of 15 μU/ml.

Diagnostic plasma levels of insulin can be obtained more rapidly by the prolongation of the overnight fast. On prolongation of the overnight fast, plasma insulin in healthy males and females declines steadily to reach levels 3–7 μU/ml from 63 through 70 hours (Fig. 4). Thus, as fasting continues in patients *without* organic hyperinsulinism, plasma insulin declines with plasma glucose. On the

Table 12. Concentrations of plasma IRI after overnight fast in 67 patients with organic hyperinsulinism

Plasma IRI	Elevated ($\geq$20 μU/ml)	Elevated ($\geq$24 μU/ml)
% of patients		
– after one overnight fast	52%	45%
– after six or more overnight fasts	88%	74%

other hand, in the patient with pancreatic islet cell disease, when plasma glucose levels fall into the hypoglycemic range on prolongation of the fast, levels of plasma insulin remain constant, may fluctuate, or rise (Fig. 5, 6). This is evidence for the presence of autonomous insulin-producing tissue. An increase or failure of decrease in IRI values in the presence of a low plasma glucose value on prolongation of the overnight fast establishes the state of insulin-mediated hypoglycemia.

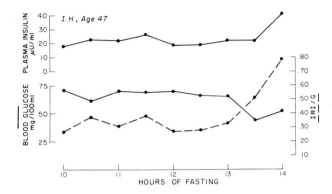

Figure 5. Levels of plasma insulin and blood glucose, and IRI/G during the last 4 hours of a 14-hour fast in a 51 year-old female with solitary islet cell adenoma. (Reprinted from Fajans, S.S., J.C. Floyd, Jr., and S.K. Vij, Endocrinol & Diabetes, Leonard J. Kryston, M.D., and Ralph A. Shaw, M.D., Ph.D., Editors, 1975, Grune & Stratton, Inc., p. 453.)

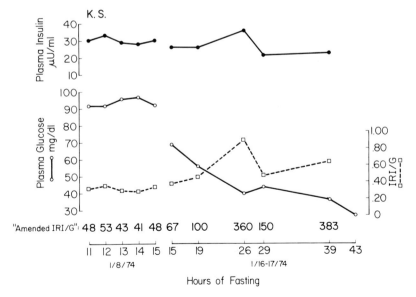

Figure 6. Levels of plasma insulin, plasma glucose, IRI/G and 'amended IRI/G' during a 15-hour fast and on another occasion during a 43-hour fast in a patient with solitary islet cell adenoma (Reprinted from Fajans, S.S., and J.C. Floyd, Jr., N Engl J Med 294: 776, 1976.)

8.1.1.3 *Ratio of immunoreactive insulin to plasma glucose (IRI/G) after overnight or more prolonged fasting.* The relationship of plasma insulin to plasma glucose can be expressed as the ratio of the plasma concentration of immunoreactive insulin (μU/ml) to the concentration of plasma glucose (G) (mg/dl). In healthy nonobese males, the normal upper limit (mean + 2 SD) of IRI/G after an overnight fast was reported by us as 0.30, based on the log of normal disribution of 412 values of IRI/G in 114 control subjects [77]. These values were based on the particular methods for plasma glucose and plasma insulin used in our laboratory. A ratio of 0.33 would be a more conservative value. As healthy subjects undergo prolonged fasting, plasma insulin declines with plasma glucose; the ratio IRI/G remains constant or declines modestly and during the 47–70 hour period becomes similar in both sexes (Fig. 4) [158]. In none of our healthy male or female subjects did the ratio exceed .24 during the 70-hour fast before exercise, or 0.31 after exercise. Even in women whose plasma glucose fell to as low as 22 mg/dl, [157] IRI/G was normal and in the range of 0.03–0.15 (T. Merimee, pers. commun.).

The application of the IRI/G ratio provides reliable data to confirm or establish a diagnosis of insulinoma in patient with mild abnormalities. A plasma insulin level in the 'normal' range and an associated fasting plasma glucose level in the hypoglycemic range constitute evidence that the secretion of insulin is excessive. This is made readily apparent by an elevated IRI/G ratio. In patients with pancreatic islet cell disease in whom fasting plasma glucose (or IRI/G) is within the normal range after a 10-hour fast, prolongation of the fast for four hours or more causes IRI/G to rise into the abnormal range (Fig. 5 and 6 and Table 13). After 14 hours of fasting, 56 of our 67 patients had abnormal ratios, and after 18 hours 61 had abnormal ratios. Another four had an abnormal ratio at 24 hours of the fast (Fig. 6). One patient had an abnormal ratio only at 32 hours of the fast (no symptoms until 40 hours), while another one did develop an abnormal ratio even though the fast had to be discontinued at 28 hours because of symptomatic hypoglycemia (Table 13). In the course of a 72-hour fast, a slight elevation of the IRI/G ratio at one or two time points of the fast are not significant. In patients with pancreatic islet cell disease the elevations in the ratios are continuous and significant [77, 158, 163].

In normal obese subjects, becaue of hyperinsulinemia due to insulin resistance, basal IRI/G may be elevated as compared to ratios of healthy nonobese subjects and therefore may simulate the ratios of patients with insulinoma. Since, in such patients, fasting plasma glucose is normal and does not fall below 55 mg/dl on prolonged fasting, there is no problem in differential diagnosis. The pattern of change of the IRI/G ratio at progressive time intervals of fasting provides the best distinction between patients with pancreatic islet cell disease and patients, nonobese or obese, without autonomous hyperinsulinism [77, 158, 163]. In patients with organic hyperinsulinism the ratio rises with prolongation of the fast while it stays constant or falls in patients without hyperinsulinism. The numerical value of the IRI/G ratio depends upon the techniques employed for measuring plasma

Table 13. Time of appearance of elevated IRI/G with fasting in 67 patients with organic hyperinsulinism

IRI/G Elevated at Time of Fast	Plasma IRI After Overnigh Fast	
	Elevated ($\geq$20 μU/ml)	Not Elevated (<20 μU/ml)
$\leq$ 14 hours	35 Pts.	21 Pts.
15–18 hours	2 Pts.	3 Pts.
19–24 hours	2 Pts.	2 Pts.
> 24 hours		1 (32 hours)
Totals	39 Patients	27 Patients

In one patient with single adenoma IRI/G not elevated within 28 hours (IRI <5 μU/ml). Fast discontinued as patient had biochemical and symptomatic hypoglycemia.

glucose and insulin, but the change in the ratio with time is independent of these variables [77, 158, 163].

Service et al. [160] have reported that a concentration of plasma IRI over 6 μU/ml in the presence of hypoglycemia (plasma glucose of <40 mg/dl) is diagnostic of insulin-mediated hypoglycemia. As with any diagnostic procedure, exceptions exist. As stated above, we have seen one patient with adenomatosis and hyperinsulinemia who at one time point had a concentration of plasma insulin below 6 μU/ml in the presence of severe hypoglycemia. Another patient with a single adenoma tolerated a 28-hour fast (Table 13). Six consecutive levels of plasma insulin between 10 and 28 hours of fasting were 4, 4, 4, 2, 5, 2 μU/ml with plasma glucose levels below 45 mg/dl. On the other hand, one female without fasting hypoglycemia and hyperinsulinism, had plasma levels of insulin of 8 and 9 μU/ml with plasma glucose levels of 36 and 39 mg/dl at 63 and 70 hours of the fast. The ratio of IRI to glucose was normal (0.22 and 0.23).

8.1.1.4 *'Amended IRI/G' after overnight or more prolonged fasting.* The 'amended' IRI/G ratio (plasma IRI (μU/ml) $\times$ 100 divided by plasma glucose (mg/dl) -30) has been reported to discriminate better abnormal from normal ratios [164]. The rationale for subtracting 30 mg/dl from the plasma glucose level is that in healthy subjects at a plasma glucose level of 30 mg/dl, secretion of insulin would be reduced sufficiently so that plasma insulin in peripheral blood measured with a sensitive radioimmunoassay for insulin would fall in the range of 0–1 μU/ml in healthy subjects (see 5.1). We found a range of 'amended' IRI/G ratios in our healthy control subjects [77] similar to that found by Turner et al. in theirs [164]. In only one of our healthy subjects or patients without fasting hypoglycemia did the 'amended ratio' exceed 52 during the 72-hour fast before exercise or 55 after exercise. In that patient the slightly elevated 'amended ratio' was not consistently elevated at subsequent time points. In patients with organic hyperinsulinism the amended ratio is elevated or rises with fasting. In only a few patients did the amended ratio became positive several hours before the IRI/G ratio [77]. Again, the change in the ratio during more prolonged fasting (ratio rises) gives a better diagnostic confirmation of the presence of inappropriate islet cell secretion [77, 158], than does a single observation during fasting.

The patient in whom pancreatic islet cell disease is strongly suspected should be studied as an inpatient. On the other hand, if suspicion is not strong, the patient can be studied as an outpatient. Under these circumstances we instruct the patient to have his last meal at 5–6 p.m. the night before and to come to the laboratory in the fasting state at 8 a.m. the following morning. Hourly or bi-hourly plasma samples for determination of glucose and insulin are obtained in the morning and throughout the afternoon unless clear-cut symptoms of hypoglycemia become apparent and the test is terminated. If fasting is prolonged to 18–22 hours and IRI/G remains in the normal range, the diagnosis of pancreatic islet cell disease with hyperinsulinism is ruled out for practical purposes. In some patients with organic hyperinsulinism after an overnight fast, pathologially elevated levels of immunoreactive insulin are not associated with a hypoglycemic level of plasma glucose. This may be due to a reduction in the number and/or affinity of insulin receptors observed in patients with insulinoma and may constitute a protective mechanism against excessive hypoglycemia [27].

8.1.2 *Additional tests and procedures.* Although inappropriate elevation of concentration of plasma insulin in the presence of hypoglycemia after overnight or more prolonged fasting remains the basis for the diagnosis of pancreatic islet cell disease, additional tests can confirm the diagnosis when fasting hypoglycemia is mild or absent. Measurement of insulin secretory products (proinsulin, C-peptide, and free insulin) in the peripheral circulation provide additional means of measuring beta cell secretion and prove useful in the study of islet cell function in patients with hypoglycemic disorders [141]. Elevation of the concentration of basal proinsulin is used for a confirming test in patients with insulinoma. Suppression tests and provocative stimulation tests are rarely employed today because of the accuracy of the evaluation of the insulin to glucose ratio during fasting.

8.1.2.1 *Basal proinsulin.* Small amounts of proinsulin, the single-chain precursor of insulin, are found in normal plasma (usually 10–15% and always less than 22% of total immunoreactive insulin). Insulin and connecting peptide (C-peptide) generated from cleavage of proinsulin are secreted in equimolar concentrations [141]. As compared to normal pancreatic tissue, insulin-producing neoplastic tissue typically releases excessive amounts of proinsulin into the blood. The estimation of fasting plasma levels of proinsulin and 'proinsulin-like components' may be helpful therefore in diagnosis of islet cell tumors. In 82% of our patients with organic hyperinsulinism, the proinsulin component was clearly elevated and exceeded 22% of fasting total IRI [77, 165]. A raised proinsulin concentration is a particularly helpful finding in establishing the diagnosis of insulinoma in patients who have low plasma concentrations of immunoreactive insulin [165, 166]. There is insufficient evidence to indicate whether proinsulin is elevated in patients with islet cell hyperplasia or nesidioblastosis, but preliminary experience indicates that it is not. In patients with undifferentiated tumors, particularly with islet cell carcinoma, very high proportions of proinsulin are found in plasma. In an individual patient the percentage of insulin immunoreactivity found in the proinsulin fraction does not differentiate malignant from benign insulinomas.

8.1.2.2 *Basal C-peptide.* Since insulin and connecting peptide (C-peptide) are released into the circulation from cleavage of proinsulin in the pancreas, the plasma concentration of C-peptide will be elevated when insulin is elevated [141]. Because clearance of C-peptide from plasma is considerably slower than that of insulin, C-peptide with its longer plasma half-life is less likely to show marked variation in concentration and should be a valuable adjunct in ascertaining the status of insulin secretion in patients with suspected insulinoma. The most useful application of the C-peptide assay is the situation in which the measurement of insulin is interfered with by the presence of circulating insulin and proinsulin antibodies from administration of insulin in diabetic patients and in its differentiation of states of hypersecretion of insulin from patients with fasting hypoglycemia due to surreptitious administration of insulin [141]. A patient with insulin-requiring diabetes who developed spontaneous hypoglycemia illustrates this technique [167]. Endogenous hyperinsulinism was confirmed by the measurement of high levels of C-peptide reactivity (CPR). Subtotal pancreatectomy was associated with a marked fall in CPR and relief of fasting hypoglycemia. Pancreatic histology showed nesidioblastosis (reported as hyperplasia).

8.1.2.3 *Suppression test – insulin infusion with C-peptide suppression.* Suppression of endogenous secretion of insulin, C-peptide, and proinsulin by hypoglycemia induced by exogenous insulin has been used to differentiate between insulin-producing tissue under normal physiological control and autonomous insulin-producing tissue. The test is performed in patients who do not have diagnostic fasting hypoglycemia. When compared with normal subjects, most patients with islet cell tumors show diminished or absent insulin, C-peptide, or proinsulin suppression. The infusion of pork insulin with simultaneous measurements of plasma levels of C-peptide at frequent intervals caused suppression of C-peptide in healthy control subjects but not in the majority of patients with insulin-secreting pancreatic islet cell disease [168, 169]. Probably because there is a long half-life of C-peptide in, as well as biological variability among normal control subjects, this test is not 100% reliable. In patients with proven islet cell adenoma, normal or near normal suppression of C-peptide has been reported [168, 169].

8.1.2.4 *Provocative tests.* In general, provocative tests are less reliable in the diagnosis of islet cell tumors than are determination of the ratio of immunoreactive insulin to plasma glucose, determination of basal proinsulin concentration or the suppression test. Provocative tests of insulin secretion (tolbutamide, leucine, glucagon tests) in patients with suspected islet cell disease are rarely necessary in the differential diagnosis of fasting hypoglycemia. They may be useful, if positive, in some rare insulinoma patients who do not have hypoglycemia after an overnight fast, who can tolerate prolonged fasts without symptoms, and whose levels of serum insulin are not consistently elevated. Examples have been given in recent publications [77, 158].

8.1.2.5 *Tolbutamide tests.* The tolbutamide test as an adjunct in the recognition of insulinoma was first described in 1960 before the availability of the immunoassay for insulin [170]. Plasma glucose criteria were employed for the interpretation of the test. By the completion of the 3-hour test a normal blood glucose response to tolbutamide consists in the return of blood glucose to 70% or more of fasting levels after the initial drop. In patients with islet cell disease, tolbutamide induces a greater reduction in blood glucose and persistence of hypoglycemia. Tolbutamide-induced hypoglycemia persisted for three hours in 50 of 55 patients subsequently proved to have insulinoma. In these patients, fasting plasma glucose levels were 50 mg/dl or above before administration of tolbutamide. The lower the fasting blood glucose, the more frequently will the test have to be terminated before its conclusion. The assay of plasma insulin in conjunction with blood glucose determination during the intravenous tolbutamide test has greatly increased the value of the test. In nonobese subjects, a maximal increase in plasma insulin above 195 μU/ml within the first 15 minutes and/or more importantly, subsequently prolonged elevation of plasma insulin (increments above basal levels of 45 μU/ml at 30 minutes, 25 μU/ml at 45 minutes, and 15 μU/ml at 60 minutes) were considered abnormal [77]. These levels are the mean + 2 standard deviation of the values obtained in 25 nonobese control subjects. In obese subjects, greater maximal increases in plasma insulin may be found, but, in the absence of islet cell disease, an abnormal blood glucose response would not be expected. Using maximal increases and values at 30, 45, and 60 minutes for interpreting insulin responses, 86% of 29 patients had abnormal tolbutamide tests. If severe hypoglycemia should occur during the test, intravenous glucose should be given and continued for several hours after the test. Service et al. have employed the tolbutamide test as a screening test to rule out insulinoma [160]. Criteria employed by Service et al. are simpler and may be more discriminating. During the last hour of the test (120–180 minutes) only one of 22 controls had blood glucose values below 50 mg/dl and only one of the insulinoma patients had values above 50 mg/dl. For plasma glucose values the value of 57 mg/dl was used; again there was only one overlap between the two groups. Utilizing plasma insulin as well, Service et al. used a linear discriminant approach [160]. Glucose minus 0.5 IRI = 42.5 at the 150 minute point provided complete separation of the control subjects and 18 insulinoma patients. Insulinoma patients had differences of less than 43 and controls had differences of greater than 43. However there was no discrimination for noninsulinoma patients, lean or obese, who were taking a variety of drugs, including phenytoin. Also, in many patients with insulinoma, the tolbutamide test has to be terminated before 150 minutes of the test because of the occurrence of severe symptoms of neuroglucopenia.

8.1.2.6 Other provocative tests. In our experience other provocative tests are less reliable. Only 74% of proven insulinomas had abnormal leucine tests and 58% had abnormal glucagon tests [77]. The stimulation of insulin secretion by calcium infusion in patients with insulinomas has been suggested as another provocative test [171, 172, 173]. Because of inconsistent results with calcium infusion, its value in the diagnosis of insulin-secreting islet cell tumors of the pancreas is also limited [174, 175, 176, 177].

8.1.3 Associated hormone secretion from islet cell tumors. The insulin-secreting pancreatic islet cell tumors of some patients with organic hyperinsulinism may also secrete glucagon, somatostatin, hPP or gastrin, one or in combination [178, 179, 180]. These may be demonstrated by elevated plasma levels of these hormones or by immunofluorescent staining of the islet cells of the tumor. The likelihood of such an occurrence is greater in patients who have islet microadenomatosis or carcinoma, especially if they also have multiple endocrine adenomatosis. The clinical manifestations in these patients are due to the dominant effect of the hyperinsulinism without any biological consequences of the secretion of other hormones.

8.1.4 Tests for malignancy. HCG and subunits. In patients with malignant insulinoma, increased plasma levels of hCG-α, hCG-β, or immunoreactive hCG were found. Plasma levels of hCG and its subunits were not elevated in any of 41 benign insulinomas [181]. Thus an elevated level of hCG or its subunits in a patient diagnosed as having insulinoma will indicate preoperatively the presence of malignant insulinoma. However a low level of hCG and its subunits does not exclude malignancy.

Liver scanning. External scanning of the liver following the intravenous administration of technetium sulfur colloid can detect evidence (cold areas) of hepatic metastases of malignant insulinomas. Such findings help confirm the diagnosis of malignancy and provide objective assessment of the effect of anti-cancer chemotherapy.

8.1.5 Test for multiple endocrine neoplasia, Type I. In all patients with proven autonomous hyperinsulinism, a search for the possible presence of sporadic or familial MEN Type I should be performed. When hyperinsulinism is accompanied by hyperfunction of other endocrine glands or elevated concentrations of other hormones (i.e., elevated concentration of serum calcium, depressed serum phosphorus, elevated serum concentration of PTH; enlargement of the sella turcica, elevated concentration of serum prolactin; elevated plasma concentration of hydrocortisone, aldosterone; elevated concentration of gastrin, etc.), it should be assumed that the source of the hyperinsulinism is diffuse (macroadenomas and/or microadenomatosis, nesidioblastosis, hyperplasia) rather than focal.

8.2 Test for other types of fasting hypoglycemia

8.2.1 *Tests to rule out factitious hypoglycemia.* The association of an increase in plasma immunoreactive insulin with a low level of plasma glucose is diagnostic of insulin-mediated hypoglycemia. Except in the neonate, this association indicates the presence of pancreatic islet cell disease provided that the surreptitious self-administration of insulin or sulfonylureas has been ruled out. Patient with factitious hypoglycemia deny the misuse of these agents, and discovery of insulin, pills or syringes used may prove difficult.

8.2.1.1 *Insulin antibodies.* If insulin has been administered for several weeks or more, it has usually been possible to demonstrate circulating antibodies to insulin. When insulin has been administered for short terms (one day to 5 weeks) antibody may not be detectable in the face of severe hypoglycemia due to surreptitious administration of insulin. With the introduction of highly purified porcine insulin and human recombinant DNA synthetic insulin, which are less antigenic, detectable levels of antibodies may be delayed or absent.

8.2.1.2 *C-peptide.* The radioimmunoassay of serum C-peptide has facilitated the detection of factitious hypoglycemia. The demonstration simultaneously of low plasma glucose, high immunoreactive insulin levels, and suppressed, low or undetectable levels of C-peptide immunoreactivity is characteristic of factitious hypoglycemia or hyperinsulinism due to administration of insulin [142]. In endogenous hyperinsulinism, on the other hand, insulin and C-peptide are secreted and therefore plasma levels of both are elevated. Determination of plasma free C-peptide and free insulin permits patients with high titers of insulin antibodies, including those with history of insulin-treated diabetes, to be studied and diagnosed in a way similar to that in subjects who have no circulating insulin antibodies [143, 167]. Sulfonylurea-induced factitious hypoglycemia can masquerade as an insulinoma both clinically and biochemically, and its incidence may be increasing [140]. Hypoglycemia may be accompanied by normal or elevated serum levels of immunoreactive insulin and C-peptide.

8.2.1.3 *Plasma sulfonylurea and urinary excretion product.* The similarity between sulfonylurea-induced hypoglycemia and the insulinoma syndrome emphasizes the importance of screening the blood and urine for sulfonylurea agents prior to diagnosis of insulinoma and abdominal exploration, as appropriate. A white precipitate, carboxytolbutamide, which appears in urine when it is acidified, points to the ingestion of tolbutamide [182].

8.2.2 *Tests for insulin autoimmune syndrome.* Patients with autoimmune hypoglycemia have very high total insulin levels on standard immunoassay. The circulating antibodies to bovine and porcine proinsulin are absent, whereas they have been present in almost all patients who have been treated with exogenous insulin, not highly purified [183]. A normal or increased amount of free C-peptide immunoreactivity indicates that the patient's beta cells are responsive rather than suppressed as by exogenous insulin taken surreptitiously [135]. Although the presence of bovine-porcine C-peptide or proinsulin antibodies provide certain evidence for exogenous insulin administration, their absence does not rule out autoimmune antibodies. With the use of highly purified insulin or synthetic human insulin, proinsulin antibodies will not be expected to be found.

8.2.3 *Tests to characterize patients with nonislet cell tumor and hypoglycemia.* Plasma NSILA-S (nonsuppressible insulin-like activity, soluble in acid alcohol) or insulin-like growth factors (IGF) measured by radioreceptor assay has been found to be elevated in approximately one-third of such patients [13, 14, 15, 118]. This finding is controversial [119, 120].

In patients with nonpancreatic tumors associated with hypoglycemia, plasma insulin concentrations decline to levels appropriate to the degree of hypoglycemia; the IRI/G or amended IRI/G ratio is normal except in the very rare patient with associated hyperinsulinism.

8.2.4 *Test for hypoglycemia due to antibodies to the insulin receptor.* These patients have slightly elevated or 'normal' levels of plasma insulin, or levels which are inappropriate for the degree of fasting hypoglycemia, similar to the situation seen in patients with insulinoma. Unlike patients with insulin autoimmune hypoglycemia, they do not have very high total insulin levels on standard immunoassay. Circulating autoantibodies to the insulin receptor can be demonstrated. Other serological evidence of autoimmunity may be found such as antibodies to extractable nuclear antigen, rheumatoid factor and antimicrosomal thyroid antibodies [137].

8.2.5 *Other endocrine disease with deficiency of counterregulatory hormones.* When deficiency of hormones that modulate the rate of gluconeogenesis or glycogenolysis is suspected as a cause of fasting hypoglycemia, the deficiency can be demonstrated by analyses of body fluids obtained when the patient is in the basal or stimulated state. In the presence of primary or secondary adrenal insufficiency, immunoassay of plasma ACTH, and/or cortisol during the ACTH test, is indicated. For growth hormone deficiency, immunoassay of plasma growth hormone before and after insulin-induced hypoglycemia, arginine infusion or exercise is performed. Glucagon deficiency is detected by immunoassay of glucagon before and after the infusion of arginine. To rule out epinephrine deficiency, measurements of plasma epinephrine and urinary excretion of catecholamines and their metabolites after insulin-induced hypoglycemia are performed.

8.2.6 Liver function test. If severe liver disease is suspected as the cause of fasting hypoglycemia the diagnosis is usually obvious. Routine liver function tests will give the appropriate confirmation.

8.2.7 Alanine test. In severe starvation, fasting hypoglycemia is thought to be due to substrate deficiency. Measurement of plasma level of alanine and the hyperglycemic response to alanine infusion are measured. A hyperglycemic response to the infusion of alanine implies that the liver can convert alanine to glucose. This conclusion is not valid if glycogen storage has not been depleted by a prior fast, since administration of alanine results in release of glucagon which can effect glycogenolysis. Failure of plasma glucose to rise during intravenous administration of alanine indicates that gluconeogenesis is impaired, presumably because of a deficiency in activity of a rate limiting hepatic enzyme.

8.2.8 Alcohol infusion test. If alcohol hypoglycemia is suspected, an alcohol infusion after a 12-hour fast can be performed to test gluconeogenic reserve [184].

8.3 Test for postprandial hypoglycemia

The oral glucose tolerance test will distinguish between the three types of postprandial hypoglycemia, alimentary hyperinsulinism, diabetes and reactive hypoglycemia, and reactive functional hypoglycemia (see Fig. 3).

9. Localization of insulin-secreting tumors and differentiation from diffuse hyperinsulinism

Accurate preoperative localization of the source of hyperinsulinism is desirable to ensure the appropriate surgical treatment in many patients. However, before attempting to 'localize an insulinoma' within the pancreas three factors should be considered. 1) Has the diagnosis been made with complete confidence? 2) Should localization procedure be used routinely preoperatively? 3) Which of the available methods for localization can be relied upon to get the correct answer? There is a high chance of an experienced surgeon being able to feel an insulinoma at operation and in the series reported by LeQuesne et al. [185] and Daggett et al. [186] this was the case in 26 of 27 tumors. However, Stefanini et al. [110], who reviewed the problem based on a questionnaire submitted to physicians caring for 1067 patients, suggested that in up to 10% of patients either tumors may be impalpable or diffuse islet cell disease exists. Based upon this and similar experience the recommendation has been made that preoperative localization should always be attempted [110, 187].

The argument raised against localization procedures [186] is that they carry a failure rate of 10–70%, which, even in the best hands, does not compare with the ability of an experienced surgeon who has a 90% chance of feeling a tumor at operation.

Most insulinomas are small (0.5 to 3.0 cm diameter) and may not be readily palpable at operation if located deep within the pancreatic parenchyma [110, 188] and/or if they have the same consistency as the rest of the pancreas. In these instances it has been the usual practice to perform a blind distal pancreatectomy without actual demonstration of the tumor. Unnecessary dissection or resection of the pancreas increases operative morbidity, and blind pancreatic resection may leave tumors in the head of the pancreas requiring re-exploration or total pancreatectomy, and increased patient morbidity and mortality [110, 160]. Furthermore, diffuse hyperinsulinism due to nesidioblastosis is being recognized with increasing frequency in adults [106, 108, 109] (see 6.1.1.1).

9.1 *Arteriography*

Arteriography was first used by Olsson in 1963 [189], and since then there have been a number of reports both for and against its efficacy. When injections of contrast are made by hand or hydraulic pump into the celiac artery between 38% and 50% of tumors will be shown [185, 190]. It is, however, clear that radiographic technique is all important and that when injections of contrast are made into more distal radicals of the celiac trunk as many as eight out of ten insulinomas may be shown in relatively small series [191, 192]. Results as good as this are exceptional and involve the use of high resolution X-ray equipment and insertion of a cathether into the pancreatico-duodenal arteries. This requires time and great expertise and carries the risk of extravasation of dye and the induction of pancreatitis. Nonetheless, a high rate of success has been reported using pancreatic angiography as the most accurate method for localization. In 88% or more of cases, successful demonstration of an insulinoma often occurred with simple injection of contrast material into the celiac artery [193, 194, 195]. We have carried out angiography in 55 patients with organic hyperinsulinism. Twenty-nine had evidence of a tumor by angiography. Localization was correct in 23, however in 6 patients the localization did not correspond to the tumor found at operation. Of the 26 negative angiograms, 3 patients were found to have nesidioblastosis. Thus, in our hands the overall success rate was 44% and the false positive rate was 21%. Often, it was found necessary to inject the materials selectively into the major arteries supplying the pancreas or even into the smaller branch vessels supplying some segments of the organ. The radiographic techniques were improved upon by the use of sterioscopy, magnification and subtraction, especially in the case of small tumors and those obscured by overlying structures such as bone or the vertebral bodies, bowel and bowel gas. When the angiogram is positive an insulinoma appears as a homogeneous, intensely vascular, sharply circumscribed mass within the substance of the pancreas. The vascular blush often persists well into the venous phase and disappears slowly (Fig. 7). A nutrient arteriole to the tumor may be identified.

Nevertheless, small insulinomas may not be readily visible because their density is similar to that of normal pancreatic tissue [188, 192, 196–198]. In our last 18 patients with organic hyperinsulinism due to an islet cell adenoma, angiography located a tumor in only 2 patients (Table 14). Furthermore, angiographs may falsely localize lesions and in unusual cases demonstrate only one tumor when multiple tumors are present [193, 199]. We have encountered two patients in whom false localization of tumors was due to peculiar opacifications in the area of the duodenal bulb in one and to what was in fact an accessory spleen in the other. False localization was found in 4 of 18 (22%) patients with insulinomas reported by Dagget et al. [186].

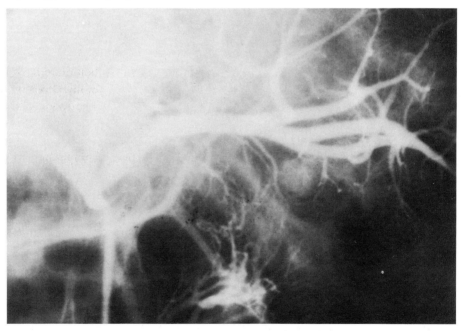

Figure 7. Celiac axis angiography illustrating visualization of an islet cell tumor.

Table 14. Insulin concentrations and gradients in portal venous system in patients with insulin-producing islet cell tumors

Patient	Tumor site	Tumor size (cm)	Tumor site			Non-tumor site	
			Max. insulin level in PVS (μU/ml)	Simultaneous arterial insulin (μU/ml)	P-A gradient (μU/ml)	Levels of insulin (mean (μU/ml)	P-A gradient (μU/ml)
EV	Head	2 × 1	64	25	39	20	− 2
DS	Neck/body	0.8 × 1	941	43	898	36	− 8
NH	Body	1 × 1	690	22	668	37	+ 8
RS	Neck	2.5 × 2	240	69	171	55	− 8
AB[a]	Tail	2 × 3	292	41	251	31	− 7
AS[b]	Neck	1.9 × 7	868	80	783	61	− 8
SP[c]	Head	7 × 5	73	21	52	17	− 1
DT	Head	2.5 × 2.1	2600	53	2547	65	+ 7
JS	Head	2 × 2	1290	204	1086	198	− 8
BT	Head	1.7 × .5	482	18	464	26	+ 8
RD	Head	1.5 × 1.5	84	16	68	20	+ 4
MS	Head	1.5 × 2	1430	206	1224	214	+ 8
AA	Head	1.5 × 1.5	118	18	100	12	− 2
MV	Body	1 × 1	1450	26	1424	22	− 5
MT	Head/neck	1 × 5	97	20	57	23	+ 3
DE	Head	2.5 × 1.0	127	32	96	16	− 4
SH	Head	0.5 × 1	616/284	29	587/255	45	+16
	Body/neck	1 × 1					
ASa[d]	Tail	1.5 × 1.0	217	15	202 (also hyperplasia, see text)		
Mean			648	52	595	50	0.0
(SE)			(161)	(14)	(155)	(14)	(1.8)

PVS = portal venous system; P-A gradient – difference between the PVS and celiac artery insulin concentration

[a] Received glucose during the procedure

[b] Insulinoma/glucagonoma

[c] Mixed insulinoma/somatostatinoma

[d] Positive by angiography

9.2 Computed tomography and ultrasound

So far computed tomography (CAT) and ultrasound have had limited success for the localization of insulinomas. A recent study reported that an insulinoma could be detected in 6 of 14 patients studied by CAT scan, and in three of 12 patients with the aid of ultrasound [200]. At the Mayo Clinic, Service et al. [160], found that in the first three years that CAT was available it was performed in eight patients in an attempt at localization. The tumor was identified in three, and in another, a focal enlargement of the pancreas was present in the area that contained the tumor. All eight patients had accurate localization by angiography. CAT scans were positive in only two of our 18 patients with islet cell adenomas, one of whom (SP) had a large (7×5 cm) tumor and the other (SH) had two adenomas with diameters of 1.0 cm (Table 14). In our experience we have been singularly unsuccessful in identifying pancreatic tumors by ultrasound in 18 patients, findings similar to those of Dagett et al. [186].

9.3 Percutaneous Transhepatic Portal Venous Sampling (THPVS)

Measurement of hormone concentrations in selective portal venous samples has been employed with success in localizing insulinomas [180, 201–204]. Aside from localizing tumors, the procedure can be useful for differentiating localized from diffuse hyperinsulinism as occurs in conditions such as nesidioblastosis, hyperplasia and multiple adenomatosis [180, 202]. The technique used at the University of Michigan has been described previously [180, 204] (Fig. 8).

During the procedure of portal venous sampling it is important to place a sampling catheter in the celiac artery or peripheral vein to allow simultaneous measurements of insulin concentrations. The latter samples aid in distinguishing apparent gradients in the portal venous system from what are actually spontaneous fluctuations in hormone release. All serum samples from a given patient should be assayed simultaneously and there should be an intraassay variability of less than 5%.

9.3.1 'Normal' hormone distribution. An appreciation of the 'normal' distribution of concentrations of insulin in the portal venous system (PVS) has been found in patients with single non-insulin-producing tumors [206]. This presupposes the absence of a marked paracrine effect of the hormone produced by the tumor upon insulin secretion and a correlation between the anatomy and physiological function. In addition, measurements of PVS concentrations of insulin have been made in three 'normal' patients without organic hyperinsulinism [186]. A wide range of insulin concentrations has been found at various sites in the 'normal' portal venous system. Insulin levels at some sites can be elevated in obese and in nonobese subjects without organic hyperinsulinism and can actually exceed levels measured in patients with insulin-producing tumors if only the absolute values are considered. However, in our experience, in the great majority of patients with organic hyperinsulinism a step-up at any one single site is indicative of the presence of a tumor as concentration at other sites are very similar to those found in the celiac artery (Fig. 9).

An awareness of the effects of catheter placement is necessary when interpret-

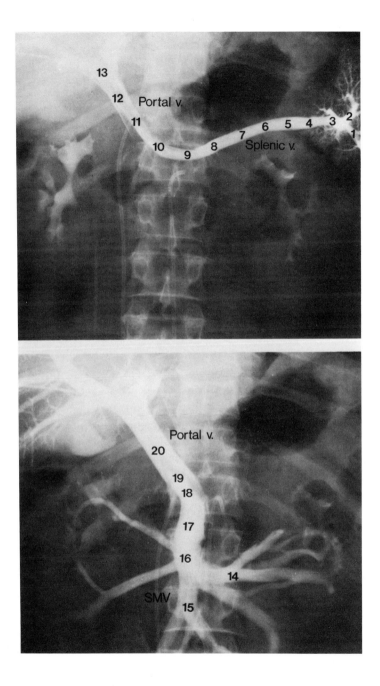

Figure 8. Venogram showing splenic, portal and superior mesenteric veins. Numbers are superimposed on the actual venogram at the time of the transhepatic study and represent sites of venous sampling for hormone assay. The catheters placed in the celiac artery and right hepatic vein are also visible.

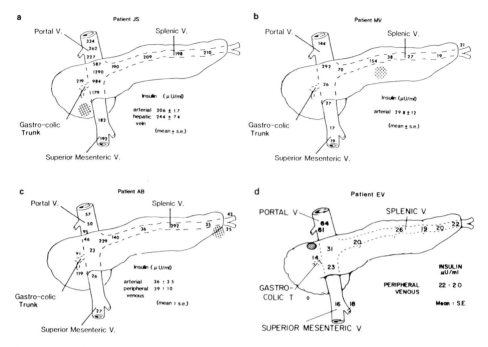

Figure 9. A collage of schematic illustrations of concentrations of insulin in the portal venous system with tumors indicated by the cross-hatched areas.

ing concentrations of hormones in the portal venous system. Insertion of the catheter tip into small tributaries and occlusion of the vessel lumen can result in falsely low or high values. For this reason we contend that superselective sampling is unneccessary and probably contraindicated. Multiple samples should be obtained at the various sites since variations of 30% or greater may occur due to streaming or laminar flow. Samples obtained through a catheter with a lateral port rotated through 360 degrees in the same site can vary widely. It is also common to find levels declining during the course of the procedure, possibly due to stress related factors.

9.3.2 *Solitary tumors.* All but one of 18 insulin-secreting tumors were localized correctly by the transhepatic portal venous sampling technique (Table 14). Figure 9 illustrates four examples of differential insulin concentrations measured in tumors of the head, body and tail of the pancreas.

Table 14 illustrates the tumor size, site and insulin concentration corresponding with the venous drainage of 17 patients with single tumors and of one patient with two tumors, and from the uninvolved pancreas in these 18 patients studied. The mean maximal insulin concentration was $648 \pm 161 \, \mu$U/ml with a mean gradient of $595 \pm 155 \, \mu$U/ml. The range of maximal concentrations varied considerably from a low of 64 (EV) to a high of $2600 \, \mu$U/ml (DT) with gradients of 39 through $2547 \, \mu$U/ml. In patients without insulinoma, the mean maximum insulin concentration in the portal venous system was 156 μU/ml in the splenic vein and 113 μU/ml in the portal vein while the mean gradient was 64 μU/ml. This overlap in findings between insulinoma and noninsulinoma patients indicates that neither the absolute value for the maximum concentration nor the gradient between portal and arterial levels distinguishes the insulinoma from noninsulinoma patients. In the patient with organic hyperinsulinism it is the step-up within the portal venous system which localizes the source of hyperinsulinism. This illustrates the importance of not performing THPVS until a diagnosis of organic hyperinsulinism has been established by rigorous criteria. Confusing results obtained in patients without organic hyperinsulinism [186] should not be a contraindication to perform this localizing procedure, when indicated in patients with true organic hyperinsulinism.

Several selected cases reveal some interesting and unusual features worthy of comment. In the patient with the largest tumor (SP), which was demonstrable angiographically, the insulin concentrations and gradients did not exceed those in one of the smallest tumors, 1 $\times$ 1.5 cm (MT). In general, there was no correlation between tumor size and the highest concentration of insulin or the gradient. Eleven of the patients had tumors correctly localized in the head of the pancreas which included the deep posterior superior position and uncinate lobe. This bias is undoubtedly due to the referral to our center of patients in whom previous localizing procedurs had been attempted and failed. NH had had repeated angiography, ultrasound and CT scan for 10 years and his tumor had not been found. RD had had a previous unsuccessful transhepatic procedure.

Certain difficulties in interpretation were encountered. Patient AB (Fig. 9) had a step-up near the junction of the body and tail of the pancreas, one at the junction of the superior mesenteric and portal vein, and one in the gastrio-colic trunk, suggestive of multicentric hyperinsulinism. At operation a single tumor was located in the tail of the pancreas. Venography and inspection at operation revealed a collateral drainage between the distal splenic and the superior mesenteric vein via the gastroepiploic vein, explaining the findings [180].

A thorough knowledge of the pancreatic venous anatomy is a prerequisite to understanding the hormone flow pattern in the portal venous system. Reichardt and Cameron [207] described the pancreatic venous anatomy on the basis of their angiographic and cadaver dissection studies. The blood from the pancreatic head drains into the superior mesenteric vein via the anterior superior and inferior pancreaticoduodenal veins, and into the portal vein via the posterior superior pancreaticoduodenal vein. The dorsal pancreatic vein receives blood from the proximal body and the head of the pancreas and enters the junction of the superior mesenteric and splenic vein. Many veins emanating from the body and tail open into the adjacent splenic vein. The transverse pancreatic vein is joined by numerous tributaries from the body while coursing along the lower border of the body and opens into the superior mesenteric, inferior mesenteric, or splenic vein.

288

Draining veins of insulinomas usually open into adjacent pancreatic and peripancreatic veins. Thus abnormal elevation of the insulin concentration will be found in the vein near the tumor. However, occasionally a second misleading step-up may be found remote from the tumor site because of free communication along pancreatic veins. Abnormal tumor vessels may also contribute to apparently aberrant drainage.

Tumors located in the head of the pancreas were associated with high insulin levels and gradients in the area of the drainage of the superior pancreaticoduodenal vein. Tumors in the uncinate lobe resulted in increased insulin values in the superior mesenteric vein close to the junction with the splenic vein. Tumors in the neck drained into the proximal portal vein [180] or near the confluence of the splenic and portal vein close to the junction of the superior mesenteric and splenic veins (Fig. 9).

When the peak level of insulin or insulin gradient is within the superior mesenteric vein, a tumor may be present in any one of three parts of the proximal pancreas; the head, uncinate lobe or neck. In such cases, if the neck and entire head of the pancreas appear to be normal, the uncinate process must be carefully explored and mobilized for palpation. Perhaps the term 'regionalization' is more accurate than 'localization' in cases where the high values of insulin are in the superior mesenteric vein [204].

Tumors in the body drained primarily into the splenic vein and those in the tail of the gland drained directly into the distal splenic vein.

9.3.3 *Diffuse insulin hypersecretion.* Of the 20 patients with organic hyperinsulinism, four had diffuse elevation of concentrations of insulin in the portal venous system. In one patient (AW) elevated insulin concentrations were found in the distal and midsplenic veins, the proximal pancreatic vein and the portal vein, suggesting multiple areas of insulin hypersecretion (Fig. 10). A 95% pancreatec-

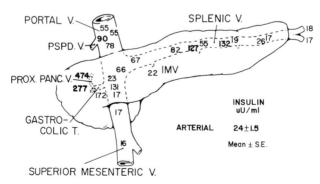

Figure 10. Portal venous insulin concentrations in a patient (AW, 20, male) with nesidioblastosis. Note the multiple areas of step-ups in insulin concentration indicative of a diffuse process. The high value in the proximal pancreatic vein could be misleading.

tomy was performed. The diagnosis of nesidioblastosis was made histologically and confirmed by immunohistochemistry. In a second patient (SH), 2 step-ups corresponded with 2 tumors (Table 14). A third patient (Asa), who had undergone surgery elsewhere for removal of a single adenoma in the tail of the pancreas one year earlier, had angiographically demonstrable 'recurrence' of a tumor in the tail. Transhepatic venous sampling showed in addiion to the gradient of $202\,\mu U/ml$ next to the tumor site identified by arteriography, gradients of $50-70\,\mu U/ml$ in the midsplenic, inferior mesenteric, posterior superior pancreaticoduodenal and dorsal pancreatic vein, which suggested a multicentric process. A distal 75% pancreatectomy was carried out and a single discrete tumor was found (as localized by angiography and THVPS) associated with diffuse islet cell hyperplasia. Since nesidioblastosis, hyperplasia or multiple adenomatosis can produce non-homogeneous elevation of insulin levels, venous sampling cannot be used to differentiate between them [180, 202]. However, these conditions can usually be distinguished from single adenomas. The apparent multicentric hyperinsulinemia in the PVS in one patient with a solidary adenoma (AB) (Fig. 9) has been discussed above.

9.3.4 Recommendation for use of transhepatic portal venous sampling. This, or any other localizing procedure should not be used unless a rigid diagnosis of organic hyperinsulinism has been made. Although an experienced surgeon has a very high probability of being able to palpate a tumor at operation [186], we and others [208] believe that transhepatic portal venous sampling and hormone measurement play an important role in the localization of symptomatic islet cell tumors which are not detectable by more conventional techniques, such as arteriography.

Although tumors in the body and tail of the pancreas can be cured by distal pancreatectomy, blind resection can no longer be justified when sophisticated means are available to localize tumors in the head or neck or body of the pancreas. Portal vein sampling, although associated with mild patient discomfort has been successful in our hands, and, apart from minimal hemobilia in one patient, has not resulted in any serious complications. THPVS also identifies patients with diffuse islet cell hyperfunction without or with specific tumor(s). It may prove to be useful in patients in whom angiography has either falsely localized a lesion or demonstrated only one of several tumors. This procedure is recommended particularly in patients with organic hyperinsulinism who have multiple endocrine neoplasia Type I or have a family history of such disease, since such patients usually harbor multiple adenomas and/or islet cell hyperplasia or nesidioblastosis. The technique may direct the attention of the surgeon to a specific region of the pancreas and may avoid blind resection of the body and tail.

10. Treatment of organic hyperinsulinism

The treatment of pancreatic islet beta cell disease is usually surgery; in the great majority of cases it provides complete cure. It should be performed only when the diagnosis is certain and only by a surgeon skilled in pancreatic surgery. When hypoglycemia can be controlled with diet alone, or with small well-tolerated doses of diazoxide, and/or when the medical condition of the patient may increase the hazard of surgery sufficiently, medical management alone may be considered. Patients for whom an operation is planned should first have a short trial of treatment with diazoxide and a naturetic benzothiadiazine. A sucessful preoperative trial allows the surgeon to be more conservative during laparotomy should there be difficulty in the identification, localization, or removal of a tumor, or if microadenomatosis, hyperplasia, or nesidioblastosis should be present or suspected, or if other complications arise. Medical treatment is required for the great majority of malignant insulinomas, since only occasionally will they be cured by operation. Medical treatment for insulinomas is antihormonal therapy and for malignant insulinoma is antihormonal and anti-tumor therapy.

10.1 Benign disease

10.1.1 Medical management
10.1.1.1 *Diet.* The cornerstone of medical management of insulinoma and other forms of hyperinsulinism is the diet. Not uncommonly, patients may avoid symptoms of hypoglycemia for variable periods of time by spacing feedings so as to shorten the number of hours between feedings. For some the inclusion of a bedtime (11:00 p.m.) feeding is sufficient; for others a midmorning, midafternoon and/or a 3:00 a.m. snack will be necessary. Even though the tumor may be stimulated to secrete insulin by the ingestion of carbohydrates, it usually is inadvisable to restrict the intake of carbohydrate. More slowly absorbable forms of carbohydrates (starches, bread, potatoes, rice, etc.) are generally preferred. During hypoglycemic episodes, rapidly absorbable forms (fruit juices with added glucose or sucrose) are indicated.

In patients with severe, refractory hypoglycemia the use of continuous intravenous infusion of glucose, coupled with increased dietary intake of carbohydrate, frequently will alleviate hypoglycemia long enough to institute additional therapy.

10.1.1.2 *Diazoxide and natriuretic benzothiadiazines.* Diazoxide, marketed as Proglycem^c, has proved to be a major advance in medical management of insulinomas, both benign and malignant [209, 210]. It owes its potent hyperglycemic properties to two effects. It directly inhibits the release of insulin by B-cells, through stimulation of alpha- adrenergic receptors, and it has an extrapancreatic hyperglycemic effect probably by inhibiting cyclic AMP phosphodi-esterase, resulting in higher plasma levels of cyclic AMP and enhanced glycogenolysis. Because diazoxide induces the retention of sodium, edema is troublesome at higher dosages. The addition of a diuretic benzothiadiazine, e.g., trichlormethiazide, not only corrects or prevents edema but synergises the hyper-glycemic effect of diazoxide. At the doses needed to counteract the higher doses of diazoxide (e.g., 450–600 mg per day) naturetic benzothiadiazines frequently induce hypokalemia. Nausea is an additional complication of higher dosages of diazoxide, and hirsutism may complicate long-term treatment. These compounds have been useful to elevate blood levels of glucose into the euglycemic range if operation must be delayed for weeks or months. Patients with benign insulinomas have been successfully managed for up to 16 or more years with diazoxide in doses of 150 to 450 mg/day in combination with trichlormethiazide in doses of 2–8 mg/day. If they can be tolerated, higher doses may be used in malignant insulinomas.

10.1.1.3 *Propranolol.* Only a few reports of the use of propranolol have appeared [211–213]. Its use has been associated with the reduction of plasma insulin levels and with the relief of hypoglycemic attacks in patients with benign or malignant insulinoma. In a patient with a benign insulinoma, 80 mg of propranolol a day was sufficient while a patient with malignant insulinoma in whom streptozotocin was no longer effective, 640 mg of propranolol orally per day was required [213].

10.1.1.4 *Dilantin.* The anticonvulsive diphenylhydantoin has been shown to in-hibit the in vitro release of insulin from both the labile and storage B-cell pools. It has been used successfully to control refractory hypoglycemia as evidenced by normal overnight fasting glucose levels and absence of hypoglycemia during total fasting for up to 24 hours [214, 215]. However, in only 1/3 or less of patients with benign insulinoma is the hyperglycemic effect of dilantin of any clinical signifi-cance. Furthermore, with the dosage required, ataxia, nystagmus, hypertrophic gums and megaloblastic anemia may be side effects. Maintenance doses of dilantin range from 300–600 mg/day. The concurrent administration of diazoxide lowers measurable blood levels of dilantin and their concurrent use is not recom-mended.

10.1.1.5 *Glucocorticoids.* The use of glucocorticoids, which increase gluconeo-genesis and cause insulin resistance, can also help stabilize blood glucose at an acceptable level. Their major indication is in the treatment of autoimmune syndromes (see 6.1.3.3 and 6.1.3.4).

10.1.1.6 *Glucagon.* Glucagon may help raise blood glucose concentrations but may simultaneously directly stimulate the release of insulin.

10.1.1.7 *Chlorpromazine.* A dosage of chlorpromazine as high as 500 mg/day was associated with a decrease in plasma IRI and an increase in plasma glucose to the euglycemic range during two months of treatment of a patient with malignant insulinoma [216].

10.1.2 *Surgical management.* When the diagnosis of functioning islet cell disease with hyperinsulinism is made, early surgery is indicated to relieve hypoglycemia and distressing symptoms, to prevent possible damage to the central nervous system, and to prevent obesity, which makes surgical management more difficult. Identification of a tumor at the time of surgery and differentiation between localized and diffuse islet cell disease may present a problem. Selective pancreatic (celiac and mesenteric) arteriography has made it possible to localize some of these tumors preoperatively. Transhepatic venous catheterization of the portal vein and measurement of plasma concentration of insulin at various sites of the venous system has the potential to differentiate between localized and diffuse hyperinsulinism and to localize a tumor (see 9.3).

The surgical approach to insulinomas may be straightforward if the tumor is visualized or palpated with ease. The surgical approach may be complicated by difficulty in identifying the tumor, particularly when the tumors are small, located deep within the pancreatic parenchyma, not detected by angiography, and when transhepatic venous catheterization has not been performed or not proved to be helpful. Moreover, multiple tumors or diffuse islet cell disease are not uncommon. If a tumor is not identified, meticulous and extensive exploration of the pancreas including the head and uncinate process should be carried out using multiple capsulotomies, if necessary, after the pancreas has been mobilized and its entire length has been palpated. In the absence of finding a definite insulinoma, resection of first the tail with the spleen and then the body of the pancreas up to the great vessels is justified since two-thirds of tumors are located in these areas. After a 70–85% pancreatectomy, the patient may be cured if the resected specimen contains an adenoma or if sufficient hyperfunctioning tissue has been removed in the case of adenomatosis, nesidioblastosis, or hyperplasia [106, 108]. In patients with unlocated tumors in the head of the pancreas or patients with microadenomatosis or nesidioblastosis who have a major amount of abnormal insulin producing tissue in the head of the pancreas, hyperinsulinism and hypoglycemia may reoccur. In this case, treatment with diazoxide and a diuretic thiazide should be employed. This has been successful in many cases.

10.2 *Malignant disease*

10.2.1 *Surgical management.* Even though it does not produce a cure, a decrease in tumor mass may alleviate symptoms and/or make medical management more effective.

10.2.2 *Medical management.* In general the intensities of application of the medical antihormonal therapy modalities discussed above must be increased when they are applied to the treatment of a malignant insulinoma. In addition, sooner or later it becomes necessary to use tumorcidal drugs.

10.2.2.1 *Streptozotocin.* Streptozotocin is the most effective anti-tumor agent to date for treating malignant insulinomas [217, 218]. It is a broad spectrum antibiotic and a naturally occurring nitrosourea that causes selected destruction of the pancreatic beta cell. It is capable of controlling hypoglycemia but also of causing measurable decrease in tumor size. It has caused objective reduction in tumor mass in approximately 50% of patients with functioning malignant insulinoma. Less than 20% were considered to have a complete remission. A favorable biochemical response was obtained in approximately 1/4 of patients. Overall, treatment significantly prolongs survival. Unfortunately, the specificity of streptozotocin for the pancreatic B-cell is relative; toxicity affects kidney, liver, and the hemapoetic system. Renal tubular toxicity is the most serious and limits the amount of drug that can be administered. It can be avoided usually by monitoring the urine for protein. The next dose should be delayed until there is a clearing of proteinuria. A weekly schedule of 0.5–2 g/m^2 intravenously administered has been used frequently [218].

10.2.2.2 *Streptozotocin plus fluorouracil.* The combination of these two drugs given intravenously has advantages over streptozotocin alone in the overall response rate (63% vs. 33%) and in rates of complete responses (33% vs. 12%) in patients with advanced islet cell carcinoma [219]. Treatment with a combination also yielded a survival advantage over treatment with streptozotocin alone. Streptozotocin was given in a dosage of 500 mg per square meter of body-surface given daily for five consecutive days in combination with 5-fluorouracil 400 mg per square meter daily for five consecutive days. Courses of therapy were repeated every six weeks if the malignant disease improved or remained objectively stable. The dosages were reduced if side effects occurred.

10.2.2.3 *Mithramycin.* A patient unresponsive to administration of streptozotocin, 5-fluorouracil, adriamycin, tubercidin, phentoin, and diazoxide was responsive to mithramycin. Plasma insulin sharply declined after one mg was given intravenously. Four additional one mg doses were followed by normoglycemia for two weeks and no symptoms of hypoglycemia for another eight weeks before the patient died of apparent congestive heart failure [220].

10.2.2.4 *Adriamycin.* Therapy with adriamycin has lead to significant decreases in insulin levels or in measurable disease; two patients had clinical remissions lasting five to seven months [221]. Cardiac toxicity and reversible myelosuppression are the main toxic effects that limit the dosage of adriamycin, but cumulative doses of less than $500\,mg/m^2$ led to congestive cardiomyopathy in only 0.3% of patients treated with adriamycin.

10.2.2.5 *L-asparaginase.* Due to its hepatic and pancreatic toxicity, use of L-asparaginase is limited to short term palliation of severe hypoglycemia [222]. It has not been shown to affect tumor mass [217].

10.2.2.6 *5-fluorouracil.* The experiences with 5-fluorouracil alone is limited to reports of therapeutic effectiveness in several case reports (see 10.2.2.2).

11. Treatment of patients with nonpancreatic tumors associated with hypoglycemia

In these patients therapy should be aimed at reducing or controlling the patient's tumor through surgery, radiation and chemotherapy. As with other functioning tumors, a decrease in tumor mass may alleviate symptoms even though it does not produce a cure. Palliative surgery, by reducing tumor mass may be extremely helpful in prolonging life and ameliorating symptoms. Radiotherapy has been of value in some patients with tumor hypoglycemia. Chemotherapy should be tried. Although streptozotocin has not been successful in the majority of patients where it has been tried, administration of streptozotocin may have produced temporary improvement of hypoglycemia and remission of symptoms (Fajans, pers. obser.).

References

1. Jaspan JB, Wollman RL, Bernstein L, Rubenstein AH: Hypoglycemic peripheral neuropathy in association with insulinoma: Implication of glucopenia rather than hyperinsulinism. Medicine 61: 33–44, 1982.
2. Cahill GF, et al.: Hormone-fuel interrelationships during fasting. J. Clin Invest 45: 1751–1766, 1966.
3. Cahill GF: Starvation in man. N Engl J Med 282: 668–675, 1970.
4. Exton JH: Gluconeogenesis. Metabolism 21: 945–989, 1972.
5. Madison L: Role of insulin in the hepatic handling of glucose. Arch Intern Med 123: 284–292, 1969.
6. Rizza RA, Mandarino L, Gerich JE: Dose-reponse characteristics for the effects of insulin on production and utilization of glucose in man. Am J Physiol 240: 630–639, 1981B.
7. Rizza RA, Haymond MW, Verdonk CA, Mandarino LJ, Miles JM, Service FJ, Gerich JE: Pathogenesis of hypoglycemia in insulinoma patients. Diabetes 30: 377–381, 1981.
8. Chiasson JL, et al.: Differential sensitivity of glycogenolysis and gluconeogenesis in insulin infusion in dogs. Diabetes 25: 283–291, 1976.
9. Chiasson JL, et al.: Effects of insulin at two dose levels on gluconeogenesis from alanine in fasting man. Metabolism 29: 810–818, 1980.
10. Zierler KL, Rabinowitz D: Roles of insulin and growth hormone, based on studies of forearm metabolism in man. Medicine 42: 385–402, 1963
11. Roth J et al.: Receptors for insulin, NSILA-S and growth hormone: Application to disease

states in man. Recent Prog Horm Res 31: 95–139, 1976.

12. Bradshaw R, Niall H: Insulin-related growth factors. Trends in Biological Science 3: 274–278, 1978.

13. Megyesi K, et al.: Hypoglycemia in association with extrapancreatic tumors: Demonstration of elevated plasma NSILAS by a new radioreceptor assay. J Clin Endocrinol Metab 38: 931–934, 1974.

14. Daughaday WH, Trivedi B, Kapadia M: Measurement of insulin-like growth factor II by a specific radioreceptor assay in serum of normal individuals, patients with abnormal growth hormone secretion, and patients with tumor-associated hypoglycemia. J Clin Endocrinol Metab 53: 289–294, 1981.

15. Gorden P, Hendricks CM, Kahn CR, Megyesi K, Roth J: Hypoglycemia associated with non-islet-cell tumor and insulin-like growth factors. New Engl J Med 305: 1452–1455, 1981.

16. Kahn CR: Membrane receptors for hormones and neutrotransmitters. J Cell Biol 70: 261–286, 1976.

17. Kahn CR, et al.: Effects of autoantibodies to the insulin receptor on isolated adipocyte. Studies of insulin binding and insulin action. J Clin Invest 60: 1094–1106, 1977.

18. Kahn CR, Rosenthal AS: Immunologic reactions to insulin: insulin allergy, insulin resistance, and the autoimmune insulin syndrome. Diabetes Care 2: 283–295, 1979.

19. Kahn CR, Baird KL, Flier JS, et al.: Insulin receptors, receptor antibodies, and the mechanism of insulin action. Recent Prog Horm Res 37: 477–538, 1981.

20. Czech MP: Molecular basis of insulin action. Ann Rev Biochem 46: 359–384, 1977.

21. DeFronzo RA, Tobin JD, Andres R: Glucose clamp technique: A method for quantifying insulin secretion and resistance. Am J Physiol 237: E214–223, 1979.

22. Gavin JR III, Roth J, Neville DM Jr, DeMeyts P, Buess DN: Insulin-dependent regulation of insulin receptor concentrations: A direct demonstration in cell culture. Proc Natl Acad Sci USA 71: 84–88, 1974.

23. Bar RS, Gorden P, Roth J, Kahn CR, DeMeyts P: Fluctuations in the affinity and concentration of insulin receptors on circulating monocytes of obese patients: Effects of starvation, refeeding, and dieting. J Clin Invest 58: 1123–1135, 1976.

24. Insel JR, Kolteran OG, Saekow M, Olefsky JM: Short-term regulation of insulin receptor affinity in man. Diabetes 29: 132–139, 1980.

25. Bar RS, Gorden P, Roth J, Kahn CR, DeMeyts P: Fluctuatons in the affinity and concentration of insuln receptors on circulating monocytes of obese patients: Effects of starvation, refeeding, and deting. J Clin Invest 58: 1123–1125, 1976.

26. Bar RS, Harrison LC, Muggeo M, Gorden P, Kahn CR, Roth J: Regulation of insulin receptor in normal and abnormal physiology in humans. Adv Intern Med 24: 23–52, 1979.

27. Bar RS, Gorden P, Roth J, Siebert CW: Insulin receptors in patients with insulinomas: Changes in receptor affinity and concentration. J Clin Endocrinol Metab 44: 1210–1213, 1977.

28. Insel JR, Kolterman OG, Saekow M, Olefsky JM: Short-term regulation of insulin receptor affinity in man. Diabetes 29: 132–139, 1980.

29. Rizza RA, Gerich JE: Persistent effect of hyperglucagonemia on glucose production in man. J Clin Endocrinol Metab 48: 352–353, 1979.

30. Cherrington AD, Liljenquist JE, Shulman GI, Williams PE, Lacy WW: Importance of hypo-glycemia-induced glucose production during isolated glucagon deficiency. Am J Physiol 236: E263–271, 1979.

31. Gerich J, Cryer P, Rizza R: Hormonal mechanisms in acute glucose counterregulation: The relative roles of glucagon, epinephrine, norepinephrine, growth hormone, and cortisol. Metabolism 29: 1164–1175, 1980.

32. Cryer PE: Hypoglycemic glucose counterregulation in patients with insulin-dependent diabetes mellitus. J Lab Clin Med 99: 451–456, 1982.

33. Sacca L, Morrone G, Cicala M, Corso G, Ungaro B: Influence of epinephrine, norepinephrine,

and isoproterenol on glucose homeostasis in normal man. J Clin Endocrinol Metab 50: 680–684, 1980.

34. Sacca L, Vigorito C, Cicala M, Ungaro B, Sherwin RS: Mechanisms of epinephrine-induced glucose intolerance in normal humans. J Clin Invest 69: 284–293, 1982.

35. Rizza RA, Cryer PE, Haymond MW, Gerich JE: Adrenergic mechanisms for the effect of epinephrine on glucose production and clearance in man. J Clin Invest 65: 682–689, 1980.

36. Adamson U, Wahren J, Cerasi E: Influence of growth hormone on splanchnic glucose production in man. Acta Endocrinol 86: 803–812, 1977.

37. MacGorman LR, Rizza RA, Gerich JE: Physiological concentrations of growth hormone exert insulin-like and insulin antagonistic effects on both hepatic and extrahepatic tissues in man. J Clin Endocrinol Metab 53: 556–559, 1981.

38. Shamoon H, Hendler R, Sherwin RS: Synergistic interactions among anti-insulin hormones in the pathogenesis of stress hyperglycemia in humans. J Clin Endocrinol Metab 52: 1235–1241, 1981.

39. Lautt W: Hepatic nerves: A review of the functions and effects. Can J Physiol Pharmacol 58: 105–123, 1980.

40. Nobin ABF, Ingemansson S, Jarhult J, Rosengren E: Organization and function of the sympathetic innervation of the human liver. Acta Physiol Scan 452: 103–106, 1977.

41. Hers HG: The control of glycogen metabolism in the liver. Ann Rev Biochem 45: 167–189, 1976.

42. Sacca L, Hendler R, Sherwin RS: Hyperglycemia inhibits glucose production in man independent of changes in glucoregulatory hormones. J Clin Endocrinol Metab 47: 1160–1163, 1979.

43. Garber AJ, Cryer PE, Santiago JV, Haymond MW, Pagliari AS, Kipnis DM: The role of adrenergic mechanisms in the substrate and hormonal response to insulin-induced hypoglycemia in man. J Clin Invest 58: 7–15, 1976.

44. Cryer PE: Glucose counterregulation in man. Diabetes 30: 261–264, 1981.

45. Clarke WL, Santiago JV, Thomas L, Haymond MW, Ben-Galim E, Cryer PE: Adrenergic mechanisms in recovery from hypoglycemia in man: Adrenergic blockage. Amer J Physiol 236: E147–152, 1979.

46. Gerich J, Davis J, Lorenzi M, Rizza R, Bohannon N, Karam J, Lewis S, Kaplan S, Schultz T, Cryer PE: Hormonal mechanisms of recovery from insulin induced hypoglycemia in man. Amer J Physiol 236: E380–385, 1979.

47. Rizza RA, Cryer PE, Gerich JE: Role of glucagon, epinephrine and growth hormone in human glucose counterregulation: Effects of somatostatin and adrenergic blockade on plasma glucose recovery and glucose flux rates following insulin induced hypoglycemia. J Clin Invest 64: 62–71, 1979.

48. Popp DA, Shah SD, Cryer PE: The role of epinephrine mediated-adrenergic mechanisms in hypoglycemic glucose counterregulation and posthypoglycemic hyperglycemia in insulin dependent diabetes mellitus. J Clin Invest 69: 315–326, 1982.

49. Voorhees ML, Jakubowski AF, MacGillivary MH: The adrenomedullary and glucagon responses of hypopituitary children to insulin induced hypoglycemia. Pediatr Res 15: 912–915, 1981.

50. Marks V, Greenwood FC, Howorth PJN, Samols E: Plasma growth hormone levels in spontaneous hypoglycemia. J Clin Endocrinol 27: 523, 1967.

51. Cloutier MG, Pek S, Crowther RL, Floyd JC Jr, Fajans SS: Glucagon-insulin interactions in patients with insulin-producing pancreatic islet lesions. J Clin Endocrinol Metab 48: 201–206, 1979.

52. Pruett EDR: Plasma insulin concentrations during prolonged work at near maximal oxygen uptake. J Appl Physiol 29: 155–158, 1970

53. DeFronzo RA, Ferrannini E, Sato Y, Felig P, Wahren J: Synergistic interaction between exercise and insulin on peripheral glucose metabolism. J Clin Invest 68: 1468–1474, 1981.

54. Felig P, Wahren J, Hendler R, et al.: Plasma glucagon levels in exercising man. N Engl J Med 287: 184–185, 1972.
55. Galbo H, Holst J, Christensen NJ: Glucagon and plasma catecholamine responses to graded and prolonged exercise in man. J Appl Physiol 38: 70–76, 1975.
56. Vranic M, Berger M: Exercise and diabetes mellitus. Diabetes 28: 147–163, 1979.
57. Christensen NJ, Alberti KGMM, Brandsborg O: Plasma catecholamines and blood substrate concentrations. Eur J Clin Invest 5: 415–423, 1975.
58. Few JD: Effect of exercise in the secretion and metabolism of cortisol in man. J Endocrinol 62: 341–353, 1974.
59. Schwartz F. Ter Haar DJ, Van Riet HG, Thijssen JHH: Response of growth hormone (GH), FFA, blood sugar and insulin to exercise in obese patients and normal subjects. Metabolism 18: 1013–1020, 1969.
60. Wahren J, Jorfeldt L: Determination of leg blood flow during exercise in man: An indicator dilution technique based on femoral venous dye infusion. Clin Sci 45: 135–145, 1973.
61. Holloszy JO, Narahara HT: Enhanced permeability to sugar associated with muscle contraction. Studies on the role of Ca++. J Gen Physiol 50: 551–562, 1967.
62. Vranic M, Wrenshall GA: Exercise, insulin and glucose turnover in dogs. Endocrinology 85: 165–171, 1969.
63. Wahren J, Felig P, Hagnefeldt L: Physical exercise and fuel homeostasis in diabetes mellitus. Diabetologia 14: 213–222, 1978.
64. Porte D Jr, Bagdade JD: Human insulin secretion: An integrated approach. Ann Rev Med 21: 219–240, 1970.
65. Gerich JE, Charles MA, Grodsky GM: Regulation of pancreatic insulin and glucagon secretion. Ann Rev Physiol 38: 353–388, 1976.
66. Hedeskov CJ: Mechanism of glucose-induced insulin secretion. Physiol Rev 60: 442–509, 1980.
67. Both JL, Vinik AI, Blake KCH, Jackson WPU: Kinetics of insulin secretion in chronic pancreatitis and mild maturity-onset diabetes (Evidence for 'gut hormone' action beyond glucoreceptor and cyclic adenosine monophosphate mediated insulin release). Europ J Clin Invest 6: 365–372, 1976.
68. Hicks BH, Taylor CI, Vij SK, Pek S, Knopf RF, Floyd JC Jr, Fajans SS: Effect of changes in plasma levels of free fatty acids on plasma glucagon, insulin, and growth hormone in man. Metabolism 26: 1011–1023, 1977.
69. Floyd JC Jr, Fajans SS, Conn JW, Knopf RF, Rull J: Stimulation of insulin secretion by amino acids. J Clin Invest 45: 1487–1502, 1966.
70. Fajans SS, Floyd JC Jr, Knopf RF, Conn JW: Effect of amino acids and proteins on insulin secretion in man. Rec Prog Hormone Res 23: 617–662, 1967.
71. Fajans SS, Floyd JC Jr Knopf RF, Pek S, Weissman PN, Conn JW: Amino acids and insulin release in vivo. Israel J Med Sci 8: 233–243, 1972.
72. Fajans SS, Knopf RF, Floyd JC Jr, Power L, Conn JW: The experimental induction in man of sensitivity to leucine-hypoglycemia. J Clin Invest 42: 216–229, 1963.
73. Floyd JC Jr, Fajans SS, Knopf RF, Conn JW: Evidence that insulin release is the mechanism for experimentally-induced leucine hypoglycemia in man. J Clin Invest 42: 1714–1719, 1963.
74. Fajans SS: Leucine-induced hypoglycemia. New Engl J Med 272: 1224–1227, 1965.
75. Fajans SS, Floyd JC Jr, Knopf RF, Guntsche E, Rull J, Thiffault CA, Conn JW: A difference in mechanism by which leucine and other amino acids induce insulin release.J Clin Endocrinol Metab 27: 1600–1606, 1967.
76. Floyd JC Jr, Fajans SS, Knopf RF, Conn JW: Plasma insulin in organic hyperinsulinism: Comparative effects of tolbutamide, leucine and glucose. J Clin Endocrinol 24: 747, 1964.
77. Fajans SS, Floyd JC Jr, Vij SK: Differential diagnosis of spontaneous hypoglycemia. In: Endocrinology & Diabetes, Kryston LJ and Shaw RA (eds). Grune & Stratton, Inc, 1975, pp 453–472.

78. Fajans SS, Quibrera R, Pek S, Floyd JC Jr, Christensen HN, Conn JW: Stimulation of insulin release in the dog by a non-metabolizable amino acid. Comparison with leucine and arginine. J Clin Endocrinol Metab 33: 35–41, 1971.

79. Fajans SS, Christensen HN Floyd JC Jr, Pek S: Stimulation of insulin and glucagon release in the dog by a nonmetabolizable arginine analog. Endocrinology 94: 230–233, 1974.

80. Floyd JC Jr, Fajans SS, Pek S, Thiffault CA, Knopf RF, Conn JW: Synergistic effects of essential amino acids and glucose upon insulin secretion in man. Diabetes 19: 109–115, 1970.

81. Dupre J, Curtis JD, Unger RH, et al.: Effects of secretin, pancreozymine or gastrin in the response of the endocrine pancreas to administration of glucose or arginine in man. J Clin Invest 68: 765–767, 1969.

82. Lerner RL, Porte D Jr,: Studies of secretin-stimulated insulin responses in man. J Clin Invest 51: 2205–2210, 1972.

83. Jensen SL, Fahrenkrug J, Holst JJ, et al.: Secretory effects of VIP on isolated perfused porcine pancreas. Am J Physiol 235: E387–391, 1978.

84. Dupre J, Ross SA, Watson D, Brown J, et al.: Stimulation of insulin secretion by gastic inhibitory polypeptide in man. J Clin Endocrinol Metab 37: 826–828, 1973.

85. Botha JL, Vinik AI, Brown JC: Gastric inhibitory polypeptide (GIP) in chronic pancreatitis. J Clin Endocrinol Metab 2: 791–797, 1976.

86. Vinik A: Gastrointestinal hormones and nutrient balance. Am J Physiol, in press 1984.

87. Unger RH: Insulin-glucagon relationships in the defence against hypoglycemia. Diabetes 32: 575–583, 1983.

88. Samols E, Marri G, Marks V: Promotion of insulin secretion by glucagon. Lancet 2: 415–416, 1965.

89. Samols E, Tyler JM, Marks V: Glucagon-insulin interrelationships. In: Glucagon: Molecular Physiology, Clinical and Therapeutic Implications, Lefebre PJ and Unger RH (eds). Oxford: Pergamon Press, 1972, pp 151–173.

90. Samols E, Weir GC: Adrenergic modulation of pancreatic A, B, and D cells. α-adrenergic suppression and α-adrenergic stimulation of somatostatin secretion, α-adrenergic stimulation of glucagon secretion in the perfused dog pancreas. J Clin Invest 63: 230–238, 1979.

91. Bonner-Weir S, Orci L: New perspectives on the microvasculature of the islets of Langerhans in the rat. Diabetes 31: 883–889, 1982.

92. Koerker DJ, Ruch W, Chideckel E, Palmer J, Goodner CJ, Ensinck J, Gale CC: Somatostatin: hypothalamic inhibitor of the endocrine pancreas. Science 184: 482–484, 1974.

93. Unger RH, Orci L: Possible roles of the pancreatic D-cell in the normal and diabetic states. Diabetes 32: 575–583, 1983.

94. Unger RH, Dobbs RE, Orci L: Insulin, glucagon, and somatostatin secretion in the regulation of metabolism. Ann Rev Physiol 40: 307–343, 1978.

95. Robertson RP: Prostaglandins, glucosehomeostatis, and diabetes mellitus. In: Annual Review of Medicine 1983, Creger WP, Coggins CH and Hancock EW (eds). Palo Alto, CA: Annual Review Inc., 1983, pp 1–21.

96. Kajinuma H, Kaneto A, Kuzuya T, et al.: Effects of methacholine on insulin secretion in man. J. Clin Invest 28: 1384–1388, 1968.

97. Halter JB, Porte Jr: Mechanisms of impaired acute insulin release in adult onset diabetes: studies with isoproterenol and secretin. J Clin Endocrinol Metab 46: 952–960, 1978.

98. Robertson RP, Halter JB, Porte D Jr: A role for alpha-adrenergic receptors in abnormal insulin secretion in diabetes mellitus. J Clin Invest 57: 791–795, 1976.

99. Ipp E, Dobbs RE, Arimura A, et al.: Release of immunoreactive somatostatin from the pancres in response to glucose, amino acids, pancreozymin-cholecystokin, and tolbutamide. J Clin Invest 60: 760–765, 1977.

100. Marco J, Calle C, Roman D, et al.: Hyperglucagonism induced by glucocorticoid treatment in man. N Engl J Med 288: 128–131, 1973.

101. Wise JK, Hendler R, Felig P: Influence of glucocorticoids on glucagon secretion and plasma amino acid concentrations in man. J Clin Invest 52: 2774–2782, 1973.

102. Berger M, Bordi C, Cuppers H-J, Berchtold P, Gries FA, Muntefering H, Sailer R, Zimmerman H, Orci L: Functional and morphological characterization of human insulinomas. Diabetes 32: 921–931, 1983.

103. Creutzfeldt W, Arnold R, Creutzfeldt C, et al.: Biochemical and morphological investigations of 30 insulinomas. Diabetologia 9: 217–231,1973.

104. Creutzfeldt W: Endocrine tumors of the pancreas. In: The Diabetic Pancreas, Volk BW and Wellman KF, (eds). New York: Plenum Press, 1977, pp 551–590.

105. Harrison TS, Child CG, Fry WJ, Floyd JC Jr Fajans SS: Current surgical management of functioning islet cell tumors of the pancreas. Ann Surg 178: 485–495, 1973.

106. Harrison TS, Fajans SS, Floyd JC Jr, Thompson NW, Rasbach DA, Santen RJ, Cohen C: Prevalence of diffuse pancreatic beta islet cell disease with hyperinsulinism – problems in recognition and management. World J Surg, in press.

107. Heitz PU, Klöppel G, Häcki WH, Polak JM, Pearse AGE: Nesidioblastosis: The pathologic basis of persistent hyperinsulinemic hypoglycemia in infants: Morphologic and quantitative analysis of seven cases based on specific immunostaining and electron microscopy. Diabetes 26: 632–642, 1977.

108. Harness JK, Geelhoed GW, Thompson NW, Nishiyama RH, Fajans SS, Kraft RO, Howard DR, Clark KA: Nesidioblastosis in adults. A surgical dilemma. Arch Surg 116: 575–580, 1981.

109. Nathan DM, Axelrod L Proppe KH, Wald R, Hirsch HJ, Martin DB: Nesidioblastosis associated with insulin-mediated hypoglycemia in an adult. Diabetes Care 4: 383–388, 1981.

110. Stefanini P, Carboni M, Patrassi N, Basoli A: Beta-islet cell tumors of the pancreas: Results of a study on 1,067 cases. Surg 75: 597–609, 1974.

111. Stefanini P, Carboni M, Patrassi N, Basoli A: Hypoglycemia and insular hyperplasia: Review of 148 cases. Ann Surg 180: 130–135, 1974.

112. Case record of the Masachusetts General Hospital, weekly clinicopathological exercises: Case 1-1983. N Engl J Med 308: 30–37, 1983.

113. Case records of the Massachusetts General Hospital, weekly clinicopathological exercises: Case 30. N Engl J Med 299: 241, 1978.

114. Jaffe R, Hashida Y, Yunis EJ: Pancreatic pathology in hyperinsulinemic hypoglycemia of infancy. Lab Invest 42: 356–365, 1980.

115. Vance JE, Stoll RW, Kitabchi AE, Williams RH, Wood FC Jr: Nesidioblastosis in familial endocrine adenomatosis. JAMA 207: 1679–1682, 1969.

116. Kahn CR: The riddle of tumour hypoglycemia revisited. Clin Endo Metab 9: 335–360, 1980.

117. Vinik AI, Pooler W: Carbohydrate metabolism in patients with primary hepatocellular carcinoma. Clin Sci Mol Med 45: 387–396, 1973.

118. Hyodo T, Megyesi K, Kahn CR, McLean JP, Friesen HG: Adrenocortical carcinoma and hypoglycemia: Evidence of production of nonsuppressible insulin-like activity by the tumor. J Clin Endocrinol Metab 44: 1175–1184, 1977.

119. Zapf J, Walter H, Froesch ER: Radioimmunological determination of insulinlike growth factors I and II in normal subjects and in patients with growth disorders and extrapancreatic tumor hypoglycemia. J Clin Invest 68: 1321–1330, 1981.

120. Froesch ER, Zapf J, Widmer U: Hypoglycemia associated with non-islet-cell tumor and insulin-like growth factors. Letter to the Editor. N Engl J Med 306: 1178, 1982.

121. Nouel O, Bernuau J, Rueff B, Benhamou J-P: Hypoglycemia. A common complication of septicema in cirrhosis. Arch Int Med 141: 1477– 1478, 1981.

122. Rutsky EA, McDaniel HG, Tharpe DL, Alred G, Pek S: Spontaneous hypoglycemia in chronic renal failure. Arch Int Med 138: 1364–1368, 1978.

123. Garber AJ, Bier DM, Cryer PE, et al.: Hypoglycemia in compensated chronic renal insufficiency: Substrate limitation of gluconeogenesis. Diabetes 23: 982–986, 1974.

124. Dusheiko G, Kew MC, Joffe BI, Lewin JR, Path FF, Mantagos S, Tanaka K: Recurrent hypoglycemia associated with glutaric aciduria type II in an adult. N Engl J Med 301: 1405–1409, 1979.

125. Bleicher SJ: Hypoglycemia. In: Diabetes Mellitus: Theory and Practise, Ellenberg M and Rifkin H (eds). New York: McGraw-Hill Book Co, 1970, pp 958–989.

126. Elias AN, Grant G: Glucose-resistant hypoglycemia in inanition. Arch Int Med 142: 743–746, 1982.

127. Hirata Y, Ishizu H, Ouchi N, et al.: Insulin autoimmunity in a case with spontaneous hypoglycemia. J Jap Diab Soc 13: 312, 1970.

128. Folling I, Norman N: Hyperglycemia, hypoglycemia attacks and production of anti-insulin antibodies without previous know immunization: Immunological and functional studies in a patient. Diabetes 21: 814, 1972.

129. Onedha A, Matsuda K, Sato M, Yamagata S, Sato T: Hypoglycemia due to apparent autoantibodies to insulin-characterization of inlusin-binding protein. Diabetes 23: 41, 1974.

130. Hirata Y, Tominaga M, Ito J, Noguchi A: Spontaneous hypoglycemia with insulin autoimmunity in Grave's disease. Ann Int Med 81: 214, 1974.

131. Hirata Y: Spontaneous insulin antibodies and hypoglycemia. In: International Congress Series #413. Amsterdam: Exerpta Medica, 1976, pp 278–284.

132. Ichihara K Shima K, Saito Y, Nonaka K, Tarui S, Nishikawa M: Mechanism of hypoglycemia observed in a patient with insulin autoimmune syndrome. Diabetes 26: 500–506, 1977.

133. Hirata Y, Methimazole and Insulin Autoimmune Syndrome with Hypoglycaemia. Lancet II: 1037, 1983.

134. Goldman J, Baldwin D, Rubenstein AH, Klink DD, Blackard WG, Fisher LK, Roe TF, Schnure JL: Characterization of circulating insulin and proinsulin-binding antibodies in autoimmune hypoglycemia. J Clin Invest 63: 1050–1059, 1979.

135. Anderson JH Jr, Blackard WG, Goldman J, Rubenstein AH: Diabetes and hypoglyceemia due to insulin antibodies. Am J Med 64: 868–873, 1978.

136. Flier JS, Bar RS, Muggeo M, Kahn CR, Roth J, Gorden P: The evolving clinical course of patients with insulin receptor antibodies: Spontaneous remission or receptor proliferation with hypoglycemia. J Clin Endocrinol Metab 47: 985–995, 1978.

137. Taylor SI, Grunberger G, Marcus-Samuels B, Underhill LH, Dons RF, Ryan J, Roddam RF, Rupe CE, Gorden P: Hypoglycemia associated with antibodies to the insulin receptor. N Engl J Med 307: 1422–1426, 1982.

138. Rosetti L, DePirro R, Lala A, et al.: Severe hypoglycemia associated with insulin receptor autoantibodies. Diabetologia 23: 303, 1982.

139. Freinkel N, Singer DL, Arky RA, et al.: Alcohol hypoglycemia. I. Carbohydrate metabolism of patients with clinical alcohol hypoglycemia and the experimental production of the syndrome with pure alcohol. J Clin Invest 42: 1112–1133, 1963.

140. Jordan RM, Krammer H, Riddle MR: Sulfonylurea-induced factitious hypoglycemia. Arch Int Med 137: 390–393, 1977.

141. Rubenstein AH, Kuzuya H, Horwitz DL: Clinical significance of circulating C-peptide in diabetes mellitus and hypoglycemic disorders. Arch Inter Med 137: 625–632, 1977.

142. Couropmitree C, Freinkel N, Nagel TC, et al.: Plasma C-peptide and diagnosis of factitious hyperinsulinism: Study of an insulin-dependent diabetic patient with 'spontaneous' hypoglycemia. Ann Int Med 82: 201–204, 1975.

143. Scarlett JA, Mako ME, Rubenstein AH, et al.: Factitious hypoglycemia: Diagnosis by measurement of C-peptide immunoreactivity and insulin-binding antibodies. N Engl J Med 297: 1029–1032, 1977.

144. Tanaka K, Kean EA, Johnson B: Jamaican vomiting sickness: Biochemical investigation of two cases. N Engl J Med 295: 461–467, 1976.

145. Seltzer HS: Drug-induced hypoglycemia: A review based on 473 cases. Diabetes 21: 955–966, 1972.

146. Quevedo SF, Krauss DS, Chazan JA, Crisafulli FS, Kahn CB: Fasting hypoglycemia secondary to disopyramide therapy. JAMA 245: 2424, 1981.
147. Goldberg I, Brown L, Rayfield E: Disopyramide (Norpace)-induced hypoglycemia. Am J Med 69: 463-466, 1980.
148. Arem R, Garber A, Field JB: Sulfanomide-induced hypoglycemia in chronic renal failure. Arch Int Med 143: 827-829, 1983.
149. Bouchard PH, Sai P, Reach G, Caubarrere I, Ganeval D, Assan R: Diabetes mellitus following pentamide-induced hypoglycemia in humans. Diabetes 31: 40–45, 1982.
150. Sharpe SM: Pentamidine and hypoglycemia. Letter to the Editor. Ann Int Med 99: 128, 1983.
151. Arena FP, Dugowson C, Saudek CD: Salicylate-induced hypoglycemia and ketoacidosis in a nondiabetic adult. Arch Int Med 138: 1153–1154, 1978.
152. Setzer HS, Fajans SS, Conn JW: Spontaneous hypoglycemia as an early manifestation of diabetes mellitus. Diabetes 5: 437–442, 1956.
153. Lev-Ran A: Nadirs of oral glucose tolerance tests are independent of age and sex. Diabetes Care 6: 405–408, 1983.
154. Permutt MA: Postprandial hypoglycemia. Diabetes 25: 719–733, 1976.
155. Cryer PE: Physiology and pathophysiology of the human sympathoadrena neuroendocrine system N Engl J Med 303: 436–444, 1980.
156. Billington CJ, Casciato DA, Choquette DL, Morley JE: Artifactual hypoglycemia associated with polycythemia vera. JAMA 249: 774–775, 1983.
157. Merimee TJ, Tyson JE: Stabilization of plasma glucose during fasting. Normal varations in two separate studies. N Engl J Med 291: 1275–1278, 1974.
158. Fajans SS, Floyd JC Jr,: Fasting hypoglycemia in adults. N Engl J Med 294: 766–772, 1976.
159. Haymond MW, Karl IE, Clarke WL, Pagliara AS, Santiago JV: Differences in circulating gluconeogenic substrates during short-term fasting in men, women, and children. Metabolism 31: 33–42, 1982.
160. Service FJ, Dale AJD, Elveback LR, Jiang N-S: Insulinoma. Clinical diagnostic features of 60 consecutive cases. Mayo Clin Proc 51: 417–429, 1976.
161. Felig P, Lynch V: Starvation in human pregnancy: Hypoglycemia, hypoinsulinemia and hyper-ketonemia. Science 170: 990–992, 1970.
162. Fajans SS, Floyd JC Jr,: Diagnosis and medical management of insulinomas. Ann Rev Med 30: 313–329, 1979.
163. Merimee TJ, Tyson JE:Hypoglycemia in man. Pathologic and physiological varients. Diabetes 26: 161–165, 1977.
164. Turner RC, Oakley NW, Nabarro JDN: Control of basal insulin secretion, with special reference to the diagnosis of insulinomas. Br Med J 2: 132–135, 1971.
165. Sherman BM, Pek S, Fajans SS, Floyd JC Jr, Conn JW: Plasma proinsulin in patients with functioning pancreatic islet cell tumors. J Clin Endocrinol Metab 35: 271–280, 1972.
166. Alsever RN, Roberts JP, Gerber JG, Mako ME, Rubenstein AH: Insulinoma with low circulating insulin levels: The diagnostic value of proinsulin measurements. Ann Int Med 82: 347–350, 1975.
167. Sandler R, Horwitz DL, Rubenstein AH, Kuzuya H: Hypoglycemia and endogenous hyperin-sulinism complicating diabetes mellitus. Application of the C-peptide assay to diagnosis and therapy. Am J Med 59: 730–736,1975.
168. Service FJ, Horwitz DL, Rubenstein AH, et al.: C-peptide suppression test for insulinoma. J Lab Clin Med 90: 180–186, 1977.
169. Turner RC, Heding LG: Plasma proinsulin, C-peptide and insulin in diagnostic suppression tests for insulinomas. Diabetologia 13: 571–577, 1977.
170. Fajans SS, Schneider JM, Schteingart DE, Conn JW: The diagnostic value of sodium tol-butamide in hypoglycemic states. J Clin Endocrinol Metab 21: 371-386, 1961.
171. Roy BK, Abuid J, Wendorff H, Nitiyanant W, De Rubertis FR, Field JB: Insulin release in

response to calcium in the diagnosis of insulinoma. Metabolism 28: 246–252, 1979.

172. Kaplan EL, Rubenstein AH, Evans R, Lee CH, Klementschitsch P: Calcium infusion: A new provocative test for insulinomas. Ann Surg 190: 501–507, 1979.

173. Harrison TS, Santen RJ: Calcium stimulation test in the evaluation of insulin-secreting pancreatic islet-cell tumors. Case report. Milit Med 146: 103–105, 1981.

174. Pointel JP, Villaume C, Gay G, Drouin P, Debry G: Absence of effect of calcium perfusion on blood sugar and plasma insulin in a patient with a benign insulinoma. Horm Metab Res 10: 572–573, 1978.

175. Kakita K, Horino M, Tenku A, Matsumura S, Matsuki M, Nishida S: Absence of insulin release in response to calcium in a patient with a benign insulinoma. Horm Metab Res 13: 237–238, 1981.

176. De Palo C, Sicolo N, Vettor R, Federspil G: Lack of effect of calcium infusion on blood glucose and plasma insulin levels in patients with insulinoma. J Clin Endocrinol Metab 52: 804–806, 1981.

177. Miller JL, Klaff LB, Abrahamson MJ, Marine N: Failure of calcium infusion as a provocative test for insulinoma. N Engl J Med 304: 1430, 1981.

178. Hayashi M, Floyd JC Jr, Pek S, Fajans SS: Insulin, proinsulin, glucagon and gastrin in pancreatic tumors and in plasma of patients with organic hyperinsulinism. J Clin Endocrinol Metab 44: 681–694, 1977.

179. Floyd JC Jr, Fajans SS, Pek S, Chance RE: A newly regognized pancreatic polypeptide: Plasma levels in health and disease. Rec Prog Horm Res 33: 519–570, 1977.

180. Glaser B, Valtysson G, Vinik AI, Fajans SS, Cho K, Thomson NW: Gastrointestinal/pancreatic hormone concentrations in the portal venous system of nine patients with organic hyperinsulism. Metabolism 30: 1001–1010, 1981.

181. Kahn CR, Rosen SW, Weintraub BD, Fajans SS, Gorden P: Ectopic production of chorionic gonadotropin and its subunits by islet-cell tumors. A specific marker for malignancy. N Engl J Med 297: 565–569, 1977.

182. Louis LH, Fajans SS, Conn JW, Struck WA, Wright JB, Johnson JL: The structure of a urinary excretion product of 1-Butyl-3-p-tolysulfonylurea (Orinase). J Am Chem Soc 78: 5701–5702, 1956.

183. Bauman WA, Yalow RS: Differential diagnoses between endogenous and exogenous insulin-induced refractory hypoglycemia in a nondiabetic patient. N Engl J Med 303: 198–199, 1980.

184. Arky RA, Freinkel N: Alcohol infusion to test gluconeogenesis in starvation, with special reference to obesity. N Engl J Med 274: 426, 1966.

185. LeQuesne LP, Nabarro JDN, Kurtz A, Zweig S: The management of insulin tumours of the pancreas. Br J Surg 66: 373–378, 1979.

186. Dagget PR, Goodburn EA, Kurtz AB, LeQuesne LP, Morris DV, Nabarro JDN, Raphael MJ: Is preoperative localisation of insulinomas necessary? Lancet 1: 484–486, 1981.

187. Turner RC, Morris PJ, Lee ECG, Harris EA: Localization of insulinomas. Lancet 1: 515–518, 1978.

188. Miller DR: Functioning adenomas of pancreas with hyperinsulinism. Arch Surg 90: 509–520, 1965.

189. Olsson O: Angiographic diagnosis of an islet cell tumor of the pancreas. Acta Chir Scand 126: 346, 1963.

190. Robins JM, Bookstein JJ, Oberman HA, Fajans SS: Selective aangiography in localizing islet-cell tumors of the pancreas. A further appraisal. Radiology 106: 525–528, 1973.

191. Clouse ME, Costello P, Legg MA: Sub-selective angiography in localizing insulinomas of the pancreas. Am J Roentg 128: 741, 1977.

192. Gray BK, Rosch J, Grollman JH: Arteriography in the diagnosis of islet-cell tumors. Radiology 97: 39–44, 1970.

193. Fulton RE, Sheedy PF, McIllrath DC, Ferris DO: Preoperative angiographic localization of

insulin producing tumors of the pancreas. Am J Roent 123: 367–377, 1975.

194. Edis AJ, McIllrath DC, Van Heerden JA, Fulton RE, Sheedy PF, Service FJ, Dale AJ: Insulinoma-current diagnosis annd surgical management. Curr Probl Surg 13. 3–45, 1976.

195. Dunnick NR, Long JA Jr, Krudy A, Shawker TH, Doppman JL: Localizing insulinomas with combined radiographic methods. Am J Roent 135: 747–752, 1980.

196. Alfidi RJ, Bhyun DS, Crile G Jr, Hawk W: Arteriography and hypoglycemia. Surg Gynec Obstet 133: 477–452, 1971.

197. Lunderquist A, Tylen U: Phlebography of the pancreatic veins. Radiologie 15: 198–202, 1975.

198. Stefanini P, Carboni M, Petrassi N, DeBernardinis G, Negro P, Blandamura V: The value of arteriography in the diagnosis and treatment of insulinomas. Am J Surg 131: 352–356,1976.

199. Korobkin MT, Palubinskas AJ, Glickman MG: Pitfalls in arteriography of islet-cell tumors of the pancreas. Radiology 100: 319–328, 1971.

200. Dunnick NR, Doppman JL, Mills SR, McCarthy DM: Computed tomographic detection of non-beta pancreatic islet cell tumors. Radiology 135: 117–120, 1980.

201. Ingemansson S, Lunderquist A, Lundquist I, Loudahl R, Tibbin S: Portal and pancreatic vein catheterization with radioimmunologic determination of insulin. Surg Synec Obstet 141: 705–711, 1975.

202. Ingemansson S, Kühl C, Larsson L-I, Lunderquist A, Lunderquist I: Localization of insulinomas and islet cell hyperplasia by pancreatic vein catheterization and insulin assay. Surg Gynecol Obstet 146: 725–734, 1978.

203. Dunn E, Stein S: Percuteous transhepatic pancreatic vein catheterization in localization of insulinoma. Arch Surg 116: 232–233, 1981.

204. Cho KJ, Vinik AI, Thompson NW, Shields JJ, Porter DJ, Brady TM, Cadavid G, Fajans SS: Localization of the source of hyperinsulinism: Percutaneous transhepatic portal and pancreatic vein catheterization with hormone assay. Am J Roentg 139: 237–245,1982.

205. Vinik AI, Strodel WE, Cho KJ, Eckhauser FE, Thompson NW: Localization of hormonally active gastrointestinal tumors. In: Endocrine Surgery Update,Thompson N, Vinik A (eds). New York: Grune and Stratton, 1983, pp 195–218.

206. Vinik AI, Strodel WE, Lloyd RV, Thompson NW: Unusual gastroenteropancreatic (GEP) tumors and their hormones. In: Endocrine Surgery Update, Thompson N, Vinik A (eds). New York: Grune and Stratton, 1983, pp 293–320.

207. Reichardt W, Cameron R: Anatomy of the pancreatic veins. A post morten and clinical phlebographic investigation. Acta Radiolo 21: 33–41, 1980.

208. Doppman JL, Brennan MF, Dunnick NR, Kahn CR, Gorden P: The role of pancreatic venous sampling in the localization of occult insulinomas. Radiology 138: 557–562, 1981.

209. Fajans SS, Floyd JC Jr, Knopf RF, Rull J, Guntsche EM, Conn JW: Benzothiadiazine suppression of insulin release from normal and abnormal islet tissue in man. J Clin Invest 45: 481, 1966.

210. Fajans SS, Floyd JC Jr, Thiffault CA, Knopf RF, Harrison TS, Conn JW: Further studies on diazoxide suppression of insulin release from abnormal and normal islet tissue in man. Ann NY Acad Sci 150: 261–280, 1968.

211. Neri V, Bartorelli A, Faglia G: Effect of propanolol on the blood sugar, immunoreactive blood insulin in a patient with insulinoma. Acta Diabetol Lat 6: 809–819, 1969.

212. Blum I, Doron M, Laron Z, et al.: Prevention of hypoglycemic attacks by propranolol in a patient suffering from insulinoma. Diabetes 24: 535–537, 1975.

213. Shaklai M, Aderka D, Blum I, et al.: Suppression of hypoglycemia attacks and insulin release by propranolol in a patient with metastatic malignant insulinoma. Diabete Metab 3: 155–158, 1977.

214. Hofeldt FD, Dippe SE, Levin SR, Karam JH, Blum MR, Forsham PH: Effects of diphenylhydantoin upon glucose-induced insulin secretion in three patients with insulinoma. Diabetes 23: 192, 1973.

304

215. Brodows RG, Campbell RG: Control of refractory fasting hypoglycemia in a patient with suspected insulinoma with diphenylhydantoin. J Clin Endocrinol Metab 38: 159–161, 1974.
216. Federspil G, Casara D, Stauffacher W: Chlorpromazine in the treatment of endogeneous organic hyperinsulinism. Diabetologia 10: 189, 1974.
217. Schein PS: Chemotherapeutic management of the hormone-secreting endocrine malignancies. Cancer 30: 1616–1626, 1972.
218. Broder LE, Carter SK: Chemotherapy of malignant insulinomas with streptozotocin. In: International Congress Series #314, Excerpta Medica,1974, pp 714–727.
219. Moertel CG, Hanley JA, Johnson LA: Streptozocin alone compared with streptozocin plus fluorouracil in the treatment of advanced islet-cell carcinoma. N Engl J Med 303: 1189–1194, 1980.
220. Kiang DT, Frenning DH, Bauer GE: Mithramycin for hypoglycemia in malignant insulinoma. N Engl J Med 299: 134–135, 1978.
221. Eastman RC, Come SE, Strewler GJ, Gorden P, Kahn CR: Adriamycin therapy for advanced insulinoma. J Clin Endocrinol Metab 44: 142–148, 1977.
222. Warne GL, Adie R, Hansky J, Martin FIR, Varigos G: Prolonged control of hypoglycemia by L-asparaginase in islet cell carcinoma producing insulin and gastrin. Aust NZJ Med 5: 466, 1975.

12. Endocrine tumors of the gastroenteropancreatic axis

AARON I. VINIK, WILLIAM E. STRODEL
and THOMAS M. O'DORISIO

1. Introduction

1.1 The endocrine tumors of the gastroenteropancreatic (GEP) axis derive from the diffuse neuroendocrine system of the gut and consist of cells capable of Amine Precursor Uptake and Decarboxylation (APUD). The tendency to label tumors of the GEP axis as APUDomas has merit in that histologic features of endocrine cells are recognized, however this practice does not embrace the clinical syndromes that derive therefrom. Although subsequently modified, the original hypothesis held that all APUD cells have a common embryological origin in the neural crest [132]. Recent experimental studies have confirmed that suprarenal chromaffin cells, C cells of the thyroid gland, and chief cells of the carotid body are indeed derivatives of the neural crest [4, 97, 134]. Current evidence suggests that the source of gut and pancreatic endocrine cells is a discrete population of endodermal stem cells different from other epithelial cells [5, 158, 172]. These cells in their primitive form appear to retain the capacity to differentiate into a number of different cell lines and function to secrete peptides normally not contained in the adult pancreas. A clear example is the gastrinoma syndrome in which the most common site of the tumor is the pancreas that, in the adult, is devoid of G cells.

Most investigators agree that tumors arising from the endocrine cells from the GEP axis should be classified by their secretory products, for example gastrinoma, glucagonoma, VIPoma, etc. Although GEP tumors are frequently composed of mixed cells, one peptide is secreted predominantly and is usually responsible for the patient's symptomology. Tumors should be referred to, not by the most prevalent cell type, but by the predominant secretory product.

1.2 The peptide and amine products of these tumors can be identified by immunocytochemical methods. An important development in this area is the use of the peroxidase-antiperoxidase (PAP) technique which allows double or even triple staining with different colors and has led to identification of more than one secretory product within a single tumor [38, 76, 103, 132]. Gold labeling combines immunocytochemistry with electronmicroscopy and antibody bound gold parti-

Santen, R.J. and Manni, A. (eds.), Diagnosis and management of endocrine-related tumors. ISBN 0-89838-636-5.
© *1984, Martinus Nijhoff Publishers, Boston. Printed in the Netherlands.*

cles can be visualized adherent to the secretory granules.

1.3 *Pathologic features common to GEP tumors.* Pathologists commonly label tumors of the GEP axis as carcinoids because of similar histologic features and the argentaffin and argyrophyllic properties [67]. The four main patterns found are: 1) cord like, 2) ribbon like, 3) alveolar acinar or rosette pattern, 4) an undifferentiated trabecular or medullary structure. The cell type may be round, ovoid, prismatic or cylindrical. When found in expected sites, e.g. pancreas, adrenal medulla or small bowel, the pathologist is often alert to the possibility of a GEP tumor. However, the features are often not sufficiently distinctive and invariably at frozen section the tumors are misdiagnosed as adenocarcinoma, or even anaplastic carcinoma. Hence the need for immunocytochemical characterization.

The tumors are proliferative in nature and may take the form of:

(1) Hyperplasia
(2) Neoplasia: adenoma
                 adenomatous hyperplasia
                 microadenamatosis
                 nesidioblastosis
                 carcinoma

Hyperplasia is relatively uncommon in benign sporadic tumors, but is the rule in MEN-syndrome. The cell type most frequently involved is reported to be the PP cell, but we are becoming increasingly aware of a high frequency of proliferation of somatostatin (SRIF) cells in many GEP tumors [47]. The secretory granules are not always characteristic of the normal cell and the tumors may be difficult to diagnose on this basis alone. The granules may be normal, abnormal or of a mixed type, or may even appear to be absent depending upon the capacity of the tumor to store its secretory product. Not uncommonly, circulating levels of a peptide may be high whereas the peptide may not be identified within the tumor by histochemical techniques. A useful marker under these circumstances appears to be the glycolytic enzyme, neuron-specific enolase (NSE) which is found in common with all tumors of the GEP axis [21, 48, 149, 162].

The tumors may be subdivided into [93]:

1. Orthoendocrine – when they secrete the normal product of the cell type.
2. Paraendocrine – when they secrete a peptide or amine product usually foreign to the organ or cell of origin.
3. Part of the MEN syndrome – when a variety of peptides or amines are secreted.

At any particular stage of tumor growth the cells appear to function autonomously with loss of the normal physiologic function.

Although a variety of peptides may be produced (Table 1) by any one tumor, the clinical syndrome generally derives from overproduction of one of the peptides or amines. Blood levels tend to be high at all times and are responsible for

Table 1. Immunohistochemical staining of islet cell tumors

Patient	Insulin	Glucagon	SRIF	Gastrin	VIP	PP
AP	−	−	−	+	−	+
TB	−	−	+	−		−
BC	−	+	−	+		−
TD(I)	+	−	−		−	−
PD(G)	−	−	+	+	−	−
RD(I)	+	−	−	−	−	−
CF(G)	−	−	+	+	−	−
HG(PP)	−	−	−	−	−	+
FH(PP)	−	−	−	−	+	+
BH(G)	−	−	−	−	−	+
SH(G)	−	−	−	+	−	+
BK(C)	−	−	−	−	−	−
CL(G)	−	−	−	−	−	−
FL(G)	+	+	−	+	−	−
BN(I)	+	+	−	−		−
SP(I)	+	−	+	+	−	+
MS(I)	+	−	+	−	−	−
ST(G)	+	−	−	+	−	+
DT(I)	+	+	+	−	−	−
MV(I)	+	−	−	−	−	−
FW(G)	+	+	+	−	−	+

I = insulinoma; G = gastrinoma; PP = PPoma; C = carcinoid.
− indicates no staining; + indicates positive staining.

the symptom complex. Some of the secretions are typically endocrine in nature, e.g. glucagon, gastrin or pancreatic polypeptide (PP) which exert uncontrolled effects in large quantities, while others derive from neurotransmitters, e.g. VIP or paracrine substances, e.g. SRIF and substance P that do not generally circulate in large quantities, but exert their actions at the local tissue level. The multipotentiality of these tumors is readily observed in longitudinal follow-up, wherein a tumor may secrete a different hormone at different times and produce a different clinical syndrome [94, 124]. The relative frequency of these tumors is difficult to estimate. A post-mortem study of 1366 cases by Grimelius estimated a prevalence of 8 cases per 1000 [67]. The following table is a rough estimate of the frequency of tumors and their manifestations (Table 2). Figure 1 shows the relative frequency of tumor location in the pancreas.

1.4 *Features common to clinical presentation of GEP tumors.* Orthoendocrine tumors secreting glucagon, somatostatin, PP, CLIP, growth hormone releasing factor (GRF), and gastrin most commonly originate from pancreatic islets or ducts. The absence of G cells in the adult human pancreas and tendency to nesidioblastosis suggest that the primitive D_1 cell lining of the pancreatic ducts

Table 2. Differentiation of Zollinger-Ellison (ZES) and WDS (Verner-Morrison; WDHA)

Feature	ZES	WDS
Diarrhea	Acid	Alkaline (HCO_3 loss)
Gastric acid	Increased	Decreased
Gastric volume	Increased	Normal or decreased
Naso-gastric suction	Diarrhea improves	Diarrhea unchanged
Motility	Increased[a]	Increased slightly[b]
Abdominal pain	Marked	Rare (initially)
Stool K$^+$ loss	Slightly	Marked
Metabolic acidosis	No (Alkalosis with gastric suction)	Yes
Lesion-location (also wall of stomach and duodenum)	Primary pancreas neuroblastoma	Primary pancreas
Mediator	Gastrin	VIP/other!

[a] Motility enhanced secondary to gastriv acid stimulation.
[b] Motility may be slightly increased secondary to direct effects of either intra arterial or intra luminal VIP (cf. ref. 10).

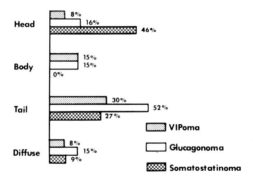

Figure 1. Relative frequencies of the location of pancreatic islet cell tumors.

may be the precursor stem cell from which the tumor cells derive [36]. What the factors are which promote the differentiation or tumor formation have not been resolved. In certain instances, e.g. VIPoma, tumors probably derive from the abundant neural elements within the pancreas [143, 145].

Paraendocrine or ectopic GEP tumors have been found in the adrenal medulla, kidney, in the peripancreatic and periaortic lymph nodes, as single intrahepatic lesions in the wall of the stomach and duedenum and small bowel, and rarely in the biliary tract or large bowel. Tumors secreting GEP peptides can occur as bronchial adenomas [79, 145].

In general these tumors are slow growing and metastasize late, if at all. It is thus critically important to make this diagnosis since the prognosis can be years of good health in contrast with the near 100% mortality within six months of the diagnosis of pancreatic adenocarcinoma. Many of these tumors have been thought to be silent symptomatically and biochemically. With the recognition of more peptides with limited biological function, for example PP, it appears that most tumors do indeed secrete but the peptides have yet to be identified.

When tumors metastasize they do so to local lymph nodes, the liver and peritoneum, rarely beyond. Even so, regression of tumors can often be achieved with cytotoxic therapy with steptozotozin and other miscellaneous agents [7, 50, 52, 66, 109, 120, 124]. Features which appear as common presentations include:

1. Pain or abdominal discomfort due to a hepatic or pancreatic mass.
2. Diarrhea due to a variety of causes.
3. Diabetes or abnormal glucose tolerance.

The occurrence of MEN syndrome may be as frequent as one third of the cases, with involvement of the parathyroids in 87% of cases and the pituitary in about one third [79, 133, 165]. It is important in all instances to 1) obtain a family history, 2) do coned down views of the pituitary sella, 3) measure serum prolactin, PP, Ca^{2+} and gastrin. If this is done, occult cases with MEN are unlikely to be missed. The secreted products, peptides or amines may be abnormal molecular forms with restricted biologic and immunologic activity. Detection of these tumors can thus be very difficult and it is important to recognize that a variety of measurements may need to be made.

2. Vipoma

2.1   In 1958, Verner and Morrison first described refractory watery diarrhea and hypokalemia associated with noninsulin-secreting tumors of the pancreatic islets [173]. Verner and Morrison [173] and Priest and Alexander [137] were among the first to note the absence of gastric hypersecretion in such patients in 1957, and in 1961, Murray, Paton and Pope [119] documented achlorhydria in a patient presenting with this tumor syndrome. Matsumoto and colleagues termed the syndrome 'pancreatic cholera' because the observed severe diarrhea resembled Vibrio cholera disease [110]. In 1967, Marks, Bank, and Louw proposed the acronym WDHA (Watery Diarrhea, Hypokalemia, Achlorhydria) [108] (Fig. 2). Since 1967, several series have been reported which have confirmed the association between certain pancreatic tumors and watery diarrhea syndrome [18, 86, 174]. It has, however, been controversial as to whether or not VIP is the causative agent.

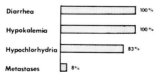

Figure 2. Relative frequency of the symptoms found in patients with VIPomas.

2.2 *The role of VIP as a neuromodular and hormone*. The role of VIP as both a normal neuromodular of intestinal secretion and an abnormal 'hormone' substance in the WDS has been recently reviewed [54, 55]. Several important in vitro and, more recently, in vivo observations have attested to a causative role for VIP in WDS. In 1974, Schwartz and colleagues reported that VIP produced net chloride secretion across rabbit and human ileal mucosa in vitro. The peptide increased short circuit current in a dose dependent manner, and produced chloride secretion in excess of sodium secretion [151]. Similar effects of VIP in the small intestine in vivo were noted in dog jejunal loops by Krejs and colleagues [87, 88]. Infusion of VIP into the superior mesenteric artery produced secretion of chloride, potassium, bicarbonate, and water into dog jejunal loops. The magnitude of the secretion suggested that VIP produced active secretion of chloride and bicarbonate, creating a favorable gradient for passive flux of potassium and perhaps sodium ions [87, 88]. Essentially the same effects on net chloride secretion as observed in vitro [151] and in vivo [87] have been observed in man [88]. Krejs and Fordtran demonstrated in normal subjects that the human jejunum secreted chloride in response to increasing doses of VIP. The process was observed to be active, but the bicarbonate flux, unlike the canine model remained unchanged. Also noted in their study, the measured plasma VIP levels (by radioimmunoassay) achieved with the VIP infusion were in the order of those observed in WDS, supporting the hypothesis that high levels of VIP could be responsible for certain secretory diarrheal states. Further, VIP has been observed to reverse net chloride absorption and cause net secretion in the rat colon in vivo [184]. In these acute experiments, as well as others [87, 88, 151], a high dose of VIP was needed to cause chloride secretion, accompanied by net sodium and potassium secretion and a fourfold enhancement of bicarbonate secretion [184].

Modlin and colleagues were amongst the first groups to recognize that acute administration of VIP for one or two hours (in pigs) did not reproduce the clinical features of WDS [114]. In contrast infusion of VIP to achieve levels slightly above the upper range of normal (i.e. 180 pg/ml of plasma) and for prolonged periods did induce cutaneous flushing and watery diarrhea. Furthermore, when VIP was infused chronically six out of eight pigs studied developed the flushing and watery diarrhea syndrome within ten hours of infusion. When VIP was given to normal subjects as a continuous intravenous infusion for 10 hours at a dose (400 pmol/kg/h) which achieved immunoassayable VIP levels within the reported tumor ranges [80], all subjects developed profuse watery diarrhea within 6.5 hours. There were statistically significant increases in fecal Na^+ and HCO_3 concentrations and pH, consistent with the active anion secretion and abolition of sodium absorption shown in previous perfusion studies [87, 88]. Also noted was the association of hyperchloremic acidosis, thought to be due to HCO_3 loss in the feces [80] and the absence of carbohydrate or fat malabsorption.

The studies demonstrating the presence of functional VIP receptors associated with adenylate cyclase on gut epithelial cells [3, 10] have established a pa-

Table 3. Clinical features of reported GEP tumors

	Glucagonoma	VIPoma	SRIFoma	PPoma
Cases (no)	80	100	15	20
Benign (%)	25	50	5–10	90
Sporadic (%)	70	70	90	50
Found in MEN (%)	5	5	(20–25)	50–75

thohumoral role of VIP in WDS and further suggest that VIP may play a physiologic role as a local neuromodulator of intestinal secretion [54, 55].

2.3 *Clinical features of VIPOMA syndrome.* In 1974, Verner and Morrison reviewed 55 patients with the syndrome [174]. In addition to diarrhea and hypokalemia, alkalosis in mild cases but acidosis in severe diarrhea with bicarbonate wasting flushing, hypercalcemia, abnormal glucose tolerance, tetany, and dilation of the gallbladder were observed. The most prominant symptom in most patients reported is profuse cholera-like diarrhea, often present for three or four years duration prior to diagnosis, with volumes usually exceeding 6 to 8 l of stool/24 h. The stools have the appearance of dilute tea and are rich in electrolytes, with an average secretion of 300 mEq of potassium/24 h. The diarrhea is always secretory in nature, will not disappear with fasting for 48 h and demonstrates an increased net secretion of electrolytes in the stool. This symptom may be confused with the diarrhea found in the ZE syndrome. The distinguishing features are shown in Table 2. Diarrhea which is not secretory is always due to causes other than endocrine tumors. However, laxative abuse may be very difficult to exclude and the measurement of stool electrolytes and osmolarity may be required. Stool electrolytes should account for the osmolarity if the condition is due to an endocrine tumor. An osmolarity that exceeds that expected from the concentration of electrolytes invariably reflects laxative abuse which must be carefully excluded.

The episodic and fulminating, secretory diarrhea in the WDS results in profound hypokalemia, hypochlorhydria (rarely achlorhydria), bicarbonate wasting, and hyperchloremic metaboic acidosis. The more commonly observed hypochlorhydria is due to the direct gastric acid inhibitory effect of VIP, a biologic property shared with other members of the secretin-glucagon family, namely, secretin, glucagon, gastric inhibitory peptide (GIP), and peptide histidine and isoleucine (PHI) [163]. The effects of VIP consistent with the signs and symptoms of WDS are shown in Table 4. In the early stage of tumor growth the predominant symptoms of diarrhea are episodic and intermittent. It is generally accepted that, as the VIP tumor enlarges, the diarrhea becomes continuous and the ensuing electrolyte abnormalities life threatening [18, 86]. Increased intestinal motility, as well as secretion, may contribute to the diarrhea [157].

Table 4. Effects of VIP consistent with signs and symptoms of WDS

Sign/Symptom
Secretory diarrhea
Hypokalemia
Hypochlorhydria
Hyperglycemia
Hypercalcemia
Flushing (vasodilation)
Atonic gallbladder

The clinical features of VIPomas are consistent with the known actions of VIP which include: stimulation of intestinal secretion, facial flushing, inhibition of gastric acid secretion, stimulation of glycogenolysis, and hypercalcemia [8, 14, 18, 63, 86, 138, 142, 174]. The structural homology between VIP and secretin, glucagon, gastric inhibitory polypeptide (GIP) and peptide histidine and iso-leucine (PHI) [138] may account for enhanced secretion of pancreatic juice and inhibition of gastric acid secretion. VIP has also been reported to cause gallbladder relaxation; a large distended gallbladder is often found in patients with the VIPoma syndrome. Hypercalcemia has been noted in nearly 50% of patients with the syndrome. The cause is not clear but may be related to dehydration, electrolyte disturbances secondary to diarrhea, to coincidental multiple endocrine neoplasia accompanied by hyperparathyroidism, or the secretion by the tumor of a calcitropic peptide. Tetany has been reported in several patients and may be due to hypomagnesemia secondary to the diarrhea. Nearly 8% of patients demonstrate facial flushing. The cause of this patchy erythematous and sometimes urticarial flushing is not clear but has been attributed to VIP or prostaglandins which may be present in the tumor.

The hyperglycemia often noted in patients with WDS is probably secondary to the profound glycogenolytic effect of high portal vein VIP on the liver [63].

2.4 *Sites of tumors secreting VIP.* VIP-secreting tumors appear to originate usually in the pancreas or along the sympathetic chain. Long reviewed a series of 62 patients [104]. Fifty-two patients (84%) had pancreatic tumors and ten patients had ganglioneuroblastomas.

Of the ten patients with ganglioneuroblastomas, seven were children. There have been 18 other case reports of elevated plasma levels of VIP which have been associated with neurogenic tumors including: ganglioneuroblastoma, ganglio-neuromas, neurofibroma, and pheochromocytoma [13, 32, 45, 77, 82, 90, 112, 166, 167, 185]. The majority of neurogenic tumors associated with the VIPoma syndrome have been found in children. Catecholamines are frequently elevated. In patients with excess catecholamine secretion, flushing, increased sweating and hypertension may occur. Hyperglycemia and hypercalcemia have not been noted in children. Plasma levels of PP are normal and it was not detected in VIP-producing ganglioneuroblastomas. Thus, it was hoped that PP levels would distinguish pancreatic and non-pancreatic sources of VIP. However, three adults with neurogenic tumors and a 64-year-old woman with a VIPoma of the lower left kidney had high serum levels of PP [68]. Excessive quantities of immunoreactive VIP and PP were found in the renal tumor tissue.

2.5 *Biochemical diagnosis and experience*. By definition, VIP levels are elevated in all patients with the VIPoma syndrome. False-positive elevations of VIP can be observed in patients with small bowel ischemia or severe low flow states caused by diarrhea and secondary dehydration not associated with VIP-producing tumors [16, 18, 113]. Bloom and co-workers contend that the measurement of plasma VIP is a useful clinical screen for detection of VIP tumors in the absence of shock, which per se may raise VIP levels [16, 18]. In addition, monitoring plasma VIP concentrations during the treatment of malignant tumors is helpful since the levels may rise detectably long before symptoms of recurrence develop. VIP is, however, not the only agent implicated in the diarrhea syndrome.

Gastrin, secretin, glucagon, enteroglucagon, gastric inhibitory polypeptide, PP, VIP, thyrocalcitonin (TCT), and prostaglandlins or any one of a number of combinations have been implicated as possible etiologic agents of the diarrhea syndrome [114]. Bloom reported 1000 patients with various forms of diarrhea [16, 17, 20]. Thirty-nine patients (3.9%) had greatly elevated levels of VIP; in each case, a tumor was found. In more than 50% of these patients the tumor was successfully removed, the symptoms remitted, and the plasma levels of VIP returned to normal. Twelve patients had diarrhea secondary to TCT-producing tumors of the thyroid; 13 patients had carcinoma of the lung; four patients had a villous adenoma of the rectum; and 24 patients had carcinoid tumors. All 53 of these patients had normal plasma VIP levels. The 11 patients who had the classic clinical features of the VIPoma syndrome in whom VIP levels were normal and no tumor was found, were probably secreting an unidentified humoral substance.

Biochemical detection of VIP secreting tumors necessitates a highly sensitive and specific VIP radioimmunoassay. Our reported range of normal VIP concentration for 100 fasting healthy control subjects is 0–170 pg/ml [54] similar to that (0–190 pg/ml) found by others [14, 45, 143].

Information gained from a single plasma VIP level may be misleading. Between periods of watery diarrhea, the VIPoma, unlike many endocrine tumors of the gut (eg insulinoma or gastrinoma) may not be actively secreting VIP; thus a 'normal' level creates a false sense of security and may delay a more vigorous search for the cause.

Between 6/79 and 5/83, we have analyzed 2908 plasma samples for VIP sent to us from Canada and the United States with the diagnosis of *presumed* WDS. Of these, 29 were found to have elevated VIP levels in their plasma and to be primary

Table 5. VIP secreting tumors and WDS (Between 6/69 and 5/83)

Patient	Age	Sex	VIP (pg/ml)[a]	Comment
1	35	M	960	VIPoma with metastasis (met)
2	2	M	1850	Ganglioneuroblastoma with met
3	46	M	640	VIPoma with met
4	40	F	1750	VIPoma with met
5	53	M	880	Pheo/ganglioneuroma
6	62	F	1150	VIPoma with met
7	36	F	280	VIPoma with met (Liver 1°?)
8	52	M	520	VIPoma
9	2	F	1700	Ganglioneuroblastoma with met
10	38	M	1200	VIPoma
11	81	F	860	VIPoma with met
12	70	F	320	VIPoma with met
13	70	M	1500	Small cell tumor of lung with met
14	64	F	540	VIPoma with met
15	3	F	960	Ganglioneuroblastma
16	3	F	225	Neuroblastoma with met[b]
17	48	F	640	VIPoma with met
18	1	F	100	Ganglioneuroblastoma
19	55	F	1250	VIPoma with met
20	5	F	900	Ganglioneuroblastoma
21	50	M	1050	VIPoma with met
22	50	M	850	VIPoma with met
23	60	F	750	VIPoma with met
24	50	F	1100	VIPoma
25	1	F	345	Mast cell tumor [c]
26	75	F	1200	VIPoma with met
27	68	M	880	VIPoma with met
28	78	M	1800	VIPoma with met
29	58	F	540	Pheo/ganglioneuroblastoma
Mean	43		956	
±SD	5		85	

[a] VIP reported was the initial sample; Normal mean: 62 (±22 SD) pg/ml.
[b] Sample drawn after surgery.
[c] See Ref. 31. Symptoms in this patient were flush and syncope – not diarrhea.

VIP secreting tumors at surgery (Table 5). The overall incidence of VIP-related tumors and WDS for all samples assayed was 1%. The mean age of our patients was 43 ± 5 years; there were 11 males and 18 females. The mean VIP values of our 29 documented VIP secreting tumors was 956 ± 85 (SE) pg/ml. The minimum initial VIP level in our 29 cases of 225 pg/ml (patient #16), was a sample drawn after the initial tumor was removed. This patient was found to have a metastatic neuroblastoma. Our highest initial VIP value was 1850 pg/ml (patient #2, with metastatic ganglioneuroblastoma). Only four of 29 patients had VIPomas *without* metastatis at the time of surgery whereas 16 or 29 (56%) were found to have gross metastasis (usually to the liver) at surgery. This finding compares with the series of Kraft and colleagues [86] and probably reflects the rather long duration between symptoms and surgery (3 years), and the unavailability of reliable and clinically useful assays for VIP. Eight ganglioneuroblastomas/pheochromo-cytoma-secreting VIP tumors and the WDS were found in our series. Six of these eight (patients 2, 9, 15, 16, 18 & 20) were children less than five years of age. The other two patients (#5 and 29) were adults and both had pheochromocytoma elements with their ganglioneuroblastoma tumors. Of interest, patient #13 had a documented small cell cancer of the lung associated with high VIP levels and the WDS as has been reported by Said [143]. Patient #25 is a patient with cutaneous mastocytoma and did not present as a classic WDS, but rather with flushing and hypotension [182]. Two patients (not shown in Table 5) with documented non-tropical sprue had elevated plasma VIP values (425 and 385 pg/ml respectively), that returned to normal on a gluten-free diet. The incidence of false negative values in our 2908 samples is uncertain. In patients without tumors, 85% of these samples had VIP levels below the limit of detection (50 pg/ml plasma).

PP was found to be elevated (i.e. 300 pg/ml) in 11 of 18 patients with tumors of the pancreas, but patients #5, 13 and 20 who also had elevated plasma levels, had extrapancreatic tumors (Table 5).

Patients #2, 14, 15 and 18 (ganglioneuroblastomas) had a mean VIP tumor level of 2.4 ng/g wet weight. The mean VIP content of fresh adrenal (predominantly medulla) from 11 normal subjects was .016 ± .005 ng/g wet weight. No PP could be detected in any of these tumors. The mean VIP tumor concentration of patients 21 and 23 (both primary pancreatic and metastatic liver tumor) was 1.3 ng/g weight, N = 4. Of interest, patients (#21 and 23) had elevated fasting PP in their plasma (1050 and 2500 pg/ml respectively); however, the PP content in their tumors was not elevated (.030 and .016 ng/g wet weight; normal mean pancreatic PP concentrations being 0.034 ng/g, N = 4).

2.6 *Treatment.* In the series reported by Long most of the solitary tumors located in the pancreas were 8 cm in size or greater [104]. In one instance three separate tumors were present in the pancreas; the incidence of nodal or hepatic metastases was 40% of this series. A patient of Verner and Morrison in 1974 had a discrete tumor of the pancreas, but diffuse hyperplasia of the non-beta islet cells and ducts was also observed [174]. Electron microscopy showed suggestive evidence of an increase in islet cells, particularly A cells. Total pancreatectomy was eventually performed on the patient who became asymptomatic.

In the series of 52 cases reported by Long, surgical excision of the primary pancreatic tumor relieved all symptoms in 17 patients (27%) [104]. No metastases were seen at operation in 15 patients but in two patients several small metastases remained. In these latter two patients, symptoms had not occurred 1.5 and 2 years postoperatively. Surgical removal of a ganglioneuroblastoma was successful in seven of their 10 patients. In two patients total excision was impossible. This experience reflects the experience reported in the world literature with VIP-omas.

We recently have had experience with a $2^1/_2$-month-old child with acidosis, flushing, and hypotension [179, 182]. A mastocytoma producing VIP was located in the child's forearm. The child was cured by resection of the tumor.

In patients who have diarrhea and no tumor is demonstratable by angiography, CAT or ultrasound or transhepatic portal venous sampling (THVS), steroids have provided some symptomatic relief. However, since other diarrheagenic agents may be implicated, a trial of inhibitors of prostaglandin synthesis, e.g. indomethacin, phenothiazines, and lithium may be warranted [11]. We do not advocate blind total pancreatectomy and have seen spontaneous remission of WDS without establishing a cause and eventual emergence of tumors in unusual sites including the kidney and skin.

In summary, when confronted with severe chronic diarrhea, it must be established that the diarrhea is secretory in nature by fasting the patient for 48 h and measuring stool volume. If diarrhea persists with fasting, VIP-producing tumors of the pancreas are frequently found, and plasma samples should be analyzed for VIP in these patients. If the VIP level is elevated, a VIP tumor should strongly be suspected. In addition, a serum pancreatic polypeptide level should be determined simultaneously. If the tumor is located in the pancreas, this peptide will almost invariably be elevated. In children catecholamine levels should also be obtained. If the serum VIP levels are normal, screening for other causative agents should be performed including gastrin, substance P, SRIF, PP, TCT, serotonin, glucagon, and prostaglandins of the E_2 series. Tumor localization should include CAT, celiac, superior mesenteric, and renal angiography and finally THVS. If a tumor is found it should be excised. We do not condone blind pancreatic resection. In the absence of finding a tumor, symptomatic therapy is warranted.

3. Somatostatinoma

3.1 *Physiological actions of somatostatin.* Somatostatin (SRIF) is a tetradecapeptide which is produced by the D cell of the pancreas and gut [95, 158], and is also found in ganglia and nerve cells in the wall of the gut [16, 150]. SRIF inhibits numerous endocrine and exocrine functions. Almost all gut hormones which have been described are inhibited by SRIF, including insulin, PP, glucagon, gastrin, secretin, GIP, and motilin [171]. Supression of both insulin and glucagon release should give rise to a syndrome of low normal fasting glucose levels with mild diabetes or impaired glucose tolerance. Because of concomitant supression of glucagon secretion neither severe endogenous hyperglycemia, or hyperketonemia occurs. In addition to the inhibition of endocrine secretion, SRIF has direct effects on a number of target organs. It is a potent inhibitor of basal and pentagastrin stimulated gastric acid secretion and it delays gastric emptying [35].

Reduced rates of gastric emptying and gastric acid production may contribute to the dyspepsia and fullness that many patients experience after meals. In the intestine, absorption of sugars, amino acids and fats are delayed [89, 95]. SRIF appears to decrease absorption of nutrients by exerting a direct effect on the mucosa that is independent of intestinal transit time. However over the entire length of the small bowel, absorption of these nutrients is still complete, although somewhat delayed [95]. Steatorrhea which may occur therefore reflects a failure of intraluminal digestion due to inhibition of pancreatic enzymes, for which more distal segments of the small intestine cannot compensate. SRIF induces an increased frequency of the interdigestive migrating complex, a decrease in gallbladder contractility, and a fall in the volume, bicarbonate and enzyme content of pancreatic secretions. Direct inhibition of gallbladder contraction and reduced pancreatic secretion may produce maldigestion and steatorrhea which may respond to enzyme treatment. In addition, stasis of bile and steatorrhea may precipitate cholelithiasis.

3.2 *Clinical presentation of patients with somatostatinomas.* The predicted presentation of patients with high circulating SRIF levels are: 1) hypochlorhydria due to the direct effects of SRIF on acid secretion and the inhibition of gastrin, 2) diabetes secondary to the inhibition of insulin secretion and, 3) malabsorption and steatorrhea due to the direct inhibitory effect of SRIF on secretion of pancreatic enzymes and absorption of fat (Fig. 3). Several other findings may be predicted on the basis of the known actions of SRIF outside the gastrointestinal tract, but in most instances these are of a secondary nature. As predicted the salient features of the somatostatinoma syndrome include diabetes, gallbladder disease, hypochlorhydria, and weight loss. Gallbladder disease including cholelithiasis, has appeared uniformly in the small number of reported cases of somatostatinoma, and is best explained by the inhibition of gallbladder contraction. Weight loss has also been a common feature and may be related to the catabolic effects of the tumor or to malabsorption.

The first case of somatostatinoma syndrome was reported in 1977 by Ganda and Larsson [59, 95] and in 1980 Krejs [89] reported another case and reviewed six other cases. There are now about 18 case reports in the literature. The majority of

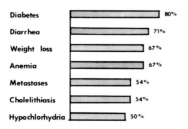

Figure 3. Relative frequency of the symptoms found in patients with somatostatinoma.

reported tumors have contained hormones other than SRIF and have been located in the pancreas. However, two tumors have been located in the small intestine, one in the duodenum and one in the jejunum. The natural history and incidence of malignancy in these tumors has not been apparent in such a small series of patients. The diagnosis can usually be suspected on the basis of the clinical syndrome and is confirmed by measurements of SRIF in the plasma. Tumors reported to date have had extremely high levels of circulating SRIF, so that the problems related to the measurement of this peptide in plasma have been of little concern. Result of treatment have been varied. In those patients who underwent total excision of the tumor, symptoms of somatostatinoma resolved and plasma SRIF levels returned to normal [16, 58, 89].

Attempts to find provocative tests to enable earlier diagnosis have met with some success. Tolbutamide has been found to stimulate SRIF release from the porcine pancreas and gastric antrum [39], but such an effect has not been detected in peripheral plasma in normal human volunteers. In the case reported by Pipeleers, tobutamide infusion induced a dramatic increase in plasma SRIF concentration and was accompanied by severe nausea and vomiting but without flushing [135]. A decrease in the response to tolbutamide infusion has been observed in patients successfully treated with streptozotocin. In the reported cases the tumors have invariably been malignant, probably related to the commonplace symptoms unrecognized until late in the disease.

We have had the experience of one unusual patient with a benign SRIF-producing tumor [179]. A thirty-two-year-old man presented with mild diarrhea and occult blood in the stool. Upper GI endoscopy was performed and demonstrated a polypoid lesion in the second portion of the duodenum. Endoscopic biopsy of this lesion was interpreted as a villous adenoma. The patient underwent operation with duodenotomy and polypectomy. Histology of the polyp demonstrated a neuroendocrine neoplasm and immunoperoxidase staining showed the presence of SRIF. Following polypectomy, the patient has remained asymptomatic and serum levels of SRIF are normal. Tolbutamide infusion did not produce an increase in peripheral venous SRIF concentration. Our experience of 14 patients with MEN-I has indicated that the commonest peptide found by immunohistochemistry of the pancreas is SRIF and not PP. However, blood levels of SRIF have not been elevated in nine of these patients studied nor have symptoms compatible with hypersecretion been evident. Elevations of SRIF levels in plasma may be found in other endocrine tumors and in family members of patients with MEN-I syndrome. In 43 patients with pheochromocytomas, five were found to have inordinately high SRIF levels without a clinical counterpart. In the results of a large family with MEN-I, of 253 members studied, seven had high levels of SRIF without the symptom complex. In future years, benign SRIF-cell hyperplasia will undoubtedly be recognized.

4. Glucagonoma

4.1 *Physiological functions of glucagon.* The pancreatic A cells produce a 29-amino acid polypeptide with a molecular weight of 3485 daltons [116]. As indicated above it shares numerous amino acid homologies with the family of secretin, VIP, and GIP [180]. Glucagon has a number of biologic actions which include relaxation of smooth muscle, inhibition of pancreatic enzyme secretion, inhibition of gastric acid secretion, stimulation of intestinal fluid and electrolyte secretion and stimulation of cardiac output. Pancreatic glucagon is stimulated primarily in response to hypoglycemia and by a number of amino acids, and its major function appears to be as a counterregulatory hormone in glucose homeostasis [176].

Enteroglucagon or glucagon-like immunoreactivity in the intestine is a term applicable to material identified in the intestine [73, 116]. Glucagon or glucagon-like immunoreactivity is found in the highest concentrations in the distal ileum in an L cell and also in the colon [117, 146]. There are a number of different molecular forms [116], one of which has been identified with an N-terminal and C-terminal extension of glucagon called glicentin. It contains 100 amino acid residues among which is the full sequence of pancreatic glucagon. Current RIA for enteroglucagon requires the measurement of total glucagon-like immunoreactivity (GLI) and the subtraction of values for pancreatic glucagon. Plasma levels rise after ingestion of a meal and these are markedly elevated in patients with intestinal hurry or the dumping syndrome [15], chronic pancreatitis and small bowel disease [26]. A single patient has been reported to have had a markedly elevated enteroglucagon level with small intestinal mucosal hyperplasia and constipation and a tumor of the kidney producing an enteroglucagon-like material [62]. It has been speculated that the major action of enteroglucagon is the growth of small intestine.

4.2 *Clinical features of glucagonoma syndrome.* In 1966, McGavran called attention to a syndrome that included acquired diabetes and glucagon-producing tumors [111]. It only became apparent later that these tumors were usually accompanied by a very characteristic skin rash described by Wilkinson in 1973 [183] and Sweet in 1974 [161]. The main features of the glucagonoma syndrome

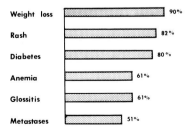

Figure 4. Relative frequency of the symptoms found in patients with glucagonoma.

include a characteristic rash termed necrolytic migratory erythema (NME), painful glossitis, angular stomatitis, normochromic normocytic anemia, weight loss, diabetes mellitus, and hypoaminoacidemia (Fig. 4).

The frequency of islet cell tumors has been estimated in autopsy series to be between 0 and 1.4% of all cases studied [67]. In a very thorough study of 1366 consecutive adult autopsies, Grimelius found a tumor frequency of 0.8% [67]. All of the tumors were adenomas and all contained histochemically defined glucagon cells. None of the tumors had been suspected during life. Although these adenomas contained glucagon it is not known whether they were overproducing or even secreting glucagon.

The rash of the glucagonoma syndrome has a characteristic distribution. It is usually widespread, but major sites of involvement are the perioral and perigenital regions along with the fingers, legs and feet. It may also occur in areas of cutaneous trauma. The basic process in the skin seems to be one of superficial epidermal necrosis, fragile blister formation, crusting and healing with hyperpigmentation. Skin biopsies usually show small bullae containing acantholytic epidermal cells as well as neutrophils and lymphocytes [161]. The adjacent epidermis is usually intact. The dermis contains a lymphocytic perivascular infiltrate. Several biopsies associated with the cutaneous lesions has been a painful glossitis manifested by an erythematous, mildly atrophic tongue. Different stages of the cutaneous lesions may be present at any single time; therefore, biopsy examination of a fresh skin lesion may be the most valuable aid in establishing the diagnosis of the glucagonoma syndrome. However repeated biopsy samples may be necessary to establish the diagnosis.

Several metabolic disorders are associated with cutaneous lesions closely resembling the NME of the glucagonoma syndrome and include acrodermatitis enteropathica, zinc deficiency induced by hyperalimentation, essential fatty acid deficiency, the dermatosis of protein calorie malnutrition or Kwashiorkor and pellagra due to niacin deficiency [11, 74, 123, 170]. Cutaneous manifestations associated with malabsorptive states are often non-specific, affecting approximately 20% of patients with steatorrhea. Improvement in the rash associated with the glucagonoma syndrome has been reported with amino acid repletion as well as with the administration of carbohydrate. The skin rash has also been shown to improve with the administration of zinc [72]. Almost invariably the dermatosis resolves after successful removal of a glucagon-producing tumor, even if the rash has been present for several years [115, 186]. In addition, in those patients who do not undergo curative resection but are treated with chemotheraputic agents, the dermatitis improves as glucagon levels decrease [98, 109, 186].

Glucose intolerance in the glucagonoma syndome has interested many investigators because of its possible relevance to the relationship between hyperglucagonemia and diabetes. Hyperglucagonemia has been observed in a number of conditions and is associated with glucose intolerance in some, such as, chronic renal failure, diabetes mellitus and Cushing's disease. The importance of hyper-glucagonemia in the etiology of glucose intolerance in these states, particularly in diabetes mellitus, is controversial [23, 71]. Glucagon is an accepted hyper-glycemic agent, which acts by stimulating hepatic glycogenolysis and gluconeo-genesis. In the glucagonoma syndrome, correlations between plasma levels of glucose and glucagon have been described, but this is not easily demonstrated in all proven cases. Massive replacement of normal pancreatic B cells with tumor may worsen glucose intolerance by diminishing insulin secretory capacity and reducing circulating levels of insulin. The size of hepatic metastases may also be a factor. Fasting plasma glucagon levels tend to be higher in patients with large hepatic metastases than in persons without hepatic metastases [115]. All patients with large hepatic metastases had glucose intolerance. Massive hepatic metas-tases may decrease the ability of the liver to metabolize splanchnic glucagon, increasing peripheral plasma glucagon levels; but glucagon may not directly induce hyperglycemia unless metabolism of glucose by the liver is directly com-promised. Another factor may be the variation in the molecular species of glucagon present in each case and the biological potency of each species [34]. A syndrome of familial hyperglucagonemia is associated with hypersecretion of pro-glucagon which has limited biologic activity [22, 37, 181]. Hyperglucagonemia is also found in cirrhosis of the liver [41], acute [42, 43] and chronic pancreatitis [26, 27] and after pancreatectomy [117] and usually derives from extrapancreatic sources of a gut pancreatic type glucagon which has little hyperglycemic activity.

Finally, other hormones secreted by these tumors may also influence glucose tolerance. Tumors that elaborate ACTH may induce hyperglycemia by causing Cushing's syndrome. VIP which may be secreted by these tumors, is a hyper-glycemic factor and may raise plasma glucose levels. The potentially complex interaction of glucagon and other hormones elaborated by glucagonomas thus altering glucose tolerance is illustrated by the possible secretion of somatostatin (SRIF) by these lesions. The effects of SRIF on plasma glucose levels have been alluded to above.

Two more features of the syndrome are worthy of mention. There is an alarmingly high rate of thromboembolic complications in patients with gluca-gonomas and many patients succumb to pulmonary embolism. Unexplained thromboembolic disease should alert one to the possibility of glucagonoma. Psychiatric disturbances including depression are characteristic and may relate in part to the chronic dermatosis [16, 83].

In previously reported cases of glucagonoma in which plasma glucagon concen-trations were measured by radioimmunoassay, fasting plasma glucagon concen-trations were $2100 \pm 334 \, \text{pg/ml}$. These levels are markedly higher than those reported in normal, fasting subjects (less than $150 \, \text{pg/ml}$), or in patients with other disorders causing hyperglucagonemia including diabetes mellitus, burn injury, acute trauma, bacteremia, cirrhosis, renal failure or Cushing's syndrome where fasting plasma glucagon concentrations are often less than $500 \, \text{pg/ml}$. More pronounced elevations in plasma glucagon concentrations may be noted occasionally in patients with cirrhosis and portacaval anastomoses.

Another syndrome of hyperglucagonemia without the chemical features of glucagonoma has been described [22]. Basal immunoreactive glucagon was elevated in four of nine asymptomatic relatives of a patient with a glucagonoma. Glucagon responses to intravenous glucose and arginine or mixed meals were abnormal, whereas glucose and insulin responses were normal. Pancreatic angiograms and hepatic scintiscans were normal in all four relatives. The data suggested an autosomal dominant pattern of transmission of hyperglucagonemia in this family. A pseudoglucagonoma syndome has also been described. NME and elevated plasma levels of glucagon were present in a patient with cirrhosis of the liver. Serum glucagon levels varied from 780 to 1000 pg/ml. Computed tomography of the liver and pancreas demonstrated a small liver with no evidence of a mass in the pancreas. A visceral angiogram also failed to demonstrate any pancreatic tumor. The dermatitis responded to topical steroid therapy. The patient eventually died of renal failure and an autopsy showed no evidence of glucagonoma.

Glucagonomas, as other islet cell neoplasms, may overproduce multiple hormones. Insulin was the most common second hormone secreted by these tumors. ACTH, pancreatic polypeptide, parathyroid hormone or substances with parathyroid hormone-like activity, gastrin, serotonin, VIP and MSH in that order of frequency.

4.3 *Treatment*. All reported glucagonomas with the cutaneous syndrome originated from single pancreatic tumors of considerable size (largest diameter 1.5 to 35 cm) [4, 74]. All tumors occurred in the tail or body of the pancreas where A cells are normally abundant and which derive from the dorsal anlage of the pancreas. At the time of diagnosis 62% of the tumors had metastases. Glucagonomas not associated with the syndrome but which are characterized by morphologic and/or chemical criteria present in various ways. First, the tumor may appear as a malignant pancreatic tumor, discovered due to local growth with or without metastases. Second, the tumor may be associated with an insulinoma or gastrinoma or as part of the MEN I syndrome. Glucagonoma may also occur as a single microadenoma found incidentally at autopsy in elderly patients [67].

If the diagnosis is made while the tumor is still localized, surgical resection can be curative [71, 170, 175]. As in other islet cell tumors, even when malignant these tumors tend to be extremely slow growing. Effective treatment with chemotherapy, using streptozotocin has been reported with increasing frequency. Surgical debulking of glucagonoma tumors has also been shown to be beneficial [115]. Another chemotherapeutic agent, DTIC, has been used successfully in a patient who showed no response to streptozotocin [7]. Even when metastases have occurred, excellent palliation with chemotherapeutic drugs has resulted in prolonged symptom-free survival [83, 106, 109].

5. Pancreatic polypeptide (PPomas)

5.1 *Physiologic functions of PP*. Pancreatic polypeptide (PP) is a 36-amino acid polypeptide with a molecular weight of 4200 daltons, isolated as a byproduct in the purification of insulin [33, 84]. It is found almost entirely in the pancreas in the D_2 cells of the islet and to a lesser extent in the acinar portion of the gland. A number of actions have been found for PP including the inhibition of pancreatic enzyme output [1, 101, 102]. At high dose levels PP exhibits a biphasic action on pancreatic bicarbonate production with initial stimulation followed by inhibition. A similar effect occurs in the stomach and PP stimulates basal acid secretion but inhibits pentagastrin-stimulated secretion [131]. The only true physiologic action of pancreatic polypeptide which has been shown is the inhibition of biliary and pancreatic exocrine secretion and even this is a weak action [1, 164]. PP is released into the circulation in large quantities after ingestion of a meal which is thought to act predominantly through a cholinergic mechanism [51]. Insulin-induced hypo-glycemia stimulates the release of PP, as do a number of hormones including CCK [117], pentagastrin, secretin [61], and bombesin [51]. Pancreatico-biliary juice also stimulates the release of PP [147, 148]. Thus, it appears that there may be a feedback loop whereby pancreatico-biliary secretions stimulate the release of PP which in turn inhibits pancreatic and biliary secretion. In almost all instances the stimulation of PP release can be blocked with atropine, suggesting that most mechanisms operate through a vagal or extravagal cholinergic mecha-nism. PP levels increase with advancing age which may be related to an alteration in vagal tone [153]. Basal PP levels have not proved of value in the diagnosis of chronic pancreatic insufficiency, but the response to meal ingestion [99], insulin-induced hypoglycemia [155], secretin [61], and CCK-OP [148] stimulation are abnormal, almost certainly in the presence of steatorrhea, and in most patients with pancreatic insufficiency without steatorrhea [61]. The inordinate sensitivity of PP responsiveness to cholinergic stimulation has suggested a usefulness for PP responsiveness to insulin-induced hypoglycemia for the diagnosis of vagal integ-rity and also of autonomic neuropathy in diabetes [100].

The PP cell has a unique distribution in the pancreas, and is found not only in the islets but also in the acinar tissue and duct epithelium. In humans, total pancreatectomy abolishes the pancreatic polypeptide response to a meal, sug-gesting that there are only insignificant amount of pancreatic polypeptide outside the pancreas. A possibility that is supported by tissue extraction studies in primates.

5.2 *Clinical features of PP hypersecretion*. Clinical interest in PP has been in-creased by the claim that an elevated basal serum human PP concentration is an important tumor marker for pancreatic neuroendocrine tumors. Taylor mea-sured basal serum PP concentration in forty-one patients with the Zollinger-Ellison syndrome and in one hundred healthy subjects [164]. Four of the patients with the Zollinger-Ellison syndrome had PP concentrations greater than 240 pg/ml. However, three of the normal subjects also had basal concentrations of PP above 240 pg/ml. Three of the four patients with the Z-E syndrome who had elevated PP concentrations had mixed tumors with high concentrations of both gastrin and PP.

Bloom recently reexamined the incidence of elevated serum human PP concentrations in gastrinomas and insulinomas using a higher upper limit of normal (300 pg/ml) and reported an incidence of 26% and 22% respectively [16, 17] However, they found a 77% incidence of elevated PP concentration in 22 patients with VIPomas. Larsson and co-workers found that three of four patients with the WDHA syndrome which included VIPomas, had elevated serum pancreatic polypeptide concentrations [96]. Three of the four tumors contained both PP and VIP cells. These workers examined a total of eighteen neuroendocrine tumors and found that ten contained more than one cell type. With the possible exception of tumors associated with WDHA syndrome, PP cells were no more frequently found as a second cell in mixed tumors then were gastrin, insulin, and glucagon cells. Apparently for neuroendocrine tumors other than VIPomas, elevated serum PP concentrations were no more a tumor marker than were insulin, gastrin, or glucagon.

The picture is further complicated by the fact that mixed tumors, PP cell hyperplasia in association with other functioning islet cell tumors, ductal hyperplasia of PP cells, nesidioblastosis, and multiple islet tumors producing PP have also been described either alone or as part of the MEN I syndrome. It appears, that many of the cases of so-called non-functional tumors are indeed PPomas. It is our experience that 50 to 75% of these tumors are associated with raised basal PP levels and in 67% the response to secretin is exaggerated. Thus, in the absence of factors which are known to cause marked elevation of PP levels such as chronic renal failure or occasionally in an older healthy patient, a markedly elevated PP level may be indictive of a non-functioning pancreatic endocrine tumor.

A few tumors have been described, composed entirely of PP cells, with PP forming the only detectable secretion. This rarity may be more apparent than real however, since these PPomas appear to be clinically silent and thus are less likely to be detected. Several patients with pure PP-secreting tumors have been described. Tomita reported two patients, one of whom had persistant watery diarrhea and the other of whom had high levels of circulating PP and PP-cell hyperplasia [168]. Bordi [25] reported a PP tumor in a patient with chronic duodenal ulcer and Ebeid reported a patient with a tumor that invaded the bile ducts, producing biliary obstruction [46]. Larsson suggested that the watery diarrhea syndrome may have its origin in PP over-production [96].

Recently Heitz performed immunocytochemical analyses on 125 pancreatic endocrine tumors [70]. In general the hormone secreted by the tumor causing clinical symptoms could be localized by immunocytochemistry. Fifty of 95 active tumors were found to contain cells immunoreactive to peptides not causing clinical symptoms. In 15 of 30 'nonsecreting' tumors, endocrine cells were none-theless found by immunocytochemistry. By electron microscopy more than one cell type could be identified in 12 tumors. Forty patients did not suffer from hormonally-induced symptoms but had an abdominal mass, pain, jaundice, or other abdominal symptoms. Ten of these patients were found to have elevated serum levels of PP and immunoreactive PP cells were found in all of them. Thirty of the 40 tumors were not found by radioimmunoassay to be actively secreting hormones and were labeled 'nonsecreting' even in the presence of immunoreac-tive cells. In five patients with PPomas, serum PP levels were determined three to fifteen weeks after surgery and were found to be within the normal range. It has been claimed that the elevated serum PP levels are due to secretion of the peptide by hyperplastic, non-tumorous PP cells. Such a mechanism may operate in some but not all patients: high numbers of PP cells, high concentration in PP tumors, and normalization of serum of PP levels after surgical excision of the tumor have been shown in five patients in Heitz's study.

5.3 *Treatment.* Our experience with PPomas reflects a spectrum of presentations including benign solitary tumors, malignant tumors with hepatic metastatases,

Table 6. Features of PPomas

Patient	Age	Sex	Duration of symptoms (mos)	Basal PP (pg/ml)	MaxPP response to secretin (pg/ml)	Findings	Results
AG	68	F	3	1480	3770	spontaneous remission	PP240
CW	53	M	2	7520	8430	5 cm tumor in head of panc.	resected PP 39
FH	74	F	3	35100	42800	7 cm tumor in body of panc.	resected PP 228
MS	48	M	24	3027	5150	4 cm tumor in tail of panc.; liver mets	Died 2 yrs + Cytotoxics
LH	67	M	9	1980–2790	7090	tumor in head of panc.; mets in liver	Died 1 yr + Cytotoxics
HG*	63	F	12	1220	1770	3 cm tumors in head, neck & tail of panc.	Resected PP450
FW*	52	M	84	890–2790	1070–3390	Multiple tumors	Died carcinoma
CS	54	M	10	1870	2400	8 cm tumor in head of panc.	Resected PP 25
TF	20	F	1	394	–	15 cm tumor in head of panc	Resected PP 15

* Associated MEN-1 syndrome.

and multiple tumors without metastases associated with the MEN I syndrome [176, 178, 179] (Table 6). One patient presented with upper gastrointestinal bleeding and was found to have a large PP-producing tumor in the head of the pancreas without evidence of metastases. He underwent successful resection of this tumor and has been asymptomatic for two years. Repeat computed abdominal tomography did not demonstrate recurrence of tumor one year after operation. Another patient had vague upper abdominal symptoms, weight loss, and a large PPoma in the body of the pancreas. At operation, no metastases were noted and the patient underwent curative resection. Serum PP levels decreased to normal after treatment and the patient remains asymptomatic without signs of recurrent tumor. Two patient developed weight loss and severe diarrhea before diagnosis. Evaluation revealed large tumor masses in the pancreas and extensive hepatic metastases. Both patients were treated with streptozotocin with modest responses and subsequently died. Two other patients in our series had PP-producing tumors in association with MEN I. One had had two parathyroid adenomas removed prior to the diagnosis of a pancreatic tumor and the other patient had multiple tumors in the pancreas including a gastrinoma. A single patient had diarrhea and elevation of serum PP concentrations, both of which resolved without treatment. Further evaluation failed to reveal a source for the elevated levels of PP. A salutary experience occurred in one patient with MEN-I whom we followed for seven years with elevated PP levels. Repeated CAT and angiography and THVS failed to define a single endocrine tumor. He ultimately succumbed with metastatic disease due to a pancreatic duct adenocarcinoma. There is one other case such as this in the literature.

In Friesen's experience, elevated serum PP levels in patients with MEN indicates one or more tumors of the pancreas [53]. He now recommends pancreatectomy for all patients with elevated PP levels because of the malignant potential of these tumors. Since it is our observation that PP levels may be raised in 50% of patients with carcinoid syndrome and VIPomas and 25% of gastrinomas and insulinomas, we prefer to define the nature of PP hypersecretion and remove or treat the offending tumor. For patients with MEN-I with elevated serum PP levels, we have recently recommended a distal 2/3 pancreatectomy as a prophylactic procedure as a compromise [160]. Total pancreatectomy with its attendant morbidity and mortality constitutes too great a risk and is in our opinion too drastic.

6. Markers of GEP tumors

Islet cell tumors, like many other endocrine tumors, are recognized during life by clinical syndromes related to hypersecretion of one or more hormones. These peptides serve as maskers for the presence of disease and after treatment allow surveillance for recurrent tumors. With a variety of techniques, some subtle differences between secretion of the benign and malignant islet cell tumor have been observed. In general however, the distinction rests on the demonstration of metastatic disease which in some cases is not possible until laparotomy. Various tumor markers apart from the peptides produced by the tumors have been described and include neuronspecific enolase (NSE), HCG and HCG subunits, S-100 protein, oncofetal antigens, and pancreatic polypeptide.

6.1 *HCG*. In 1973, Braunstein, as part of a large survey, studied serum from four patients with malignant insulinomas and found that two had an increase in plasma levels of immunoreactive HCG-beta, suggesting that this may be a useful marker is this disease [28]. In 1977, Kahn and co-workers measured HCG and its subunits in 76 patients with islet cell tumors [81]. Seventeen of 27 patients with functioning islet-cell carcinomas had elevated plasma levels of HCG or one of its subunits (HCG-alpha and HCG-beta). Secretion was often discordant; the most frequent finding was an elevated level of HCG-alpha alone. In one patient responding to streptozotocin, changes of HCG-alpha correlated with the clinical response. Studies of tumor extracts suggested that the markers observed in the circulation were being produced in the tumor itself. In contrast, none of the 43 patients with benign disease or the six patients with non-functioning malignant tumors had elevated levels of HCG, HCG-alpha or HCG-beta. Later in 1981 Oberg investigated HCG and its subunits in twenty-nine patients with APUD tumors, 16 patients with endocrine pancreatic tumors and 13 patients with carcinomas [127]. Twenty of 29 patients (69%) had elevated levels of HCG and its subunits. Among patients with endocrine pancreatic tumors, 11 of 16 had raised levels of these peptides. Three patients with benign tumors had normal concentrations. In patients with carcinoids nine of thirteen (69%) had elevated serum levels of at least one of the components. A discordance in secretion patterns between the two types of endocrine tumors was noticed. Only one patient with a carcinoid had a raised level of the complete HCG molecule. The levels of HCG-alpha were elevated in 23% of the patients with malignant endocrine pancreatic tumors and 69% of the patients with carcinoids while the corresponding frequency of raised HCG-beta levels was 69%. Three of four patients with so-called non-functioning islet cell tumors had raised levels of the subunits.

The reason for this discrepancy is not apparent. These results indicate that HCG subunits may be valuable tumor markers for both of these APUD tumors. The finding of a raised HCG subunit strongly suggests the diagnosis of malignancy but a normal level does not exclude it!

6.2 *NSE*. Neuron specific enolase (NSE) is a specific neural isomer of the glycolytic enzyme 2-phospho-D-glycerate hydrolase originally extracted from bovine tissue, and was once thought to be present only in the central nervous system [149]. Subsequent studies however have shown that NSE is present in all APUD cells. Tapia demonstrated that NSE is present in a wide variety of APUD neoplasms, including islet cell tumors of the pancreas, medullary carcinoma of the thyroid, pheochromocytoma, and small cell carcinoma of the lung [162]. In contrast, NSE is not found in any of the non-neural endocrine tumors of twenty-one patients with neuroendocrine tumors. Nine had elevated levels, four had borderline elevations and eight NSE levels were indistinguishable from control values. Two of six gastrinomas, both with hepatic metastases, had elevated levels. Two patients with metastatic glucagonomas had normal NSE levels. Each of these patients however was receiving chemotherapy and had resolution of their symptoms at the time NSE levels were determined. One malignant somato-statinoma was evaluated and NSE was abnormally high. Of three patients with medullary carcinoma of the thyroid, one had an elevated NSE level. This patient also manifested the carcinoid syndrome. Two children with neuroblastomas had abnormally elevated levels of NSE. Clear elevation of NSE was found only in patients with malignant APUD tumors and all these tumors had extensive meta-stases or local invasion. In our experience of 11 patients with APUD tumors (Table 7), NSE was uniformly found in the tumors but only in one instance of a malignant gastrinoma was the plasma level raised.

Consequently, NSE is not likely to prove useful for early diagnosis of APUD tumors. NSE may prove to be useful in monitoring the course of these tumors and assessing their response to various treatment modalities. Serum NSE was elevated before operation in one patient with a neuroblastoma but fell to within the normal range after resection of all gross tumor.

6.3 *Protein S-100* was first described as a nervous tissue specific protein by Moore in 1965 [118] and was so named because of its solubility in 100% ammonium sulfate solution at neutral pH. S-100 protein is a mixture of two similar proteins, S-100A

Table 7. Immunohistochemical staining of tumor tissue and serum NSE levels in 11 patients with islet tumors

Patient	Serum NSE (ng/dl)*	Immunohistochemical stain
RD(I)	3.0	+
DT(I)	5.3	+
FW(G)	4.5	+
SP(I)	5.	+
ST(G)	14.7	+
SH(G)	7.2	+
CL(G)	3.6	+
FH(PP)	3.9	+
PA(G)	5.2	+
BK(C)	8.1	+
MS(I)	4.3	+

I = insulinoma; G = gastrinoma; PP = PPoma; C= carcinoid.
* Normal serum NSE levels 5 ng/dl.

and S-100B. Until recently clinical diagnostic applications of S-100 protein were confined mainly to the central nervous tissue and tumors. Nakajima in 1982 determined S-100 protein in the tissues of a variety of tumors [121]. Of 22 carcinoid tumors S-100 protein was demonstrated in nine. Ten of the tumors originated from the lung and the remainder were from the gastrointestinal tract. Six of the tumors which were positive for S-100 protein were of bronchial origin. Immunoreactive products of S-100 protein were observed in tumor cells forming solid nests. Further study will be necessary to determine whether S-100 will become a useful marker for examination of neuroendocrine tumors.

6.4 *Pancreatic polypeptide* is found in endocrine cell types located in pancreatic islets and also scattered among the acini and occasionally in cells lining the ducts of the pancreas. Polak and co-workers have proposed that a high fasting serum PP concentration is an important marker for pancreatic endocrine tumors [136]. However, in 1981, Oberg determined serum levels of pancreatic polypeptide in 31 patients with endocrine tumors, 16 localized in the pancreas, 13 in the small intestine, and 2 in the respiratory tract [125]. Elevated serum levels in the peripheral circulation were noted in 56% of the patients with pancreatic tumors and 69% of those with bronchial tumors and in addition two patients with laxative abuse. This study suggested that the elevated PP concentration may originate from non-tumor PP cells and only occasionally from the tumor. Our experience of raised PP levels in 50% of patients with carcinoid syndrome supports this notion [177]. Thus, PP is a valuable tumor marker for endocrine gastrointestinal tumors but is not specific for the pancreas. Furthermore, certain inflammatory diseases, renal failure and laxative abuse must be considered when evaluating elevated PP levels. It further does not appear to be useful to monitor progress. No correlation between clinical course or tumor size and peripheral serum PP levels has been demonstrated.

7. Peptide heterogeneity as an indicator of GEP tumors

In endocrine neoplasms of pancreatic B cells the finding of an increase in the precursor proinsulin of >22% occurs in 85% or more of cases [64]. There have been few reports of the value of characterization of the molecular species of GEP hormones in GEP tumors.

7.1 *Gastrin* circulates as four main components in man [139]. Four corresponding forms have been isolated from extracts of antral mucosa and gastrinomas. The amino acid sequence of three molecular forms is known. Component I has a molecular size of 22 A Component II (big gastrin) corresponds to the tetratriacontapeptide amide, gastrin-34. Component III corresponds to the well-known heptadecapeptide amide, gastrin-17, and Component IV corresponds to the tetratriacontapeptide, gastrin-14, or 'minigastrin.' In addition to these forms, a fragment corresponding to the amino terminal tridecapeptide of gastrin-17 has been found in serum from Zollinger-Ellison syndrome patients, but this fragment has recently been demonstrated in the serum of normal subjects [139]. In addition there are paired sulfated and non sulfated variants.

A macromolecular form of gastrin, 'big, big gastrin,' may be found in some large tumors secreting gastrin. Several authors have suggested that a preponderance of G17 or its NH_2 terminal fragment is indicative of malignant disease [40]. Our studies suggest that a high NH_2-:COOH terminal ratio occurs only in metastatic disease, but this needs verification.

7.2 *Large glucagon*, or proglucagon may be found in certain GEP tumors [37, 175, 181] but this is by no means a universal finding and cannot be relied upon for diagnosis or management.

Investigations of the heterogeneity of other gut hormones are still sparse. At least two different molecular forms of gastrointestinal substance-P, somatostatin, neurotensin, and VIP have been described [6, 31, 122], but not so far related to tumor production of the peptide.

The fact that endocrine cells of the gut release several, not a single, molecular form of hormone may be of pathogenetic significance if forms of relatively low biological activity are released in abnormally large amounts. Certainly in patients with MEN syndrome, hormone levels may be very high without apparent biologic activity, which may relate to molecular heterogeneity.

In a report by Weir, five patients with glucagonomas had elevated plasma levels of total glucagon immunoreactivity [181]. Gell filtrations of plasma from samples from these patients showed that the majority of immunoreactivity eluted in the 3,500 and a larger 9,000 Dalton fraction. Thus, with conversion to a neoplastic state, the A cell of glucagonomas, much like the B cell of insulinomas may secrete an increased amount of a larger, 9,000 Dalton glucagon species which may be a pro-hormone. In another study by VonSchenck a classic case of the glucagonoma syndrome was described [186] in which gel filtration of the plasma demonstrated 60% pancreatic glucagon and 30% 'proglucagon.'

7.3 *Somatostatin*. Larsson studied a patient with a pancreatic somatostatinoma [95]. Gel chromotography of serum revealed one minor and three major fractions all of which were biologically active.

8. GEP tumors in the future

There are no data available that illustrate possible changes in the frequency of GEP tumors over the years. The fact that the majority of the cases have been reported during the last 20 years probably does not indicate an increasing frequency but rather an increased awareness of tumor-associated syndromes and, above all, the availability of radioimmunoassay techniques for the detection of tumor markers. This, in turn, means that the list of syndromes in undoubtedly incomplete. Since the secretory products of the majority of gut endocrine cells remains unknown, the possible biological consequences of overproduction cannot be entertained. The clinician who is confronted with the problem of whether a

Table 8. Indications for hormone assays

	Condition	Assays
1.	Peptic ulcer disease	gastrin
2.	Diarrhea – secretory in nature	gastrin
		VIP
		PP
		SRIF
		Calcitonin (and motilin)
		Serotonin
		PGE_2
3.	Hypoglycemia	Insulin
4.	Flushing, hypotension, wheezing and diarrhea	Serotonin (or metabolites)
		VIP
		PGE_2
		Substance P (neurotensin) (motilin)
5.	Pancreatic tumors or masses	Gastrin
		VIP
		Somatotatin
		Insulin
		Growth hormone
		ACTH
6.	Extra pancreatic tumors, small bowel, lung, kidney	Enteroglucagon
		PP
		Motilin
		Somatostatin
7.	Dermatosis – protracted and unexplained	Glucagon
8.	Diabetes – especially without a family history, presence of a skin rash, diarrhea or flushing and wheezing	Glucagon
		SRIF
		PP
		VIP
9.	Hypercalcemia – unexplained	VIP
10.	Constipation – intractable	Motilin
		Enkephalin
		Endorphin
11.	Multile endocrine neoplasia	PP
		Gastrin
		Prolactin
		PTH and Ca^{2+}

gut endocrine tumor can account for a constellation of symptoms in a particular patient may consult the incomplete list of symptoms caused by overproduction of the various gut peptides we have outlined. Alternatively an awareness of the physiologic effects of these peptides, which by excessive secretion (Table 8), may cause the symptoms may suggest a possible GEP tumor. Thus, these lists will constantly change as the number of cell types characterized by specific peptide production increases. It is only by a high index of suspicion and constant vigilance that these rare and unusual tumors, often readily treatable, will be uncovered.

9. Localization of hormonally active gastrointestinal tumors

9.1 *The need for localization.* Accurate preoperative localization of islet cell tumors is necessary to ensure the appropriate surgical treatment. Percutaneous transhepatic portal venous sampling to localize sites of hormone over-production has proved valuable for many endocrine tumors, but application of this technique to gastroentero-pancreatic (GEP) tumors is complicated by several unique problems which may be misleading.

Tumors may be mixed and produce more than one humoral agent [19, 56, 59, 75, 85, 96, 126, 144, 176–179]. In patients with multiple endocrine neoplasia (MEN), the tumors are usually multiple, although diffuse islet cell adenomatosis, hyperplasia or nesidioblastosis may be present and produce clinical syndromes [60, 69, 94].

9.2 *The normal distribution of GEP hormones.* The various hormone-secreting cells are not evenly distributed within the pancreas. Large numbers of cells producing one hormone may be found in some areas but not in others [47, 94, 129]. Thus, the peak venous concentrations of different pancreatic hormones will vary greatly depending on the location of the cells of origin. A thorough knowledge of the normal distribution of endocrinologically active cells within the pancreas and gut as well as familiarity with anomalous venous drainage of the pancreas and proximal gut is required if hormone measurements of portal venous samples in man are to be interpreted correctly.

Furthermore, venous tributaries draining tumors particularly in the body and tail of the pancreas may take a circuitous course and drain into large veins far removed from the primary neoplasm. Also, the gastroepiploic vein which receives blood from the distal pancreatic bed terminates in the superior mesenteric or portal vein, and may lead to erroneous localization of tumors in the tail or neck of the pancreas. It should also be made clear at the onset that transhepatic venous sampling requires considerable experience, is time-consuming, and expensive and should not be embarked upon without clinical and confirmatory biochemical evidence that increased hormone secretion is the cause of the patient's symptoms. The hormone assays employed must be reliable and reproducible. Simple, less invasive techniques of tumor localization should be used first.

The identification of the normal venous distribution of gut/pancreatic hormones has been studied in patients with single hormone-producing tumors by measuring the distribution or other gut hormones which are not being secreted in excess. The hormone concentrations and portal vein/systemic arterial gradients of gastrin, glucagon, hPP, somatostatin, VIP and motilin in five patients with isolated single insulinomas are summarized in Table 9. Levels of insulin, glucagon, hPP, somatostatin, VIP and motilin in five patients with the gastrinoma syndrome are shown in Table 10.

9.3 *Hypergastrinemia.* The highest PV concentration and PV/SA gradient of gastrin were found in the gastrocolic trunk, which is compatible with its origin from the gastric antrum.

A gastrin concentration of more than 300 pg/ml, a gradient of more than 200 pg/ml, and a PV/SA ratio higher than 3 between the gastrocolic trunk and the peripheral circulation suggests a gastrin-producing tumor or G cell hyperfunction. In the remainder of the portal venous system, gastrin concentrations of more than 150 pg/ml and PV/SA gradients in excess of more than 50 pg/ml are highly suggestive of a tumor. A positive hepatic vein/portal vein gradient, i.e. a value higher in the hepatic vein, suggests hepatic metastases and may preclude surgical extirpation of the tumor. In the absence of gradients elsewhere, an elevated gastrin concentration in an hepatic vein may indicate an intrahepatic gastrinoma.

Table 9. Hormone concentrations and A-V gradients in patients with organic hyperinsulinism

	Gastrin (pg/ml)	Gluagon (pg/ml)	hPP (pg/ml)	SRIF (pg/ml)	VIP (pg/ml)	Motilin (pg/ml)	SP (pg/ml)
Splenic vein	82	130	124	108	55	76	3.5
V-A	4	47	− 1	2	− 3.2	2.7	0.7
Superior mesenteric vein	83	114	96	186	59	93	3.2
V-A	− 1	25	− 6	57	5	21	− 1.2
Portal vein	85	123	164	126	58	81	3.2
V-A	5	38	49	2.4	1.6	11	0.4
Gastrocolic trunk	6	131	144	178	59	84	3.3
V-A	46	60	34	55	2.0	0.5	0
Celiac artery	90	94	95	125	58	79	3.5
Peripheral vein	76	84	114	126	56	–	–
Portal/systemic gradients	6%	31%	30%	2%	3%	14%	12%

V-A gradient = gradient measured between the vein indicated and the celiac artery.
* Portal vein gradient divided by mean portal vein concentration.

Table 10. Hormone concentrations and A-V gradients in patients with the gastrinoma syndrome

	Insulin (μU/ml)	Glucagon (pg/ml)	hPP (pg/ml)	SRIF (pg/ml)	Motilin (pg/ml)
Splenic vein	156	565	2100	126	253
V-A	112	356	1020	12	− 11
Superior mesenteric vein	70	186	1070	136	382
V-A	27	19	92	26	20
Portal vein	113	211	1640	134	366
V-A	66	60	543	23	81
Gastrocolic trunk	89	257	2640	95	258
V-A	48	− 19	1640	4.2	− 5.5
Celiac artery	41	185	1030	117	295
Hepatic vein	86	249	1610	102	347
Portal/systemic gradient*	58%	28%	33%	17%	22%

V-A = gradient measured between the vein indicated and the celiac artery.
* Portal vein gradient divided by mean portal vein concentration.

9.4 *Clinical details of patients with hypergastrinemia.* The clinical details of 15 patients with hypergastrinemia are summarized in Table 11 and the results of the venous sampling studies and operation in Table 12. Of the 15 patients, nine had MEN I, four had isolated gastrinomas, one had G cell hyperfunction and one had hepatic metastases from an unidentified primary. It would seem that localization of gastrin-secreting tumors in the patient with MEN I sydrome is of no real value since the tumors are invariably multiple and surgery is usually not curative. However, nearly 20% of patients with MEN I may have solitary gastrinomas and venous sampling may prove to be of value in these cases. At present it would seem that the major indication for venous sampling in patients with MEN with hyper-gastrinemia would be to confirm that angiographically identified single tumors are indeed solitary and thus amenable to resection.

In contrast to the patients with MEN I, a single high gastrin value is compatible with a single benign gastrinoma (Fig. 5). Single tumors were found. After excision of the tumors, basal gastrin, acid secretion, and the gastrin response to secretin returned to normal. Patient PD represents a unique case. He had symptoms for seven years and had previously undergone a Finney pyloroplasty and finally a total gastrectomy. Gastrins remained elevated and CAT, ultrasound and angiography were negative. Venous sampling revealed a raised gastrin in the right hepatic vein and a single 2.5 × 2.5 cm gastrinoma was buried deep with the right anterior portion of the liver.

Although not essential to the diagnosis, transhepatic venous sampling was performed in patient PG in whom the diagnosis of G cell hyperfunction was made (Fig. 5). The highest concentration of gastrin (810 pg/ml) was found in the

Table 11. Clinical details of 15 patients with hypergastrinemia

Patient	Age (yrs)	Sex	Duration of symptoms (years)	Basal gastrin (pg/ml)	Maximum response to secretin (pg/ml)	Findings
BE*	41	M	7	84	189	Pancreatic, duodenal tumors
FW*	53	M	0.25	150	101	Adenocarcinoma of pancreas; Islet cell adenomatosis
LS*	49	F	7	503	554	2 adenomas in tail of panc
PG+	23	M	5	336	122	Increased rugal folds with gastritis
JH*	59	F	2	1663	1083	Multiple pancr adenomas
PA**	49	F	6	810	2060	Adenoma in head of pancreas
PN*	55	F	0	520	1650	2 duodenal adenomas
SH*	33	F	3	20,000	105,000	Adenoma in proximal jejunal mesent
ST	55	M	2	561	1405	Hepatic met; no primary found
BH*	28	F	–	232	328	Microadenomatosis; 2 pancreatic adenomas
FL*	57	M	0.3	800	950	Single gastrin secreting adenoma head; multiple neoplasms secreting body & tail
CF**	10	M	1.5	434	1096	Adenoma in head of pancreas
WG*	62	M	11	83	176	Tumor in lymph node
HG*	63	F	1	55	106	7 pancreatic tumors
PD**	25	M	7	179	2334	Intrahepatic gastrinoma

* = MEN I syndrome; ** = isolated sporadic gastrinoma; + = G cell hyperfunction.

gastroepiploic vein, suggesting an antral origin. After antrectomy and truncal vagotomy, gastrin levels and acid secretion returned to normal, and a normal response to secretin was observed. Patient FW underwent venous sampling after hypergastrinemia and an abnormal response to secretin were noted. Elevated levels of gastrin in the hepatic veins suggested hepatic metatases. Hepatic angiography and abdominal CT failed to demonstrate metastases. At operation, several 0.5 to 1.0 cm metastatic nodules were present in both lobes of the liver.

Table 12. Clinical details of 15 patients with hypergastrinemia

Patient	Tumor site	Tumor size (cm)	Max IG (pg/ml)	Simultaneous arterial (pg/ml)	P-A gradient (pg/ml)	Site of max IG
BE	Head of pancreas	0.8	143	71	72	PSPD vein
	Duodenal wall	0.4				
FW	Head of pancreas	0.5	199	125	74	IPD vein
LS	Head of pancreas	–	1107	783	424	veins draining head of panc
PG	G cell hyperfunction	–	810	253	557	GE vein
JH	Multiple	–	1452	1404	48	Panc magna
PA	Head of pancreas	2.5	5380	2020	3360	Proximal SMV
PN	2 tumors in	0.25	945	333	612	Distal gastro-
	duodenal wall	0.25	543	353	190	colic trunk; proximal SMV
ST	Hepatic metastases	–	880	1063	– 183	Hepatic vein
	No primary found					
SH	Jejunal mesentery	15	25,850	20,000	5850	Mid PV
BH	Tail of pancreas	1.5	328	203	125	Mid PV
FL	Head of pancreas	2.5				High portal & SMV
CF	Head of pancreas	1.5	2198	774	1424	Low PV
WG	Lymph node	2	670	444	226	proximal splenic
HG	Multiple tumors	variable	400	48	352	Splenic PV Junction
PD	Intrahepatic	2.5×2.5	878	252	626	R hepatic vein

PSPD = posterior superior pancreatico-duodenal; IPD = inferior pancreatico-duodenal; GE = gastroenpiploic; SMV - superior mesenteric vein; PV = portal vein.

9.5 *Angiography, CAT, ultrasound.* For many years visceral angiographic studies have been the most sensitive means for localizing islet cell adenomas with success rates ranging widely among reported series [2, 78, 105, 140, 141, 156, 169]. Of the 55 cases of islet tumors we have studied by the percutaneous transhepatic route, we have been able to identify only two by CT (1%). Ultrasound has not been helpful in our experience. It must be pointed out that the cross-section of cases we see includes mainly patients referred because of failure to localize tumors at other institutions. The overall success using angiography has been reported to be 30 to 80% and should precede portal venous sampling.

Once the diagnosis of GEP tumors has been established, an experienced surgeon should be able to determine the site of the lesion at operation and perform the appropriate surgical procedure. However, to be forewarned of the site of such a lesion gives some degree of comfort, and is particularly useful for tumors in the head, neck and uncinate process of the pancreas. In many circumstances these tumors are not visualized by angiography, CT or ultrasonography, and may not be palpable at the time of operation. Venous localization has made it

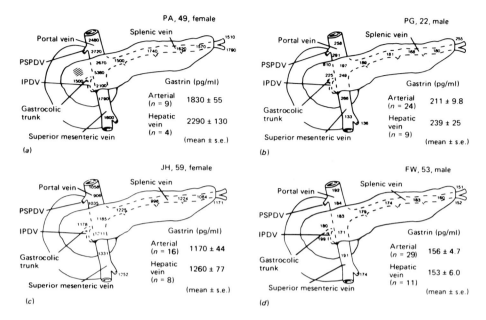

Figure 5. Patterns of gastrin concentrations in portal venous system in different conditions. (a) A solitary sporadic gastrinoma of the head of the pancreas. (b) G cell hyperfunction and high gastrin values in the gastrocolic trunk which drains the antrum. (c) This patient had two angiographically demonstrable tumors in the body of the pancreas, but diffuse hypergastrinemia compatible with diffuse disease in MEN. (d) A patient wth MEN and multiple hormone-secreting tumors and diffusely aised gastrin levels. PSPDV = posterior superior pancreatico-duodenal vein; IPDV = inferior-pancreatico-duodenal vein.

possible in these cases to identify tumors in the head, neck and uncinate process of the pancreas. This has allowed removal of the tumor with sparing of sufficient parenchyma to avoid insulin-dependent diabetes and exocrine insufficiency. The preoperative determination of islet cell hyperplasia, multiple adenomas, or nesi-dioblastosis clearly dictates a different approach from that for the single islet cell tumor. Transhepatic portal venous sampling and hormone measurement plays an important role in the localization of symptomatic islet cell tumors which are not detectable by conventional diagnostic studies. This technique also identifies patients with islet cell hyperfunction but no specific tumor and may be useful in patients in whom angiography has either falsely localized a lesion or demonstrated only one of several tumors.

References

1. Adrian TE, Greenberg GR, Bloom SR: Actions of pancreatic polypeptide in man. In: Gut Hormones, Second Edition, Bloom, SR, Polak, JM (eds). New York: Churchill Livingstone, 1981.

338

2. Alfidi RJ, Bhyun DS, Crile G, Hawk W: Arteriography and hypoglycemia. Surg Gynec Obstet 133: 477–482, 1971.

3. Amiranaff B, Laburthe M, Rosselin G: Characterization of specific binding sites for vasoactive intestinal peptide in rat intestinal epithelial cell membrane, Biochem Biophys Acta 627: 215, 1980.

4. Andrew A: An experimental investigation into the possible neural crest origin of pancreatic APUD (islet) cells. J Embryol Exp Morphol 35: 577–593, 1976.

5. Andrew A, Kramer B, Rawdon BB: Gut and pancreatic amine precursor uptake and decarboxylation cells are not neural crest derivatives. Gastroenterology 84(2): 429–431, 1983.

6. Arimura A, Sato H, Dupont H, Nishi N, Schally AV: Somatostatin: abundance of immunoreactivity in rat stomach and pancreas. Science 198: 1007–1009, 1975.

7. Awrich AE, Peetrz M, Fletcher WS: Dimethyltriazenoimidazole carboxamide therapy of islet cell carcinoma of the pancreas. J Surg Oncol 17: 321–326, 1981.

8. Barbezat GO, Grossman M: Intestinal secretion: Stimulation by peptides. Science. 174: 422, 1971.

9. Barraclough MA, Bloom SR: Vipoma of the pancreas: Observations on the diarrhea and circulatory disturbances. Arch Intern Med 139: 467–471, 1979.

10. Binder HJ, Lemp GF, Gardner JD: Receptors for vasoactive intestinal peptide and secreton on small intestinal epithelial cells. Am J Physiol, GI- Liver Physiol I: G190, 1980.

11. Binnick AN, Spencer SK, Dennison WL Jr, et al.: Glucagonoma syndrome. Arch Dermatol 113: 749–754, 1977.

12. Bisette G, Manberg P, Nemeroff CB, Prange AJ Jr: Neurotensin, a biologically active peptide. Life Sci 23: 2173, 1978.

13. Blair AW, Ahmed S: Presacral vipoma in a 16-month old child. Acta Paediatr Belg 34: 89–91, 1981.

14. Bloom SR, Polak JM: VIP measurement in distinguishing Verner-Morrison syndrome and pseudo-Verner-Morrison syndrome. Clin Endocrin (suppl) 5: 223s, 1976.

15. Bloom SR, Polak JM: In: 'Progress in Gastroenterology,' Glass BJ (ed). New York: Grune and Stratton, 1977, pp 109–151.

16. Bloom SR, Polak JM: Glucagonomas, VIPomas and somatostatinomas. Clin Endocrinology and Metabolism 9(2): 285–297, 1980.

17. Bloom SR, Polak JM: Hormone profiles. In: Gut Hormones, Bloom SR, Polak JM (eds). New York: Churchill Livingstone, 1981.

18. Bloom SR, Polak JM: Vipomas. In: Vasoactive Intestinal Peptides, Said SI (ed). New York: Raven Press, 1982.

19. Bloom SR, Polak JM, Pearse AGE: Vasoactive intestinal polypeptide and watery diarrhea syndrome. Lancet 2: 14–16, 1973.

20. Bloom SR, Mitchell SJ: Experimental evidence for VIP as the cause of the watery diarrhea syndrome. Gastroenterology 75: 101, 1978.

21. Bock KW, Dissing J: Demonstration of enolase activity connected to the brain specific protein. Scand J Immunol 4: 31, 1975.

22. Boden G, Owen OE: Familial hyperglucagonemia-An autosomal doninant disorder. N Engl J Med 196(10): 534–538, 1977.

23. Boden G, Owen OE, Rezvani I, et al.: An islet cell carcinoma containing glucagon and insulin. Chronic glucagon excess and glucose homeostatis. Diabetes 26(2): 128–137, 1977.

24. Bordi C, Ravazzola M, Baetens D, et al.: A study of glucagonomas by light and electron microscopy and immunofluorescence. Diabetes 28: 925–936, 1979.

25. Bordi C, Rogni R, BVaetens D, et al.: Human islet cell tumor storing pancreatic polypeptide: A light and electron microscopic study. J Cli Endocrinol Metab 46: 215–19, 1977.

26. Botha JL, Vinik AI, Child PT Jackson WPU: Inhibition of exaggerated gastrointestinal glucagon responses in chronic pancreatitis by somatostatin. J Clin Endocrinol Metabol 45: 1265–1270, 1977.

27. Botha JL, Vinik AI, Child PT: Gastric inhibitory polypeptide in acquired pancreatic diabetes: effects of insulin treatment. J Clin Endocrinol Mebabol 47: 543–549, 1978.

28. Braunstein GD, Vaitukaitis JL, Carbone PP, Ross GT: Ectopic production of human chorionic gonadotropin by neoplasms. Ann Int Med 78: 39–45, 1973.

29. Broor SL, Soergel KH, Garancis JC, et al.: Hormone producing pancreatic islet cell carcinoma: changing clinical presentation. Am J Med Sci 278(3): 229–233, 1979.

30. Burcharth F, Stage JG, Stadil F, Jensen LI, Fischermann K: Localization of gastrinomas by transhepatic portal catheterization and gastrin assay. Gastroenterology 77: 444–450, 1979.

31. Carraway R, Leeman SE: Characterization of radioimmunoassayable neurotensin in the rat. Its differential distribution in the central nervous system, small intestine and stomach. J Biol Chem 251: 7045–7052, 1976.

32. Carson DJ, Glasgow JFT, Ardill J: Watery diarrhea and elevated vasoactive intestinal polypeptide associated with a massive neurofibroma in early childhood. J Royal Soc Med 73: 69–72, 1980.

33. Chance RE, Moon NE, Johnson MG: Human pancreatic polypeptide (HPP) and bovine pancreatic polypeptide (BPP). In: Methods of Hormone Radioimmunoassay, Jaffe BM, Behrman HR (eds). New York: Academic Press, 1978.

34. Conlon JM: The glucagon-like polypeptides – order out of chaos? Diabetologia 18: 85–88, 1980.

35. Creutzfeldt W, Arnold R: Somatostatin and the stomach: Exocrine and andocrine aspects. Metabolism 27(9 Suppl 1): 1309, 1978.

36. Creutzfeldt W, Arnold R, Frerich H: Insulinomas and gastrinomas. In: Gut Hormones, Bloom, SR (ed). Edinburgh, New York: Churchill Livingstone, 1978.

37. Danforth DN Jr, Triche T, Doppman JL, et al.: Elevated plasma proglucagon-like component with a glucagon-secreting tumor. N Engl J Med 295–245, 1976.

38. DeLellis RA, Wolfe HJ: Contributions of immunohistochemistry to to clinical endocrinology and endocrine pathology. J Histochem Cytochem 31: 187, 1983.

39. deNutte N, Somers G, Gepts W, et al.: Pancreatic hormone release in tumor-associated hypersomatostinemia. Diabetologia 14: 227, 1978.

40. Dockray GJ, Walsh JF: Amino terminal gastrin fragment in serum of Zollinger-Ellison syndrome patients. Gastroenterology 68: 222–230, 1975.

41. Doyle JA, Schroeter AL, Rogers RS: Hyperglucagonaemia and necrolytic migratory erythema in cirrhosis – possible pseudoglucagonoma syndrome. Brit J Dermatology 100: 581–587, 1979.

42. Drew SI, Joffee B, Vinik AI, Seftel H, Singer F: The first 24 hours of acute pancreatitis: changes in biochemical and endocrine homeostasis in patients with pancreatitis compared with those in control subjects undergoing stress for reasons other than pancreatitis. Am J Med 64: 795–803, 1978.

43. Drew SI, Joffee BI, Vinik AI, Seftel H, Singer F: First 24 hours of acute pancreatitis. Am J Gastroenterol 79(1): 66–72, 1978.

44. Dunn E, Stein S: Percutaneous transhepatic pancreatic vein catheterization in localization of insulinomas. Arch Surg 116: 232–233, 1981.

45. Ebeid AM, Murray PD, Fisher JE: Vasoactive intestinal peptide and the watery diarrhea syndrome. Ann Surg 187: 411, 1978.

46. Ebeid AM, Dragon R, Brand D, et al.: Clinical and pathological considerations in apudomas (in press).

47. Erlandsen SL, Hegre OD, Parsons JA, McEroy RC, Elde RP: Pancreatic islet cell hormones: Distribution of cell types in the islet and the evidence for the presence of somatostatin and gastrin within the D cell. J Histochem Cytochem 24: 883–897, 1976.

48. Facer P, Polak JM, Maangos PJ, et al.: Immunocytochemical localization of neurone specific enolase (NSE) in the gastrointestinal tract. Proc Ray Microscop 15: 133, 1980.

49. Faurel JP, Bernard P, Saigot Th, et al.: A case of VIP and somatostatin-secreting phaeochromocytoma. Nouv Presse Med 11: 1483–1485, 1982.

50. Fennelly JJ, Cantwell B, Fielding J, et al.: Metastatic pancreatic vipoma: A case report of clinical response following treatment with corticosteroids and actinomycin D. Clin Onc 8: 167–170, 1982.

51. Floyd JC, Vinik AI: Pancreatic polypeptide. In: Gut Hormones, Bloom SR, Polak JM (eds), 2nd ed. New York: Churchill Livingstone, 195–205, 1981.

52. Friesen SR, Stephens RL, Huard GS II: Effective streptozotocin therapy for metastatic pancreatic polypeptide apudoma. Arch Surg 116: 1090–1092, 1981.

53. Freisen SR: Pancreatic polypeptide in the detection of the MEA I syndrome: Islet apudomas and hyperplasias. In: Endocrine Surgery Update, Thompson NW, Vinik AI (eds). New York: Grune and Stratton, 1983.

54. Gaginella TS, O'Dorisio TM: Vasoactive intestinal polypeptide. In: Neuromodulators of Intestinal Secretion on Mechanisms of Intestinal Secretion, Binder HJ (ed). New York: Alan R. Liss, Inc., 1979.

55. Gaginella TS, O'Dorisio TM. Effects of vasoactive intestinal peptide on intestinal chloride secretion. In: Vasoactive Intestinal Peptides, Said (SI (ed). New York: Raven Press, 1982.

56. Gahniche JP, Conlin R, Dubois PM, Chayvialle JA, Descos F, Paulin C, Geffory Y: Calcitonin secretion by a pancreatic somatostatinoma. N Eng J Med 299: 1252, 1978.

57. Galmiche JP, Chayvialle JA, Dubois PM, et al.: Calcitonin-producing pancreatic somato-statinoma. Gastroenterology 78: 1577–1583, 1980.

58. Ganda OP, Soeldner JS: 'Somatostatinoma': Follow-up studies. N Engl J Med 297(24): 1352–1353, 1977.

59. Ganda OP, Weir GC, Soeldner JS, et al.: 'Somatostatinoma': A somatostatin-containing tumor of the endocrine pancreas. N Engl J Med 296(17): 963–967, 1977.

60. Glaser B, Valtysson G, Fajans SS, Vinik AI, Cho K, Thompson N: Gastrointestinal/pancreatic hormone concentration in the portal venous system of nine patients with organic hyperinsuli-nism. Metabolism 30(10): 1001–1010, 1981.

61. Glaser B, Vinik AI, Sive AA, Floyd JC Jr: Plasma human pancreatic polypeptide responses to administered secretin (effects of surgical vagotomy, cholinergic blockade and chronic pan-creatitis). J Clin Endocrinol Metabol 50(6): 1094–1099, 1980.

62. Gleeson MH, Bloom SR, Polak JM, Henry K, Dowling RH: Endocrine tumor in kidney affecting small bowel structure, motility, and absorptive function. Gut 12: 773, 1971.

63. Go VLW, Korinek JK: Effect of vasoactive intestinal polypeptide on hepatic glucose release. In: Vasoactive Intestinal Peptide, Said SI (ed). New York: Raven Press, 1982.

64. Gorden P, Sherman B, Roth J: Proinsulin-like component of circulating insulin in the basal state and in patients and hamsters with islet-cell tumors. J Clin Invest 50: 2113–2120, 1971.

65. Gray RK, Rosch J, Grollman JH: Arteriography in the diagnosis of islet cell tumors. Radiology 97: 39–44, 1970.

66. Granuci P, Mahler RJ: Streptozotocin treatment of a juvenile onset type diabetic patient with Verner-Morrison syndrome and multi hormonal probable malignant islet cell carcinoma with liver metastases. Horm Metabol Res 14: 327–328, 1982.

67. Grimelius L, Wilander E: Silver stains in the study of endocrine cells of the gut and pancreas. Invest Cell Pathol 3: 3, 1980.

68. Hamilton I, Reis L, Bilimoria S, Lang RG: A renal vipoma. Br Med J 281: 1323–1324, 1980.

69. Hayashi M, Floyd JC Jr, Pek S, Fajans SS: Insulin, proinsulin, glucagon and gastrin in pancreatic tumors and in plasma of patients with organic hyperinsulinism. J Clin Endocrin Metab 44: 681–694, 1977.

70. Heitz PU, Kasper M, Polak JM, Kloppel G: Pancreatic endocrine tumors: Immunocytochemi-cal analysis of 125 tumors. Human Pathol 13: 263–271, 1982.

71. Higgins GA, Recant L, Fischman AB: The glucagonoma syndrome: Surgical curable diabetes. Am J Surg 137: 142–148, 1979.

72. Hoitsma HFW, Cuesta MA, Starink ThM, et al.: Zinc deficiency syndrome versus

glucagonoma syndrome. Arch Chir Neerlandicum 13(3): 131–139, 1979.

73. Holst JJ: Physiology of enteric glucagon-like substances. In: Gut Hormones, Bloom SR (ed). Edinburgh: Churchill Livingstone, 1978.

74. Holst JJ: Possible entries to the diagnosis of a glucagon-producing tumour. Scand J Gastroent Suppl 53: 53–56, 1979.

75. Holst JJ, Hellend S, Ingemannson S, Bang Petersen N, Von Schenck H: Functional studies in patients with glucagonoma syndrome. Diabetologic 17: 151–156, 1979.

76. Hsu SM, Raine H, Fanger J: A comparative study of the peroxidase-antiperoxidase method and the avidin-biotin complex method for studying polypeptide hormones with radioimmunoassay antibodies. J Histochem Cytochem 29: 77, 1981.

77. Iida Y, Nose O, Kai H, et al.: Watery diarrhoea with a vasoactive intestinal peptide-producing ganglioneuroblastoma. Arch Dis Child 55: 929–936, 1980.

78. Ingemansson S, Holst J, Larsson L-I, et al.: Localization of glucagonomas by catheterization of the pancreatic veins and with glucagon assay. Surg Gynecol Obstet 145: 509–516, 1977.

79. Jones RA, Dawson IMP: Morphology and staining pattern of endocrine cell tumors in the gut, pancreas and bronchus and their possible significance. Histopathology 1: 137–150, 1977.

80. Kane MG, O'Dorisio TM, Krejs GJ: Intravenous VIP infusion causes secretory diarrhea in man. Gastroenterology 84: 1202 (A), 1983.

81. Kahn CR, Rosen SW, Weintraub BD, Fajans SS, Gorden P: Ectopic production of chorionic gonadotropin and its subunits by islet cell tumours; a specific marker for malignancy. N Engl J Med 297: 565–569, 1977.

82. Kaplan SJ, Holbrook CT, McDaniel HG, et al.: Vasoactive intestinal peptide secreting tumors of childhood. Am J Dis Child 134: 21–24, 1980.

83. Khandekar JD, Oyer D, Miller HJ, et al.: Neurologic involvement in glucagonoma syndrome. Response to combination chemotherapy with 5-flurouracil and streptozotocin. Cancer: 44: 2014–2016, 1979.

84. Kimmel JR, Hayden LJ, Pollock HG: Isolation and characterization of a new pancreatic polypeptide hormone. J Biol Chem 250: 9369, 1975.

85. Kovacs K, Horvath E, Ezrin C. Immunoreactive somatostatin in pancreati islet-cell carcinoma accompanied by ectopic ACTH syndrome. Lancet 25: 1365–1366, 1977.

86. Kraft AR, Tompkins RK, Zollinger R: Recognition and management of the diarrheal syndrome caused by non-beta cell tumors of the pancreas. Am J Surg 119: 163, 1970.

87. Krejs GJ, Barkey RM, Read NW, Fordtran JS: Intestinal secretion induced by vasoactive intestinal polypeptide. J Clin Invest 61: 1337, 1978.

88. Krejs GJ, Fordtran JS, Fischer JE, et al.: Effect of CIP infusion on water and ion transport in the human jejunum. Gastroenterology 78: 722–727, 1980.

89. Krejs GJ, Orci L, Conlon JM, et al.: Somatostatinoma syndrome. Biochemical, morphologic and clinical features. N Engl J Med 30: 285–292, 1979.

90. Kudo K, Kitajima S, Munakata H, et al.: WDHA syndrome caused by VIP-producing ganglioneuroblastoma. J Ped Surg 17: 426–428, 1982.

91. Larsson LI: Two distinct types of islet abnormalities associated with endocrine pancreatic tumors. Virchows Arch (Pathol Anat) 376: 209–219, 1977.

92. Larsson LI: Pathology of gastrointestinal endocrine cells. Scand J Gastroent 14(Suppl 53): 1–8, 1979.

93. Larsson LI: Gastrointestinal cells producing endocrine, neurocrine and paracrine messengers. Clin Gastroent 9: 485–615, 1980.

94. Larsson LI, Grimelius L, Hakanson R, et al.: Mixed endocrine pancreatic tumors producing several peptide hormones. Am J Pathol 79: 271–284, 1975.

95. Larsson LI, Holst JJ, Kuhl C, et al.: Pancreatic somatostatinoma. Clinical features and physiological implications. Lancet 26: 666–668, 1977.

96. Larsson LI, Schwartz T, Lundqvist G, et al.: Pancreatic polypeptide in pancreatic endocrine

tumors, possible implication in watery diarrhea syndrome. Am J Path 85: 675–682, 1979.

97. LeDouarin N: The migration of neural crest to the wall of the digestive tract in avian embryo. J Embryol Exp Morphol 30(1): 31, 1973.

98. Leichter SB: Clinical and metabolic aspects of glucagonoma. Medicine 59(2): 100–113, 1980.

99. Levitt NS, Vinik AI, Child PT: Glucose-dependent insulin-releasing peptide in noninsulin-dependent maturity-onset diabetes: effects of autonomic neuropathy. J Clin Endocrinol Metab 51(2): 254–258, 1980.

100. Levitt NS, Vinik AI, Sive AA, Van Tonder S, Lund A: Impaired pancreatic polypeptide responses to insulin-induced hypoglycemia in diabetic autonomic neuropathy. J Clin Endocrinol Metabol 50(3): 445–449, 1980.

101. Lin TM: Actions of gastrointestinal hormones and related peptides on the motor function of the biliary tract. Gastroenterology 69: 1006, 1975.

102. Lin TM, Evans DC, Chance RE, Spray GF: Bovine pancreatic polypeptide action on gastric and pancreatic secretion in dogs. Am J Physiol 232: E311, 1977.

103. Lloyd RV, Fruhman J: Comparison of peroxidase-antiperoxidase and avidin-biotin methods with radioimmunoassay antibodies. Am J Clin Pathol 86: 795, 1982.

104. Long RG, Byrant MG, Mitchell SJ, et al.: Clinicopathological study of pancreatic and ganglioneuroblastoma tumours secreting vasoactive intestinal polypeptide (vipomas). Br Med J 282: 1767–1771, 1981.

105. Lunderqvist A, Tylen U: Phlebography of the pancreatic veins. Radiologie 15: 198–202, 1975.

106. Machina T, Marcus R, Levin SR: Inhibition of glucagon secretion by diphenylhydantoin in a patient with glucagonoma. West J Med 132(4): 357–360, 1980.

107. Mallinson CN, Bloom SR, Warin AP, et al.: A glucagonoma syndrome. Lancet 6: 1–5, 1974.

108. Marks IN, Bank S, Louw JH: Islet cell tumor of the pancreas with reversible watery diarrhea and achlorhydria. Gastroenterology 52: 695–708, 1967.

109. Marynick SP, Fagadau WR, Duncan LA: Malignant glucagonoma syndrome: Response to chemotherapy. Ann Int Med 93(3): 453–454, 1980.

110. Matsumoto KD, Peter JB, Schultze RG, Hakin AA, Frank PT: Watery diarrhea and hypokalemia associated with pancreatic islet cell adenoma. Gastroenterology 52: 695, 1967.

111. McGavran MH, Unger RH, Recant L, et al.: A glucagon-secreting alpha-cell carcinoma of the pancreas. N Engl J Med 274: 1408–1413, 1966.

112. Modlin IM, Bloom SR: VIPomas and the watery diarrhoea syndrome. S Afr Med J 54: 53–56, 1978.

113. Modlin IM, Bloom SR, Mitchell JJ: Plasma vasoactive intestinal polypeptide (VIP) levels and intestinal ischemia. Experientia 34: 535, 1978.

114. Modlin IM, Mitchell ST, Bloom SR: The systemic release and pharmacokinetics of VIP. In: Gut Hormones, Bloom SR (ed). Edinburgh, New York: Churchill Livingstone, 1978.

115. Montenegro F, Lawrence GD, Macon W, et al.: Metastatic glucagonoma. Improvement after surgical debulking. Am J Surg 139: 424–427, 1980.

116. Moody AJ, Frandsen EK, Jacobsen H, Sundby F, Baetens D, Orci L: Heterogeneity of gut glucagon-like immunoreactivity (GLI). In: Glucagon. Its Role in Physiology and Clinical Medicine, Foa PP, Bajaj JS, Foa NL (eds). Amsterdam: Excerpta Medica, 1978.

117. Moody AJ, Sundby F, Jacobsen H, Lauritsen KB: The tissue distribution and plasma levels of glicentin (gut GLI-1). Scand J Gastroenterol 13(suppl 49): 127, 1978.

118. Moore BW: A soluble protein characteristic of the nervous system. Biochem Biophys Res Commun 19: 739–744, 1965.

119. Murray JS, Paton RR, Pope CE: Pancreatic tumor associated with flushing and diarrhea. Report of a case. N Engl J Med 264: 436, 1961.

120. Murray-Lyon IM, Cassar J, Coulson R, et al.: Further studies on streptozotocin therapy for a multiple-hormone producing islet cell carcinoma. Gut 12: 717–720, 1971.

121. Nakajima T, Watanabe S, Sato Y, Kameya T, Hirota T, Shimosato: An immunoperoxidase

study of S-100 protein distribution in normal and neoplastic tissues. Am J Surg Pathol 6: 715–727, 1982.

122. Nilsson G, Brodin E: Tissue distribution of substance-P-like immunoreactivity in dog, cat, rat and mouse. In: Substance P, van Euler US, Pernow B (eds). New York: Raven Press, 1977.

123. Norton JA, Kahn CR, Schiebinger R, et al.: Acid deficiency and the skin rash associated with glucagonoma. Ann Int Med 91: 213–215, 1979.

124. Oberg K, Boistrom H, Fahrenkrug J, et al.: Streptozotocin treatment of pancreatic tumour producing VIP and gastrin associated with Verner-Morrison syndrome. Actra Med Scand 206: 223–227, 1979.

125. Oberg K, Grimelius, Lundqvist, et al.: Update on pancreatic polypeptide as a specific marker for endocrine tumours of the pancreas and gut. Act Med Scand 210: 145–152, 1981.

126. Oberg K, Loof L, Bostrom H, Grimelius L, Fahrenkrug J, Lundquist G: A hypersecretion of calcitonin in patients with the Verner-Morrison syndrome. Scand J Gastroent 16: 135–144, 1981.

127. Oberg K, Wide L: hCG and hCG subunits as tumour markers in patients with endocrine pancreatic tumours and carcinoids. Acta Endocrinol 98: 256–260, 1981.

128. Ohneda A, Otsuki M, Fujiya H, et al.: A malignant insulinoma transformed into a glucagonoma syndrome. Diabetes 28: 962–969, 1979.

129. Orci L, Malaisse-Lagae F, Baeteus D, Panelent A: Pancreatic polypeptide-rich regions in human pancreas. Lancet 2: 1200–1201, 1978.

130. Panman E, Lowry PJ, Wass JAH, et al.: Molecular forms of somatstatin in normal subjects and in patients with pancreatic somatostatinoma. Clin Endocrinology 12: 611–620, 1980.

131. Parks D, Gingerich R, Jaffe BM, Akande B: Role of pancreatic polypeptide in canine gastric acid secretion. Am J Physiol 236(4): E488, 1979.

132. Pearse AGE: The cytochemistry and ultra-structure of polypeptide hormone producing cells of APUD series and embryologic, physiologic and pathologic implications of the concept. J Histochem Cytochem 17: 303–313, 1969.

133. Pearse AGE, Takor T: Neuroendocrine embryology and the APUD concept. Clin Endocrinol (suppl) 5: 229S, 1976.

134. Pictct RL, Rall LB, Phelps P, Rutter WJ: The neural crest and the origin of the insulin-producing and other gastrointestinal hormone-producing cells. Science 191: 191, 1976.

135. Pipeleers D, Somers G, Gepts W, et al.: Plasma pancreatic hormone levels in a case of somato-statinoma: Diagnostic and therapeutic implications. J Clin Endocrinol Metab 49(4): 572–579, 1979.

136. Polak JM, Adrian TE, Bryant MG, et al.: Pancreatic polypeptide in insulinomas, gastrinomas, vipomas, and glucagonomas. Lancet 14: 328–330, 1976.

137. Priest WM, Alexander MK: Islet-cell tumor of the pancreas with peptic ulceration, diarrhea, and hypokalemia. Lancet 2: 1145, 1957.

138. Rambaud JD, Modiglioni R, Matuchansky C, Bloom S, Said SI, Pessayre D, Bernier JJ: Pancreatic cholera. Gastroenterology 69: 110, 1975.

139. Rehfeld JF, Stadil F, Vikelsoe J: Immunoreactive gastrin components in human serum. Gut 15: 102–111, 1974.

140. Rehfeld JF: Radioimmunoassay in diagnosis, localization and treatment of endocrine tumours in gut and pancreas. Scand J Gastroenterol 14(Suppl 53): 33–38, 1979.

141. Robins JM, Bookstein JJ, Oberman HA, Fajans SS: Selective arteriography in localizing islet cell tumors of the pancreas. Radiology 106: 525–528, 1973.

142. Said SI, Mutt V: Isolation from porcine intestinal wall of a vasoactive ocatcospeptide related to secretin and to glucagon. Eur J Biochem 28: 129, 1972.

143. Said SI: Vasoactive intestinal polypeptide: Elevated plasma and tissue levels in the watery-diarrhea syndrome due to pancreatic and other tumors. (From the VA Hospital and Dept of Internal Med and Pharm, Univ of Texas Southwestern Med School, Dallas, Texas.)

144. Said SI, Faloona GR: Elevated plasma and tissue levels of vasoactive intestinal polypeptide in

the watery diarrhea syndrome due to pancreatic, bronchogenic and other tumors. N Eng J Med 293: 155–160, 1975.

145. Said SI: Evidence for secretion of vasoactive intestinal peptide by tumours of pancreas, adrenal, medulla, thyroid and lung: Support for the unifying apud concept. Clin Endocrin 5 (Suppl): 201s–204s, 1976.

146. Sasaki H, Rubacalva B, Baetens D, Blasquez E, Srikant CB, Orci L, Unger RH: Identification of glucagon in the gastrointestinal tract. J Clin Invest 56: 135, 1975.

147. Scarpello JH, Vinik AI, Owyang C: The intestinal phase of pancreatic polypeptide release. Gastroenterology 82: 406–12, 1982.

148. Scarpello JH, Vinik AI, Rader D, et al.: Correlation between duodenal trypsin and plasma pancreatic polypeptide: evidence for modulation of human pancreatic polypeptide (hPP) responses to secretin by duodenal luminal factors. Gastroenterology 78: 1252, 1980.

149. Schmechel D, Marangfos PJ, Brightman M: Neurone-specific enolase as a molecular marker for peripheral and central neuroendocrine cells. Nature 276: 834, 1978.

150. Schusdziarra V, Unger RH: Physiology and pathophysiology of circulating somatostatin in dogs. In: Gut Hormones, Second Edition, Bloom SR, Polak JM (eds): New York, Churchill Livingstone, 1981.

151. Schwartz CJ, Kimberg DV, Sheerin HE, Field M, Said SI: Vasoactive intestinal peptide stimulation of adenylate cyclase and active electrolyte secretion in intestinal mucosa. J Clin Invest 54: 536, 1974.

152. Schwartz TW: Pancreatic-polypeptide (PP) and endocrine tumours of the pancreas. Scand J Gastroenterol 14(Suppl 53): 93–100, 1979.

153. Schwartz TW: Pancreatic polypeptide as indicator of vagal activity. In Gastrin and the Vagus, Rehfeld JH, Amdrup E (eds): New York, Academic Press, 1979.

154. Shield CF, Haff RD: The VIPoma: Further confirmation of CIP as the hormonal agent in the WDHA syndrome. Am J Surg 132: 784–786, 1976.

155. Sive A, Vinik AI, Van Tonder S, Lund A: Impaired pancreatic polypeptide secretion in chronic pancreatitis. J Clin Endocrinol Metab 47: 556–559, 1978.

156. Smith FR, Rogers AI: Localization of a vasoactive intestinal peptide-producing tumor with selective venous sampling. Am J Gastroenterol 74: 282–284, 1980.

157. Snisky CA, Wolfe MM, Martin JL, Howe BA, O'Dorisio TM, McGuigan JE, Mathias JR: Effect of intravenous and intraluminal infusions of vasoactive intestinal peptide on myoelectric activity of rabbit small intestine. Am J Physiol 244: G46, 1983.

158. Solcia E, Capella C, Buffa R, et al.: Endocrine cells of the gastrointestinal tract and related tumors. Pathobiology Annual 9: 163–204, 1979.

159. Stacpoole PW, Jaspan J, Kasselbery AG, et al.: A familial glucagonoma syndrome. Genetic, clinical and biochemical features. Am J Med 70: 1017–1026, 1981.

160. Strodel WE, Vinik AI, Lloyd RV, Glaser B, Eckhauser FE, Fiddian-Green RG, Turcotte JG, Thompson NW: Pancreatic polypeptide-producing tumors: silent lesions of the pancreas? Arch Surg (in press).

161. Sweet RD: A dermatosis specifically associated with a tumour of pancreatic alpha cells. Br J Dermatology 90: 301–308, 1974.

162. Tapia FJ, Barbosa AJA, Marangos PJ, et al.: Neuron-specific enolase is produced by neuroendocrine tumours. Lancet 1: 808, 1981.

163. Tatemoto K, Mutt V: Isolation of two novel candidate hormones using chemical method for finding naturally occurring polypeptide. Nature 285: 417, 1980.

164. Taylor IL, Solomon TE, Walsh JH, Grossman MI: Pancreatic polypeptide: metabolism and effect on pancreatic secretion in dogs. Am J Gastroenterol 76(3): 524, 1979.

165. Thompson NW: Surgical considerations in the MEA I syndrome. In: Endocrine Surgery, Johnston DA, Thompson NW (eds). London: Butterworth 1983.

166. Tiedemann K, Long RG, Pritchard J, et al.: Plasma vasoactive intestinal polypeptide and other

regulatory peptides in children with neurogenic tumours. Eur J Pediatr 137: 147–150, 1981.

167. Tiedemann K, Pritchard J, Long R, et al.: Intractable diarrhoea in a patient with vasoactive intestinal peptide-secreting neuroblastoma. Eur J Pediatr 137: 217–219, 1981.

168. Tomita T, Kimmel JR, Friesen SR, et al.: Pancreatic polypeptide cell hyperplasia with and without watery diarrhea syndrome. J Surg Oncolog 14: 11–20, 1980.

169. Trimble MR: Vipoma: localisation by percutaneous transhepatic portal venous sampling. Br Med J 16: 1682–168, 1978.

170. Unger RH, Orci L: Glucagon and the A cell. Physiology and pathophysiology. N Engl J Med 304: 1518–1580, 1981.

171. Vale W, Rivier C, Brown M: Regulatory peptides of the hypothalamus Ann Rev Physiol 39: 473, 1977.

172. van Bogaert LJ: The diffuse endocrine system and derived tumours. Histological and histo-chemical characteristics. Acta Histochem 70: 122–129, 1982.

173. Verner JV, Morrison AB: Islet cell tumor and a syndrome of refractory watery diarrhea and hypokalemia. Am J med 25: 374–380, 1958.

174. Verner JV, Morrison AB: Endocrine pancreatic islet disease with diarrhea. Arch Intern Med 133: 492–500, 1974.

175. Villar HV, Johnson DG, Lynch PJ, et al.: Pattern of immunoreactive glucagon in portal, arterial and peripheral plasma before and after removal of glucagonoma. Am J Surg 141: 48–152, 1981.

176. Vinik AI, Achem-Karam S, Owyang C: Gastrointestinal hormones in clinical medicine. In: Special Topics in Endocrinology and Metabolism, Cohen MP, Foa PP (eds). Volume 4. New York: Alan R. Liss, Inc., 1983.

177. Vinik AI, Glaser B: Pancreatic endocrine tumors. In: Pancreatic Disease, Diagnosis and Therapy, T. Dent (ed). New York: Grune and Stratton, 1981.

178. Vinik AI, Glowniak J, Glaser B, Shapiro B, Funakoshi A, Cho KJ, Thompson NW, Fajans SS: Localization of gastroenteropancreatic (GEP) tumors. In: Surgery 2, Endocrine Surgery, Johnston IDA, Thompson NW (eds). Chapter 6, Butterworth's International Medical Reviews. London, 1983, pp 76–103.

179. Vinik AI, Strodel WE, Lloyd RV, Thompson NW: Unusual Gastroenteropancreatic (GEP) tumors and their hormones, Chapter 25. In: Endocrine Surgery Update, Thompson NW, Vinik AI (eds).New York: Grune & Stratton, 1983.

180. Walsh JH: Gastrointestinal peptide hormones and other biologically active peptides. In Gastrointestinal Disease: Pathophysiology, Diagnosis, Management, Sleisenger MH, Fordtran JS (eds). Philadelphia: Saunders, 1978.

181. Weir GC, Horton ES, Aoki TT, et al.: Secretion by glucagonomas of a possible glucagon precursor. J Clin Investigation 59: 325–330, 1977.

182. Wesley JR, Vinik AI, O'Dorisio TM, Glaser B, Fink A: A new syndrome of symptomatic cutaneous mastocytoma producing vasoactive intestinal polypeptide (VIP). Gastroenterology 82: 963–967, 1982.

183. Wilkinson DS: Necrolytic migratory erythema with carcinoma of the pancreas. Trans St. Johns Hosp Dermatol Soc 59: 244, 1973.

184. Wu ZC, O'Dorisio TM, Cataland S, Mekhjian HS, Gaginella TS: Effects of pancreatic polypeptide and vasoactive intestinal polypeptide on rat ileal and colonic water and electrolyte transport in vivo. Dig Dis Sci 24: 625, 1979.

185. Yamaguchi K, Abe K, Adachi I, et al.: Clinical and hormonal aspects of the watery diarrhea-hypokalemia-achlorhydria (WGHA) syndrome due to vasoactive intestinal polypeptide (VIP)-producing tumor. Endocrinol Japan 1: 79–86, 1980.

186. von Schenck H, Thorell JI, Berg J, et al.: Metabolic studies and glucagon gel filtration pattern before and after surgery in a case of glucagonoma syndrome. Acta Med Scand 205: 155–162, 1979.

13. The diagnosis and treatment of gastrinoma and Zollinger-Ellison syndrome

DENIS M. McCARTHY

1. Introduction

Twenty-eight years ago, Robert Zollinger and Edwin Ellison described the syndrome which now bears their names [1]. The Zollinger-Ellison syndrome (ZES) consisted of fulminant peptic ulcer disease not relieved by the usual gastric surgical procedures, accompanied by severe hypersecretion of gastric acid and associated with the presence of nonspecific islet cell tumors in the pancreas. While not the first to note the association between ulcers and pancreatic endocrine tumors, they were the first to document the massive hypersecretion of gastric acid which linked the conditions and which remains the essential requirement for diagnosis. They suggested that a hormone released by the tumor caused the stomach to secrete acid. This inspired guess was followed within five years by extraction from the tumor of a 'gastrin-like' substance active on bioassay [2], and later by demonstration that the material was identical to gastrin in its chemical structure [3]. This led to the tumor being designated 'gastrinoma,' and to the short-lived belief that solitary gastrinomas, often benign, were the main cause of the syndrome. Within two years of its first description, the association of ZES with multiple endocrine neoplasia – type I (MEN-I) was recognized [4], though much remains unclear as to the precise nature of the association.

The pioneering work of Yalow and Berson on radioimmunoassay of insulin [5] led Stremple and Meade [6] and McGuigan and Trudeau [7] in 1968 to the development of radioimmunoassays (RIA) for gastrin in human serum. This crucial development transformed the diagnosis of ZES and made it possible for the nonspecialist or primary care doctor to diagnose the condition, and to screen for it in the relatives of affected subjects. Within five years of the development of RIA, diagnosis of the syndrome had been confirmed in over 1,000 cases in North America alone, compared to about 150 cases detected world-wide between 1955 and 1960 [8, 9]. While the diagnosis of existing cases has become more common, the condition itself remains rare and accounts for less than 1 percent of peptic ulcers [10].

The essential features of ZES are hypersecretion of gastric acid and inappropriate hypergastrinemia: gastric hyperacidity should diminish gastrin release from

Santen, R.J. and Manni, A. (eds.), Diagnosis and management of endocrine-related tumors. ISBN 0-89838-636-5.
© *1984, Martinus Nijhoff Publishers, Boston. Printed in the Netherlands.*

the gastric antrum and lower serum gastrin. It can not be overstressed that both findings must be present before any serious attempts to establish the presence of ZES are undertaken. Hypergastrinemia without high basal gastric acidity is no more relevant to ZES than is raised serum concentrations of parathyroid hormone (PTH) in the absence of hypercalcemia to hyperparathyroidism.

Initially, it was thought that the combination of hypergastrinemia and hypersecretion of gastric acid was diagnostic of ZES, that the syndrome always arose from the presence in the pancreas of an adenomatous tumor which released only gastrin, that deaths occurred largely from acid-peptic disease, that medical therapy played no part in treating this, that total gastrectomy was the best and almost the sole therapy, and that growth or progression of the tumor was invariably very slow. All of these assumptions are now known to be incorrect to varying degrees, and much current controversy surrounds the syndrome, its diagnosis, and its clinical management.

2. Clinical features

Clinical features of ZES have been reviewed by many authors [8–17] and will not be discussed exhaustively in this article, other than to focus some attention on and to summarize those aspects of more contemporary relevance. In the years following its description, ZES was thought of as a highly symptomatic clinical disorder at the core of which was the triad of hyperacidity, hypergastrinemia and ulcers. Many of the early descriptions stressed the atypical features of the ulcers describing them as 'post-bulbar,' 'jejunal,' 'distal duodenal,' 'chronic,' 'recurrent,' 'rapidly recurring following gastric surgery,' 'fulminant' (implying high complication rate), 'multiple,' etc. While atypical ulcers, when present, strongly suggest the diagnosis, today the large majority of ulcers in ZES are typical duodenal ulcers, and 18–25 percent of patients have no ulcers at the time of diagnosis; erosions are common [14, 15]. It used to be almost characteristic for this diagnosis to be delayed for very long periods, with total gastrectomy being done in 52 percent of cases only at the fifth exploratory operation [11]. Nowadays, most patients have symptoms not different from conventional duodenal ulcer (DU) for 3–5 years before diagnosis which, in the majority of cases, is established prior to surgery [16]. Surgical mortality is also much reduced.

Thus, the disease is being encountered at an earlier stage in its natural history and is not infrequently seen at a subclinical or latent stage, either unmasked by hyperparathyroidism and ameliorated by parathyroidectomy, or detected in asymptomatic subjects during screening of relatives of ZES patients or of kindreds with MEN-I [18, 19]. Finally, in the past five years, we have had available powerful drugs, e.g. Cimetidine, Ranitidine, and Pirenzepine, etc., many of which are prescribed for dyspeptic patients who have not been investigated. Use of these drugs may lead to delay in diagnosis. However, having ulcers refractory to such forms of therapy is an increasingly common reason why patients are referred for investigation. Occasionally, ulcer symptoms may be absent or easily controlled. Patients may present with diarrhea or steatorrhea [17, 20], weight loss [21], esophageal disease [22], accelerated gastric emptying or rapid intestinal transit [23–25], hyperparathyroidism [26–30], or other manifestations of MEN-I ([31] and see Chapter 12 of this volume). Additional clinical findings in ZES cannot all be explained by the action of gastrin or by the presence of MEN-I. For example, the increase in fractional rate of gastric emptying and the fast transit seen on fluoroscopy do not appear to be due to gastrin [23–25]. The possible existence of additional gastric or pituitary hormonal factors in ZES has been raised from time to time [32, 33] but without convincing evidence. Histological and histochemical similarities between islet cell and carcinoid tumors [34–36] and the known capacity of such tumors to produce multiple hormones, e.g. histamine, motilin, 5HT, substance P, makes it possible that additional hormonal or neuro-humoral factors are involved. Of itself, hypergastrinemia due to pancreatic gastrinoma [34], atrophic gastritis or pernicious anemia [35], is known to stimulate argyrophil cells in the fundic mucosa causing hyperplasia of such cells or the formation of gastric carcinoids with additional hormone production [34].

More controversial and more important is our understanding of the relationship between ZES and disturbances of other endocrine glands, principally parathyroids, adrenals, and pituitary in patients with MEN-I. The dominant pathological finding in these glands is not adenoma formation but rather diffuse, bilateral hyperplasia of hormone-producing cells identical to that seen in these glands in states of secondary hyperfunction [37, 28]. The pathogenic mechanisms leading to such hyperplasias have not been elucidated. In contrast, the clinical picture may be complicated rarely by hypofunction of an endocrine organ regulated by the pituitary when the pituitary suffers compressive destruction of one or more of its parts during expansion of the gland within bony confines. Whether pituitary involvement is primary and independent of other lesions or is secondary and develops only in response to other systemic endocrine stresses has not been adequately studied.

3. Pathology

3.1 Subgroups of gastrinoma

Initial descriptions of islet cell tumors of the pancreas as the sole cause of hypergastrinemic hyperchlorhydria have been modified considerably. It is now clear that the majority of the tumors are malignant, that they can occur in sites other than the pancreas, that they can make other hormones in addition to gastrin, especially insulin and 5HT, and that they can be difficult if not impossible to find at surgery. Furthermore, the clinical features of hypergastrinemia, hyper-

Table 1. Types of gastrinoma

Type I	Sporadic (non-familial) Gastrinoma with ZES
	a) Pancreatic
	b) Extrapancreatic
Type II	Genetic Gastrinoma with ZES *or*
	Multiple Endocrine Neoplasia – Type I (MEN-I) with ZES
	a) Familial
	b) Sporadic
Type III	Malignant tumors containing gastrin on immunohistochemistry or on extraction with or without other hormones but not accompanied by hypergastrinemia or Clinical ZES

chorhydria and peptic ulcer disease may have causes other than tumor. In the light of current knowledge [16, 39, 40, 41], the relationship of ZES to gastrinoma of various types may be summarized as in Table 1.

Exact information as to how much each type contributes to the total number of gastrinoma patients is currently unknown and likely to remain so for some time. The proportion of MEN-I patients depends on the accuracy of family history and on how it was obtained. The yield of affected cases on screening is highly dependent on the ages of screened subjects, the intensity and methodology of screening, the number of times rescreened and the duration of follow-up (see below). Similar problems surround the evaluation of claims that there are patients with familial ZES who have no other demonstrated evidence of MEN-I and also patients with non-familial sporadic ZES with other glandular involvement [42]. In various series [8, 10, 21, 26, 29, 39], from 10–60 percent of patients with ZES have features of MEN-I, but on the average two-thirds appear 'sporadic' and one-third 'genetic.' Whether the existence of these two subgroups represents a variation in genetic penetrance or the existence of basically different diseases or mutations is not known. Most of the non-pancreatic tumors are associated with sporadic gastrinoma (Type I), and most of the tumors in MEN-I patients (Type II) will be found in the pancreas or exceptionally in the duodenal wall. According to Friesen, antral G-cell hyperplasia (AGCH) may also be found in MEN-I cases [38, 43], but this does not appear specific or to have been much studied by others. AGCH may be a consequence of the hyperparathyroidism [44, 45] commonly seen in these patients and may have little to do with the presence or absence of pancreatic tumors or the MEN-I trait. Most of the sporadic tumors are malignant and solitary, while tumors in MEN-I are small and multiple but generally benign. At the time of first diagnosis (often the 3rd or 4th decade), MEN-I tumors usually appear 'benign', but with prolonged follow-up some prove metastatic. The incidence of malignancy has not been examined in the two groups matched for age. It is possible that by the time MEN-I patients reach the age when most sporadic tumors occur (fifth to eight decades), the incidence of malignancy is similar in both groups. However, survival may be reduced when other glands are involved, especially adrenal and pituitary, and in the past life expectancy has been foreshortened in MEN-I patients more than in those with sporadic gastrinoma [8].

Some authors [43, 46] would include the various syndromes of antral dysfunction [47] as causes of Zollinger-Ellison Syndrome. I prefer to retain this title (ZES) for patients who have severe acid peptic disease associated with high acid secretion, fasting hypergastrinemia, and the presence of a tumor not necessarily in the pancreas. I readily concede that other entities (described below) may resemble ZES in their presentation. I use the term 'gastrinoma' to describe a tumor which contains gastrin, as demonstrated by immunohistochemistry or by extraction and radioimmunoassay. I recognize that there are tumors in many sites, including the pancreas, which contain gastrin alone or in the company of other hormones [48], which might qualify under this definition of 'gastrinoma' but which are not associated with the clinical illness of ZES. This is most commonly the case with ovarian malignancies [49], bronchial carcinoids [34], and small-cell carcinoma of the lung [50]. In what follows, I shall be discussing only those gastrinomas which are functional, which have been associated with hypergastrinemia and hypersecretion of acid, and which are included as Type I or Type II in Table I above.

3.2 Type I gastrinoma: Sporadic gastrinoma

Gastrinomas most commonly occur in the pancreas [8, 10, 34, 36, 49, 41], but in recent years an increasing number of reports have documented the presence of functioning tumors outside the pancreas, especially in the duodenal wall, stomach, and jejunum [15, 16, 34, 39–41, 51–54], with duodenal tumors accounting for 6–23 percent of tumors found at surgery [16]. Gastrinomas may be considered ectopic in the adult pancreas, since no gastrin producing cells are demonstrable there beyond fetal life [34, 41]; the other three locations normally possess G-cells and tumors in these may be considered entopic [36]. The incidence of malignant change seems appreciably lower (38 percent) when tumors occur in entopic locations, and the behavior of such tumors seems to differ from that of ectopic and generally more malignant (60–70 percent) tumors [34]. For instance, dominantly typical G-cells have been seen in gastric, duodenal and jejunal gastrinomas, whereas such cells are rare in pancreatic gastrinomas [34, 39–41]. In the opinion of Solcia [34], duodenal gastrinomas can be diagnosed both immunohistochemically and ultrastructurally, and the tumors probably arise from G-cells in duodenal crypts and Brunner's glands. Patients with such tumors may show a large increase in serum gastrin following a meal [55], although post-prandial acid output may be inhibited [56]. Furthermore, on challenge with calcium or bombesin in patients with pancreatic gastrinoma (ectopic), calcium infusion is more potent than bombesin in raising serum gastrin, whereas the opposite appears true in patients with duodenal (entopic) gastrinomas [57]. These interesting observations require further confirmation.

An additional important location for gastrinomas is in lymph glands [12, 33, 40, 58, 59]. While the demonstration of tumor in areas adjacent to the pancreas was traditionally regarded as evidence of metastasis even when no primary tumor site was identified, extrapancreatic location of primary tumors is being increasingly recognized [40, 58, 59]. Earlier ZES cases were subjected to total gastrectomy during which the surgeon sometimes removed lymph nodes containing islet cell tumor believed to be metastatic in nature. Some such cases have been followed by apparent 'cure' [12, 58, 59] possibly because of the inadvertent removal of primary tumors in lymph nodes. Such tumors may be found adjacent to the pancreas, stomach, and duodenum, in the hilum of the spleen, in the mesentery, or in the omentum [59]. Whether or not congenital rests of multipotent endocrine cells occur in peripancreatic regions, including lymph nodes, and later became overactive [33] developing into primary tumors with malignant potential remains unknown. Additional extrapancreatic primary gastrinomas not in lymphoid tissue also occur in these locations and can occasionally be found within the liver [40, 59] and biliary system [60, 61]. Not more than 50 percent of ZES patients are found to have tumors in the pancreas, stomach, or duodenum at surgery. While this has been attributed to misdiagnosis, antral hyperfunction, very small tumors, islet cell hyperplasia and other such causes, there is a real possibility that ectopic location contributes significantly to the surgical failure to locate primary tumors. ZES has been described in association with ovarian cancer in four cases [49, 62–64] and with a gastrin-containing parathyroid adenoma in one additional case [65].

In the case of pancreatic gastrinomas, most authors [35, 36, 39–41] agree that ultrastructural appearances are not uniform, that cell types are mixed (A, B, EC, D, PP, etc.), that tumor cells may contain more than one hormone and more than one kind of secretory granule, and that the tumors derive from multipotent, endocrine cells, probably of ductular rather than islet cell origin. Such 'pseudo-glandular' or 'tubuloacinar' tumors may be difficult to distinguish from ade-nomas, adenocarcinomas, hyperplasias, nesidioblastosis, or other 'pseudoneo-plastic reactions" to ductular obstruction [66]. Occasionally, ZES has been described in a patient with what appears to be a gastrin-secreting ductular adenocarcinoma of the pancreas [67].

A final distinct group of functioning tumors associated with ZES is that of carcinoid-islet tumors (atypical carcinoid syndrome). These for the most part derive from non-argentaffin endocrine multipotent foregut cells which have APUD characteristics [36] but which are almost certainly endodermal in origin [34, 40]. These tumors may secrete any of the polypeptides or other biologically active agents associated with the APUD system, including serotonin, 5HTP, substance P, prostaglandins, and kallikreins. True gastric carcinoid tumors of EC-cell origin, or diffuse 'carcinoidosis,' or 'microcarcinoidosis' of the stomach, can also arise in association with pancreatic gastrinoma or other causes of prolonged hypergastrinemia [34] giving rise to mixed clinical syndromes, but these are not to be confused with carcinoid-islet tumors. Carcinoid-islet tumors at the time of diagnosis may present with secretion of more than one hormone by the same tumor [68], e.g. gastrin and insulin [69, 70], gastrin, insulin and ACTH [71] gastrin, ACTH, and MSH [72], insulin and ACTH [68, 73] gastrin and VIP [74], insulin and 5H1AA [75], gastrin, VIP, and PGE [76], and many other combinations [77–79]. These tumors may be regarded as variants of Type I (d or G) gastrinoma (Table 1).

While the tumor may synthesize and release more than one hormone, it is usual for one clinical syndrome to predominate, the other features being silent and overlooked unless the patient is investigated in detail. Occasionally, the patient will have features of more than one clinical syndrome. More rarely still, the clinical manifestation of the tumor-related illness will alter with time, e.g. Cushing's syndrome to ZES [80], ZES to insulinoma [81], insulinoma to ZES and hyperglucagonism [82], ZES to carcinoid syndrome [83] and hypoglycemia to ZES with increased motilin and GIP [84]. Sequential chemotherapy with different drugs may be associated with this kind of progression of illness, each drug therapy being followed by the emergence of clones of endocrine-active cells whose presence was not appreciated prior to treatment. While I am assigning to these tumors the 'carcinoid-islet' designation, it must be acknowledged that the histochemical and ultrastructural features of the tissues may be pleomorphic, and that when poorly-differentiated carcinomas arising in the same tissues are studied ultrastructually, many show similar abortive attempts at endocrine differentiation [34].

It is important to recall that other tumors which are not gastrinomas can also be associated with moderate hypergastrinemia [47] but not with hyperacidity and ZES. This can occur in cases of phaeochromocytoma [85], gastric carcinoidosis [86], or in hypochlorhydric or achlorhydric patients with gastric cancers [87], or Verner-Morrison syndrome [47, 74]. 'Islet-cell-type' or 'carcinoid-type' histology in a patient with hypergastrinemia does not establish the diagnosis of gastrinoma unless the tumor is shown to contain gastrin. The diagnosis of ZES is not established without evidence of hypersecretion of gastric acid.

3.3 Type II gastrinoma: multiple endocrine neoplasia – Type I

The precise cause of MEN-I is not understood. Wermer [8] proposed that it is due to the inheritance of a pleiotropic genetic defect which directly stimulates growth in each of the affected glands (pancreas, pituitary, parathyoid, adrenal, etc.). However, Vance and colleagues have argued [38, 89] with some opposition [27] that the basic genetic defect involves primarily nesidioblastotic overgrowth of the multipotent ductular cells of the pancreas. In this model other endocrine dysfunction is seen as resulting secondarily, in response to chronic hypersecretion of one or more islet hormones. This model is quite compatible with the multicentric nature of the pathological findings in the pancreas in MEN-I [36–40] and with the generalized involvement of other endocrine organs. In these organs, secondary-appearing, diffuse 'hyperplasias' are the usual finding [37–40], although less commonly and unpredictably other processes, e.g. 'microadenoma,' 'adenoma,' 'carcinoma' or 'carcinoid' may also be identified. These latter too could arise from glandular foci during sustained hyperplastic responses [40, 86, 90]. The MEN-I syndrome accounts for about one-third of all cases of ZES (see above).

ZES occurs in 52–61 percent of affected MEN-I subjects [18, 29, 38]. ZES may present clinically somewhat later in life than the hyperparathyroidism which occurs in 90 percent of cases [18, 38]. Among MEN-I kindreds, the absence of hyperparathyroidism almost abolishes the chances of detection of subclinical gastrinoma by screening with serum gastrin [30] or even with secretin tests [18], but it does not abolish the chances of detecting other pancreatic tumors commonly associated with the MEN-I syndrome, e.g. insulinoma, glucagonoma or carcinoid. Pancreatic tumors releasing pancreatic polypeptide (hPP) must now be added to this list [19], though tumor cells are not the sole source of high plasma hPP in MEN-I or ZES. Pancreatic endocrine cell proliferations in MEN-I patients may contain and release pancreatic polypeptide (hPP), somatostatin, vasoactive intestinal polypeptide (VIP), ACTH, growth hormone, calcitonin and, rarely, parathormone or ADH. Release of these hormones may or may not be accompanied by related clinical syndromes.

Hypergastrinemia leads to parathyroid hyperplasia in experimental animals [91]. Vance and colleagues have pointed out [37] that sustained high serum levels of insulin, glucagon or calcitonin may also lead to parathyroid hyperplasia [37], so that it is not surprising that hyperparathyroidism is more common than ZES in MEN-I. In affected kindreds, the majority of subjects have abnormalities on screening but do not suffer from overt endocrine disease [18, 38]. Only with prolonged follow-up, and the increased manifestation of the syndrome with age, does the underlying pancreatic abnormality (not necessarily ZES) become apparent [29, 38, 92]. About 20 percent of patients with parathyroid hyperplasia have MEN-I which is discussed in detail in Chapter 12. In patients with MEN-I, gastrinomas are usually located in the pancreas or, more rarely, in the duodenal wall, are less commonly malignant than sporadic gastrinomas, and nowadays appear associated with better survival [20]. However, the tumors are usually multiple and often very small and are, therefore, hard to find or remove [93, 94]. This, together with the general lack of success of conservative pancreatic surgery in MEN-I patients with identifiable and resectable gastrinoma, suggests that only radical excision of the pancreas, duodenum and adjacent nodes could offer any real hope of surgical cure of ZES in MEN-I patients. There is a clear need for surgical research in this area and additionally, for clearly separating in future publications, the results of surgery for gastrinoma in MEN-I patients from the results in patients with sporadic tumors. Paradoxically, there may be more rationale for radical surgery in those with benign but multifocal disease, and a liability to develop many different kinds of largely pancreatic tumors than in those with sporadic gastrinomas which, though solitary, run a much higher chance of being extrapancreatic, malignant and metastasized at the time of surgery [95]. In the case of sporadic gastrinoma, a good case can be made for local excision of tumor with preservation of much of the pancreas [94, 95]. In patients whose tumors cannot be found at surgery, there is no pathological basis for blind partial pancreatectomy, with excision of the tail or distal half of the gland, since many sporadic gastrinomas occur in extrapancreatic locations.

3.4 *Islet-cell hyperplasia – nesidioblastosis – Microadenomatosis*

Human pancreatic islets contain four major cell types – A-cells containing glucagon, B-cells containing insulin, D-cells containing somatostatin or bombesin-like material, and PP- or F-cells containing pancreatic polypeptide. The proportions of these cells making up the islets are different in the two functionally distinct components of the pancreas, derived from dorsal and ventral primordial buds [97–99]. No gastrin-containing cells are found in normal human islets, in adult life, or in the fetus prior to the 22nd week of gestation. If G-cells are present at any later time, their numbers must be very small [39, 40].

The number of islets/section seen microscopically may give an erroneous impression of islet hyperplasia due to selective loss of acinar tissue and other sampling artifacts. Islet size is the most objective measure of hyperplasia. Most normal islets are less than $150\,\mu$ in diameter; size greater than $250\,\mu$ is a reliable index of hyperplasia [100]. Islet-cell hyperplasia has been observed in ZES patients with sporadic gastrinomas in the gut or pancreas or with MEN-I [40], but the islets have not contained gastrin as judged by immunoperoxidase, immunofluorescent or electromicroscopic techniques or by radioimmunoassay of tissue extracts [39, 40]. In fact, on immunohistochemical staining, most hyperplastic endocrine tissues contain glucagon A-cells, insulin B-cells, somatostatin D-cells and pancreatic polypeptide PP-cells [39, 40]. Thus, the hyperplasia of islets seen in ZES is regarded, by most authorities, not as a cause of the disease but rather as its consequence, analogous to the hyperplasias of parietal, argentaffin, and perhaps parathyroid chief cells [40, 91, 101] found in hypergastrinemic states.

Some authorities distinguish between 'simple' islet hypertrophy or hyperplasia, usually with selective involvement of a particular cell type, and 'nesidioblastosis,' where islet proliferation appears to occur in response to ductular obstruction and acinar fibrosis, perhaps because of increased blood flow through the islets [41, 66]. There seems little doubt that the pancreas possesses the capacity for islet or tubuloislet proliferation following a variety of insults [102–104] or as a consequence of hypergastrinemia [103], but, again, there is little evidence that such proliferation results in the synthesis or release of gastrin. Islet hyperplasia has been described in pernicious anemia or achlorhydria presumably as a consequence of hypergastrinemia [103]. Since such proliferation can also occur in the presence of pancreatitis or neoplastic obstruction of ducts [66], it is difficult to exclude the possibility that it occurs in the pancreas of ZES patients as a consequence of obstructive pathology. Furthermore, as pointed out by Creutzfeldt and colleagues [39], glands demonstrated to contain tumors almost invariably contain areas of hyperplasia or nesidioblastosis. Hence, in the 10 percent of cases in the older literature where 'islet-cell hyperplasia' appears to be the sole cause of ZES, it is difficult to be sure that glands reported as 'hyperplastic' or 'nesidioblastotic' did not contain a tumor, of such small size that it would have been detected only if the whole pancreas had been sectioned or, perhaps, located in an extrapancreatic site and causing secondary hyperplasia in the islets. The available literature does not allow a comment on whether or not 'islet cell hyperplasia' is found more frequently in MEN-I patients than in patients with sporadic gastrinoma. Neither do most series offer criteria which define the differences between 'simple islet cell hyperplasia' and 'nesidioblastosis' clearly enough to allow us to draw a conclusion as to which type of islet proliferation is associated with which type of ZES. The pioneering work of Larsson [103] offers hope that in the future immunochemical methods may lend themselves to the unraveling of this problem. There is a great shortage of data from such investigations, where the immunohistochemical characteristics of islets in adjacent nontumorous pancreatic tissue have been studied in clearly separated MEN-I and sporadic gastrinoma patients.

There are additional semantic problems surrounding the description of very large islets or small tumors. When islets of diameter of 500–600 μ are seen, the decision as to whether they should be called 'hyperplastic islets' or 'microadenomata' seems to be subjective. This leads to conceptual confusion as to whether or not 'microadenomata' can result from hyperplasia or can cause ZES, and uncertainty as to the possible development of larger and potentially malignant gastrinomata from 'microadenomata.' This is particularly important in MEN-I where 'nesidioblastosis' and 'islet-cell hyperplasia' are both described, and where multifocal tumors producing a variety of hormones are commonly encountered [37]. In very rare cases of nesidioblastosis associated with neonatal hypoglycemia, there is some evidence of increased release of gastrin from the pancreas, but so far there has not been a satisfactory direct demonstration of gastrin-containing cells in the pancreas in this condition [103, 104]. There are other very rare but well-described instances where ZES has been caused by a variety of rare lesions, 'nesidioblastosis with antropyloric gastrinoma' [107], 'poorly-defined infiltrative G-cell containing tumor of the stomach' [108], 'solitary G-cell tumor of stomach' [40], 'G-cell micronodules' [40], and 'gigantic islets or nesidioblastoma' [109]. Incomplete descriptions and lack of clear nomenclature and pathological criteria deprive us of adequate understanding of these entities and of the opportunity to examine their possible interrelationships.

Beyond this, complexity of the pathology is not simply semantic; it also arises from the pleomorphic manifestations of islet-cell dysplasias and tumors. As pointed out by Bartow et al. [64], 'Between obvious regeneration and *de novo* neoplasm, there exists a morphological spectrum in which the distinction between neoplasia and hyperplasia is difficult, even for the experienced observer.' This highlights an additional difficulty, i.e. distinguishing histologically between hyperplastic, nesidioblastotic, adenomatous, carcinomatous, carcinoid, and islet-cell carcinomatous tissues. This is particularly important when dealing with frozen sections at the time of surgery. For the diagnosis of malignancy, only direct extension of tumor through the capsule or the finding of non-lymphoidal distant metastases (e.g. in the liver, lung, bone, etc.) justify the term 'malignant.' In addition, the histological finding of neurovascular invasion, though less reliable [66], generally indicates the presence of malignant disease. Clinically, the detection of micrometastases, commonly present, is quite difficult, and serological indications of dissemination, e.g. high G17/G34 ratio in serum [110, 111] or high α- or β-hCG in serum [112, 113], may be more valuable than angiographic, tomographic or other methods. As a final observation, it should be pointed out that islet-cell hyperplasia may have many other causes. For all of these reasons, the finding of islet-cell hyperplasia or 'nesidioblastosis' must be regarded as doubtful causes of ZES and, in my opinion, should not be used to justify the surgical removal of all or part of the pancreas when no tumor has been found.

4. Epidemiology

The incidence and prevalence of ZES are unknown, but it is estimated that there are between 250–500 cases in the U.S.A., an approximate prevalence of 2–4 cases per million of population. These crude figures are for all clinical types of ZES who have overt disease, including MEN-I patients. To date, screening of relatives of ZES or MEN-I patients for subclinical disease has been haphazard. No standards for the methodology, extent or frequency of screening have been developed or generally accepted, probably because of the rarity of the condition. Ongoing studies in Holland in time may yield valuable insights, but MEN-I appears more common in the Dutch population, and results from Holland may not apply generally. While serum gastrin measurements remain very important in screening, a total serum gastrin includes in the measurement various species of the hormone from several anatomical sites. Isolation and purification of a tumor-specific, antigenic form of gastrin or gastrin precursor, and use of monoclonal-antibody production techniques, may soon allow development of an RIA more useful in detecting the presence of tumors. Furthermore, as discussed above, there are at least two distinct types of the disease – the 'sporadic' and the 'familial' (MEN-I). When both variants are included, the male-to-female ratio is 3:2. The gene frequency for MEN-I is unknown, and whether the sex difference arises from patients with sporadic disease or MEN-I has not been studied.

5. Pathogenesis

The clinical features of the disease, other than those arising from the spread of malignant tumor, mostly arise from the presence of excess acid in the lumen of the gut; removal or neutralization of gastric acid abolishes most symptoms. Acid secretion in turn derives from the action of excessive amounts of various types of circulating gastrin (G14, G17, G34, Component-I, and the NH_2-terminal fragment of G17, which contains 13 amino acid residues) released by the tumor [114]. Tumor-derived gastrin potentiates the background, calcium-dependent secretion mediated by the endogenous agonists, e.g. antroduodenal gastrin, histamine and acetylcholine. Rarely 'big-big' gastrin, considered an artifact in normals, may be found in sera of patients with gastrinoma [115]. C-terminally extended gastrins have also been described [116]; these would not be detected with conventional RIA using antibody directed against the C-terminus of G17. Because of gastrin heterogeneity in serum, correlation between basal acid output (BAO) and serum gastrin is generally poor.

Chronic hypersecretion over long periods is associated with the development of parietal and chief cell hyperplasia, and prominent mucosal folds in the body and fundus of the stomach. In intact patients, the basal hypersecretion occuring during sleep, in late postprandial and in interdigestive phases, is probably the key to damaging the mucosa of the esophagus, stomach, and small intestine. Gastric emptying is generally enhanced [23, 24], but feeding generally results in a paradoxical inhibition of both secretion [55] and emptying [115]; serum gastrin generally shows little change but may rise to very high levels. Delivery of large quantities of acid into the duodenum releases mucosal secretin, increases serum secretin [118, 119], and may further enhance release of gastrin from the tumor. Occasionally, continuous aspiration of gastric juice, or gastrectomy without excision of tumor, have been observed to result in a fall in serum gastrin, possibly by removing and diminishing release of secretin; data on this point are incomplete. Enhanced release of secretin is probably responsible for the enhanced pancreatic secretion observed in the condition [120].

In addition to gastrin and secretin, many other hormones are commonly found in increased concentrations in serum. These include parathormone [121], calcitonin [122], human pancreatic polypeptide [19, 123], prolactin [124], and α- or β-subunits of hCG [112, 113]; their pathogenetic significance is unknown, but they may be important. If the tumor is of the carcinoid-islet type, a considerable number of other hormones (reviewed above) may also be found and may result in the development of additional clinical syndromes, but this is exceptional.

6. Diagnosis

The diagnosis of ZES involves identification of the secretory diathesis, confirmation of the presence of tumor, location of the site of the neoplasm, and determination of the extent of spread. Since the physician usually encounters this problem in an elderly patient with probably malignant disease, it is most important that the patient receive a very careful assessment of his overall health, including cardiac, renal, pulmonary and intellectual status and social resources. Long-term management plans must be specific for that individual, and key decisions as to his care must be taken with truly informed consent. Once the diagnosis is confirmed, all available first-degree relatives should be screened, at least with a fasting serum gastrin, calcium and hPP [19]. If there is evidence of MEN-I, particularly if the relatives are young, screening should include a secretin test (see below), and this should be repeated at regular intervals even in asymptomatic cases [29].

6.1 *Basic tests*

Most patients with ZES present with a typical duodenal ulcer (DU) plus additional symptomatology. DU patients with features listed in Table 2 should first have a serum gastrin and, if elevated, an acid secretory study, at least a determination of BAO. If gastrin and BAO are elevated, this should lead to additional tests. Such screening of DU patients may increase the detection of ZES early in its progression [125]. Many ZES patients have no ulcer but may have erosive duodenitis. They may present with or without ulcer symptoms and few or no radiographic findings [52, 53].

The diagnosis rests on finding simultaneous hypergastrinemia and hypersecretion of gastric acid. As will be seen under differential diagnosis (below), the combination, while highly suggestive of ZES, is not peculiar to it. Practical points about making the diagnosis have recently been discussed in more depth elsewhere [47], and only the diagnostic criteria (serum gastrin > upper limit of normal and BAO >15 mEq/h for an unoperated patient or >5 mEq/h for those with prior gastric surgery) will be discussed here. There is considerable overlap

Table 2. Indications for measurement of serum gastrin in subjects with peptic ulcer

---

a) Ulcers that are:
   Familial, multiple, ectopic, chronic, recurrent, refractory to therapy, following previous surgery, being considered for future surgery or found at extremes of age.
b) Ulcers accompanied by:
   Hypercalcemia, hypophosphatemia, alkalosis, diarrhea, weight loss, nephrolithiasis, endocrinopathy, prior endocrine surgery.
c) Ulcers with x-ray or other evidence of:
   Gastric hypersecretion, prominent folds which do not efface on distension, rapid emptying, outlet obstruction, multiple duodenal erosions, Brunner's Gland hypertrophy
d) Ulcer resistant to conventional therapy

---

between values at the low end of the gastrinoma range and those at the high end of the DU range. It has been argued that provided hypochlorhydria has been excluded, the addition of acid studies to a serum gastrin adds nothing of discriminative value to the latter, especially when gastrin concentration is between the upper limit of normal and about 1000 pg/ml, and that it is better therefore to proceed immediately from a high serum gastrin to a provocative test (see below) without detailed acid studies [126, 127]. This may be true in special centers where specimen collection, RIA, avoidance of patient and assay artifacts, and interpretation of results, are all undertaken by experienced workers; in most hospitals such expertise cannot be assumed. Measurement of BAO remains an essential step and is quick, cheap and generally easy to perform. False positive diagnoses of ZES are common, and most occur in cases with no or low acid output. Provocative tests are generally much more expensive and should be performed only when BAO is elevated >10 mEq/h. There are many falsely low estimates of BAO in hospitals where acids are infrequently measured. The decision to proceed with a provocative test should thus be taken on the basis of an output of >10 mEq/h, accepting that many such cases will have negative provocative studies and will not have ZES.

6.2 Provocative tests

Because of the degree of overlap between ZES patients and DU patients with high acid output and/or hypergastrinemia, there have been many attempts to devise provocative tests that would be sensitive and specific for ZES. The most useful of these tests is the secretin (bolus) test, recently reviewed by McGuigan and Wolfe [128] and by Lamers [129]. Others have studied the effect on serum gastrin of infusions of secretin [53, 130], calcium [131], theophylline ethylenediamine [132] or injections of glucagon [133], bombesin [57] or somatostatin, or of meals [39, 55, 56, 134]. With the exception of calcium infusion, none of these are of established value in the diagnosis of ZES, though bombesin may be useful in the diagnosis of incomplete antrectomy [135]. Calcium infusion tests are difficult to perform, associated with side effects, hazardous in the presence of hypercalcemia, and unpopular with patients. Comparative studies of the various tests [39, 53, 55, 56, 127, 136, 137, 138] suggest that the secretin test is the most specific, the simplest, the quickest, and safest. However, false negative and rare false positive tests are reported. The latter are hard to evaluate since very small or ectopic tumors may easily be missed at surgery. Furthermore, there continue to be differences in what investigators regard as a positive response, with various groups advocating increments of 110 pg/ml [136], 200 pg/ml [128], 50 percent increased above basal [55], 100 percent above basal [139], 300 percent increased above basal [140], and peak concentration [127]. An increment of >200 pg/ml following 2 IU/kg GIH secretin [128] is the best supported. At this time it would appear that most centers must develop their own norms for the test, a real problem given the rarity of ZES and the difficulty of assembling a patient group. Finally, there is a notable shortage of data on the outcome of secretin tests in disease controls with conditions such as gastric outlet obstruction, antral hyperfunction, anastomotic ulcer, retained and excluded antrum, proximal Crohn's disease and other uncommon conditions likely to be confused with ZES. All groups agree that provocative tests are unnecessary in patients with hypersecretion of acid >15 mEq/h., and serum gastrin >1000 pg/ml. Outside of centers where RIA for gastrin is subject to rigorous quality control, assay variation is a major problem with the secretin test, and fluctuations in basal values may exceed the local criterion for a positive response. For these reasons, the test is best done in special centers interested in ZES.

Personal experience has been similar to that of Stage and Stadil [53], who note that 'ZES can be diagnosed in most cases by combining symptomatology with measurements of acid and gastrin.' In view of the existence of false negative results, some of which may be due to hypocalcemia [141], a positive test while helpful, is not a diagnostic requirement. A recent study has combined secretin bolus injection with rapid calcium infusion and found no false positive or false negative results [138]. If this can be established in larger series with adequate numbers of disease controls, it may in time prove to be the best test. Long-duration calcium infusions (12 mgCa^{++}/kg/3 h), while sensitive, are lacking in specificity, and positive calcium infusion tests on their own should not be used to justify explorative surgery. Equally, total gastrectomy should not be performed on secretin negative subjects, without other strong evidence of ZES.

6.3 Localization of tumor

Locating the primary tumor continues to be a major problem. Selective angiography leads to its detection in 10–30 percent of cases [15, 142–145] and is one of the better techniques for detecting hepatic metastases. Two selective hepatic arterial injections should always be performed prior to surgery. CT scanning is somewhat better [16, 146, 147], but because ZES patients have little peripancreatic fat and because the x-ray absorption coefficient of tumor tissue does not differ appreciably from that of surrounding pancreas [146], results have been generally disappointing. CT scan results may be improved by cholegrafin infusion [16]. The best imaging technique has been grey-scale ultrasound [148, 149] leading to location of the tumor in about 50 percent of cases.

Technical factors relating to performance and interpretation of these tests frequently result in rather 'soft' findings, and additional problems arise when the various tests are 'positive' in the same patient but point to different regions of the pancreas as the site of the primary. An exciting new development, from surgeons at the University of Illinois, has been intraoperative ultrasonic assessment of the exposed pancreas for detection of the tumor [150]. ZES tumors appear relatively sonolucent. Unpublished studies are underway at Seattle, NIH and other centers, and preliminary results appear most encouraging. This promises to be a major advance, and because of its simplicity and the immediate availability of results, its usefulness is likely to greatly exceed that of percutaneous retrograde transhepatic venous sampling (described below).

Simpler tests, such as barium meal or hypotonic duodenography, occasionally lead to localization of a primary tumor, especially if large and located in the duodenal wall, but more often they show other nonspecific features suggestive of the diagnosis of ZES and helpful to its management but not to its localization. Upper G.I. endoscopy is indicated in all cases. Performed in undiagnosed cases, endoscopic findings suggestive of ZES include extreme gastric hypersecretion – the walls dripping constantly 'like a tropical forest' – and necessitating almost constant suction of material whose pH is close to 1.0, very prominent folds in the corpus and fundus of the stomach, marked increase in the motility of both stomach and duodenum, and multiple erosions on otherwise prominent and often nodular-appearing duodenal folds. Endoscopy has resulted in location and removal of primary tumors in a number of cases [151–153]. For this reason, diagnosed patients should be subjected to very careful endoscopy, after preinjection I.V. with cimetidine and an anticholinergic and with an additional injection of glucagon (1 mg) when the scope is in the duodenum. This drug therapy greatly reduces hypersecretion and hypermotility and allows 1–3 minutes to search behind generally prominent folds for a small tumor. Without drug therapy, visualization of anything in this area is haphazard. As many as 20 percent of locatable tumors may be in the duodenal wall [93]. Detection of metastases will not be discussed in detail here but is alluded to throughout the text. Radionucleide scanning of liver, spleen and bone, and liver biopsy are all useful in some cases.

Recently, the technique of percutaneous transhepatic portal venous sampling (PTPVS) has been used to detect gastrinomas but only in small numbers of patients [16, 94, 145, 154–157]. The procedure is technically difficult, takes much time and effort, and a number of problems are already apparent [94, 155, 157], so that its use will probably be confined to special centers. In the presence of large gradients (Δ gastrin > 1000 pg/ml), confined to a single vein, the technique may be very helpful, but smaller gradients may be found in more than one vein simultaneously, and in some patients large amounts of antral gastrin may also enter the drainage area. False negative results are common [157]. Preliminary evidence suggests that the technique may be valuable in sporadic gastrinoma (solitary tumor) but of little help in MEN-I patients (multiple tumors) who are unlikely to be helped even when tumors are located and excised [94]. Hence, some groups [93, 94] are abandoning attempts at local excision of tumor in MEN-I, though for various reasons this decision seems premature. The alternative approach, i.e. total pancreatectomy, carries a high morbidity but may merit consideration in the younger MEN-I patient. Intraoperative ultrasound seems likely to supercede PTPVS in the localization of tumors within the pancreas, but PTPVS may continue to be of occasional use in the preoperative detection of ectopic tumors, provided all accessible veins are sampled. The use of nuclear magnetic resonance scanners is currently being evaluated.

7. Differential diagnosis

Overdiagnosis of ZES is relatively common with many physicians getting into difficulty by proceeding from the finding of marginal or moderate fasting hyper-gastrinemia to the often equivocal results of provocative tests, without carrying out the essential intermediate step of demonstrating elevation of BAO. How-ever, assuming that hypergastrinemias associated with hypo- or achlorhydria have been excluded, there are still a number of situations where both gastrin and acid may be elevated, for reasons other than the presence of gastrinoma.

7.1 Isolated retained antrum syndrome (IRAS)

Failure to excise all antral tissue from the duodenal stump created during a Billroth II gastrectomy may very rarely leave the patient with antral G-cells chronically exposed to an alkaline medium and, therefore, stimulated to release gastrin. The action of gastrin leads to sustained gastric hypersecretion of acid similar to that seen in ZES [158, 159, 160]. The acid diverted by normal peristalsis out of the afferent and into the efferent loop never reaches the antral tissue, and normal feedback inhibition of gastrin release does not occur, leading to moderate hypergastrinemia [161, 162]. The secretin bolus test results in a fall in serum gastrin [163–165], as does injection of bombesin [135, 166]. Other provocative tests employing meals or calcium infusion are unhelpful [165–167]. If IRAS is suspected, endoscopic biopsies of the stump will show gastric tissue, and isotopic scanning with ^{99m}Tc-labeled sodium pertechnetate may demonstrate increased uptake by the stump [165–168]. The number of documented cases in the world literature is small and the number who have had secretin tests or other physiologi-cal studies even smaller [163–165]. Today, IRAS is rarely observed. Because of the very high frequency of recurrent ulceration [160], surgeons became aware of this entity prior to widespread availability of gastrin RIA and have been checking operative margins histologically since about 1965. However, when it does occur, the resemblance to ZES can be striking and only the secretin test seems of established value in differential diagnosis at this time.

7.2 Chronic gastric outlet obstruction

This is the clinical situation in which a false positive diagnosis of ZES is most likely to be made. Affected patients have hypergastrinemia, hyperchlorhydria, radiological abnormalities of the stomach and duodenum, and impaired gastric emptying. There are several other features which increase the confusion. The first is that underlying ZES may cause and co-exist with impaired gastric empty- ing and outlet obstruction, although in ZES patients without obstruction, gastric emptying is very rapid [23, 25]. Other causes of incomplete obstruction include Crohn's disease, ectopic gastric mucosa, annular pancreas, vascular obstructions, pancreatic tumors, and severe peptic ulcer disease, especially that occuring in young people who have channel ulcers. Serum gastrin, while apparently 'fasting', may not be close to basal levels, since the stomach may contain food several days old and may also be distended. In man, acute distension of the normal stomach has little or no effect on serum gastrin, but patients with prepyloric ulcer and pyloric obstruction may meet the diagnostic criteria for ZES [169]. Up to 7–14 days of cleansing and continuous aspiration of the stomach may be needed to return the patient to the basal state. In DU subjects, MAO may take 30 days to return to normal [170]. The obstruction does not have to be 'complete' or radiologically obvious for confusion to occur (personal observations). This is supported by animal studies which show that the amount of parietal cell hyper- plasia, and the accompanying hypersecretion of acid, are functions of the degree of obstruction and the duration for which it has existed [171]. The results of secretin tests in such patients are unknown but important, and should be exam- ined in patients with impaired drainage of variable severity and duration. Rapid or increased rates of gastric emptying, as measured by isotopic scintiscans follow- ing solid phase labelling of gastric contents, are the best evidence that impaired drainage can be ignored as the cause of hypergastrinemic hyperchlorhydria in the patient [23–25]. However, if emptying is slow, the differential diagnosis is diffi- cult and rests on a minimum amount of data. Radiographic estimates of adequacy of drainage are unreliable.

7.3 Ulcer following previous surgery

Not infrequently, ulcers are encountered in patients who have already had one or more gastric operations, usually without serum gastrin or acid secretory rate measured prior to surgery. The patient may have 'prominent gastric folds' and be 'doing poorly with medical therapy', and his 'serum gastrin may be minimally or moderately elevated.' This is a common and potentially difficult clinical situation, but with careful attention to acid secretion, it is resolved readily in most cases. First, ulcers associated with hypersecretion of acid are almost always on the jejunal side of the anastomosis or in the efferent loop, and ulcers on the gastric side of the anastomosis are more likely due to 'alkaline reflux' than to ZES patients unless the patient is taking aspirin. Secondly, difficulties of measuring acid output in such patients have been exaggerated. If the tube is placed $1\frac{1}{2}''-3''$ distal to the LES, the patient laid in the left lateral position with the foot of the bed elevated, and if the first 30 minutes of aspirate are discarded, acid secretory studies can be performed in most cases. If BAO >5 mEq/h, the diagnosis of ZES should be suspected. Against this in true ZES, 70 percent of such cases will exceed 15 mEq/h, unless the gastric remnant is very small. Aspiration should be manual, constantly attended to, and the tube position checked again at the end of the procedure. The causes of hypergastrinemia in such patients include vagotomy (especially truncal), obstructed drainage (see above), stasis with retention of food (i.e. not truly fasting), and isolated retained antrum (7.2 above). Most subjects are hypochlorhydric. There is a shortage of studies in this area, but it has often appeared to this author that the above factors may be additive, and serum gastrins of up to 500 pg/ml in such patients are usually due to causes other than ZES. Secretin stimulation tests are negative or equivocal. This particular problem should now be preventable by the simple step of obtaining a fasting serum gastrin, followed if elevated by acid secretory studies, in every patient scheduled for elective gastric surgery and by delaying surgery until the results have been inspected.

7.4 Syndromes of antral hyperfunction

In ZES, the concentration of gastrin in antral mucosa is significantly lower than that in controls [172], and the antral G-cell population appears to be normal [173]. However, occasional patients with duodenal or anastomotic ulcer disease have disturbances of G-cell regulation which may give rise to borderline or slightly elevated serum concentrations of gastrin and be confused with ZES on superficial examination. Such cases are apparently rare, mild, and not seen in association with severe disease such as that observed in ZES. The clinical syndrome has been variously described as Zollinger-Ellison syndrome – Type I [46, 174] Antral G-cell Hyperplasia [44, 175–178], Nontumorous Hypergastrinemic Hyperchlorhydria [161], Hypergastrinemia of Antral Origin [179], Pseudo-ZES [180] and Antral G-cell Hyperfunction [181]. It is by no means clear that all of these titles describe the same entity, and most experienced workers have either not encountered it at all [15, 16, 47, 127, 145, 178, 182] or have seen it only very rarely [55, 178, 179]. At present, Antral G-cell Hyperfunction (AGCH) has much to recommend it as a title, since the syndrome is diagnosed by its advocates on the basis of functional changes which, when combined, may be characteristic. A critical review of all the data is beyond the scope of this chapter but has been dealt with at some length elsewhere [47]. For the moment, it is perhaps best to summarize the situation by stating that there are a small number of patients reported in the literature who presented with peptic ulcer, marginal serum gastrin elevation, BAO >15 mEq/h, and who, in the face of surgery at which no tumor could be found, were treated with antrectomy (with or without vagotomy) and resolved their problems: postoperative acid and gastrin concentrations were within the normal range. The question that preoccupies gastroenterologists is whether or not these patients can be recognized prior to surgery. Affirmative claims to this effect [178–180] state that the combination of a negative secretin response, a large increase in serum gastrin following a meal, and a failure to find tumor at a carefully performed laparotomy [145], allow confident identification of patients best treated by antrectomy. This may be true; however, this reviewer's reservations with the claim derive from the known existence of false negative secretin tests in patients with proven tumors, the documented existence of ectopic tumors generally missed at surgery, the finding of low basal and marked post-prandial increases in serum gastrin, in proven cases of gastrinoma [39, 55, 56, 134], especially in those who have had previous gastric surgery [55], and the general lack of any long-term follow-up information on cases allegedly cured by antrectomy. All of the so called 'characteristics' are thus nonspecific findings. Their combination might be specific, but this has not been studied in disease controls, e.g. outlet obstruction or antacid-treated DU patients. More information is needed to be certain about these points, but in the meantime most authorities agree that AGCH must be very rare, if the criterion of BAO >15 mEq/h is strictly enforced and if cases with previous gastric surgery are excluded.

7.5 Syndromes of hypergastrinemia

There are many causes of serum gastrin elevations [47, 183]. Only those associated with elevated BAO merit investigation for ZES. IF BAO cannot be measured, patients with anastomotic ulcers on the jeunal side of their anastomosis or with histological evidence of islet cell tumors also merit investigation. Many of these patients, if they have ZES, will have diarrhea which can be abolished by therapy with H_2-blocking drugs.

7.6 Syndromes of hyperacidity

Patients with high BAO and severe ulcer disease are more likely not to have ZES than to have it [184]. In the absence of serum gastrin elevations, and rare conditions such as systemic mastocytosis or foregut carcinoids, such patients should be managed with highly selective vagotomy and not investigated for ZES.

In summary, with the exception of rare conditions, e.g. IRAS and syndromes where both criteria for ZES have usually not been met, differential diagnosis comes down to rigorous clinical exclusion of hypersecretory conditions associated with impaired gastric drainage, antral dysfunction, and a variety of gastric/vagal malfunctions following previous gastric surgery; these three areas frequently overlap. Studies of acid secretion, gastric emptying, and the effects of prolonged aspiration of gastric contents, on secretion of acid and on serum gastrin, are most helpful in excluding these confusing conditions.

8. Management

8.1 *Therapy of acute disease*

Much controversy surrounds the long-term management of ZES, but few would disagree that the potent antisecretory drugs developed in recent years should be used initially in virtually all cases. About 30 percent of ZES patients present with complications of ulcer disease, e.g. perforation, hemorrhage, obstruction, alkalosis, and dehydration. Except in rare cases, there is no need to perform total gastrectomy on these cases in an emergency setting. Patients should be stabilized using I.V. cimetidine (loading dose plus infusion), supplemented if necessary with potent anticholinergic drugs, e.g. Pirenzepine, Isopropamide or Glycopyrrolate, while on continuous nasogastric suction with a Salem Sump tube. When the clinical condition is stabilized, the patient can be taken to surgery for conservative management of the complication, e.g. closure of perforation. A careful search for primary gastrinoma, perhaps followed by highly selective vagotomy (see later) and excision of obvious resectable tumor, can be done at that time if the situation permits: most cases should have minimal surgery prior to careful assessment of their disease. The volume and acid content of the aspirate can be used to determine adequate dosage of drugs. Acid secretion should be reduced to 10 mEq/h or less, and serum calcium, electrolytes and blood gases require careful monitoring. Plasma volume should be expanded until urinary specific gravity is <1.020 and plasma chloride >100 mEq/l.

8.2 *Long-term therapy*

8.2.1 *Selection of patients.* Although total gastrectomy continues to be a viable alternative to long-term medical control of the hypersecretory disorder [145], it is unnecessary in most cases [16, 47, 93]. H_2-blocking antihistamine therapy has been carried out successfully in many departments, though considerable expertise and careful supervision of cases are required. The most common problems attending medical therapy are inadequate dosage of drug, lack of monitoring for altered drug requirement with progression of the disease, and poor patient compliance. Patients who are not intelligent, careful, and strongly motivated towards medical therapy should have elective total gastrectomy, combined when feasible with excision of their tumor. They should not be considered for long-term medical therapy. This is particularly true of alcoholics. On the other hand, many patients are elderly and debilitated and may have little to gain from surgery [93, 95] especially when evidence of metastatic disease is present. Between these two extremes are patients in whom the choice of medical or surgical therapy must be based on the specific findings in the individual case with many patients needing combinations of medical and surgical therapy over the years [16, 93, 96, 185–187].

8.2.2 *Drug therapy.* Both Cimetidine [16, 21, 93, 188–191] and Ranitidine [192, 193] alone or in combination with anticholinergics [194, 195] have been succesfully used in the long-term treatment of ZES. There is no recommended dose of any drug in ZES. The dose of drug required to control acid secretion and heal ulcers must be determined in each case by measuring acid secretory rates, for two hours prior to the next dose of drug [196], and by endoscopic confirmation of ulcer healing. These assessments must be repeated at least yearly and more often if patients are symptomatic [191, 196]. However, relief of symptoms is an unreliable guide to the adequacy of therapy in the opinion of most observers [96, 190, 191, 196]. Prolonged maintenance of acid secretory rates, at less than 10 mEq/h. is generally associated with absence of endoscopic abnormality or complications of acid-peptic disease [196, 197]. Failure to abolish diarrhea is the best clinical indicator of inadequate dosage of drug [21, 190, 197].

When these principles have not been rigidly adhered to, failure rates have been unacceptably high. Inspection reveals in many cases that inadequate dosage or failure to demonstrate the adequacy of dosage are commonly followed by claims that 'medical therapy has failed' [54, 96, 191, 198]. However, in medical units where control is tight, failure of drugs to control the disease is much less common and does not occur in more than 20 percent of cases [16, 93, 198, 199]. Since the disease is relentless and progressive and since the dose of drug required for control, rises with time and may be unacceptably high to the patient either because of cost, side effects or inconvenience, the decision to abandon medical therapy may be fully justified, though not based on pharmacological failure. Reports of 'failure of medical therapy' should clearly distinguish between loss of drug efficacy and the exercise by the patient or his doctor of a choice or preference for total gastrectomy. To date the 'failures of medical therapy' have included several different kinds of patients: those who continued to have symptoms or developed complications of acid-peptic disease while noncompliant or on inadequate dosage, others whose doses were rising and unacceptably high to their physicians but in whom hypersecretion was not necessarily demonstrated, or who developed side effects or toxic effects of drugs, and patients who opted to be explored for gastrinoma while under good control pharmacologically. Comments about 'cimetidine resistance' are equally confusing. The implication of 'resistance' implies that tachyphylaxis develops with prolonged use of the drug in a patient who was initially sensitive or responsive. Such 'resistance' or tachyphylaxis to cimetidine has never been documented in situations where secretory drive may be presumed to be relatively constant, i.e. DU. On the other hand, ZES is a progressive condition in which secretory drive increases with growth of the tumor, with increasing G_{17}/G_{34} gastrin species ratio in plasma, and with progressive hyperplasia of parietal cells from the sustained action of gastrin.

Since gastrin potentiates the response to endogenous agonists – e.g. histamine and acetylcholine (Ach) – if follows that no amount of any H_2-blocking drug on its own can totally abolish acid secretion. Gastrin-mediated drive increases with progression of the tumor. Since many species of gastrin are detected by RIA at the same time, there is no way to correlate secretory drive with total serum gastrin. Furthermore, within ZES there are marked interpatient differences making it difficult to pool cases for statistical comparison. Thus, when 'resistant' ZES patients were compared with 'sensitive' ones, there was 'no significant difference' between the groups, but mean BAO was almost twice, and mean serum gastrin about three times, as high in 'resistant' cases [200]. In some cases, drug resistance may be present from diagnosis and may increase gradually with time accompanied by up to 10-fold increases in the plasma concentration of drug needed to cause a 50 percent inhibition (IC_{50}) of BAO. The problem is thus one of altered parietal cell responsiveness and not simply of reduced bioavailability. Patients whose IC_{50} for Cimetidine is raised, all have closely comparable elevations in IC_{50} for Ranitidine or other H_2-blockers. Because of such problems, newer H^+/K^+ ATP-ase inhibitor drugs, e.g. Omeprazole [201], currently on trial, seem far more suited to the long-term therapy of ZES. By acting on the final step, transport of H^+ out of the cell, they avoid all the problems of potentiation and receptor interaction. Data on their long-term safety and efficacy is awaited with great interest.

At the present time, the most widely studied drug is Cimetidine, and this should be used initially in most cases. If the dose required exceeds 2.4 g/day, anticholinergic therapy should be added using a potent long-acting anticholinergic drug. The selective antimuscarinic drug Pirenzepine is the drug of choice and is devoid of many of the side effects of classical anticholinergics. While probably the most useful supplementary agent, Pirenzepine is still investigational in the USA (protocol available from Boehringer-Ingelheim Corp., Ridgefield, CONN). In the absence of Pirenzepine, Isopropamide ('Darbid,' Smith-Kline-French, 1600 Spring Garden, Philadelphia, PA) may be given in doses of 5–20 mg/q8h to good effect [195]. Male patients given Cimetidine in higher dosage over prolonged periods develop gynecomastia, loss of libido, and impotence in a significant proportion of cases [202], but in studies using lower doses this problem has been much less common [21, 93]. Patients developing these side effects should be switched to the more expensive but more potent drug Ranitidine. When the problem of rising dose requirement is encountered, with frequent administration of large amounts of Cimetidine, one can either switch the patient to Ranitidine, increase the dose of anticholinergic, or lower the H_2-blocking requirement by performing a proximal gastric vagotomy (PGV) [203, 204]. The comparative potency of Ranitidine in ZES is 2.5–3 times that of Cimetidine [193], and in many cases the drug can be given twice or three times daily, simplifying therapy and improving compliance. However, its long-term safety or the risks of other side effects are not well established. Ranitidine requirements also rise with time in some cases [192], and Ranitidine 'failures' have also been reported rarely [205]. When patients unsuited to medical therapy from the beginning are combined with those who later fail on therapy, it seems that about two-thirds of ZES patients can be managed medically for at least 5–8 years; no follow-up data are available beyond this point. When unsuitable cases are excluded, the failure rate due to lack of acceptable pharmacological control appears to be about 15–20 percent. This figure is likely to decline with the development of a number of new drugs which include several new H_2-blockers, synthetic prostaglandins, substituted benzimidazoles, somatostatin analogs, carbonic anhydrase inhibitors, and competitive inhibitors of gastrin. A review of all these is beyond the scope of the present work.

8.2.3 *Surgical management.* The role of surgery in ZES has received much attention in recent years [16, 93, 95, 96, 145, 182, 186, 191, 198, 199, 205]. The development of this debate has been made possible by the availability of medical therapy far more effective than that which existed from 1955–65 when initial surgical policy was defined. More recently, the emergence of new diagnostic technology, such as CT-scanning, PTPVS, grey scale and now intraoperative ultrasound, is continuing to improve the surgeon's chance of finding gastrinoma at surgery. Hormone assays, angiography, and other preoperative assessments are frequently able to demonstrate the presence or probable presence of metastases prior to exploration of the patient. All of these developments have greatly increased the data base available for decisions in each patient and have highlighted the need for flexibility in serving the needs of the individual. Today, no one solution is universally applicable in ZES. Total gastrectomy is needed in a minority of cases irrespective of the presence or absence of metastases, and should certainly be combined with local excision of tumor whenever possible. Children have done especially well with this approach [206]. However, the need for total gastrectomy appears overstated in some [96, 145, 191, 198] but not all [93, 182, 187, 199] surgical circles. This derives partly from preselection of cases but perhaps also from less willingness on the part of some surgeons to undertake the close monitoring of drug dosage and drug responsiveness necessary for the success of medical therapy. The recent study from the Mayo Clinic [93] found that 44 of 53 patients were fit for surgery and were explored but that no gastrectomies had been performed since 1976.

This contemporary study shows several additional important points. First, the general condition of these patients seemed to be much better than that of patients included in the first U.S. Cimetidine study [21] which probably preselected poor surgical candidates. Secondly, the purpose of surgery in all cases since 1976 was to attempt curative excision of gastrinoma whenever possible and not routinely to excise the stomach. Third, if patients with MEN-I were included, surgical 'cure' rate among those explored was about 20 percent, as judged by normalization of serum gastrin post-operatively, and negative secretin challenge tests. Similar, secretin-negative 'cures' have now been reported from several other centers. The frequency with which apparent 'cure' is achieved continues to be low except in the case of duodenal wall tumors which accounted for 5 of the 7 'cures' in the Mayo Clinic series. In general, duodenal wall tumors account for between 6 and 23 percent of all tumors found at surgery [16] with approximately half of them free of metastases and curatively resectable [95]. In the various surgical series reported since 1975, overall apparent 'cure' rates, from excision of gastrinoma from all sites (follow-up <5 years in most), have been 10 of 23 [187], 2 of 7 [190], 2 of 8 [94], 7 of 44 [93], 1 of 34 [53], 3 of 27 [145], 4 of 69 [15]. When these figures are combined, 29/202 or 14 percent appear cured. From theoretical considerations, this figure can probably not exceed 20 percent [15]. Seven additional cures have been reported [59, 207] without definition of the sample size from which they were drawn. A reasonable expectation of patient 'cure' by surgery thus appears to be about 1 in 6 for all tumor sites and about 1 in 2 for duodenal wall tumors. Beyond 'cure,' the data of Zollinger et al. [182] suggest that removal of all resectable tumor, performable in about 50 percent of cases and often combined with gastrectomy, prolongs life expectancy by over 6 years. Finally, several series have suggested that surgical failure to find tumor is associated with a particularly good prognosis [54, 93].

Not addressed separately in most of these papers is the surgical prognosis in MEN-I patients. Although these patients seem to have a lower incidence of malignancy, they appear more likely to have multiple small tumors which are often hard to find on exploration. When located, removal of tumor is rarely followed by 'cure', and at least two centers are abandoning pancreatic surgery in MEN-I [93, 94]. Against this, overall surgical results from other centers, where MEN-I patients are repeatedly explored for local excision of pancreatic and other tumors [19, 36, 38], are among the best in the literature [187]. These patients are subjected to prolonged follow-up and careful monitoring with serum gastrin, hPP, and secretin tests, and re-explored aggressively when there is evidence either that previous surgical removal was incomplete or that a new tumor has developed. Whether or not MEN-I patients need total gastrectomy more frequently than other ZES patients remains controversial [198]. Personal experience suggests that their disease is easily managed provided that their parathyroid function is tightly controlled [197]. In my opinion, there are simply not enough data on MEN-I patients treated and analyzed as a separate group for a clear policy to be developed at this time. While they should theoretically be 'cured' in most cases by total excision of the pancreas and adjacent duodenum, the morbidity and mortality attending this policy appears unacceptably high to most surgeons. Repeated enucleation of tumors as detected during careful screening [19] may be the better approach.

A final surgical question surrounds the use of 'Highly Selective,' 'Parietal Cell,' or 'Proximal Gastric' vagotomy (PGV) in ZES patients. There are initial reports that this operation markedly lowers both BAO and PAO in ZES patients who have no other surgical procedure [203, 204]. PGV also renders the patients much more easily controlled with H_2-blockers, such as Cimetidine, and none of the vagotomized cases require more than 3.0 gm/day for control in contrast to the much higher doses required in some non-vagotomized patients [202]. While vagotomy may not prevent the ultimate development of 'resistance' to H_2-blockers [191] due to progressive increase of gastrin-mediated potentiation of acid secretion, it presumably delays for many years the need for high doses of drugs or gastrectomy, and allows much additional time for the localization and excision of gastrinoma and the development of better drug therapy. Surgical concerns that PGV may lead to esophageal reflux or make subsequent total gastrectomy very difficult, have limited its acceptance in some centers. Furthermore, there are some anecdotal reports of cases in which the operation did not lower BAO or the patient's required dose of H_2-blocker [191, 199]. For these reasons, results of ongoing, long-term trials of PGV are awaited with great interest.

In summary, if patients who either need, or are totally unfit for, total gastrectomy are treated separately, there are a number of surgical options in the remaining cases especially when patients are young and fit. Excision of gastrinoma offers the only hope of cure, but the chance of cure is small. Tumor removal short of cure significantly prolongs life expectancy [182]. In patients treated medically or solely with total gastrectomy, tumor growth is slow in most cases, with 5–10 year survival rates of 42 percent and 30 percent respectively even in patients with hepatic metastases at the time of diagnosis [208]. PGV may be useful in many patients when tumor is removed, not found, or nonresectable [95], but needs more evaluation. The various management options should be discussed with the patient as the basis of informed consent, and the final decisions should relate to the findings in the individual case. Given these data, it seems likely that many patients will choose to have a diagnostic laparotomy in the hope of cure, and will agree to the surgeon proceeding with more radical operations, including tumor excision, only if cure seems possible.

8.2.4 *Management of metastatic disease.* Patients with tumor involving local peripancreatic nodes, which are excised at surgery, generally do well if the primary tumor is removed and need no special therapy [187]. Most metastatic disease is found in the liver, though more rarely deposits may be found in the lung, bone and other sites. Radiotherapy may be useful in managing lung and bone lesions or in dealing with unresectable primary tumors [209]. For the most part, management problems center around the treatment of metastatic liver disease with chemotherapeutic agents. Many drugs have been tried and not found useful, though much of the information is unpublished. These include Adriamycin, Mitomycin-C, Chlorozotocin, Chromomycin A3, and Methothrexate, used I.V. as single agents, often after more common drugs have failed. The main drugs associated with clinical responses or remissions are Streptozotocin [78, 81, 209–212] and 5-Fluorouracil [134, 213–215] used either singly or in combination [216]. About 30–50 percent of patients show worthwhile responses when these drugs are given I.V. Experience in the treatment of a small number of ZES patients [212, 217] and Verner-Morrison syndrome patients given repeated intra-arterial administration of drug [218], suggests that intra-arterial therapy may be less toxic and more effective, but this has not been shown in controlled trials. Such therapy is facilitated by removal of the primary tumor and adjacent lymph nodes, allowing all the drug to be infused into the hepatic artery. Chemotherapy is most helpful in patients with rapidly growing tumors but often seems of marginal benefit in those with slowly progressive disease.

References

1. Zollinger RM, Ellison EH: Primary peptic ulcerations of the jejunum associated with islet cell tumors. Ann Surg 142: 709–728, 1955.
2. Gregory RA, Tracy HJ, French JM, Sircus W: Extraction of a gastrin-like substance from a pancreatic tumor in case of Zollinger-Ellison Syndrome. Lancet (i): 1045–1048, 1960.
3. Gregory RA, Grossman MI, Tracy HJ, Bentley PH: Nature of gastric secretagogue in Zollinger-Ellison tumors. Lancet (ii): 543–546, 1967.
4. Ellison EH: The ulcerogenic tumor of the pancreas. Surgery 40: 147–170, 1956.
5. Yalow RS, Berson SA: Immunoassay of endogenous plasma insulin in man. J Clin Invest 89, 1157–1175, 1960.
6. Stremple JF, Meade RC: Production of antibodies to synthetic human gastrin I and radio-immunoassay of gastrin in the serum of patients with the Zollinger-Ellison syndrome. Surgery 64: 165–174, 1968.
7. McGuigan JE, Trudeau WL: Immunochemical measurements of elevated levels of gastrin in the serum of patients with pancreatic tumors of the Zollinger-Ellison variety. N Engl J Med 278: 1038–1042, 1968.
8. Wilson SD: Ulcerogenic tumors of the pancreas: The Zollinger-Ellison syndrome. In: The Pancreas, Carey LC (ed). St. Louis: C.V. Mosby Co., 1973, pp 295–218.
9. Ellison EH, Wilson SD: The Zollinger-Ellison syndrome updated. Surg Clin N Amer 47(5): 115–1124, 1967.
10. Isenberg JI, Walsh JH, Grossman MI: Zollinger-Ellison syndrome. Gastroenterol 65: 140–164, 1973.
11. Ellison EE, Wilson SD: The Zollinger-Ellison syndrome: Reappraisal and evaluation of 260 registered cases. Ann Surg 160(3): 512–530, 1964.
12. Fox PS, Hoffman JW, DeCosse JJ, Wilson SD: The influence of total gastrectomy on survival in malignant Zollinger-Ellison tumors. Ann Surg 180: 558–566, 1974.
13. Friesen SR: The Zollinger-Ellison syndrome. In: Current Problems in Surgery, Ravitch MM (ed). Chicago: Year Book Medical, 1972, pp 1–52.
14. Regan PT, Malagelada JR: A reappraisal of clinical, roentgenographic and endoscopic features of the Zollinger-Ellison syndrome. Mayo Clin Proc 53: 19–23, 1978.
15. Deveney CW, Deveney KS, Way LW: The Zollinger-Ellison syndrome – 23 years later. Ann Surg 188: 384–393, 1978.
16. Jensen RT, moderator: Zollinger-Ellison syndrome: Curret concepts and management. Ann Int Med 98: 59–75, 1983.

17. Fang M, Ginsberg AL, Glassman L, McCarthy DM, Cohen P, Geelhoed G, Dobbins WO: Zollinger-Ellison syndrome with diarrhea as the predominant clinical feature. Gastroenterol 76(2): 378–387, 1979.

18. Lamers CB, Buis JT, Van Tongeren JH: Secretin-stimulated serum gastrin levels in hyperparathyroid patients from families with multiple endocrine adenomatosis – type I. Ann Int Med 86: 719–724, 1977.

19. Friesen SR, Kimmel JR, Tomita T: Pancreatic polypeptide as a screening marker for pancreatic polypeptide tumors in multiple endocrinopathies. Am J Surg 139: 61–72, 1980.

20. Rambaud JC, Matuchansky C: Diarrhea in digestive endocrine tumors. Clin Gastroenterol 3: 657–669, 1974.

21. McCarthy DM: Report on the U.S. experience with Cimetidine in Zollinger-Ellison syndrome and other hypersecretory states. Gastroenterol 74: 453–458, 1978.

22. Richter JE, Pandol SJ, Castell DO, McCarthy DM: Esophageal abnormalities in the Zollinger-Ellison syndrome. Ann Int Med 95: 47–43, 1981.

23. Dubois A, Van Eerdewegh P, Gardner JD: Gastric emptying and secretion in the Zollinger-Ellison syndrome. J Clin Invest 59:255–263, 1977.

24. Dubois A, McCarthy DM. Cholinergic influence on gastric emptying in the Zollinger-Ellison syndrome. Gastroenterol 80: 1139, 1981.

25. Harrison A, Ippoliti A, Cullison R: Rapid gastric emptying in Zollinger-Ellison syndrome (ZES). Gastroenterol 78:1180, 1980.

26. Kaplan EL, Peskin GW, Deveney C, Way L, Jaffe B: Ulcer disease, metabolic alkalosis, and hyperparathyroidism: A mechanism of interrelationship? Ann Surg 180(4): 549–557, 1974.

27. Axelrod L: Case Records of the Massachusetts General Hospital – Case 47–1974. N Engl J Med 291: 1179–1186, 1974.

28. Mommens JP, Limet R, Vosse-Matague G, Heynem G, Franchimont P, Epstein S, Honore D: Role of calcitonin in the Zollinger-Ellison syndrome combined with hyperparathyroidism. Acta Chir Belg 75: 606–611, 1976.

29. Lamers CB, Stadil F, Van Tongeren JH: Prevalence of endocrine abnormalities in patients with the Zollinger-Ellison syndrome and their families. Am J Med 64: 607–612, 1978.

30. Betts JB, O'Malley BP, Rosenthal FB: Hyperparathyroidism: A prerequisite for Zollinger-Ellison syndrome in MEA-I: Report of the further family and a review of the literature. Quart J Med Ns XLIX 193: 69–76, 1980.

31. Ballard HS, Frame B, Hartsock RJ: Familial multiple endocrine adenoma-peptide ulcer complex. Medicine (Baltimore) 43: 481–516, 1964.

32. Friesen SR: A gastric factor in the pathogenesis of Zollinger-Ellison syndrome. Ann Surg 168: 483–501, 1968.

33. Friesen SR, Bolinger RE, Pearse AGE, McGuigan JE: Serum gastrin levels in malignant Zollinger-Ellison syndrome after total gastrectomy and hypophysectomy. Ann Surg 172: 504–521, 1970.

34. Solcia E, Capello C, Buffa R, Usellini L, Frigerio B, Fontana P: Endocrine cells of the gastrointestinal tract and related tumors. Pathobiology Annual 9: 163–204, 1979.

35. Larsson LI: Pathology of gastrointestinal endocrine cells. Scand J Gastroent 14 (supp. 53): 1–8, 1979.

36. Friesen SR: Tumors of the endocrine pancreas. N Engl J Med 306: 58–590, 1982.

37. Vance JE, Stoll RW, Kitabchi AE, Buchanan KD, Hollander D, Williams RH: Familial nesidioblastosis as the predominant manifestation of multiple endocrine adenomatosis. Am J Med 52: 211–227, 1972.

38. Friesen SR: The development of endocrinopathies in the prospective screening of two families with MEA-I. World J Surg 3: 753–764, 1979.

39. Creutzfeldt W, Arnold R, Creutzfeldt C, Track N: Pathomorphologic, biochemical, and diagnostic aspects of gastrinomas. Human Pathol 6: 47–75, 1975.

40. Solcia E, Capella C, Buffa R, Frigerio B, Fiocca R: Pathology of the Zollinger-Ellison syndrome. Prog in Surg Path 1: 119–133, 1980.
41. Solcia E, Capello C, Buffa R, Frigerio B, Sessa F, Tenti T: Histopathology and cytology of gastroenteropancreatic endocrine tumors. In: Diagnosis and Treatment of Upper Gastrointestinal Tumors. Amsterdam – Oxford: Excerpta Media – Elsevier North Holland, Princeton, International Congress Series, 1980, pp 32–51.
42. Newsome HH: Multiple endocrine adenomatosis. Surg Clin N Amer 54(2): 389–393, 1974.
43. Driesen SR, Schimke RN, Pearse AGE: Genetic aspects of Z-E syndrome: Prospective studies in two kindreds: Antral gastrin cell hyperplasia. Ann Surg 176:370–383, 1972.
44. Creutzfeldt WR, Arnold C, Creutzfeldt C, Feurle G, Kelterer H: Gastrin and G-cells in the antral mucosa of patients with pernicious anemia, acromegaly, and hyperparathyroidism and in a Zollinger-Ellison tumor of the pancreas. Euro J Clin Invest 1: 461–479, 1971.
45. Polak JM, Bussolati G, Pearse AGE: Cytochemical, immunofluorescence and ultrastructural investigations of the antral G-cells in hyperparathyroidism. Virchows Archives, ABT B Zelipath 9: 187–197, 1971.
46. Polak JM, Stagg B, Pearse AGE: Two types of Zollinger-Ellison syndrome: Immunofluorescent, cytochemical and ultrastructural studies of the antral and pancreatic gastrin cells in different clinical states. Gut 13: 501–512, 1972.
47. McCarthy DM: Zollinger-Ellison syndrome. Annual Review of Medicine 33: 197–215, 1982.
48. Haverback BJ, Dyce BJ: Gastrins, multiple endocrine adenomatous and the Zollinger-Ellison syndrome. Annal NY Acta Sci 230: 297–305, 1974.
49. Sporrong B, Alumets J, Clase L, Falkmer S, Hakanson R, Ljungberg O, Sundler F: Neurohormonal peptide immuno-reactive cells in mucous cystadenomas and cystadenocarcinomas of the ovary. Virchows Archives (Pathol Anat.) 392: 271–280, 1981.
50. Hattori M, Imura H, Matsukura S, Yoshimoto Y, Sekita K, Tomomatsu T, Kyogoku M, Kameya T: Multiple-hormone producing lung carcinoma. Cancer 43: 2429–2437, 1979.
51. Hoffman JW, Fox PS, Wilson SD: Duodenal wall tumors and the Zollinger-Ellison syndrome. Arch Surg 107: 334–339, 1973.
52. Regan PT, Malagelada JR: A reappraisal of clinical roentgenographic and endoscopic features of the Zollinger-Ellison syndrome. Mayo Clin Proc 53: 19–23, 1978.
53. Stage JG, Stadil F: The clinical diagnosis of Zollinger-Ellison syndrome. Scan J Gastroent 14 (supp. 53): 79–91, 1979.
54. Bonfils S, Landor JH, Mignon M, Hervoir R: Results of surgical management of 92 consecutive patients with Zollinger-Ellison syndrome. Annal Surg 194(6): 692–697, 1981.
55. Lamers CBH, Van Tongeren JHM: Comparative study of the value of the calcium, secretin and meal-stimulated increase in serum gastrin to the diagnosis of the Zollinger-Ellison syndrome. Gut 18: 128–134, 1977.
56. Malagelada JR: Pathophysiological responses to meals in the Zollinger-Ellison syndrome: 1. Paradoxical postprandial inhibition of gastric secretion. But 19: 284–289, 1978.
57. Basso N, Lezoche E, Materia A, Passaro E, Speranza V: Studies with bombesin in Zollinger-Ellison syndrome. Brit J Surg 68: 97–100, 1981.
58. Sircus W: Vagotomy in Z.E. syndrome. Gastroenterol 79: 607–608, 1979.
59. Wolfe MM, Alexander RW, McGuigan JE: Extrapancreatic, extraintestinal gastrinoma. N Engl J Med 306: 1533–1536, 1982.
60. Ratzenhoffer M: Lokalisation, morphologie, und biologie der desseminierten endokrinen zeller des verdauungstraktes. Z Int Med 26: 21–29, 1971.
61. Bernades P, Bonneford A, Martin E, Bonfils S: Syndrome de Zollinger-Ellison avec tumeur endocrine carcinoide insulaire de siege vesciculaire primitif. Arch Fr Mal App Dig 61: 759–766, 1972.
62. Cocco AE, Conway SJ: Zollinger-Ellison syndrome associated with ovarian mucinous cystadenocarcinoma. N Engl J Med 293: 485–486, 1975.

63. Long TT III, Barton TK, Draffin R, Reeves WJ, McCarty KS: Conservative management of Zollinger-Ellison syndrome: Ectopic gastrin production by ovarian cystadenoma. JAMA 243: 1837–1839, 1980.

64. Julkunen R, Partanen S, Salaspuro M: Gastrin-producing ovarian mucinous cystadenoma. J Clin Gastroenterol 5: 67–70, 1983.

65. Stremple JF, Watson CG: Serum calcium, serum gastrin, and gastric acid secretion before and after parathyroidectomy for hyperparathyroidism. Surgery 75: 841–852, 1974.

66. Bartow SA, Mukai K, Rosai J: Pseudoneoplastic proliferation of endocrine cells in pancreatic fibrosis. Cancer 47: 2627–2633, 1981.

67. Mihas AA, Ceballos R, Mihas A, Gibson RG: Zollinger-Ellison syndrome associated with ductal adenocarcinoma of the pancreas. N Engl J Med 298: 144–146, 1978.

68. Hammar S, Sales G: Multiple hormone-producing islet-cell carcinomas of the pancreas: A morphological and biochemical investigation. Human Pathol 6: 349–362, 1975.

69. Sheiber W: Insulin-producing Zollinger-Ellison syndrome. Surgery 54: 448–450, 1963.

70. Bozmyski EM, Woodruff K, Sessions JT: Zollinger-Ellison syndrome with hypoglycemia associated with calcification of the tumor and its metastases. Gastroenterology 65: 658–661, 1973.

71. Meador CK, Liddle GW, Island DR, Nicholson EW, Lucas CP, Nucton JP, Luetscher JA: Causes of Cushing's syndrome in patients with tumors arising from non-endocrine tissues. J Clin Endocrinol Metab 22: 693–701, 1962.

72. Shimizu N, Ogata E, Nicholson EW, Island DP, Ivey RL, Liddle GW: Studies on the melanotropic activity of human plasma and tissues. J Clin Endocrinol Metab 25: 984–990, 1965.

73. Walter RM, Ensinck JW, Ricketts H: Insulin and ACTH production by a streptozotocin responsive islet-cell carcinoma. Am J Med 55: 667–670.

74. Graham DY, Johnson CD, Benflit PS: Islet cell carcinoma, pancreatic cholera and vasoactive intestinal peptide. Ann Int Med 83: 782–785, 1975.

75. Van Der Sluys Veer JS, Chonfoer JC, Wurtifo S, Van Der Heul RO, Hollander CF, Van Rijssel TG: Metastasizing islet cell tumor of the pancreas associated with hypoglycemia and the carcinoid syndrome. Lancet (i), 1416–1418, 1964.

76. Judge DM, Demers LM, Nahrwold DL: Vasoactive intestinal polypeptide and gastrin-producing islet cell carcinoma. Arch Pathol Lab Med 101: 262–265, 1977.

77. Bloom SR, West AM, Polak JM: New view of pancreatic endocrine tumors. Gut 18: 983, 1977.

78. Broder LE, Carter SK: Pancreatic islet cell carcinoma: I – Clinical features of 52 patients. Ann Int Med 79: 108–118, 1973.

79. Soergel KH: Hormonally mediated diarrhea. N Engl J Med 292: 970–972, 1975.

80. Law DH, Liddle GW, Scott WH, Tauber SD: Ectopic production of multiple hormones (ACTH, MSH and gastrin) by a single malignant tumor. N Engl J Med 273: 393, 395, 1965.

81. Murray Lyon IM, Cassar J, Coulson RC, Williams, R, Ganguli PC, Edwards JC, Taylor KW: Treatment of multiple hormonal producing malignant islet cell tumor with streptozotocin. Lancet 2: 895–898, 1968.

82. Vance JE, Kitabchi AE, Buchanan KD, Stoll RW, Hollander D, Wood FC: Hypersecretion of insulin, glucagon and gastrin in a kindred with MEA. Diabetes 17: 299–210, 1968.

83. Block MA, Kelly AR, Aorn RC: Elevation of multiple hormonal substaces in Zollinger-Ellison syndrome. Arch Surg 98: 734–738, 1969.

84. Broor SL, Soergel KH, Garancis JC, Wilson SD: Hormonal producing pancreatic islet cell carcinoma: Changing clinical presentation. Am J Med Sciences 273(3): 229–233, 1979.

85. Hayes JR, Ardill J, Kennedy TL: Stimulation of gastrin release by catecholamines. Lancet (1): 819–821, 1972.

86. Capella C, Polak JM, Timson CM, Frigerio B, Solcia E: Gastric carcinoids of argyrophil ECL cells. Ultra-structural Pathology 1: 411–418, 1980.

87. McGuigan JE, Trudeau WL: Serum and tissue gastrin concentrations in patients with car-

cinoma of the stomach. Gastroenterology 64: 22–25, 1973.

88. Wermer P: Endocrine adenomatosis and peptic ulcer in a large kindred: Inherited multiple tumors and mosaic pleiotropism in man. Am J Med 35: 205–212, 1963.

89. Vance JE, Stoll RW, Kitabchi AE, Williams RH, Wood FC: Nesiodioblastosis in familial endocrine adenomatosis. JAMA 207: 1679–1682, 1969.

90. Russo A, Buffa R, Grasso G, Giannone G, Sanfilippo G, Sessa F, Solcia E: Gastric carcinoma and diffuse G-cell hyperplasia associated with chronic atrophic gastritis. Digestion 20: 416–419, 1980.

91. Grimelius L, Johansson H, Lundquist G, Olazabal A, Polak JH, Pearse AGE: The parathyroid glands in experimentally induced hypergastrinemia in the rat. Scand J Gastro 12: 739–744, 1977.

92. Johnson GJ, Summerskill WHJ, Anderson VE: Clinical and genetic investigation of a large kindred with multiple endocrine adenomatosis. N Engl J Med 277: 1379–1385, 1967.

93. Malagelada JR, Edis AJ, Adson MA, Van Heerden JA, Go VLW: Medical and surgical options in the management of patients with gastrinoma. Gastroenterol 94: 1524–1532, 1983.

94. Glowniak JV, Shapiro B, Vinik AI: Percutaneous transhepatic venous sampling of gastrin. N Engl J Med 307: 293–297, 1983.

95. McCarthy DM: The place of surgery in the Zollinger-Ellison syndrome. N Engl J Med 302: 344–348 and 942–943, 1980.

96. Passaro EP, Stabile BE: Of gastrinomas and their management. Gastroenterol 84: 1621–1623, 1983.

97. Orci L, Malaisse-Lagae F, Baltens D, Perrelet A: Pancreatic polypeptide-rich regions in human pancreas. Lancet ii:1200–1201, 1978.

98. Rahier J, Wallon J, Gepts W, Haot J: Localization of pancreatic polypeptide cells in a limited lobe of the human neonate pancreas: Remnant of the ventral primordium? Cell Tissue Res 200: 359–366, 1979.

99. Bommer G, Friedl U, Heitz Ph.U., Kloppel G: Pancreatic PP-cell distribution and hyperplasia. Virchows Arch A 387: 319, 1980.

100. Bloodworth JMB, Elliott DW: The histochemistry of pancreatic islet cell lesions. J Am Med Assoc 183: 1011–1015, 1963.

101. Pearse AGE, Polak JM, Bloom SR: The newer gut hormones, cellular sources, physiology, pathology and clinical aspects. Gastroenterol 72: 746–761, 1977.

102. Boquist L, Edstrom C: Ultrastructure of pancreatic acinar and islet parenchyma in rats at various intervals after duct ligation. Virchows Arch A 349: 69–79, 1970.

103. Larsson LI: Two distinct types of islet abnormalities associated with endocrine pancreatic tumors. Virchows Arch A 376: 209, 219, 1977.

104. Kloppel G, Bommer G, Commandeur G, Heitz P: The endocrine pancreas in chronic pancreatitis: Immunocytochemical and ultrastructural studies. Virchows Arch A 357: 157–174, 1977–78.

105 Holland E, Giron B, Lehy T, Accary JP, Roze MD: *In vitro* secretion of gastrin, insulin, and glucagon in tissue cultures of pancreas from a child with neonatal, intractable hypoglycemia. Gastroenterol 71: 255–262, 1976.

106. Larsson LI, Rehfeld JF, Gottermann N: Gastrin in the human fetus. Distribution and molecular forms of gastrin in the antropyloric gland area, duodenum, and pancreas. Scand J Gastroent 12: 869–872, 1977.

107. Larsson LI, Ljungberg O, Sundler F: Antropyloric gastrinoma associated with pancreatic nesidioblastosis and proliferation of islets. Virchows Arch (Pathol Anat) 360: 305–314, 1973.

108. Royston CMS, Brew DSJ, Garrham JR, Staff BH, Polak J: The Zollinger-Ellison syndrome due to an infiltrating tumor of the stomach. Gut 13: 638–642, 1972.

109. Laidlaw GF: Nesidioblastoma, the islet cell tumor of the pancreas. Am J Path 14: 125–134, 1938.

110. Johnson JA, Fabri PJ, Lott JA: Serum gastrins in Zollinger- Ellison syndrome – identification of localized disease. Clin Chem 26: 867–970, 1980.

111. Fabri PJ, Johnson JA, Ellison EC: Prediction of progressive disease in Zollinger-Ellison syndrome – comparison of available preoperative tests. Surg Research 31: 93–97, 1981.

112. McCarthy DM, Weintraub B, Rosen S: Subunits of human chorionic gonadotropin in the Zollinger-Ellison syndrome. Gastroenterol 76: 1198, 1979.

113. Stabile BE, Braunstein G, Passaro E: Serum gastrin and human chorionic gonadotropin in the Zollinger-Ellison syndrome. Arch Surg 115: 1090–1095, 1980.

114. Gregory RA: A review of some recent developments in the chemistry of the gastrins. Bio-organic Chemistry 8: 497–511, 1979.

115. Rehfeld JF, Schwartz TW, Stadil F: Immunochemical studies on macromolecular gastrins. Evidence that 'big-big gastrins' are artifacts in blood and mucosa but truly present in some large gastrinomas. Gastroenterol 73: 469–477, 1979.

116. Rehfeld JF: COOH-terminally extended endogenous gastrins. Biochem Biophys Res Comm 92: 811–818, 1980.

117. Malagelada JR: Pathophysiological responses to meals in the Zollinger-Ellison syndrome: 2. Gastric emptying and its effect on duodenal function. Gut 21: 98–104, 1980.

118. Strauss E, Greenstein RJ, Yallow RS: Plasma secretin in the management of Cimetidine therapy for Zollinger Ellison syndrome. Lancet (ii): 73–75, 1978.

119. Chey WY, Hamilton DL: Endocrinopathies of the gastrointestinal tract. Curr Concepts Gastroenterol 4: 3–12, 1979.

120. Dreiling DA, Greenstein A: Pancreatic function in patients with Zollinger-Ellison syndrome: Observations concerning acid-bicarbonate secretion ratios. Am J Gastroenterol 58: 66–72, 1972.

121. Jaffe BM, Peskin GW, Kaplan EL: Serum levels of parathyroid hormone in the Zollinger-Ellison syndrome. Surgery 74: 621–625, 1973.

122. Sizemore G, Go VLW, Kaplan EL, Sanzenbacher LJ, Holtermuller KH, Arnaud CD: Relations of calcitonin and gastrin in the Zollinger-Ellison syndrome and medullary carcinoma of the thyroid. N Eng J Med 288: 641–644, 1973.

123. Taylor IL, Walsh JH, Rotter J, Passaro E: Is pancreatic polypeptide a marker for Zollinger-Ellison syndrome? Lancet (i): 845–848, 1978 and (ii): 43–44, 1978.

124. Stabile BE, Passaro E, Carlson HE: Elevated serum prolactin level in the Zollinger-Ellison syndrome. Arch Surg 116: 49–453, 1981.

125. Modlin IM, Jaffe BM, Sank A, Albert D: The early diagnosis of gastrinoma. Ann Surg 196: 512–517, 1982.

126. Malegalada JR, Davis CE, O'Fallon WM, Go VLW: Laboratory diagnosis of gastrinoma. I. A prospective evaluation of gastric analysis and fasting serum gastrin levels. Mayo Clin Proc 57: 211–218, 1982.

127. Malagelada, JR, Glanzman SL, Go VLW: Laboratory studies of gastrinoma. II. A prospective study of gastrin challenge tests. Mayo Clin Proc 57: 219–226, 1982.

128. McGuigan JE, Wolfe MM: Secretin injection test in the diagnosis of gastrinoma. Gastroenterol 79: 1324–1331, 1980.

129. Lamers CB: Clinical usefulness of the secretin provocation test. J Clin Gastroenterol 3: 255–259, 1981.

130. Thompson JC, Reeder DD, Bunchman HH, Becker HD, Brandt EN: Effect of secretin on circulating gastrin. Ann Surg 176: 384–393, 1972.

131. Lamers CBH, Van Tongeren JHM: Serum gastrin response to acute and chronic hypercalcemia in man: Studies on the value of calcium stimulated serum gastrin levels in the diagnosis of Zollinger-Ellison syndrome. Euro J Clin Invest 7: 315–317, 1977.

132. Feurle G, Arnold R, Helmstadter V, Creutzfeldt W: The effect of intravenous theopylline ethylenediamine on serum gastrin concentrations in control subjects and patients with duodenal ulcers and Zollinger-Ellison syndrome. Digestion 14: 227–231, 1976.

133. Hansky J, Soveny C, Korman MG: The effect of glucagon on serum gastrin. Gut 14: 457–461, 1973.

134. Thompson JC, Reeder DD, Villar HV, Fender HR: Natural history and experience with diagnosis and treatment of the Zollinger-Ellison syndrome. Surg Gynecol Obstet 14: 721–739, 1975.

135. Basso N, Lezoche E, Ciri S, Percoco M, Speranza V: Acid and gastrin levels after bombesin and calcium infusion in patients with incomplete antrectomy. Dig Dis 22: 125–128, 1977.

136. Deveney CW, Deveney KS, Jaffe BM, Jones RS, Way LW: Use of calcium and secretin in the diagnosis of gastrinoma. Ann Int Med 87: 680–686, 1977.

137. Ippoliti AF: Zollinger-Ellison syndrome: Provocative diagnostic tests. Ann Int Med 87: 787–788, 1977.

138. Romanus ME, Neal JA, Dilley WG, Leight GS, Linehan WM, Santen RJ, Farndon JR, Jones RS, Wells SA: Comparison of four provocative tests for the diagnosis of gastrinoma. Ann Surg 197: 608–617, 1983.

139. Creutzfeldt W, Arnold R: Endocrinology of duodenal ulcer. Worl J Surg 3: 605–613, 1979.

140. Strauss E, Yalow RS: Differential diagnosis in hyperchlorhydric hypergastrinemia. Gastroenterol 66: 867, 1974.

141. Jansen JBMJ, Lamers CBHW: Effect of changes in serum calcium on secretin-stimulated serum gastrin in patients with Zollinger-Ellison syndrome. Gastroenterol 83: 173–178, 1982.

142. Fox PS, Hoffman JW, DeCosse JJ, Wilson SD: The influence of total gastrectomy on survival in malignant Zollinger-Ellison tumors. Ann Surg 180: 538–566, 1974.

143. Giacobazzi P, Passaro E: Preoperative angiography in the Zollinger-Ellison syndrome. Ann J Surg 126: 74–76, 1973.

144. Mills SR, Doppman JL, Dunnick NR, McCarthy DM: The evaluation of angiography in Zollinger-Ellison syndrome. Radiology 131: 317–320, 1979.

145. Thompson JC, Lewis BG, Weiner I, Townsend CM: The role of surgery in the Zollinger-Ellison syndrome. Ann Surg 197: 594–607, 1983.

146. Damgaard-Petersen K, Stage JG: CT-scanning in patients with Zollinger-Ellison syndrome and carcinoid syndrome. Scan J Gastroent 14 (supp. 53): 117–122, 1979.

147. Dunnick NR, Doppman J, Mills S, McCarthy DM: Computed tomographic appearance of non-beta (or non-insulin producing) pancreatic islet cell tumors. Radiology 135: 117–120, 1980.

148. Hancke S: Localization of hormone-producing gastrointestinal tumors by ultrasonic scanning. Scand J Gastroenterol 14 (suppl. 53): 115–116, 1979.

149. Shawker T, Doppman J, Dunnick NR, McCarthy DM: Ultrasonic investigation of pancreatic islet cell tumors. J Ultrasound in Medicine 1: 193–200, 1982.

150. Sigel B, Coelho JCU, Nyhus LM, Velasco JM, Donohue PM, Wood DK, Spigos DG: Detection of pancreatic tumors by ultrasound during surgery. Arch Surg 117: 1058–1061, 1982.

151. Wu WC, Kengis J, Whalen GE, Schulte WJ, Unger CF, Classen M: Endoscopic localization of a duodenal wall tumor in Zollinger-Ellison syndrome. Gastroenterology 66: 1237–1239, 1974.

152. Otten MH, Bitkenhager JC, Van Blankenstein M: Zollinger-Ellison syndrome treated by endoscopic removal of a duodenal wall gastrinoma. Neth J Med 21: 248–251, 1978.

153. Donovan DC, Dureza R, Jain U: Gastrinoma of the duodenum: Diagnosis by endoscopy. NY State J Med 79: 1766–1768, 1979.

154. Burcharth F, Stage JG, Stadil F, Jensen LI, Fischerman K: Localization of gastrinomas by transhepatic portal catheterization and gastrin assay. Gastroenterol 77: 444–450, 1979.

155. Passaro, E: Localization of pancreatic endocrine tumors by selective portal vein catheterization and radioimmunoassay. Gastroenterol 77: 806–807, 1979.

156. Ingemansson S: Biochemical localization of pancreaticoenteric endocrine tumors. Scand J Gastroenterol 14 (supp. 53): 131–132, 1979.

157. Feurle GE, Helmstadter V, Hoevels J, Wenzel-Herzer G, Klempa I: Wandel von diagnose und therapie beim Zollinger-Ellison syndrom. Dtsch Med Wschr 107: 697–704, 1982.

158. Woodward ER, Robertson C, Fried W: Further studies on the isolated retained gastric antrum. Gastroenterol 32: 868–877, 1957.

159. Scobie BA, McGill DB, Priestly JT, Rovelstad RA: Excluded gastric antrum simulating the Zollinger-Ellison syndrome. Gastroenterol 47: 184–187, 1964.

160. Van Heerden JA, Bernatz PE, Rovelstad RA: The retained gastric antrum. Mayo Clin Proc 46: 25–28, 1971.

161. Strauss E, Yalow RS: Differential diagnosis of hypergastrinemia. In: Gastrointestinal Hormones, Thompson JC (ed). Austin and London. Univ. of Texas Press, 1975, pp 99–113.

162. Pedersen JH, Wille-Jorgensen P: Secretion of gastric acid and serum gastrin following antral exclusion in man. Acta Chir Scand 146: 615–617, 1980.

163. Korman MG, Scott DF, Hansky J, Wilson H: Hypergastrinemia due to an excluded antrum: A proposed method for differentiation from the Zollinger-Ellison syndrome. Aust N Z J Med 3: 266–271, 1972.

164. Webster MW, Barnes EL, Stremple JF: Serum gastrin in the differential diagnosis of recurrent peptic ulceration due to retained gastric antrum. Am J Surg 135: 248–252, 1978.

165. Cortot A, Fleming R, Brown ML, Go VRW, Malagelada JR: Isolated retained antrum: Diagnosis by gastrin challenge tests and radioscintillation scanning. Dig Dis and Sci 26: 748–751, 1981.

166. Speranza V, Basso N, Lezoche E: Effects of bombesin and calcium on serum gastrin levels in patients with retained or excluded antral mucosa. Adv Exp Med Biol 106: 319, 1978.

167. Strauss E, Yalow RS: Differential diagnosis in hyperchlorhydric hypergastrinemia. Gastroenterol 66: 867A, 1974.

168. Sciarretta G, Malguti P, Turba E, Fini A, Verri A, Garagnani B, Cacciari C: Retained gastric antrum syndrome diagnosed by (^{99M}Tc-) pertechnitate scintiphotography in man: Hormonal and radioistopic study of two cases. J Nucl Med 19: 377–380, 1978.

169. Feurle G, Ketter H, Becker HD, Creutzfeldt: Circadian serum gastrin concentrations in control persons and in patients with ulcer disease. Scand J Gastroenterol 7: 177–183, 1972.

170. Sircus W: Gastric secretion in peptic ulcer disease with special reference to the influence of body weight, duration of disease and stenosis. In: The Physiology of Gastric Secretion. Semb LS, Myren J (eds). Oslo Univ. – Williams Wilkins, Baltimore, 1968, pp 581–591.

171. Crean GP, Hogg DF, Ramsay RDE: Hyperplasia of the gastric mucosa produced by duodenal obstruction. Gastroenterol 56: 193–199, 1969.

172. Hughes WS, Snyder N, Hernandez A: Antral gastrin concentration in upper gastrointestinal disease. Am J Dig Dis NS 22: 201–208, 1977.

173. Voillemot N, Potet F, Mary JY, Lewin MJM: Gastrin cell distribution in normal human stomachs and in patients with Zollinger-Ellison syndrome. Gastroenterol 75: 61–65, 1978.

174. Royston CMS, Polak J, Bloom SR, Cooke WM, Russell RC, Pearse AGE, Spencer J, Welbourn RB, Baron JH: G-cell population of the gastric antrum, plasma gastrin and gastric acid secretion in patients with and without duodenal ulcer. Gut 19: 689–698, 1978.

175. Ganguli PC, Polak JM, Pearse AGE, Elder JB, Hegarty M: Antral-gastrin-cell hyperplasia in peptic ulcer disease. Lancet (i): 583–586, 1974.

176. Lam SK, Sircus W: Antral-gastrin-cell hyperplasia in peptic ulcer disease. Lancet (1): 939–940, 1974.

177. Ganguli PC, Elder JB, Polak JM, Pearse AGE: Antral-gastrin-cell hyperplasia in peptic ulcer disease. Lancet (i): 1288–1289, 1974.

178. Hansky J: Antral-gastrin-cell hyperplasia in peptic ulcer disease. Lancet (i): 1344–1345, 1974.

179. Lamers CBH, Ruland CM, Joosten HJM, Verkooyen HCM, Van Tongeren JHM, Rehfeld JF: Hypergastrinemia of antral origin in duodenal ulcer. Dig Dis 23: 998–1002, 1978.

180. Friesen SR, Tomita T: Pseudo-Zollinger-Ellison tumor. Ann Surg 194: 481–493, 1981.

181. Taylor IL, Calam J, Rotter JI, Vaillant C, Samloff MD, Cook A, Simkin E, Dockray GJ: Family studies of hypergastrinemic, hyperpepsinogenemic 1 duodenal ulcer. Annals Int Med 95: 421–425, 1981.

182. Zollinger RM, Ellison C, Fabri PJ, Johnson J, Sparks J, Carey LC: Primary peptic ulcerations

of the jejunum associated with islet cell tumors. Ann Surg 192: 422–430, 1980.

183. Walsh JH, Grossman MI: Gastrin. N Engl J Med 292: 1324–1334 and 1377–1384, 1975.

184. Kirkpatrick PM, Hirschowitz BI: Duodenal ulcer with unexplained marked basal gastric acid hypersecretion. Gastroenterol 79: 4–10, 1980.

185. Clain JE: Diagnosis and management of gastrinoma. Mayo Clin Proc 57: 265–267, 1982.

186. Malagelada JR: Uncertainties in the management of the Zollinger-Ellison syndrome. Gastroenterol 84: 188–189, 1983.

187. Freisen SR: Treatment of Zollinger-Ellison syndrome: A 25-year assessment. Am J Surg 143: 331–338, 1982.

188. Stadil F, Stage JGF: Cimetidine and the Zollinger-Ellison syndrome. In: Cimetidine: The Westminster Hospital Symposium, Waste C, Lance P (eds). Edinburg: Churchill Livingston, 1978, pp 91–104.

189. McCarthy DM, Collins SM, Korman LY, Jensen RT, Gardner JD: Long-term medical therapy in Zollinger-Ellison syndrome. Gastroenterol 80: 1227, 1981.

190. Bonfils S, Mignon M, Gratton J: Cimetidine treatment of acute and chronic Zollinger-Ellison syndrome. World J Surg 3: 587–604, 1979.

191. Deveney C, Stein S, Way LW: Cimetidine in the treatment of Zollinger-Ellison syndrome. Am J Surg 146: 116–123, 1983.

192. Bonfils S, Mignon M, Vallot T, Mayeur S: Use of Ranitidine in the medical treatment of Zollinger-Ellison syndrome. Scand J Gastroenterol 16 (supp. 69): 119–123, 1981.

193. Collen MJ, Howard JM, McArthur KE, Raufman JP, Gardner JD, Jensen RT: Long-term therapy with Ranitidine in patients with Zollinger-Ellison syndrome. Gastroenterol 84: 1127A, 1983.

194. Mignon M, Vallot T, Calmiche JP, Dupas JL, Bonfils S: Interest of a combined anti-secretory treatment, Cimetidine and Pirenzepine in the management of severe forms of Zollinger-Ellison syndrome. Digestion 20: 56–61, 1981.

195. McCarthy DM, Hyman P: Effect of isopropamide on response to oral Cimetidine in patients with Zollinger-Ellison syndrome. Dig Dis and Sci 27: 353–359, 1982.

196. Raufman JP, Collins SM, Pandol SJ, Korman LY, Collen MJ, Cornelius MJ, Feld MK, McCarthy DM, Gardner JD, Jensen RT: Reliability of symptoms in assessing control of gastric acid secretion in patients with Zollinger-Ellison syndrome. Gastroenterol 84: 108–113, 1983.

197. McCarthy DM, Peikin SR, Lopatin RN, Crossley RJ, Harpel HS: H-Receptor antagonists in gastric hypersecretoy states. Excerpta Medica, International Congress Series 443: 153–164, 1978.

198. Stabile BE, Ippoliti AF, Walsh JH, Passaro E: Failure of histamine H_2-receptor antagonist therapy in Zollinger-Ellison syndrome. Am J Surg 145: 17–23, 1983.

199. Brennan MF, Jensen RT, Wesley RA, Doppman JL, McCarthy DM: The role of surgery in patients with Zollinger-Ellison syndrome (ZES) managed medically. Ann Surg 196: 239–245, 1982.

200. Raufman JP, Collen MJ, Howard JM, McArthur KE, Gardner JD, Jensen RT: Decreased parietal cell responsiveness to Cimetidine in some patients with ZES. Gastroenterol 84: 1281A, 1983 (presented more fully at Amer Gastroenterol Assoc, Wash, DC, May 1983).

201. Lamers CBH, Lind T, Moberg S, Jansen JBMJ, Olbe L: Omeprazole in Zollinger-Ellison Syndrome: Effects of a single dose and of long-term treatment in patients resistant to histamine H_2-receptor antagonists. N Engl J Med 310: 758–761, 1984.

202. Jensen RT, Collen MJ, Pandol SJ, Allende HD, Raufmann JP, Bissonnette BM, Duncan WC, Durgin PL, Gillin JC, Gardner JD: Cimetidine-induced impotence and breast changes in patients with gastric hypersecretory states. N. Engl J Med 308: 883–887, 1983.

203. Richardson CT, Feldman M, McClelland RN, Dickerman RM, Kumpuris D, Fordtran JS: Effect of Vagotomy in Zollinger-Ellison syndrome. Gastroenterol 77: 682–686, 1979.

204. Peters MN, Richardson CT, Feldman M, McClelland R, Willeford G, Dickerman R, Fordtran

382

JS: Exploratory laparotomy, vagotomy, and Cimetidine treatment of Zollinger-Ellison syndrome. Gastroenterol 82: 1149, 1982.

205. Bonfils S, Mignon M, Landor J: Management of Zollinger-Ellison syndrome. N Engl J Med 303: 942–943, 1980.

206. Wilson SD: The role of surgery in children with the Zollinger-Ellison syndrome. Surgery 92: 682–692, 1982.

207. Barreras RF, Mack E, Goodfriend T, Damm M: Resection of gastrinoma in the Zollinger-Ellison syndrome. Gastroenterol 82: 953–956, 1982.

208. Fox PS, Hoffman JW, De Cosse JJ, Wilson SD: The influence of total gastrectomy on survival in malignant Zollinger-Ellison tumors. Ann Surg 180: 558–566, 1974.

209. Passaro E, Gordon HE: Malignant gastrinoma following total gastrectomy. Arch Surg 108: 444–448, 1974.

210. Sadoff L, Franklin D: Streptozotocin in the Zollinger-Ellison syndrome. Lancet (ii): 504–505, 1975.

211. Lamers CBH, Van Tongeren JH: Streptozotocin in the Zollinger-Ellison syndrome. Lancet (ii): 1150–1151, 1975.

212. Hayes JR, O'Connell N, O'Neill T, Fenelly JJ, Weir DG. Successful treatment of malignant gastrinoma with streptozotocin. Gut 17:285–288, 1976.

213. Gallitano A, Fransen H, Martin RG: Carcinoma of the pancreas: Results of treatment. Cancer 22: 939–944, 1968.

214. Earle E, Butts D, Hoaglin LL: Metabolically active liver metastases treated by 5-fluorouracil hepatic artery infusion. Cancer 25: 1170–1173, 1970.

215. Massey WH, Fletcher WS, Judkins MP, Dennis DL: Hepatic Artery infusion for metastatic malignancy using percutaneously placed catheters. Am J Surg 121: 160–164, 1971.

216. Moertel CG, Hanley JA, Johnson LA: Streptozotocin alone compared with streptozotocin plus fluorouracil in the treatment of advanced islet cell carcinoma. N Engl J Med 303: 1189–1194, 1980.

217. Stadil F, Stage G, Rehfeld JF, Efsen F, Fischerman K: Treatment of Zollinger-Ellison syndrome with streptozotocin. N Engl J Med 294: 1440–1442, 1976.

218. Kahn CR, Levy AG, Gardner JD, Miller JV, Gorden P, Schein P: Pancreatic cholera: Beneficial effects of treatment with streptozotocin. N Engl J Med 282: 941–943, 1975.

14. The syndrome of multiple endocrine neoplasia type I

J.D. VELDHUIS

1. Introduction

Multiple endocrine tumors can occur in diverse clinical settings and exhibit varied and challenging clinical features. In some cases, the presentation of individual patients with solitary endocrine tumors has prompted the subsequent elucidation of extensive pedigrees which manifest pluriglandular tumors over several generations. Conversely, the prior identification of a kindred with established multiple endocrine tumors has permitted the timely recognition and detection of emerging neoplasms in other family members at genetic risk.

Our understanding of multiple endocrine neoplasia has been enhanced in the past decade. For example, although the nosologic classification of these endocrine neoplasms was initially unambiguous, more recent reports of ostensibly incongruous patterns of glandular involvement suggest a broader overlap between the two principal entities (MEN I and II), which were previously regarded as distinct. Moreover, with increasingly precise biochemical markers of endocrine disease, the screening of affected pedigrees and the longitudinal assessment of affected individuals has been improved substantially. With the advent of effective forms of pharmacologic treatment, surgical intervention can be supplemented with appropriate medical therapy.

In this chapter we will examine the clinical, biochemical and pathological features of multiple endocrine neoplasia type I (MEN I). For this purpose we will review pragmatic aspects of the clinical presentation, biochemical features, and pathological attributes of these tumors. In addition, we will explore some of the unresolved problems in evaluation and management.

2. Historical perspectives

The occurrence of multiple adenomas of endocrine glands in man has been recognized since at least 1903, when Erdheim described a pituitary adenoma associated with parathyroid disease and thyroid nodules in an acromegalic electrician [1]. In 1953, Underdahl, Woolner and Black at the Mayo Clinic reported 8

Santen, R.J. and Manni, A. (eds.), Diagnosis and management of endocrine-related tumors. ISBN 0-89838-636-5.
© 1984, Martinus Nijhoff Publishers, Boston. Printed in the Netherlands.

cases of multiple endocrine tumors, in which the parathyroid glands, pituitary, and pancreatic islets were involved [2]. In addition, these workers reviewed 14 other cases, in which two endocrine glands were affected by adenomas. Affected patients had clinical acromegaly, pathological hyperplasia of the parathyroid glands, and symptomatic hypoglycemia or perforating duodenal-ulcer disease [2]. A year later, Paul Wermer identified genetic aspects of diffuse adenomatosis of endocrine glands, and emphasized the association of pluri-glandular endocrine tumors with ulcer disease in a large kindred [3]. In this study, a father and four daughters were affected with primary hyperparathyroidism. ulcers, hypoglycemia, and chromophobic pituitary adenomas. The subject was sporadically discussed [4] and then further reviewed extensively by Wermer in 1963 [5] and Ballard in 1964 [6], both writers emphasizing the association of familial endocrine tumors with severe peptic ulcer disease [6]. A somewhat enlightened understanding of the pathophysiological basis for the peptic ulcerations had become possible in view of the observations of Robert Zollinger and Edwin Ellison in 1955, who discerned an association between islet-cell tumors and intractable ulcers [7]. The later work of Johnson, Summerskill, Anderson and Keating at the Mayo Clinic in 1967 meticulously described 134 members of a 5-generation family with multiple endocrine adenomas comprising pituitary tumors, hyperparathyroidism and so-called ulcerogenic islet-cell tumors [8]. (Table 1).

Since these pivotal initial observations by various clinical investigators, there has been a progressive expansion in our understanding of multiple endocrine tumor syndromes. This refinement in pathophysiological concepts reflects largely the development of precise radioimmunoassay methodology to detect an increasing variety of peptide hormones produced e.g. by islet cell tumors, as well as the emergence of pharmacologic agents that are effective in the medical therapy of these secretory endocrine tumors. In the remaining sections, we will focus on these recent developments in the concepts of pathophysiology, diagnosis and treatment.

Table 1. Key historical observations in the MEN I syndrome

Year	Author	Observations
1903	Erdheim [1]	Parathyroid and pituitary tumors coexisted in an acromegalic man.
1953	Underdahl *et al.* [2]	Pituitary, parathyroids, and pancreatic islets are involved.
1954	Wermer [3]	Genetic analyses suggest autosomal dominance.
1955	Zollinger & Ellison [7]	Islet-cell tumors are associated with peptic ulcers.
1966–68	Pearse [9, 11]	Neuroectodermal origin of APUD cells suggested.

Corresponding references are given in brackets.

3. Clinical features

3.1 *Nosologic classification*

The common cytochemical characteristics of cells producing polypeptide hormones was enunciated by Pearse in the course of his studies of the properties of thyroid C-cells [9, 10]. These studies initially delineated the neural crest origin of ultimobranchial C-cells, using cytochemical markers such as amines (catecholamines or 5 hydroxytryptamine) or amine precursors (dopamine or 5 hydroxytryptophan), and the functional capacity of tissues to take up amino acids and decarboxylate them [11,12]. The neural ectodermal cells with these characteristics are ubiquitous, notably comprising enterochromaffin cells, thyroidal C-cells, pancreatic islet cells, bronchial epithelium (in its degenerative state, the carcinoid tumor or the oatcell carcinoma), and according to some studies the anterior pituitary gland [13–20]. All of these glands are believed to contain APUD cells, so designated for their capacity for 'amine precursor uptake and decarboxylation'. This concept has provided some unification of the apparently diverse syndrome of multiple endocrine tumors. Thus, dysplasia of derivatives of neural crest cells might produce a constellation of geographically remote individual tumors, connected by their common derivative from rhombencephalic, mesencephalic or spinal neural-crest origins [9–21]. (Table 2).

On the basis of site of pluriglandular endocrine tumors, two predominant syndromes have been described. In so-called multiple endocrine adenomatosis (or neoplasia) type I [MEA I or MEN I], tumors typically involve the pituitary gland, the islet cells of the pancreas, and the parathyroid glands. This pattern of tumor involvement has also been refered to as Wermer's Syndrome [3, 5]. The second major category, namely Sipple's Syndrome or multiple endocrine ade-

Table 2. Classification of MEN syndromes

	Tumors of hyperplasia of:
Type I:	1. Pituitary gland 2. Parathyroid glands 3. Pancreatic islets
Type II (a and b):	1. *Parathyroid glands 2. Thyroidal C-cells 3. Adrenal medulla
Unclassified or 'Overlap' Syndromes:	1. Acromegaly + pheochromocytoma 2. Prolactinoma + aldosteronoma 3. Zollinger-Ellison syndrome + carcinoid tumor 4. Others (see text)

* NOT affected in IIb.

nomas type II, embraces medullary carcinoma of the thyroid in conjunction with pheochromocytoma or carotid body tumors, and parathyroid disease [22]. These two principal syndromes were initially regarded as distinct and separable, but substantial overlap has been recognized more recently. These so-called overlap syndromes are reviewed briefly (vide infra). The remainder and majority of this chapter will focus on the classical MEN I syndrome, emphasizing its varied clinical manifestations and its diverse biochemical features. Some of these comments have been presented in other recent reviews [23–29].

3.2 Spectrum of clinical presentations

Because tumors may develop in the pituitary gland, parathyroid gland, or pancreatic islet cells, patients may present a diverse spectrum of initial manifestations. For example, large pedigrees of patients with multiple endocrine tumors have been discovered after initial presentation of the propositus with primary amenorrhea, nephrolithiasis, duodenal ulcer disease, hypoglycemic symptoms, or acromegaly [23–30]. This heterogeneity of presenting complaints may lead to an under-estimation of the detection and prevalence of familial MEN I, as emphasized by several investigators recently [25, 31–33]. In addition, the varied age of presentation may be confounding, since propositi range in age from the first to the eight decade of life [24–29].

3.2.1 *Pituitary tumors.* Secretory pituitary tumors may be the first manifestation of MEN I, with concurrent or sequential evolution of extrapituitary endocrine neoplasia [24–33]. Approximately 15% of patients with subsequently diagnosed MEN I have presented with pituitary tumors [25, 32]. Moreover, in MEN I kindreds, patients with at least one tumor but no initial evidence for pituitary involvement have approximately a 50% risk of developing intra-sellar tumors subsequently.

Pituitary disease in MEN I typically involves the hypersecretion of prolactin or growth hormone [25, 32, 33]. In the case of hyperprolactinemia, primary or secondary amenorrhea, galactorrhea, or infertility are recognized in the female [33–48] and clinical hypogonadism associated with infertility or impotence is apparent in the male [49, 50]. In some patients, the first indication of pituitary disease can be attributed to mass lesion effects [51], including visual field loss, headaches, ocular nerve paresis, or more rarely pituitary apoplexy [25] (Table 3).

Acromegalic patients from kindreds with documented MEN I do not appear to differ in clinical presentation from patiens with sporadically occuring growth-hormone secreting tumors [25, 32]. Thus, symptoms and signs are attributable to local mass-lesion effects, excessive acral growth, nerve entrapment (e.g. carpal tunnel syndrome), prognathism, hyperhidrosis, night sweats, soft tissue pharyngotracheal obstruction (e.g. sleep apnea), and possibly hypertension, con-

Table 3. Cardinal clinical symptoms and signs in MEN I

Glandular involvement	Hormone secreted	Endocrine symptoms and signs
Pituitary	Prolactin	Galactorrhea, amenorrhea, infertility in women
	Prolactin	Impotence and diminished libido in men. Mass-lesion effects
	Growth hormone	Features of acromegaly: acral growth, hyperhidrosis, carpal-tunnel syndrome, etc.
Parathyroids	Parathormone	Commonly asymptomatic
Pancreas	Insulin	Hypoglycemia-neuropsychiatric presentations
	Gastrin	Zollinger-Ellison syndrome (peptic ulcers, diarrhea)
	Glucagon	Eczymatous dermatitis, stomatitis, etc.
	Vasoactive intestinal peptide	Diarrhea

gestive cardiac failure, or osteoporosis [25]. These observations support the argument that recognition of the MEN syndrome in patients with secretory pituitary tumors may be delayed, because there are no characteristic clinical features of the MEN I-associated pituitary tumors compared with sporadic adenomas. As discussed further under Endocrine Pathology, at present, there is no singular identifying feature histopathologically of MEN I-associated pituitary tumors, although the possibility of diffuse pituitary hyperplasia has been considered in these individuals [25].

Given a patient with hyperprolactinemia or acromegaly, one would wish to know what the patient's risk was for MEN I. Unfortunately, such information is not readily available. On the one hand, surveys of more than 600 patients presenting with suspected or proven prolactinomas have only revealed five or six patients with subsequently demonstrated familial MEN I [25, 33, 38, 42]. On the other hand, the true prevalence of this association may be underestimated because of lack of physician awareness, or infrequent reporting of small pedigrees.

Given a patient with MEN I, what is the exact risk of pituitary tumor? Although such data in patients with established MEN I are not precisely defined, hyperprolactinemia may represent the single most useful biochemical marker. In sporadic 'chromophobic' pituitary tumors, increased serum prolactin concentrations occur in 30–70% of cases [30–35]. Hyperprolactinemia is also commonly present in acromegaly [36, 37]. Thus, serum concentrations of prolactin should be measured in patients from kindreds with known MEN I affecting extrapituitary sites, or whenever intrasellar disease is suspected.

Although in principle anterior pituitary tumors could be also secrete ACTH, beta lipotropin, LH, FSH, or TSH, to the author's knowledge hypersecretion of these polypeptide hormones has not yet been described in kindred with established MEN I. Nonetheless, there is currently no pathogenetic basis for excluding the possibility that patients would manifest hypersecretion of these hormones. Thus, a clinical presentation of Cushing's Syndrome, hyperpigmentation, hypogonadism, apparently functionless pituitary tumors, or hyperthyroidism would point to the need for more detailed evaluation of pituitary secretory status. In summary, patients with MEN I who have pituitary disease generally will manifest biochemical or clinical evidence of prolactin or growth-hormone hypersecretion, but the possibility of hypersecretion of other anterior-pituitary hormones must be considered when clinically indicated.

3.2.2 *Parathyroid disease.* Parathyroid disease is generally regarded as the most common single manifestation of endocrine gland hypersecretion in MEN I [25–32]. In patients with initial hyperparathyroidism, pituitary and/or pancreatic islet disease may be delayed for many years, or appear only in other members of the kindred [25, 52–54]. Thus, the demonstration of familial hyperparathyroidism due to chief-cell hyperplasia requires long-term family surveillance for the emergence of other endocrine tumors. The possibility of other endocrine tumors is particularly suggested by the presence of multiple adenomas or diffuse microscopic hyperplasia in individuals with verified (familial) primary hyperparathyroidism, in whom 5–50% of patients have had MEN I or MEN II [52–56].

The clinical manifestations of parathyroid disease are typically those observed in sporadic cases. Patients may have renal lithiasis, peptic ulcer disease, pancreatitis, osteoporosis and skeletal fractures, disturbances in mental clarity, constipation, anorexia, or other less common clinical manifestations of hypercalcemia [55] (Table 3).

The hallmark of the parathyroid disease in MEN I is multiple gland involvement histopathologically or on gross examination. Thus, for individuals (not in identified MEN I kindred) discovered to have diffuse hyperplasia of the parathyroid glands, there is some need to consider risk of associated or delayed non-parathyroid endocrine tumors [52–56].

3.2.3 *Pancreatic neoplasms.* In MEN I kindred, disease of the panreatic islet cells is recognized in approximately one third of the patients [25]. Conversely, in a review of 1,067 cases of documented islet cell tumors, 4% of patients had MEN I [57]. When pancreatic islet cells are involved in MEN I, the typical products of secretion are gastrin, insulin and more recently recognized, glucagon [58–60]. The clinical presentations corresponding to hypersecretion of these and other polypeptides in MEN I do not appear to differ from those in sporadic cases (*vide infra*, and Table 3).

Hypersecretion of gastrin has been recognized in the classical Zollinger-Ellison syndrome [7, 58–63]. As originally described, this syndrome comprised patients with multiple and refractory ulcerations [7], but more recent clinical observations indicate that there is a wide spectrum of disease severity, with the majority of patients exhibiting symptoms of unifocal duodenal ulcer disease [64,65]. Nonetheless, in some patients with Zollinger-Ellison syndrome, additional symptoms and signs, such as diarrhea, reversible enteropathy (principally malabsorption) and intestinal perforation have been recognized [61–63]. The extent to which some of these patients' tumors secreted multiple enterically active peptides which contributed to additional symptoms has not been completely clarified, although severe diarrhea associated with vasoactive intestinal peptide production has been reported in MEN I (discussed further below).

Since acute elevations in serum calcium concentrations are known to stimulate gastrin release, serum gastrin and calcium concentrations have been evaluated in patients with chronic hypercalcemia associated with primary hyperparathyroidism in MEN I. In general, these studies have indicated that *chronic* elevations in serum calcium are not sufficient to produce pathological hypergastrinemia [66–69]. Moreover, appropriate diagostic procedures (such as secretin infusion, *vide infra*) will generally distinguish patients with underlying Z-E from those with minimally elevated serum gastrin concentrations associated with primary hyperparathyroidism [66–69]. Recently, studies have also indicated that *chronically* elevated serum gastrin levels do not result in hypercalcitoninemia [68], although infusion of pentagastrin is a potent stimulus for calcitonin release acutely. Thus, in MEN I (or II) patients with primary hyperparathyroidism, basal gastrin (and calcitonin) measurements are useful in an initial search for associated gastrinoma (in MEN I) or medullary carcinoma of the thyroid (in MEN II).

Secretion of insulin by beta-cell adenomas is also prevelent in MEN I, and may be the dominant presentation of this syndrome [70–73]. In general, fasting hypoglycemia, late afternoon 'spells', or other neuropsychiatric features may herald the presence of underlying beta-cell hypersecretion. Plurihormonal secretion is also recognized, for example with simultaneous production of gastrin and insulin in some individuals [70, 71, 72]. Thus, clinical manifestations may be complex, including symptoms associated with hypergastrinemia, as well as those attributable to insulin excess.

Most recently, hypersecretion of glucagon has been described, initially sporadically [74–76], and subsequently also in families with MEN I syndrome [77]. Patients with glucagonomas typically have glucose intolerance (although not frank insulin-dependent diabetes mellitus), a characteristic migratory necrolytic erythema, glossitis or stomatitis, anemia and unexplained weight loss [74–77]. A small number of these patients also have diarrhea, vaginitis, and thromboembolic disease. The characteristic eczymatous dermatitis is the clinical hallmark of this syndrome.

Hormonally mediated watery diarrhea sometimes associated with hypokalemia and hypochlorhydria may be caused by multiple islet-cell adenomas in the MEN I syndrome [78–80]. In some cases, high concentrations of vasoactive peptide have been assayed in tumor or plasma, but some of these patients also exhibited increased gastrin concentrations which could contribute to the diarrhea [78, 80].

In summary, one should expect that most or all of the recognized islet-cell peptides could be produced in excess in patients with MEN I. To date, most clinical presentations have emphasized hypersecretion of gastin, insulin, and less often glucagon.

3.3 *Overlap syndromes*

Although the earlier nosological classification of multiple endocrine tumors seemed straight forward, an increasing number of patients have been recognized who share features of MEN I and MEN II. These conditions comprise a growing group of diverse syndromes. Such possible syndromes include acromegaly associated with pheochromocytomas [81], uterine tumors and MEN I [82–84], mediastinal neoplasms (presumptively of carcinoid type [85]), pheochromocytoma and islet cell tumors of the pancreas [86–90], and MEN I or II associated with Cushing's disease [91, 92], or with multiple fibromas and possibly von Recklinghausen's disease [93, 94]. More unusual combinations have included Zollinger-Ellison syndrome with thyroid adenomas, adrenal cortical adenoma and duodenal carcinoid [95]; familial islet cell tumors in von Hippel-Lindau's disease [96]; MEN I with skeletal dyschondroplasia and cutaneous hemangiomas [97], the Maffucci syndrome); MEN I with familial multiple colonic polyps [98, 99]; MEN I and an ovarian thecoma or testicular tumors [100, 101]. Because some of these ostensible syndromes have been described in only single or occasional case reports, the persuasiveness of their integral association with MEN I remains to be established. Nonetheless, such associations underscore the clinical admonition that new clinical symptoms or signs developing in a patient with one or more recognized endocrine tumors requires a consideration of additional co-existent endocrine and non-endocrine neoplasms.

3.4 *Diagnostic approaches*

3.4.1 *General assessment.* Each patient must provide a detailed account of symptoms that could be associated with hyperinsulinism, hypergastrinemia, hypercalcemia, hyperprolactinemia, excess growth-hormone secretion, or the production of other polypeptides and amines. In general, a thorough knowledge of the spectrum of clinical presentations (reviewed in detail in 3.2 Spectrum of clinical presentations) will permit one to undertake this inventory of systemic complaints. The enumeration of significant clinical complaints requires one to proceed with appropriately focused biochemical testing [25]. In other cases, symptoms suggestive of local mass-lesion effects (for example in the sella turcica) make radiographic studies also mandatory [51].

The physical examination in MEN I is not distinctive, in contrast to certain phenotypic features recognized for MEN II [22]. However, in rare individuals, there are stigmata of the underlying disorders e.g. visual field deficit associated with pituitary tumor, galactorrhea in association with prolactin excess, migratory necrolytic erythema in glucagonoma patients, epigastric tenderness related to duodenal ulcer disease, or dehydration attributable to severe diarrhea in gastrin/vasoactive intestinal peptide-secreting islet cell tumors.

3.4.2 *Biochemical.* The salient diagnostic tests are generally biochemical in nature in MEN I [25,26, 29]. Tumors of the pituitary gland are likely to secrete prolactin or growth hormone (or less often TSH, LH, FSH orACTH). Given a history of infertility, amenorrhea, galactorrhea [45–48] or hypogonadism (impotence or diminished libido in a male [49]), a sellar abnormality on skull radiograms, or a history suggesting mass-lesion effects in the region of the pituitary, the physician should measure the serum prolactin concentration [25, 33, 34]. If acromegaly is suspected clinically, serum growth hormone concentrations should also be determined in the fasting state and after oral glucose loading to demonstrate pathological nonsuppression or paradoxical stimulation [1–8, 25, 32]. Increasing experience with serum somatomedin C determinations suggests that this peptide product of growth-hormone action should also be measured in the serum of patients with suspected or proven acromegaly as an estimate of metabolic activity of the disease. In general, unless a pituitary tumor is known to be present, the serum levels of the other anterior pituitary hormones need not be measured. However, whenever a pituitary tumor is recognized, its secretory products should be identified (which will be possible in the majority of pituitary adenomas [25, 32, 34]), and pituitary reserve should be assessed. For this purpose, a measurement of serum thyroid hormone concentrations (e.g. free T_4 index) and an assessment of ACTH-adrenal responsivity (e.g. insulin-induced hypoglycemia) is needed. If the reserve capacity of adrenal glucocorticoid secretion is uncertain prior to a major radiographic (for example, cerebral angiography) or surgical procedure, the patient should receive immediate pre-operative and peri-operative parenteral supplementation with hydrocortisone or its equivalent.

The diagnosis of primary hyperparathyroidism is ordinarily accomplished by the demonstration of increased serum total or ionized calcium concentrations, in the absence of local or metastatic malignant disease, exposure to vitamin D or vitamin A, acute renal failure, or history of granulomatous disease (such as sarcoidosis, berylliosis or histoplasmosis). Radioimmunoassay of circulating parathyroid concentrations can be used to judge the relative 'inappropriateness' of the serum parathyroid level for the corresponding degree of hypercalcemia. Although radioimmunoassay of parathyroid hormone is an imperfect procedure, the demonstration of inappropriate serum concentrations of parathyroid hormone in the presence of sustained hypercalcemia without other disease argues for primary hyperparathyroidism [53–55]. In questionable cases, additional assays of serum, 1,25-dihydroxycholecalciferol, fasting fractional urinary calcium excretion, and urinary nephrogenous cAMP determinations may be required. However, in an otherwise healthy member of a family with established MEN I, the demonstration of sustained elevations in serum calcium concentrations must be regarded as highly suspicious for primary parathyroid disease [25, 53–55].

The presence of islet-cell disease is confirmed biochemically by the demonstration of inappropriate secretion of one or more peptides. In general, significant fasting hyperinsulinemia or hypergastrinemia in the context of corresponding clinical symptomatology provides evidence for insulinoma/β-islet cell hyperplasia, or gastrinoma, respectively [57–69]. When serum concentrations of insulin are only minimally elevated in the fasting rate, an assessment of the insulin/glucose ratio may help demonstrate the inappropriateness of the insulin level. Alternatively, a more prolonged fast with serial serum insulin and glucose determinations performed every 8–12 hours for 72 hours may be necessary [58]. Normal individuals have a progressive and appropriate decline in serum insulin levels as glucose concentrations fall during the fast, but patients with insulinomas typically maintain inappropriate insulin secretion. A 2-hour interval of physical exercise at the end of the fast may help further discriminate the presence of insulinoma, which tends to promote a decline in plasma glucose levels with exercise.

In some patients, the serum concentrations of insulin or gastrin remain in an indeterminate range that is non-diagnostic for islet cell disease. In this circumstance, provocative tests are sometimes helpful to delineate underlying hypersecretion. For example, in the case of suspected gastrinomas, the rapid infusion of secretin can elicit a striking increase in serum gastrin concentrations in individuals with MEN I who harbor pancreatic non-beta islet cell tumors, but not in sibling controls [102–105]. The rapid infusion of calcium also provokes gastrin release within 2–5 minutes in gastrinoma patients. Gastrin levels generally increase ≥ 50% of basal or in excess of 110 pg/ml, in contrast to normal individuals in whom gastrin concentrations decrease or minimally increase in response to calcium or secretin [105–107]. Nonetheless, neither the secretin test nor the calcium infusion may be completely reliable in individuals with active symptomatic peptic ulcer disease, patients who are asymptomatic following surgery for duodenal ulcers [104, 108], or who have retained gastric antrum, pernicious anemia, renal failure, or possibly G-cell hyperplasia [104]. In summary, if basal gastrin concentrations are only moderately increased (100–500 pg/ml), a secretin or calcium infusion test may be helpful to confirm one's clinical impression of Zollinger-Ellison Syndrome due to gastrinoma in MEN I. In the experience of some authors, the occurrence of Zollinger-Ellison syndrome in MEN I is generally associated with co-existant hyperparathyroidism [109], so that a serum calcium concentration should be checked before infusing additional calcium.

In patients with borderline fasting serum insulin concentrations, the rapid infusion of calcium may also discriminate between normal subjects and those with islet-cell tumors. Acute infusion of calcium promotes very minimal insulin release in normal subjects, but a more striking and rapid (within 1–5 minutes) secretion in patients with insulinomas [110–113]. Such testing can be done on an outpatient basis, requiring less than an hour. After calcium infusion and blood sampling, the patient can be fed to avoid delayed hypoglycemia. If the efficacy of this provacative test is additionally confirmed, it may provide a useful and practical approach to the diagnosis and follow-up of beta-cell disease in MEN I.

Other tumor markers have also been suggested to aid in the diagnosis of MEN I. Serum concentrations of pancreatic polypeptide, a 36-amino acid hormone isolated from islet cells, were initially put forward as a useful marker of endocrine pancreatic tumors in families with MEN I [113–118]. However, studies of larger kindreds with MEN I indicate that measurement of serum pancreatic polypeptide levels is an insensitive indicator of endocrine pancreatic tumors [119–120]. Moreover, a variety of other conditions can be associated with apparent elevation in serum pancreatic polypeptide concentrations [119–121]. Thus, despite initial enthusiasm for pancreatic polypeptide as a unique and specific marker for pancreatic tumors in MEN I, this polypeptide cannot be regarded as a diagnostic panacea in this setting.

Islet cell tumors may also secrete peptides other than gastrin and insulin, notably glucagon or vasoactive intestinal peptide. In patients with MEN I who have appropriate clinical manifestations (see Clinical features 3.2.3 Pancreatic neoplasms), serum concentrations of glucagon and vasoactive intestinal polypeptide should be assayed. However, elevated levels of glucagon may occur in an autosomal dominant fashion in asymptomatic individuals [122], and vasoactive intestinal polypeptide secreton may be a reflection of non-islet cell disease in some patients [123]. More recently, radioimmunoassay of human chorionic gonadotropin subunits in peripheral serum has been proposed to identify the presence of pancreatic islet cell disease, which may be malignant, or carry a poorer prognosis [124, 125]. As yet, the value of alpha or beta subunit determinations in the *initial* diagnosis of pancreatic islet cell disease in MEN I kindreds is not certain. Nonetheless, in patients with known islet cell disease, measurements of chorionic gonadotropin subunits may provide an additional marker to evaluate disease progression or response to therapy longitudinally.

3.4.3 *Radiographic approaches.* In patients with pituitary tumors, skull radiographs and computerized axial tomography to search for suprasellar disease (in conjunction with visual field and neurological examinations) are appropriate [25, 51, 126]. If surgery is indicated, additional invasive neuroradiographic studies are usually requested by the neurosurgeon, including arteriography to define vascular anatomy in the region of the sella and pneumoencephalography to exclude the presence of an empty sella.

In general, radiological studies have not been helpful in the initial evaluation of primary hyperparathyroidism, but can be employed in selected patients for whom further localization of residual parathyroid tissue is required after unseccessful primary surgery. The role of computerized axial tomography in neck disease is still uncertain.

Angiographic localization of beta cell and non-beta cell tumors in *sporadic* cases has been generally effective. The radiologist must be familiar with subtle pitfalls in the arteriography of islet cell tumors of the pancreas [127–129]. Unfortunately, the preponderance of experience has to date been obtained in sporadic islet-cell tumors, for which there seems to be a higher probability of isolated tumors. In MEN I, the source of gastrin hypersecretion may be diffuse, so that attempts at discrete localization are of limited value [130, 131]. At present, the value of arteriography in pancreatic islet cell disease associated with MEN I is not known to be the same as in sporadic disease. In addition, further experience is required in pancreatic venous catherization with hormone sampling in MEN I as an alternative localizing procedure. Pancreatic vein sampling has demonstrated a generalized increase in pancreatic secretion of insulin in some patients with islet cell hyperplasia [130], and obviated a need for surgical exploration. Thus, in the author's opinion, computerized axial tomography of the pancreas should be performed first (if ultrasonography is negative) to assess tumor bulk and localization. In selected cases, arteriography may be useful to demostrate highly vascular extra-pancreatic metastases (e.g. in the hepatic bed). Venous sampling may confirm the site(s) of involvement.

4. Endocrine pathology

Knowledge of the spectrum of histopathological changes in pituitary adenomas associated with MEN I is incomplete. Studies from the laboratory of Kovacs have revealed sparsely granulated, prolactin- and growth-hormone secreting adenomas in MEN I patients, but to date no workers have disclosed any unusual or characteristic cyto-architectural features of these tumors [31]. The possibility that specifically prolactin and growth-hormone secreting cells of the anterior pituitary are more prone to neoplastic transformation than other pituitary cell types in the MEN I syndrome has been raised by both clinical observations and histopathological examination [25, 31, 132–134]. As illustrated in Fig. 1, prolactin producing tumors in MEN I tend to be sparsely granulated, containing dense particles that are pleomorphic, and exhibit misplaced exocytosis. These features are also common to sporadically occuring prolactinomas [31, 132–134].

Diffuse hyperplasia of the parathyroid glands is recognized in MEN I, but distinguishing multiple adenomas or microadenomatosis from diffuse hyperplasia can be very difficult on pathological bases [1–8,135]. Moreover, no studies have revealed distinctive histopathophysiological features of hyperparathyroidism associated with MEN I compared with sporadic cases, some of which also exhibit diffuse or multiple glandular involvement.

The gastrin-secreting neoplasms in MEN I vary in structural appearance, with

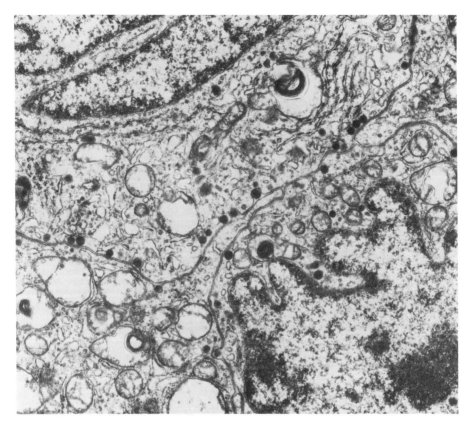

Figure 1. Electron micrograph showing the typical features of sparsely granulated prolactin-cell adenoma in a patient with MEN I syndrome. Note the abundance of rough endoplasmic reticulum and prominence of Golgi apparatus. Magnification ×9,300, reduced by 34 per cent. This patient's pedigree is depicted in Fig. 2.

the majority of cells containing electron-dense granules resembling those of G-cells of the gastric antrum [135]. The presumptively delta cells of pancreatic-islet gastrinomas contain cytoplasmic secretory granules with appropriate immunofluorescent activity against gastrin [136, 137]. In hyperinsulinemic patients with MEN I, beta cells are involved, whereas in glucagonomas, the alpha cell is affected. Specific immunologic stains or assays are required to characterize islet-cell neoplasms precisely, because in many instances, the granules of neoplasms lose their characteristic ultrastructural appearance [135, 137]. Although not rigorously demonstrated to date, one would expect that islet cell disease in patients with MEN I is diffuse or multifocal in nature. This expectation was fulfilled in some familial islet-cell tumors associated with hyperinsulism or hypergastrinemia (71, 73, 131), but not all [70].

5. Treatment

5.1 *Surgical*

Large pituitary tumors with compressive effects are susceptible to initial surgical treatment, followed by appropriate suppressive medical therapy. In the case of prolactin-secreting pituitary tumors, the possibility of preoperative reduction of tumor size through medical therapy should be considered (see part 5.2 below). When pituitary adenomas are relatively small (less than 10 mm) in sporadically occurring cases, trans-sphenoidal microneurosurgery has been effective in apparently curing hypersecretion and preserving anterior pituitary function [35, 45, 51, 138–140]. However, in individuals with MEN I, the long-term follow-up and the prospects of surgical cure by subtotal hypophysectomy (i.e. selective adenomectomy) remain uncertain. At present, there is insufficient experience to claim that the efficacy of surgical treatment of pituitary tumors in MEN I will equal that in sporadically occurring disease. Since other endocrine glands affected in MEN I commonly exhibit multifocal hyperplasia of adenomatosis, the possibility that surgical treatment of pituitary disease would be difficult to cure short of total hypophysectomy must be borne in mind at present [138–140].

Because of the prevalence of diffuse parathyroid hyperplasia and of postoperative recurrent hyperparathyroidism in patients with MEN I, operable hyperparathyroidism requires subtotal ($3^1/_2$ gland) or total parathyroidectomy, preferably with heterotopic autotransplantation into the forearm [141–143]. However, patients with generalized primary parathyroid hyperplasia are still difficult to cure. Moreover the heterotopic graft tissue may also contribute to hyperparathyroidism, but surgical accessibility of this tissue offers advantages over re-exploration of the neck [143, 144]. In view of these difficulties, the intraoperative measurement of urinary cyclic AMP has been suggested as a guide to completeness of parathyroidectomy in patients with primary hyperparathyroidism [145]. At present, surgical management is important because there are no alternative medical therapies available for outpatient treatment of parathyroid disease, and because the risks of sustained hyperparathyroidism include osteoporosis developing overtly or subclinically, and symptomatic hypercalcemia with hypercalcemic crisis [146]. Although the exact natural history of primary hyperparathyroidism in MEN I has not been defined, surgical intervention is appropriate in the presence of hypercalcemic symptoms, osteoporosis, and possibly asymptomatic but progressive hypercalcemia.

Surgical treatment of choice for hypergastrinemic islet cell disease was gastrectomy in the past, but the advent of effective medical therapy has obviated the need for immediate surgery in the Zollinger-Ellison syndrome. The current role of surgery in islet cell hyperplasia associated with hyperinsulinism is also difficult to define. For example, because of the expectation of diffuse pancreatic involvement in gastrinomas or insulinomas in MEN I, surgery would require near total

Table 4. Principal treatment modalities in the MEN I syndrome

1. Surgical	– Principally for pituitary and parathyroid disease
2. Medical	– Bromergocryptine for prolactinomas (and some growth-hormone secreting tumors)
	– Cimetidine to suppress ulcer diathesis associated with gastrinomas
	– Diazoxide to block insulin secretion in β-cell disease.
3. Chemotherapeutic	– Streptozotocin and 5-fluorouracil in islet-cell carcinoma (possibly adriamycin, or mithramycin).

pancreatectomy [147–150]. In contrast, in sporadically occurring cases, 13% of patients with Zollinger-Ellison syndrome have duodenal wall tumors, although only 2.5% of these are surgically curable [147]. Thus, in the author's opinion, there is a very limited role for surgery in islet cell-disease associated with MEN I. A possible exception to this might be the appearance of mass effects attributible to a slowly growning apudoma of the pancreas (see summary in Table 4).

5.2 *Medical*

Medical therapy of endocrine tumors has improved substantially in the last decade. In particular, the advent of potent and orally effective dopamine agonists has permitted effective therapy of pituitary tumors that secrete prolactin, and, to a lesser degree, tumors that secrete growth hormone [151–154]. Therapy with bromergocryptine is effective in suppressing hyperprolactinemia and galactorrhea with consequent restoration of menstrual cycles in the majority of women, and can produce improvement in clinical hypogonadism in men. When large invasive pituitary tumors are present, surgical and radiation therapy are generally indicated, but these modalities can be applied simultaneous with or after initial administration of a dopamine agonist, in an effort to achieve pharmacologically induced tumor shrinkage.

Therapy of the Zollinger-Ellison syndrome has been remarkably improved by the advent of potent and selective H-2 receptor antagonists, such as cimetidine or metiamide [155–157]. The H-2 receptor antagonists provide a compelling alternative to total gastrectomy, and have relatively few side-effects (occasional gynecomastia or liver dysfunction have been described in patients with Zollinger-Ellison syndrome under chronic treatment [156]). In some patients, cimetidine combined with antacid therapy may be required for symptomatic relief. Although cimetidine was considered to affect parathyroid hormone secretion, more recent studies indicate that it does not alter calcium homeostasis in the MEN I patients with primary hyperparathyroidism [158]. The medical therapy of insulin-secreting islet cell tumors comprises diazoxide usually combined with a diuretic benzothiazide [159]. Dilantin, propranolol, and chlorpromazine have been less effective in suppressing insulin hypersecretion.

398

When malignant islet cell disease is present, chemotherapy with streptozotocin plus 5-fluorouracil appears to be valuable with a possible survival advantage [160]. Occasional favorable reports exist for therapy with adriamycin, mithramycin, or streptozotocin [161–165]. Because these tumors secrete peptide products, some assessment of chemotherapeutic response can be obtained by serial measurements of the appropriate secreted hormone (see Diagnostic approaches, 3.4.2 Biochemical detection).

6. Patterns of Heritability

In most studies to date, heritable forms of MEN I partake of an autosomal dominant mode of inheritance, with virtually complete penetrance, but variable expressivity [25,166]. As shown in Fig. 2, large pedigrees with multiple endocrine tumors can be identified. The families exhibit a highly penetrant transmission of risk for glandular tumors. A similar pattern of inheritance of multiple adenomas restricted solely to the beta cells of the pancreas has also been described recently [167]. The relation of the latter condition to MEN I is not clear.

7. Screening for multiple endocrine tumors

In established pedigrees, the determination of serum calcium, prolactin and fasting gastrin concentrations will provide an initial assessment of early endocrine

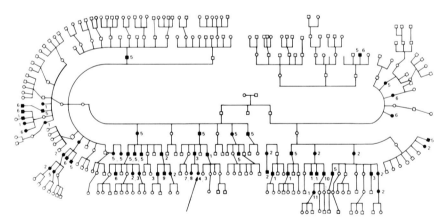

Figure 2. Six-generation kindred affected in an autosomal dominant fashion with tumors of the parathyroids, pancreatic islet cells, and anterior pituitary gland. Arrow designates propositus: (1) 1° HPT; (2) Zollinger-Elllison syndrome; (3) 1° HPT and ZE; (4) prolactinoma; (5) peptic ulcers; (6) renal lithiasis; (7) hypercalcemia; (8) hyperprolactinemia, amenorrhea, galactorrhea, asymmetric sella; (9) Grave's disease; (10) bronchial carcinoid; (11) insulinoma. Reprinted from the American Journal of Medicine with permission by Veldhuis et al. [25] and Technical Publishing.

Table 5. Screening for MEN I

Gland involvement	Test
1. Pituitary	*Prolactin* – growth hormone, if indicated by acromegalic signs or symptoms. – Other anterior pituitary hormones, if clinically suggested.
2. Parathyroid	*Serum calcium* – PTH level if hypercalcemia is present
3. Pancreas	*Serum gastrin* – Fasting serum insulin level if any hypoglycemic symptoms exist. – hCG subunits if malignant disease of the islets is suspected. – Serum glucagon if eczymatous skin lesions are present.

gland involvement in an asymptomatic subject. The relatively uninformative value of serum pancreatic polypeptide levels has been discussed above (Diagnostic approaches: 3.4.2 Biochemical). In individuals with specific symptoms, appropriate laboratory determinations should be made to search for corresponding hypersecretion of one or more peptides. More extensive screening procedures have not yet been validated for their cost: benefit ratios (Table 5).

8. Longitudinal assessment of affected individuals

Affected patients within an MEN I kindred must be followed longitudinally for the evolution of pluriglandular tumors. Symptomatic follow-up in conjunction with perhaps yearly assays of serum calcium, prolactin, and possibly gastrin (and insulin) would provide an initial estimate of progressive endocrine gland involvement. Other tests are pursued in greater detail if focal or specific symptoms evolve.

Unlike kindred with MEN II and medullary carcinoma of the thyroid [168], provocative tests for the early detection of pituitary, parathyroid or pancreatic tumors have not yet been validated in the MEN I syndrome. However, the possibility that acute calcium infusion could be used to identify early pancreatic islet cell disease is being evaluated in several institutions. In MEN I, asymptomatic children below the age of 10 years have endocrine tumors uncommonly, but nesidioblastosis with severe hyperinsulinism occurs sporadically in children [169]. Thus, proper longitudinal evaluation of the time-dependent risk for development of hyperparathyroidism or other endocrine gland hyperplasias in MEN I must be sought. The author believes that any child with symptoms presumptively attributable to endocrine tumors in such pedigrees must have appropriate laboratory tests performed to clarify the etiology of the symptoms.

9. Unresolved problems in evaluation and management

Several significant problems remain in the evaluation and management of MEN I. First, there does not appear to be a single marker that can be used to detect the genetic risk for MEN I within a pedigree. For example, more recent studies of pancreatic polypeptide concentrations reveal that it is not a useful tumor marker [170]. On the other hand, elevated serum prolactin levels in patients with the Zollinger-Ellison syndrome seem to occur more commonly than anticipated [171], but whether all patients with hyperprolactinemia and Zollinger-Ellison syndrome have a partial MEN I syndrome cannot be resolved from available reports. Moreover, prolactinomas and carcinoid tumors in MEN I appear to be associated with certain histocompatiability antigens (HLA haplotypes) at least in some pedigrees [172]. A clear relation to HLA haplotype within pedigrees would provide a useful genetic marker of risk for endocrine tumors.

The pathology of the endocrine tumors in MEN I is not distinctive. Thus, there is an unresolved problem: how does one identify a patient at risk for pluriglandular endocrine tumors, when an individual presents with a single endocrine tumor? In additon, the tendency for diffuse hyperplasia or multiple adenomatoses of the endocrine glands involved in MEN I raises important questions regarding theories of pathogenesis. For example, the possibiliy that certain of these tumors produce multiple releasing factors (such as somatostatin, luteinizing-hormone releasing factor, or growth hormone relasing factor [173–176]) that induce the development of remote tumors has not been thoroughly evaluated.

Long-term therapy in MEN I remains somewhat unclear, because of the limitations of definitive surgical cure in this condition. The safety of chronic medical therapy remains to be fully ascertained. In additon, the most cost-effective means of initial screening and longitudinal assessment of affected individuals must be clarified further.

After surgical therapy, the risk of recurrent endocrine gland hypersecretion is presumed to be increased in the MEN I syndrome, particularly in the case of parathyroid disease. Further follow-up regarding curability and risk of recurrence not only after subtotal parathyroidectomy with autotransplantation but also after pituitary surgery must be evaluated.

10. Summary and Conclusions

MEN I comprises a syndrome of pluriglandular endocrine tumors typically involving the pituitary, parathyroid and pancreatic islets. Because of the diversity of the secreted products, there is a broad spectrum of initial clinical presentations. Moreover, patients presenting with an ostensibly single tumor may have unrecognized concurrent disease in other remote endocrine glands, or may sequentially manifest pluriglandular disease. The highly penetrant autosomal dominant inheritance pattern of MEN I places affected kindreds at high risk. Nonetheless, recent improvements in effective medical (and surgical) therapy permit rational treatment directed at hormonal hypersecretion or target tissue responsivity in the MEN I syndrome.

Acknowledgements

The author gratefully acknowledges the skilled assistance of Maureen Schandert in the preparation of the manuscript. This work was supported in part by NIH Biochemical Research Support Award 5S07RR05431-21.

References

1. Erdheim J: Zur normalen und pathologischen Histologie der Glandula Thyreoides, Para-thyreoides, und Hypophysis Beitrage Path Anat 33: 158–169,1903.
2. Underdahl LO, Woolner LB, Black BM: Multiple endocrine adenomas. Report of 8 cases in which parathyroids, pituitary and pancreatic islets were involved. J Clin Endocrinol Metab 13: 20–29, 1953.
3. Wermer P: Genetic aspects of adenomatosis of endocrine glands. Am J Med 16: 363–371, 1954.
4. Moldawer MP, Nardi GL, Raker JW: Concomitance of multiple adenomas of the parathyroids and pancreatic islets with tumor of the pituitary. A syndrome with familial incidence. Am J Med Sci 228: 190–196, 1954.
5. Wermer P: Endocrine adenomatosis and peptic ulcer in a large kindred. Inherited multiple tumors and mosaic pleiotropism in man. Am J Med 35 (2): 205-212, 1963.
6. Ballard HS, Frame B, Hartsock RJ: Familial multiple endocrine adenoma peptic-ulcer complex. Medicine 43: 381–388, 1964.
7. Zollinger RM, Ellison EH: Primary peptic ulceration of the jejunum associated with islet-cell tumors of the pancreas. Am J Surg 142: 709–713, 1955.
8. Johnson GJ, Summerskill WHJ, Anderson VE, Keating FR: Clinical and genetic investigation of a large kindred with multiple endocrine adenomatosis. N Engl J Med 277: 1330–1335, 1967.
9. Pearse AGE: 5-Hydroxytryptophan uptake by dog thyroid C cells and its possible significance in polypeptide hormone production. Nature (Lond) 211: 588–599, 1966.
10. Pearse AGE: Common cytochemical properties of cells producing polypeptide hormones, with particular reference to calcitonin and the thyroid C cells. Vet Rec 79: 587–590, 1966.
11. Pearse AGE: Common cytochemical and ultrastructural characteristics of cells producing polypeptide hormones (the APUD seried) and their relevance to thyroid and ultimobranchial C cells and calcitonin. Proc Roy Soc B 170: 71–75, 1968.
12. Pearse AGE: The cytochemisty and ultrastructure of polypeptide hormone producing cells (the APUD series) and the embryologic, physiologic and pathologic implications of the concept. J Histochem Cytochem 17: 303–308, 1969.
13. Tischler AS.Dichter MA, Biales B, Greene LA: Neuroendocrine neoplasms and their cells of origin. N Engl J Med 296: 919–925, 1977.
14. Pearse AGE, Polak JM: Cytochemical evidence for the neural crest origin of mammalian ultimobranchial C cells. Histochemie 27: 96–99, 1971.
15. Pearse AGE, Polak JM: Neural crest origin of the endocrine polypeptide (APUD) cells of the gastrointestinal tract and pancreas. Gut 12: 783–787, 1971.

16. Pearse AGE, Polak JM,Rost FWD, et al: Demonstration of the neural crest origin of Type 1 (APUD) cells in the avian carotid body, using a cytochemical marker system. Histochemie 34: 191–197, 1973.

17. Polak JM, Rost FWD, Pearse AGE: Fluorogenic amine tracing of neural crest derivatives forming the adrenal medulla. Gen Comp Endocrinol 16: 132–137, 1971.

18. Polak JM, Stagg B, Pearse AGE: Two types of Zollinger-Ellison syndrome. Immunofluorescent, cytochemical and ultrastructural studies of the antral and pancreatic gastrin cells in different clinical states. Gut 13: 501–504, 1972.

19. Weichert RF: The neural ectodermal origin of the peptide-secreting endocrine glands. Am J Med 49: 233–242, 1970.

20. Case reports of the Massachusetts General Hospital. Weekly Clinocopathological Exercises. N Engl J Med 294 (1): 37–42, 1976.

21. Sziji I, Csapó Z, Lászlo FA, Kovács K: Medullary cancer of the thyroid gland associated with hypercorticism. Cancer 24: 167, 1969.

22. Sipple JH: The association of pheochromocytoma with carcinoma of the thyroid gland. Am J Med 31: 163–175, 1961.

23. Haverback BJ, Dycc BJ: Gastrointestinal cancer syndromes. Gastrins, multiple endocrine adenomatosis, and the Zollinger-Ellison syndrome. Ann NY Acad Sci 230: 297–305, 1976.

24. Schimke FN: Multiple Endocrine Adenomatosis Syndromes. Adv Intern Med 21: 249–265, 1976.

25. Veldhuis JD, Green JE, Kovacs E, Worgul TJ, Murray FT, Hammond JM: Prolactin-secreting pituitary adenomas: association with multiple endocrine neoplasia, Type I. Am J Med 67: 830–837,1979.

26. Harrison RS, Thompson NW: Multiple Endocrine Adenomatosis I and II. Curr Probl Surg 12(8): 1–51, 1975.

27. Bouzaglou A, HerskovicA, Lipsett J, George RW. Sellar tumors with clinical syndromes. Int J Radiat Oncol Biol Phys 2 (Suppl 1): 60–81,1977.

28. Gelston AL, Delisle MB, Patel YC: Multiple endocrine adenomatosis type I. Occurence in an octogenarian with high levels of circulating pancreatic polypeptide. JAMA 247 (5): 665–666, 1982.

29. Newsome HH: Multiple Endocrine Adenomatosis. Surg Clin North Am 54: 387–393,1974.

30. Tournaiaire J, Trouillas J, Maillet P, David L, Pallo D, Minh VT, Bressot C: Polyadenomatose endocrinienne associant un adenome hypophysaire à prolactine et un adenome parathyroidien intrathyroidien. Annales d'Endocrinologie (Paris) 37: 465–466, 1976.

31. Kovacs K, Horvath E, Kerenyi NA: Prolactin cell adenomas associated with the multiple endocrine adenomatosis syndrome. Pathology 5: 466–477, 1977.

32. Crosier JC, Azerad E. Lubetzki J: L'adenomatose polyendocrienne (syndrome de Wermer): a propos d'une observation personnelle. Revue de la littérature. Sem Hop Paris 47: 494–501, 1971.

33. Levine JJ, Sagel J, Rosenbrock GL, et al: Hyperprolactinemia and the MEN I syndrome (editorial). Arch Intern Med 138: 1777–1778, 1978.

34. Franks S, Nabarro JDN, Jacobs HS: Prevalence and presentations of hyperprolactinemia in patients with functionless pituitary tumors. Lancet 1: 778–780, 1977.

35. Friesen H, Tolis G, Shin R, et al: Human Prolactin. In: Excerpta Medica, Pasteels JL, Robyn C (eds). Amsterdam, 1973, pp 11–40.

36. Franks S, Jacobs HS, Nabarro JDN: Prolactin concentrations in patients with acromegaly: clinical significance and response to surgery. Clin Endocrinol (Oxf) 5: 63–67, 1976.

37. Tolis G, Bertrand G, Carpenter S, et al: Acromagaly and galactorrhea-amenorrhea with two pituitary adenomas secreting growth hormone or prolactin. Ann Intern Med 89: 345–348, 1978.

38. Carlson HE, Levine GA, Goldberg NJ, et al: Hyperprolactinemia in multiple endocrine adenomatosis, type I. Arch Intern Med 138: 1807–1810, 1978.

39. Vandeweghe M, Braxel K, Schutyser J, et al: A case of multiple endocrine adenomatosis with primary amenorrhea. Postrad Med J 54: 618–620,1978.

40. Snyder N, Scury MT, Deiss WP: Five families with multiple endocrine adenomatosis. Ann Intern Med 76: 53–58, 1972.

41. Wieland RG, O'Dea JP: Hyperprolactinemia Associated with Familial Multiple Endocrine Neoplasia Type I (MEN-I). Diabetes 27 (Suppl 2): 512–514, 1978.

42. Prosser PR, Karam JH, Townsend JJ, Forsham PH: Prolactin- secreting pituitary adenomas in multiple endocrine adenomatosis, Type I. Ann Intern Med 91 (1): 41–44, 1979.

43. Gray PI, Botha AP, Nel CJ, Potsieter GM, Rohm GF, Steyn AF, van den Heever CM: Wermer's syndrome. A case report. S Afr Med J 59: 497–498, 1981.

44. Le Briggs R, Rowell, JR: Chiari-Frommel syndrome as a part of the Zollinger-Ellison multiple endocrine adenomatosis complex. Calif Med 111 (2): 92–96, 1969.

45. Boyd III AD, Reichlin S, Turksoy RN: Galactorrhea-Amenorrhea Syndrome: Diagnosis and therapy. Ann Int Med 87: 165–175, 1977.

46. Kleinberg DL, Noel GL Frantz AG: Galactorrhea: A study of 235 cases, including 48 with pituitary tumors. N Engl J Med 296: 589–600, 1977.

47. Dolman LI, Toberts TS, Poulson Jr AM, Tyler FH: Infertility in patients with hyperprolactinemia from a pituitary adenoma. Arch Intern Med 137: 1161–1164, 1977.

48. Malarkey WB, Johnson JC: Pituitary tumors and hyperprolactinemia. Arch Intern Med 136: 40–44, 1976.

49. Franks S, Jacobs HS, Martin N, Nabarro JDN: Hyperprolactinaemia and impotence. Clin Endocrinol 8: 277–287,, 1978.

50. Carter JN, Tyson JE, Tolis G, van Vliet S, Faiman C, Friesen HG: Prolactin-secreting tumors and hypogonadism in 22 men. N Engl J Med 299(16): 847–852, 1978.

51. Kurnick JE, Hartman CR, Lufkin EG, Hofeldt FD: Abnormal sella turcica. Arch Intern Med 137: 111–117, 1977.

52. Block MA, Frame B, Jackson CE, Parfitt AM, Horn RC: Primary diffuse micro-scopical hyperplasia of the parathyroid glands. Surgical Importance. Arch Surg 111(4): 348–354, 1976.

53. Jung RT, Davie M, Grant AM, Jenkins D, Chalmers TM: Multiple endocrine adenomatosis (Type I) and familial hyperparathyroidism. Postgrad Med J 54: 92–94, 1978.

54. Wells SA, Leicht GS, Ross AJ: Primary hyperparathyroidism. Curr Probl Surg 17(8): 398–463.

55. Reynolds LR, Flueck JA: Evaluation of the hypercalcemic patient. Am Fam Physician 23(4): 105–111, 1981.

56. Verdonk CA, Edis AJ: Parathyroid double adenomas: fact or fiction? Surgery 90(3): 523–526, 1981.

57. Stefanini P, Carboni M, Patrassi N, Basoli A: Beta-islet cell tumors of the pancreas: Results of a study on 1,067 cases. Surgery 75(4): 597–609, 1974.

58. Friesen SR: Tumors of the endocrine pancreas. N Engl J Med 306(10): 580–590, 1982.

59. Modlin IM: Endocrine tumors of the pancreas. Surg Gynecol Obstet 149: 751–769, 1979.

60. Track NS: The gastrointestinal endocrine system. Can Med Assoc J 122: 287–292, 1980.

61. Kingham JG, Levison DA, Fairclough PD: Diarrhoea and reversible enteropathy in Zollinger-Ellison syndrome. Lancet 2: 610–612, 1981.

62. Ptak T, Kirsner JB: The Zollinger-Ellison syndrome, polyendocrine adenomatosis and other endocrine associations with peptic ulcer. Adv Intern Med 16: 213–242, 1970.

63. Liu DH, Crastnopol P, Phillips W: Perforation of a gastrojejunal ulcer into the pericardium. Complication of Wermer's disease (Zollinger-Ellison syndrome). Arch Surg 94(2): 294–298, 1967.

64. Cameron AJ, Hoffman II HN: Zollinger-Ellison syndrome. Clinical features and long-term follow-up. Mayo Clin Proc 48: 44–51, 1974.

65. Regan PT, Malagelada J-R: A reappraisal of clinical, roentgenographic and endoscopic features of the Zollinger-Ellison syndrome. Mayo Clin Proc 53: 19–23, 1978.

66. Thompson MH: The relationship of the serum gastrin and calcium concentrations in patients with multiple endocrine neoplasia Type I. Br J Surg 63(10): 779–783, 1976.

67. Nakanome C, Ishimori A, Goto Y, Yamazaki T, Kameyama J, Sasaki I, Inui M, Furukawa Y, Komatsu K: Clinical significance of glucagon provocation test in the diagnosis of hypergastrinemia. Gastroenterol Jpn 16(3): 213–222, 1981.

68. Lamers CB, Hackens WH, Thien T, van Tongeren JH: Serum concentrations of immunoreactive calcitonin in patients with hypergastrinaemia. Digestion 20(6): 379–382, 1980.

69. Snyder N, Scurry M, Hughes W: Hypergastrinemia in familial multiple endocrine adenomatosis. Ann Int Med 80: 321–325, 1974.

70. Peurifoy JT, Gomez LG, Thompson JC: Separate pancreatic gastrin cell and betacell adenomas. Report of a patient with multiple endocrine adenomatosis Type 1. Arch Surg 114(8): 956–958, 1979.

71. Vance JE, Stoll RW, Kitabchi AE, Buchanan DD, Hollander D, Williams RH: Familial nesidioblastosis as the predominant manifestation of multiple endocrine adenomatosis. Am J Med 52(2): 211–217, 1972.

72. Vance JE, Kitabchi AE, Buchanan KD, Stoli RW, Hollander D, Wood Jr FC: Hypersecretion of insulin, glucagon and gastrin in a kindred with multiple adenomatosis. Diabetes 17: 299–303, 1968.

73. Larsson LI, Ljungberg O, Sundler F, Svensson SO, Rehfeld J, Stadil F, Holst J: Antro-pyloric gastrinoma associated with pancreatic nesidioblastosis and proliferation of islets. Virchows Arch Abt A Path Anat 360: 305–314, 1973.

74. McGavran MH, Unger RH, Recant L, Polk HC, Kilo C, Levin ME: A glucagon-secreting alpha-cell carcinoma of the pancreas. N Engl J Med 274: 1408–1413, 1966.

75. Higgins GA, Recant L, Fischman AB: The glucagonoma syndrome: surgically curable diabetes. Am J Surg 137: 142–150, 1979.

76. Leichter SB: Clinical and metabolic aspects of glucagonoma. Medicine 59: 100–113, 1980.

77. Stacpoole PW, Jaspan J, Kasselberg AG, Halter SA, Polonsky K, Gluck FW, Liljenquist JE, Rabin D: A familial glucagonoma syndrome. Genetic, clinical and biochemical features. Am J Med 70: 1017–1026, 1981.

78. Hutcheon DF, Bayless TM, Cameron JL, Beylin SB: Watery diarrhea mediated by different hormones in a multiple endocrine neoplasis type I kindred. Gastroenterol 74: 1047–1051, 1978.

79. Hutcheon DF, Bayless TM, Cameron JL, Baylin SB: Hormone-mediated watery diarrhea in a family with multiple endocrine neoplasms. Ann Intern Med 90(6): 932–934, 1979.

80. Croizier JC, Lehy T, Zeitoun P: A2 cell pancreatic microadenomas in a case of multiple endocrine adenomatosis. Cancer 28(3): 707–713, 1971.

81. Anderson RJ, Lufkin EG, Sizemore GW, Carney JA, Sheps SG, Sillman YE: Acromegaly and pituitary adenoma with phaeochromocytoma: A variant of multiple endocrine neoplasia. Clin Endocrinol 14: 605–612, 1981.

82. Dehner LP, Prem KA, Delaney JP, Weber WR, Najarian J: Primary uterine tumors and multiple endocrine adenomatosis, type I. Obstet Gynecol [Suppl] 49(1): 41s–45s, 1977.

83. Hansen OP, Hansen M, Hansen HH, Rose B: Multiple endocrine adenomatosis of mixed type. Acta Med Scand 200(4): 327–331, 1976.

84. Sanmarti A, Tresanchez JM, Fox M, Bonnin J: Endocrine polyadenomatosis type 1. Med Clin 63(5): 246–250, 1974.

85. Rosai J, Higa E, Davie J: Mediastinal endocrine neoplasm in patients with multiple endocrine adenomatosis. A previously unrecognized association. Cancer 29(4): 1075–1083, 1972.

86. Zeller JR, Kauffman HM, Komorowske RA, Itskovitz HD: Bilateral pheochromocytoma and islet cell adenoma of the pancreas. Arch Surg 117: 827–830, 1982

87. Taleishi R, Wada A, Ishiguro S, Ehara M, Sakamoto H, Miki T, Mori Y, Matsui Y, Ishikawa O: Coexistence of bilateral pheochromocytoma and pancreatic islet cell tumor. Cancer 42(6): 2928–2934, 1978.

88. Carney JA, Go VL, Gordon H, Northcutt RC, Pearce AG, Sheps SG: Familial pheochromocytoma and islet cell tumor of the pancreas. Am J Med 68(4): 515–521, 1980.

89. Popa M: Familial polyadenomatoses of the endocrine glands. Endocrinologie 18(1): 61–63, 1980.

90. Nathan DM, Daniels GH, Ridgway EC: Gastrinoma and phaeochromocytoma: is there a mixed multiple endocrine adenoma syndrome? Acta Endocrinol (Copenh) 93(1): 91–93, 1980.

91. Steiner AL, Goodman AD, Powers SR: Multiple endocrine neoplasia type 2, and Cushing's disease. Medicine 47: 371–409, 1968.

92. Vesely DL, Faas FH: Multiple endocrine adenomatosis with Cushing's disease and the amenorrhea-galactorrhea syndrome responsive to proton beam irradiation. South Med J 74(9): 1147–1149, 1981.

93. Franksson C, Alveryd A, Brismar B, Ostman J: Neural crest tumour syndromes. Acta Chir Scand 147(2): 105–107, 1981.

94. Farhi F, Dikman SH, Lawson W, Cobin RH, Zak FG: Paragangliomatosis associated with multiple endocrine adenomas. Arch Pathol 100(9): 495–498, 1976.

95. Yamaguchi K, Abe K, Zeze F, Adachi I, Tanaka M, Kameya T, Kitaoka H, Kobayashi K, Sasagawa M: A case of Zollinger-Ellison syndrome associated with thyroid adenomata, adrenocortical adenoma and duodenal carcinoid. Jpn J Clin Oncol 6(2): 83–89, 1976.

96. Hull MT, Warfel KA, Muller J, Higgins JT: Familial islet cell tumors in von Hippel-Lindau's disease. Cancer 44(4): 1523–1526, 1979.

97. Schnall AM, Genuth SM: Multiple endocrine adenomas in a patient with the Maffucci syndrome. Am J Med 61(6): 952–956, 1976.

98. Doumith R, deGennes JL, Cabane JP, Zygelman N: Pituitary prolactinoma, adrenal aldosterone-producing adenomas, gastric schwannoma and colonic polyadenomas: a possible variant of multiple endocrine neoplasia (MEN) type I. Acta Endocrinol 100: 189–195, 1982.

99. Schneider NR, Cubilla AL, Chaganti RS: Association of endocrine neoplasia with familial multiple colon polyps. Am J Hum Genet 32(6): 128A, 1980.

100. Borit A, Blanshard TP: Sphenoidal pituitary adenoma. Hum Pathol 10(1): 93–96, 1979.

101. Rosenzweig JL, Lawrence DA, Vogel DL, Costa J, Gordon P: Adrenocorticotropin-independent hypercortisolemia and testicular tumors in a patient with a pituitary tumor and gigantism. J Clin Endocrinol 55: 421–427, 1982.

102. Ippoliti AF: Zollinger-Ellison syndrome: provocative diagnostic tests. Ann Intern Med 81: 758–762, 1974.

103. Lamers CB, Buis JT, vanTongeren J: Secretin-stimulated serum gastrin levels in hyperparathyroid patients from families with multiple endocrine adenomatosis type I. Ann Intern Med 86: 719–724, 1977.

104. Primrose JN, Ratcliffe JG, Joffe SN: Assessment of the secretin provocation test in the diagnosis of gastrinoma. Br J Surg 67: 744–746, 1980.

105. Tiengo A. Fedele D, Marchiori E, Nosadini R, Muggeo M: Suppression and stimulation mechanisms controlling glucagon secretion in a case of islet cell tumor producing glucagon, insulin and gastrin. Diabetes 25(5): 408. 1976.

106. Lamers CBH, vanTongeren JHM: A comparative study of the value of calcium secretion and meal-stimulated increase in serum gastrin to a diagnosis of Zollinger-Ellison syndrome. Gut 18: 128–134, 1977.

107. Deveney CW, Deveney KS, Jaffe BM, et al: Use of calcium and secretin in the diagnosis of gastrinoma (Zollinger-Ellison syndrome). Ann Intern Med 87: 680–686, 1977.

108. Stage JG, Stadil F, Rehefeld JF, et al: Secretin and the Zollinger-Ellison syndrome. Reliability of secretin tests and pathogenetic role of secretin. Scand. J Gastroenterol 13: 501–511, 1978.

109. Betts JB, O'Malley BP, Rosenthal FD: Hyperparathyroidism: a prerequisite for Zollinger-Ellison syndrome in multiple endocrine adenomatosis Type 1 – report of a further family and a review of the literature. Q J Med 49(193): 69–76, 1980.

406

110. Gaeke RF, Kaplan EL, Rubenstein A: Insulin and proinsulin release during calcium infusion in a patient with islet cell tumor. Metabolism 24: 1029–1034, 1975.

111. Kaplan GL, Rubenstein AH, Evans R: Calcium stimulation: a new provocative test for insulinomas. Ann Surg 190: 501–507, 1979.

112. Roy BK, Abuid J, Wendorff H, Nitiyanant W, DeRubertis FR, Field JB: Insulin release in response to calcium in the diagnosis of insulinoma. Metabolism 28: 246–252, 1979.

113. Romanus ME, Dilley WG, Leight GS, Wells SA: Insulin release from human and hamster insulinomas stimulated by rapid calcium infusion. Surg Forum 32: 207–209, 1981.

113. Floyd JD, Fajans SS, Pek S, Chance RE: A newly recognized pancreatic polypeptide; plasma levels in health and disease. Recent Prog Horm Res 33: 519, 1977.

144. Bloom SR, Adrian TE, Bryant MG, Polak JM: Pancreatic polypeptide: a marker for Zollinger-Ellison syndrome: Lancet 1: 1155, 1978.

115. Taylor Il, Walsh JH, Rotter J, Passaro E: Is pancreatic polypeptide a marker for Zollinger-Ellison syndrome? Lancet 1: 845, 1978

116. Schwartz TW: Pancreatic-polypeptide (PP) and endocrine tumours of the pancreas. Scand J Gastroenterol [Suppl 53] 14: 93–120, 1979.

117. Friesen SR, Kimmel JR, Tomita T: Pancreatic polypeptide as screening marker for pancreatic polypeptide apudomas in multiple endocrinopathies. Am J Surg 139: 60–66, 1980.

119. Lamers CBHW, Diemel CM: Basal and postatropine serum pancreatic polypeptide concentrations in familial multiple endocrine neoplasia type 1. J Clin Endocrinol Met 55(4): 774–778, 1982.

120. Nelson RL, Service FJ, Ilstrup DM, Go VLW: Are elevated pancreatic polypeptide levels in patients with insulinoma secondary to hypoglycaemia? Lancet 2: 659–661, 1980.

121. Skare S, Hanssen KF, Lundqvist G: Increased plasma pancreatic polypeptide (PP) in diabetic ketoacidosis; normalization following treatment. Acta Endocronologica 93: 466–469, 1980.

122. Boden G, Owen OE: Familial hyperglucagonemia – an autosomal dominant disorder. N Engl J Med 296(10): 534–538, 1977

123. Hansen LP, Lund HT, Fahrenkrug J, Sogaard H: Vasoactive intestinal polypeptide (VIP)-producing ganglioneuroma in a child with chronic diarrhea. Acta Paediatr Scand 69: 419–424, 1980.

124. McCarthy DM, Weintraub BD, Rosen SW: Subunits of human chorionic gonadotropin in malignant gastrinoma. Gastroenterology 67: 1198, 1979.

125. Stock JL, Weintraub BD, Rosen SW, Aurbach GD, Spiegel AM, Marx SJ: Human chorionic gonadotropin subunit measurement in primary hyperparathyroidism. J Clin Endocrinol Metab 54(1): 57–63, 1982.

126. Teal JS, Tsai FY, Ahmadi J, Becker TB, Segall HD: CT in the evaluation of pituitary microadenoma. J Computer Assit Tomography 3(4): 565–570, 1979.

127. Damgaard-Petersen K, Stage JG: CT scanning in patients with Zollinger-Ellison syndrome and carcinoid syndrome. Scand J Gastroenterol [Suppl] 14(53): 117–122, 1979

128. Madsen B: Angiographic localization of beta cell tumors. Scand J Gastroenterol 14(53): 101–109, 1979.

129. Korobkin MT, Palubinskas AJ, Glickman MG: Pitfalls in arteriography of islet cell tumors of the pancreas. Radiology 100(2): 319–28, 1971.

130. Ingemansson S, Kuhl C, Larsson L-I, Lunderquist A, Lundquist I: Localization of insulinomas and islet cell hyperplasias by pancreatic vein catheterization and insulin assay. Surg Gynecol Obstet 146: 725–734, 1978.

131. Glowniak JV, Shapiro B, Vinik AI, Glaser B, Thompson NW, Cho KJ: Percutaneous transhepatic venous sampling of gastrin. Value in sporadic and familial islet-cell tumors and G-cell hyperfunction. N Engl J Med 307(5): 293–297, 1982.

132. Horvath E, Kovacs K: Histologic, immunocytologic and fine structural findings in pituitary adenomas associated with the multiple endocrine neoplasia syndrome (MENS). Lab Invest 40(2): 261, 1979.

133. Kovacs K: Morphology of prolactin producing adenomas. Clin Endocrinol 6: 71s–79s, 1977.
134. Horvath E, Kovacs K: Ultrastructural classification of pituitary adenomas. Can J Neurol Sci 3(1): 9–21, 1976.
135. Scully RE, Galdabini JJ, McNeely BU: Case records of the Massachusetts General Hospital (Case 1-1976). N Engl J Med 294(1): 37–42, 1976.
136. Cruetzfeldt W, Arnold R, Creutzfeldt C: Pathomorphologic, histochemical and diagnostic aspects of gastrinomas (Zollinger-Ellison syndrome). Human Pathol 6: 47–76, 1975.
137. Greider MH, Rosai H, McGuigan JE: The human pancreatic islet cells and their tumors. II. Ulcerogenic and diarrheogenic tumors. Cancer 33: 1423–1443, 1974.
138. Carmalt MHB, Dalton GA, Fletcher RF, Smith WT: The treatment of Cushing's Disease by trans-sphenoidal hypophysectomy. Q J Med (New series XLVI) 181: 119–134, 1977.
139. Ludecke D, Kautzky R, Saeger W, Schrader D: Selective removal of hypersecreting pituitary adenomas? An analysis of endocrine function, operative and microscopical findings in 101 cases. Acta Neurochirurgica 35: 27–42, 1976.
140. Ludecke DK, Herrmann HD, Saeger W: Mode of therapy of endocrine active pituitary adenomas. Acta Neurochir (Wein) 56: 118, 1981.
141. Scholz DA, Purnell DC, Edis AJ, vanHeerden JA, Woolner LB: Primary hyperparathyroidism with multiple parathyroid gland enlargement. Review of 53 cases. Mayo Clin Proc 53: 792–797, 1978.
142. Prinz RA, Gamvros OI, Sellu D, Lynn JA: Subtotal parathyroidectomy for primary chief cell hyperplasia of the multiple endocrine neoplasia type I syndrome. Ann Surg 193(1): 26–29, 1981.
143. Wells RA, Farndon JR, Dale JK, Leight GS, Dilley WG: Long-term evaluation of patients with primary parathyroid hyperplasia managed by total parathyroidectomy and heterotpoic auto-transplantation. Ann Surg 192: 451–458, 1980.
144. Esselstyn CB: Parathyroid surgery. How many glands should be excised? Is there still a controversy? Surg Clin North Am 59: 77–81, 1979.
145. Spiegel AM, Eastman ST, Attie MF, Downs RW, Levine MA, Marx SJ, Stock JL, Saxe AW, Brennan MF, Aurback GD: Intraoperative measurements of urinary cyclic AMP to guide surgery for primary hyperparathyroidism. N Engl J Med 303(25): 1457–1460, 1980.
146. Friesen SR, Hermreck AS, Brackett CE, Schimke RN: Case reports; Cimetidine in the management of synchronous crises of MEA I. World J Surg 4(1): 123–129, 1980.
147. McCarthy DM: The place of surgery in the Zollinger-Ellison syndrome. N Engl J Med 302(24): 1344–1347, 1980.
148. Harrison TS, Child III CG, Fry WJ, Floyd Jr JC, Fajans SS: Current surgical management of functioning islet cell tumors of the pancreas. Ann Surg 178(4): 485–495, 1973.
149. Hofmann JW, Fox PS, Wilson SD: Duodenal wall tumors and the Zollinger-Ellison syndrome. Arch Surg 107: 334–339, 1973.
150. Schein PS, deLellis RA, Kahn CR, Gorden P, Kraft AR: Islet cell tumors: current concepts and management. Ann Intern Med 79: 239–257, 1973.
151. Thorner MO, McNeilly AS, Hagan C, Besser GM: Long-term treatment of galactorrhea and hypogonadism with bromocriptine. Br Med J ii: 419–422, 1974.
152. Thorner MO, Besser GM, Jones A, Dacie J, Jones AE: Bromocriptine treatment of female infertility: report of 13 pregnancies. Br Med J iv: 694–697, 1975.
153. Nagulesparen M, Ang V, Jenkins JS: Bromocriptine treatment of males with pituitary tumours, hyperprolactinaemia, and hypogonadism. Clin Endocrinol 9: 73–79, 1978.
154. Zarate A, Canales ES, Forsbach G, Fernandez-Lazala R: Bromocriptine. Clinical experience in the induction of pregnancy in amenorrhea-galactorrhea syndrome. Obstet Gynecol 52(4): 442–444, 1978.
155. Halloran LG, Swank M, Haynes BW: Metamide in Zollinger-Ellison syndrome. Lancet I: 281, 1975.
156. McCarthy DM: Report on the United States experience with cimetidine in Zollinger-Ellison

408

syndrome and other hypersecretory states. Gastroenterology 74: 453–458, 1978.

157. Code CF: Reflections on histamine, gastric secretion and the H_2 receptor. N Engl J Med 296(25): 1459–1462, 1977.

158. Robinson MF, Hayles AB, Heath H: Failure of cimetidine to affect calcium homeostasis in familial primary hyperparathyroidism (multiple endocrine neoplasia, type 1). J Clin Endocrinol Metab 51(4): 912–914, 1980.

159. Ensinck JW, Williams RH: Disorders causing hypoglycemia. In:Textbook of Endocrinology, Williams RH (ed), Philadelpia: W.B. Saunders, Co., 1981, p. 844–876.

160. Moertel CG, Hanley JA, Johnson LA: Streptozocin alone compared with streptozocin plus fluorouracil in the treatment of advanced islet-cell carcinoma. N Engl J Med 303(21): 1189, 1980.

161. Hansen M, Hansen HH, Hansen OP, Hainau B: Combination chemotherapy of an apudoma. With special reference to the therapeutic value of monitoring hormonal substances. Acta Med Scand 202: 139–144, 1977.

162. Bunick EM, Rose LI, Haegele LA: Endocrine neoplasia. In: Cancer Chemotherapy III. The forty-sixth Hahnemann Symposium, Brodsky I, Kahn SB, Conroy JF (eds), New York: Grune & Stratton, 1978, p 493.

163. Eastman RC, Come SE, Strewler GJ, Gorden P, Kahn CR: Adriamycin therapy for advanced insulinoma. J Clin Endocrinol Metab 44(1): 142, 1977.

164. Kiang DT, Frenning DH, Bauer GE: Mithramycin for hypoglycemia in malignant insulinoma. N Engl J Med 299(3): 134–135, 1978.

165. Murray-Lyon IM, Eddleston ALWF, Williams R, Brown M, Hogbin BM, Bennet A, Edwards JC, Taylor KW: Treatment of multiple-hormone-producing malignant islet-cell tumour with streptozotocin. Lancet 2: 895–898, 1968.

166. Reimer D, Sins SM: A kindred with 5 cases of multiple endocrine adenomatosis type I. Hum Hered 31(2): 84–88, 1981.

167. Tragl K-H, Mayr WR: Familial islet-cell adenomatosis. Lancet 2: 426–428, 1977.

168. Sizemore GW, Go VLW: Stimulation tests for diagnosis of medullary thyroid carcinoma. Mayo Clin Proc 50: 53–56, 1975.

169. Knight J, Garvin PJ, Danis RK, Lewis Jr JE, Willman VL: Nesidioblastosis in children. Arch Surg 115: 880–882, 1980.

170. Taylor IL, Walsh JH, Rotter J, Passaro Jr E: Is pancreatic polypeptide a marker for Zollinger-Ellison syndrome? Lancet 1: 845–848, 1978.

171. Stabile BE, Passaro E, Carlson HE: Elevated serum prolactin level in the Zollinger-Ellison syndrome. Arch Surg 116(4): 449–453, 1981.

172. Farid NR, Buehler S, Russell NA, Maroun FB, Allerdice P, Smyth HS: Prolactinomas in familial multiple endocrine neoplasia syndrome type I. Relationship to HLA and carcinoid tumors. Am J Med 69(6): 874–880, 1969.

173. Wahlstrom T, Seppala M: Luteinizing hormone-releasing factor-like immunoreactivity in islet cells and insulomas of the human pancreas. Int J Cancer 24: 744–748, 1979.

174. Krejs GJ, Orci L, Conlon JM, Ravazzola M, Davis GR, Raskin P, Collins SM, McCarthy DM, Baetens D, Rubenstein A, Aldor RAM, Unger RH: Somatostatinoma syndrome. N Engl J Med 301(6): 285–292, 1979.

175. Wright J, Abolfathi A, Penman E, Marks V: Pancreatic somatostatinoma presenting with hypoglycaemia. Clin Endocrinol 12: 603–608, 1980.

176. Frohman LA, Szabo M, Stachura ME, Berelowitz M: Growth hormone-releasing activity (GHRA) in extracts of bronchial carcinoid (BC) and pancreatic islet cell (PI) tumors associated with acromegaly. Clin Res 27(2): 505A, 1979.

15. Endocrine neoplasms: pheochromocytoma

TIMOTHY S. HARRISON

1. Pheochromocytoma

1.1 Historical background

That adrenal tumors could be associated with violent attacks of high blood pressure, anxiety, sweating, tachycardia, prostration, and death was first appreciated at the postmortem table by Labbé Tinel and Doumer [1]. Their patient was a woman of 23 who died in acute pulmonary edema and at her autopsy they found a single adrenal tumor. Labbé, Tinel, and Doumer wondered if the adrenal tumor might be responsible for the violent, fatal attacks.

In March and October of 1926, Prof. César Roux of Lausanne, Switzerland and Dr. Charles Mayo, Sr. in Rochester, Minnesota removed adrenal tumors associated with violent hypertension, alarming tachycardia, and cardiovascular instability. At the time he operated, Mayo was unaware of Roux's success. Roux's case, described by Roland von der Muhl [2] in 1929 in his Pathology thesis on chromaffin cell tumors, was notable because the tumor was palpable, 'the diameter of a croquet ball' (probably about 10.0 cm in diameter) according to the pathologist's description. Mayo's case was that of Sister Joachim, a Canadian music teacher whose condition so perplexed her referring physician, a Dr. Duncan of Chatham, Ontario, that he claimed in his letter about her to Dr. Mayo that 'I feel much as Festus must have felt when he summoned Paul to Rome, I have no accusation against this (man)' [3]. Mayo and his colleagues were equally perplexed and decided to section the splanchnic nerves to control the blood pressure. During the exposure of the left splanchnic nerve, a tumor was felt near but not in the left adrenal. The tumor was removed, the splanchnic nerves left undisturbed, and the patient's attacks cured. Following Mayo's report cases followed in steady succcession, that of Pincoffs and Shipley being notable in 1929 because they not only made the correct diagnosis preoperatively but attempted to secure it by measuring increased circulating epinephrine [4]. The results of the epinephrine analysis were uncertain probably because the available analytical techniques were crude and not sensitive enough to show changes in epinephrine and related compounds in pheochromocytoma.

Santen, R.J. and Manni, A. (eds.), Diagnosis and management of endocrine-related tumors. ISBN 0-89838-636-5.
© 1984, Martinus Nijhoff Publishers, Boston. Printed in the Netherlands.

1.2 *Incidence*

In unselected autopsy populations, the incidence of pheochromocytoma has been estimated as high as 0.1% [5]. Other suggestions vary, some placing the incidence as high as 1% of the hypertensive population and still others quoting 0.1% of the hypertensive population as harboring pheochromocytoma. Differing patient clienteles and varying surveillance techniques probably account for such seemingly diverse incidences of pheochromocytoma.

Probably a more useful perspective of pheochromocytoma is gained by realizing that in years just passed the diagnosis is still overlooked in patients eventually dying from fatal complications of the tumor; in three such patients, death was caused by ventricular tachycardia, profound irreversible hypotension associated with hemorrhage into a pheochromocytoma, and the third from a violent hypertensive crisis under general anesthesia for an unrelated condition. Many other cases can be cited; suffice it to say here that each of these patients had been known to be hypertensive for 3, 6 and 12 years respectively but their physicians failed to investigate the cause. In a typical pheochromocytoma series in the United States, for every 10 patients succesfully treated, one could be found dying in the same hospital with the tumor undiagnosed and untreated. In a hospital specializing in endocrinologic problems in England's National Health Service, 1 in 4 pheochromocytoma patients die from fatal complications of undiagnosed pheochromocytoma.

In our view these realizations make the succesful screening of populations at risk for pheochromocytoma an urgent concern. Unfortunately, there is no ideal screening technique available since neither cost effectiveness or simplicity of technique is possible with the analytical methods available today for determining endogenous catecholamines or their major metabolites in urine or plasma.

1.3 *Pathophysiology of pheochromocytoma*

Within the chromaffin cells comprising them, pheochromocytomas relentlessly biosynthesize and uncontrollably release varying but often huge quantities of the catecholamines, Dopamine, Norepinephrine and Epinephrine. Physiologic rate limitation of tyrosine hydroxylase by Norepinephrine and Epinephrine, well-recognized in normal functioning adrenergic nerves, simply do not operate in pheochromocytoma. A few clues exist to suggest that tumor prostaglandins, cytolysis of infarcted tumor cells and physical manipulation of the tumor all may cause exaggerated release of catecholamines from pheochromocytomas.

A direct consequence of increased biosynthesis and release is that plasma catecholamines and urinary excretion rates of catecholamines are increased in pheochromocytoma. Later we will describe the diagnostic advantage of the increased catecholamines. A more immediate consequence to be emphasized is that increased circulating catecholamines in pheochromocytoma are taken up by active transport from the circulation and stored in increased quantities in adrenergic nerve storage granules distributed throughout the body, including the opposite adrenal gland. Exaggerated reflex release of these increased stored catecholamines does occcur in pheochromocytoma [6]. Whether or not the brain's catecholamine stores are increased in pheochromocytoma is not known and it would be extremely valuable to have insight into this important question.

1.4 *Symptoms of pheochromocytoma*

Although understandable because of its dramatic life threatening features, in a sense it is unfortunate that the episodic hypertensive attacks originally leading to recognition of pheochromocytoma receive such heavy emphasis today. Fifty percent of pheochromocytoma patients have sustained hypertension and rare pheochromocytoma patients have normal blood pressures and present with cardiac or metabolic consequences of the disease such as diarrhea, a variety of ectopic cardiac arrythmias, ranging from occasional extraventricular beats to complete heart block. It is a good idea to be broadly aware of these various clinical possibilities before deciding a given patient need not be studied for the possibility of pheochromocytoma.

In their marvelously complete monograph on the symptomatology of pheochromocytoma, Hermann and Mornex place excessive sweating as the second most frequent symptom after hypertension itself [7]. While I am personally unaware of any pheochromocytoma patient in whom sweating was the only symptom, it is possible and should not be ignored as a possible presenting complaint.

One of the most demanding presentations of pheochromocytoma is unexpected hypertensive crisis on the operating table during surgery for some other condition. Opinions vary on how to deal with this problem; if the unrelated operation is in the abdomen and an adrenal tumor can be felt, it is certainly tempting to remove the tumor and solve the problem of the pheochromocytoma by taking it out. My view is that this is unnecessarily dangerous in a patient without any prior adrenergic receptor blockade. In one patient extremely ill from prior negative laparotomy for a presumed carcinoid, we had to be sure there was no pelvic sepsis from a related appendectomy. We felt her right adrenal tumor but delayed removing the pheochromocytoma for several more days during which we confirmed the diagnosis biochemically and then instituted partial alpha and beta receptor blockade. Her pheochromocytoma excision went smoothly and her convalescence though prolonged was uncomplicated and we were glad in retrospect that we staged the removal of her pheocchromocytoma rathe than attempting to remove it in unstable conditions.

1.5 *Diagnosis of pheochromocytoma*

While the presence of pheochromocytoma can be suspected from its more overt symptoms, there are, as mentioned already, as many patients whose hypertension is sustained. For this reason, the diagnosis is made securely by measuring increased quantities of catecholamines or metabolites in the urine or plasma of pheochromocytoma patients. First appreciated by the late U.S. von Euler of the Karolinska Institute's Department of Physiology, critical catecholamine analysis now underlies diagnostic precision for making the diagnosis of pheochromocytoma quickly and accurately.

We mention in passing a variety of tests of historical interest, useful at the time they were designed but whose obsolescence was inevitable given the greater precision for diagnosis of catecholamine analysis. The cold pressor test, the Histamine Stimulation Test, the Tyramine Test, a blocking test with regitine all are unnecessarily dangerous and have appreciable false negative and false positive reactivity associated with them. The glucagon stimulation test is better but for utmost accuracy depends on catecholamine measurement and is a more powerful stimulus than sometimes seems safe in pheochromocytoma. I am unaware of any deaths from the glucagon test.

Free urinary excretion rates of norepinephrine, epinephrine, and their primary 3-0-methyl metabolites normetanephrine and metanephrine, when used for the diagnosis of symptomatic pheochromocytoma patients with high blood pressure was, in our hands, 93% accurate for the diagnosis of pheochromocytoma when only epinephrine and norepinephrine excretion were determined and 100% accurate when normetanephrine and metanephrine urinary excretion rates were calculated [8]. Rarely false-positive values are seen for metanephrine and normetanephrine excretion rates but these could be resolved generally with scrupulous dietary control removing foods containing catecholamines and metabolites such as bananas and avocados. Repeated study easily resolves these rare false positives. A more troublesome false positive urinary catecholamine elevation is seen with alpha-methyl-(α-cH$_3$)-dopa, a commonly used anti-hypertensive. This compound is metabolized to α-cH$_3$-Norepinephrine. These α-cH$_3$ compounds form a trihydroxy-indole ring on which urinary catecholamine determinations depend. The problem can be overcome by high performance liquid chromatography [9] which is preferable to removing patients from their Aldomet treatment for 3 or 4 weeks [9]. A smoother baseline excretion of urinary catecholamines occurs at night and this is the reason we rely on 12 hour overnight excretion rates of catecholamines rather than 24-hour collections. Other laboratories emphasize other biochemical approaches to the diagnosis of pheochromocytoma. The combination of metanephrine and normetanephrine excretion with Vanillyl Mandelic (VMA) secretion is used in one respected and experienced laboratory. The diagnostic accuracy is comparable with the two approaches. It is important to measure epinephrine and norepinephrine and metanephrine and normetanephrine individually rather than adding them together for convenience as 'total' catecholamines or total metanephrines. An epinephrine secreting pheochromocytoma was overlooked by another laboratory using total catecholamines and easily diagnosed when epinephrine and metanephrine urinary excretion rates were determined individually by us.

Others have emphasized plasma catecholamine detemination for diagnosis [10] and there is no question that this is accurate most of the time but is more expensive and time consuming for most laboratories. Recent reports identify a small group (3 or 4) of sporadic pheochromocytoma patients in whom urinary catecholamine, metanephrine, and other metabolites were persistently normal but plasma catecholamines were elevated. Obviously, this requires astute awareness and persistence on the part of the diagnostician. Equally certain is that a small number of patients exist with falsely positive plasma catecholamines whose values revert to normal with repeated study and insistence on ideal resting conditions for sampling, i.e. patients resting, supine wth an indwelling venous catheter placed 30 minutes before sampling.

The recently described Clonidine test is commendably safe and currently interests us not so much for helping secure the diagnosis of pheochromocytoma but as a sensitive additional method of following patients postoperatively for early recurrences of the tumor [11]. Clonidine, a centrally acting alpha adrenergic agonist, inhibits central nervous system mediated reflex catecholamine release and consequently decreases plasma catecholamine levels in normal subjects. Pheochromocytoma patients fail to suppress and generally have high resting plasma catecholamine levels. In a recent patient with dopamine and norepinephrine secreting malignant pheochromocytoma, we found plasma norepinephrine did not return all the way to normal postoperatively even though plasma norepinephrine suppressed in the early postoperative period. Urinary catecholamines and metanephrines became normal but within six months increased non-suppressible plasma norepinephrine levels recurred as did flagrant elevations of norepinephrine and normetanephrine excretion. Recurrent tumor disseminated to palpable supraclavicular lymph nodes and the patient died at home, six months after excision of her malignant pheocromocytoma.

The most difficult diagnostic problems are in MEN-II kindreds at risk not only for bilateral pheochromocytoma but also for subtle nodular and diffuse adrenal medullary hyperplasia. The hyperplasia may have normal or only slightly increased catecholamine excretion associated with it and the decision of when to remove these glands requires careful judgment. It is wise to follow MEN-II patients with medullary hyperplasia for a long time with repeated urinary catecholamine measurement to learn the trend of their catecholamine excretion rates.

2. Treatment

2.1 *Preoperative*

2.1.1 *Partial alpha and beta adrenergic receptor blockade.* Unquestionably the single feature making contemporary care of pheochromocytoma patients safe as opposed to the hazards of 20 years ago, is the availability of newer adrenergic receptor blocking agents. Intelligently administered partial alpha and beta adrenergic receptor blockade preoperatively [12] helps prevent excessively dangerous adrenergic agonist effects of increased circulating catecholamines.

For alpha adrenergic blockade, the most frequently used agent for most physicians is phenoxybenzamine; 'Dibenzyline', generally given in a total daily dose of approximately 1 mgm/kg/24° divided into 3 smaller ses given orally at widely spaced intervals during the patient's waking hours. A most convenient index for judging the effectiveness of Dibenzyline has been with serial hematocrits which often show, as the blockade becomes effective, drops of 4 to 8 volumes percent as the patient re-expand their plasma volume. The pheochromocytoma patient with a full, expanded plasma volume has a more stable blood pressure, is a safer surgical risk and is better able to tolerate invasive localization procedures such as retrograde venography and selective arteriography.

Many centers advocate preoperative phenoxybenzamine for all pheochromocytoma patients regardless of their cardiovascular status. With thoughtful help from our pharmacologists, we adopted a selective approach but find as our experience deepens we use preoperative alpha receptor blockade in almost all patients. Adverse effects of preoperative alpha receptor blockade are rare [12].

For beta receptor blockade sensitive selection of patients is, we believe, wise. We know of 3 deaths from refractory cardiac standstill during anesthesia induction in pheochromocytoma patients too aggressively medicated with propranolol. We usually use propranolol for beta receptor blockade in pheochromocytoma and our criteria for it are give in Table 1. Surprisingly, small doses of propranolol, 20 mgm, t.i.d. by mouth can be effective in many pheochromocytoma patients as judged by resolution of tachycardia to 80–90 beats/minute. We think the reason for this extreme beta receptor sensitivity is that myocardial beta receptor populations are diminished in pheochromocytoma with excessive circulating catecholamine levels. In dogs implanted successfully with human pheochromo-

Table 1. Criteria for using beta receptor blockade in pheochromocytoma. Reprinted by permission from Harrison TS, Gann DS, Edis AJ, Egdahl RH: Surgical Disorders of the Adrenal Gland. New York: Grune & Stratton, 1975, 150 pp, p. 93.

1. Resting pulse rate greater than 100 beats/min.
2. Any cardiac arrhythmia
3. Tumors secreting 75% or more epinephrine.

cytoma, there is experimental confirmation of this interesting pheonemon.

In isolated pheochromocytoma cases with especially chaotic circulations, occasionally brilliant success can result with other specific drugs used to correct a life-threatening problem. Thus, intravenous phenoxybenzamine and beta receptor blockade were life saving in a 70-year-old with complete heart block and cardiac arrest. Parenthetically her heart block completely reversed after her pheochromocytoma removal. Graceful management of many profound hypertensive crises is possible with intravenous sodium nitroprusside, an agent also useful during surgery as I discuss subsequently.

2.1.2 *Preoperative localization of pheochromocytoma.* Surgeons removing pheochromocytomas not only seek a safe and stable patient on whom to operate, but they wish to know the number, size and complexity of the vasculature of the lesions before surgery in order to be able to proceed with safe and efficient removal of pheochromocytomas.

There are many localization techniques and more are evolving rapidly; palpation (rarely possible), plain abdominal X-rays, excretory nephrotomography (often disappointing), abdominal laminograms with pre-sacral CO_2 insufflation, regional venous sampling (with or without retrograde venography), computerized tomography (with or without enhancement), selective arteriography, and most recently of all meta-mono-iodo-benzylguanidine (MIBG) photo-emission scanning. Hardly ever will a given patient require more than one or two of these techniques and there are special situations in which each is uniquely helpful. It is not our purpose to go into this in depth but perhaps it will suffice to emphasize again that accurate knowledge of the number and location of the tumors is indispensably helpful to the surgeon.

The recent brilliant development of successful meta-mono-iodo-benzylguanidine (MIBG) scanning by William Beierwaltes and his colleagues in the Division of Nuclear Medicine at the University of Michigan Hospital requires special comment and the interested attention of all physicians caring for pheochromocytoma patients [13]. Fifteen years ago Beierwaltes began to survey suitably radioactive compounds potentially helpful as additional treatment in incurable neuroblastoma. Concomitantly at the University of Michigan as experience was gained with pheochromocytoma it was obvious that the localization of disseminated pheochromocytoma recurrences was not possible and small multiple sequestered pheochromocytomas often could not be located by available techniques. This led 5 and 20 years postoperatively to injudicious surgery in two patients with diffusse, undetectable pulmonary metastases of originally solitary pheochromocytomas. A steady succession of catecholamines and their analogs, enzyme inhibitors and other compounds were surveyed by Beierwaltes et al, with no enduring success until the guanethidine analog, meta-mono-iodo-benzyl guanidine was tried. Successful imaging of dog adrenals and human pheochromocytoma quickly followed and the technique now emerges as remarkably versatile and accurate in disclosing tumors overlooked by all the techniques we have mentioned and rarely by surgical exploration as well. At present, MIBG scanning is just beginning to be generally available to the profession and although there have been some tumors not visualized with it, there is nevertheless little question that it is the most important localizing technique for pheochromocytoma yet developed. We can also hope that kinetic analysis of MIBG scanning will give us new insights into the remarkable ability of pheochromocytoma tissue to take up, biosynthesize, and release the prodigious quantities of endogenous catecholamines that can be life threatening in pheochromocytoma.

3. Principles in the treatment of pheochromocytoma

3.1 *Pathology*

That microscopic morphology of most endocrine neoplasms is not helpful in deciding whether or not they are malignant is certainly true and is particularly troublesome in pheochromocytoma. The incidence of malignant pheochromocytoma is low, probably less than the often quoted 10%, and within the realm of pheochromocytomas that metastasize, there is huge variation in the agressiveness of the tumor.

Our two patients with diffuse pulmonary implants of pheochromocytoma occurring 5 and 20 years after their primary operation had absolutely no other tumor present except in one of them, a few cells embedded in the operative dissection. No nodules were visible on routine chest X-rays but doubtless MIBG scanning would have imaged the pulmonary implants successfully.

At the other extreme a farmer's elderly wife had a solitary right adrenal tumor with diarrhea, weight loss, and high Dopamine and Norepinephrine excretion. Removal of her tumor was difficult but possible – we used 12 pints of blood. Postoperatively catecholamine and metanephrine excretion rates returned to normal as did her clonidine suppression of mildly elevated plasma catecholamines. The pathologist could not be certain that her pheochromocytoma was malignant. Six months later she was dead from disseminated tumor, including supra-clavicular lymph nodes and a large recurrence in the site of her original tumor.

Some hope has been raised that malignant pheochromocytomas might have associated with them release of higher quantities of catecholamine precursors such as dopamine or its metabolite, Homovanillic Acid (HVA) or any of several other intervening dopamine metabolites. This is often true, but many patients with benign pheochromocytoma also excrete increased dopamine and a careful statistical comparison of dopamine excretion in benign and malignant pheochromocytoma has to our knowledge, not yet been done.

3.2 *Surgical removal and early postoperative care of pheochromocytoma*

Thoughtful collaboration between anesthesiologist, surgeon, and an endocrinologically-oriented internist is essential for modern operative removal of pheochromocytoma. Ideally, all three should be in the Operating Room during the tumor removal. An intra-arterial catheter, pulmonary artery catheter and large bore intravenous catheter should be in place and the pressures displayed where easily seen by all. An indwelling bladder catheter should be in place.

If the patient is well blocked by Dibenzyline and Propranolol preoperatively, the surgery itself proceeds smoothly. Available for immediate use should be sodium nitroprusside, norepinephrine, epinephrine, hydrocortisone, propranolol and regitine. Several liters of blood should be directly available even though most of the time it is not necessary to give blood. Pheochromocytoma patients tolerate blood loss poorly, particularly if partial alpha adrenergic blockade is effective and blood pressure will fall dramatically with minimal volume loss. Even with the low blood pressure, tissue perfusion is good but crystalloid solution and blood considerably in excess of the volume originally lost is required to restore the blood pressure back to normal. It is better not to lose blood but this is not always possible.

If the blood volume is full, very seldom are special drugs required after tumor removal or postoperatively to support the blood pressure.

The special problem of epinephrine shock should be mentioned. In rare patients with tumors secreting predominantly epinephrine, hypotension refractory to all measures may develop 24–36 hours postoperativly. If volume replacement is adequate and neo-synephrine and norepinephrine are ineffective, large doses, 500 to 1000 mg, of intravenous hydroccortisone should be given within 20 minutes. Life-saving reversal of the epinephrine shock has followed. Although rare, this syndrom of epinephrine shock is well documented investigatively and is reversible by steroids, both in the experimental laboratory in dogs as well as in the rare postoperative pheochromocytoma patient exhibiting the problem.

3.3 *Followup*

Roughly 10 percent of pheochromocytoma patients will require more than one operation to control their disease. There are a variety of reasons for this, multiple primary pheochromocytomas spread out through time, tumors overlooked at the initial surgery, and recurrences of the variety we already mentioned. For these reasons it is wise that post-operative pheochromocytoma patients have catecholamine excretion rates checked every two years after their operation and obviously have their blood pressure checked carefully whenever they are seeing a doctor. In MEN-II kindreds closer surveillance is wise since these patients are at a greater risk for development of bilateral tumors than are patients with sporadic pheochromocytoma.

418

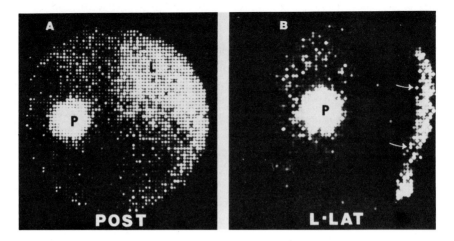

Figure 1. A. A left adrenal pheochromocytoma (P) is localized by [131I] mono-meta-iodo-benzyl-quanidine. Liver (L) uptake is present on this posterior projection. B. In a left lateral projection the arrows identify a radioactive marker on the patient's back. Reprinted by permission from Sisson et al. [13].

References

1. Labbé M, Tinel J, Doumer E: Crises solaires et hypertension paroxystique en rapport avec une tumeur surrénale. Bull Soc Méd Hôp 46: 982–990, 1922.
2. von der Muhl R: Contribution a l'étude paragangliones de la Surrenale, Thesé, Universite de Lausanne, Imprimie C. Vanzy, Burnier, S.A. Lausanne, 1928.
3. Mayo C: Paroxysmal hypertension with tumor of retroperitoneal nerve, report of a case. J Am Med Assoc 89: 1047–1050, 1927.
4. Pincoffs, MC: A case of paroxysmal hypertension associated with suprarenal tumor. Trans Assoc Am Physicians 44: 295–299, 1929.
5. St. John Sutton MC, Sheps SG, Lie JT: Prevalence of clinically unsuspected pheochromocytoma. Mayo Clin Proc 56: 354, 1981.
6. Harrison TS, Bartlett JD Jr, Seaton JF: Exaggerated urinary norepinephrine response to tilt in pheochromocytoma. N Engl J Med 277: 725, 1967.
7. Hermann H, Mornex R: Human tumors secreting catecholamines: clinical and physiopathological study of the pheochromocytomas. Oxford, New York: Pergamon Press, 1964, 207 pp.
8. Freier DT, Harrison TS: Rigorous biochemical criteria for the diagnosis of pheochromocytoma. J Surg Res 14: 177, 1973,
9. Munion GL, Seaton JF, Harrison TS: HPLC for urinary catecholamines and metanephrines with alpha-methyldopa. J Surg Res (in press).
10. Bravo EL, Tarazi RL, Gifford RW, Stewart BH: Circulating and urinary catecholamines in pheochromocytoma: diagnostic and pathophysiologic implicatons. N Engl J Med 301: 682–686, 1979.
11. Bravo EL, Tarazi RL, Fouad FM: Clonidine suppression test. N Engl J Med 305: 623, 1981.
12. Harrison TS, Bartlett JD Jr, Seaton JF: Current evaluation and management of pheochromocytoma. Ann Surg 168: 701–713, 1968.
13. Sisson JL, Farger MS, Valk TW: Et Al. Scintigraphic localization of pheochromocytoma. N Engl J Med 305: 1217, 1981.

16. Controversies in the treatment of endocrine tumors: medical and surgical management of prolactinomas, acromegaly and thyroid cancer

RICHARD J. SANTEN and ANDREA MANNI

1. Pituitary tumors

Controversy arises in medicine with regard to therapy whenever multiple effective treatments have not been rigorously compared in a controlled fashion. For this reason, various investigators advocate surgery [1, 2], radiation [3, 4], or medical therapy [5, 6] (at least for prolactinomas), as the initial treatment of choice of functioning pituitary tumors. Controlled, prospective clinical trials comparing the relative efficacy and safety of these treatments do not currently exist to guide the choice of therapy for pituitary tumors. Consequently, therapeutic decisions remain subjective and frequently reflect the background training of the physician.

The preceding chapters in this volume were designed to detail various approaches to treatment of pituitary tumors. It is our goal here to focus on concepts developed from available data which may help the physician in making rational choices between these therapies for individual patients.

1.1 Prolactin secreting tumors

The first principle regarding management of this entity is to be certain of the diagnosis. Since the introduction of specific radioimmunoassay for prolactin [7], hyperprolactinemia from a variety of causes has been recognized [8–12]. Once hypothyroidism, pregnancy, suprasellar tumors and the use of psychotropic drugs and oral contraceptives are excluded, the differential diagnosis of elevated serum prolactin is between a pituitary tumor and 'idiopathic' hyperprolactinemia. Sophisticated dynamic tests of prolactin secretion such as those described by Arafah et al. [8] in their chapter are not helpful in distinguishing between these two entities. The degree of elevation of prolactin and high resolution computed tomography are the best tools available to identify which patients with hyperprolactinemia have a pituitary tumor.

Improved understanding of the natural history of these tumors will probably help in the future in the selection of appropriate therapy. Longitudinal studies of

Santen, R.J. and Manni, A. (eds.), Diagnosis and management of endocrine-related tumors. ISBN 0-89838-636-5.
© *1984, Martinus Nijhoff Publishers, Boston. Printed in the Netherlands.*

420

women harboring clinically significant, prolactin-secreting adenomas reveal that the vast majority of them, probably around 80%, remain stationary [13, 14]. The identification of a large number of microadenomas of the pituitary at autopsy in patients who were not known to have symptoms of a pituitary tumor [15] provided further evidence that many microadenomas remain quiescent clinically.

A small but significant proportion of patients, around 10%, may actually show signs of spontaneous improvement with time and some of them, particularly after an induced pregnancy, may have complete normalization of serum prolactin and resumption of menses [16]. On the other hand, a similar small fraction of patients manifests unequivocal evidence of tumor progression [13, 14]. Obviously, all tumors detected as macroadenomas must have been once microadenomas.

Since the natural history of most prolactin-secreting tumors is very benign, it is essential that the physician does not indiscriminantly use potentially hazardous treatments in a group of patients who are usually young and in an excellent state of health. Specific goals should instead dictate whether to choose any treatment at all in an individual patient and what form of therapy to employ.

A question to ask in this regard is whether the hyperprolactinemia per se represents a hazard to health. Existing evidence suggests that hyperprolactinemic women may be at an increased risk of developing osteoporosis, related either to the associated estrogen deficiency or to an effect of prolactin itself on bones [17, 18]. This potential risk may constitute a reason to institute therapy, particularly in the very young patient. On the other hand, in a woman older than 40 years of age, this consideration would be much less important in the choice of therapy. Outside the possible risk of osteoporosis, there appears to be no other harmful effect to the general state of health from elevation of serum prolactin. Thus, it can be seen how the best therapeutic decision for an older woman not interested in having children and without signs or symptoms of mechanical compression from the tumor may simply be periodic follow up without any treatment.

Restoration of fertility is probably the most common indication for treatment of women with prolactin secreting tumors. Both transsphenoidal microsurgery [1, 8] and dopaminergic drugs such as bromocriptine [5, 6] are highly successful in achieving this goal. In selecting between these forms of treatment, two important considerations have to be kept in mind. One is the availability of an experienced neurosurgeon. It is of critical importance that the physician refers the suitable patient to a medical center where there is a proven record of success in performing transsphenoidal microsurgery. Such a procedure, if performed by an inexperienced neurosurgeon, may not only be ineffective but also associated with significant morbidity and mortality. The other factor to take into account in the selection of therapy is the size of the tumor. As clearly shown by Arafah et al. [8] in their chapter as well as other investigators [1], the smaller the tumor the greater the chance of cure with transsphenoidal microsurgery.

Perhaps, the age of the patient and the duration of symptoms may be additional factors (far less important in our opinion) which predict the outcome of surgery.

A recent study suggested that the long-term cure rate may be higher in younger women with amenorrhea of shorter duration [19]. Thus, based on the available information, the ideal circumstances to recommend surgery would be in the case of a young woman who wishes to become pregnant, is less than 25 years old, has amenorrhea of short duration, and radiologic evidence of a microadenoma. An experienced neurosurgeon must be available if this course is chosen. Furthermore, an additional consideration in the selection of therapy should be that transsphenoidal microsurgery probably offers the best chance of 'long-term' and perhaps 'permanent cure'. Although, unquestionably, some patients relapse following what initially seemed to be a successful surgery, a significant fraction of women remain free of disease after several years of follow up [8, 20]. Recently, Dr. Reichlin has reviewed the literature regarding the relapse rate of hyperprolactinemia following an initially successful transsphenoidal surgery. Of 248 patients, in whom serum prolactin was restored to normal by surgery, 41 (17%) have relapsed after an average follow up of 50 ± 3 months (personal communication). Most importantly, it seems possible to identify those patients likely to be cured by the demonstration of a 'suppressed' serum prolactin level in the immediate postoperative period [8, 20] and the restoration of normal dynamic prolactin secretion 3 months after surgery [8].

The introduction of dopamine agonists such as bromocriptine has been a major advance in the treatment of hyperprolactinemia. When all prolactin secreting tumors are included, there is no other therapy alone that can match the effectiveness of bromocriptine in normalizing serum prolactin levels (over 95% of the cases) and restoring fertility (80–90%). It is probably universally agreed upon that, in the patient with normal radiologic findings, bromocriptine is the initial treatment of choice to lower prolactin in the attempt to restore fertility. Controversy on the use of bromocriptine versus surgery as initial treatment arises in the patient with radiologic evidence of a pituitary tumor. In my opinion, the data available in the literature indicate that the use of bromocriptine in this setting is probably acceptable, provided that the patient has a microadenoma. It is now, in fact, well established that bromocriptine, when taken in the early weeks of pregnancy, has no teratogenic effect [21]. Furthermore, in the case of a microadenoma, the risk of symptomatic tumor enlargement during pregnancy is small, at most 5% [22]. Finally, following delivery, the physician may elect to discontinue bromocriptine treatment and follow the patient for evidence of resolution of the hyperprolactinemia, which has been reported to occur in up to 10% of the patients [16].

On the other hand, if a woman has a large pituitary tumor, particularly with suprasellar extension, and desires fertility, I do not think that bromocriptine alone should be used. Under these circumstances, in fact, it has been shown that the likelihood of significant tumor enlargement during pregnancy is much higher, reaching 35% [22]. Under these circumstances, it is preferable to treat the patient surgically first. Some patients will be cured by surgery alone despite the large size of their tumors [8]. If the hyperprolactinemia persists, it is probably safe to induce pregnancy with bromocriptine, since the large bulk of the tumor has been removed. As an alternative to surgery, the physician may elect to use radiation prior to conception, since it has been shown to reduce the likelihood of tumor enlargement during pregnancy [23]. Incidentally, whenever tumor enlargement has occurred in this setting, the outcome has been favorable. Prompt regression of the symptoms has occurred following delivery, surgery [24], or bromocriptine [25].

Neither surgery nor bromocriptine are optimal treatments of large prolactin secreting tumors with or without extrasellar extension when fertility is not desired. Under these circumstances, the primary concern of the physician is the local growth of the tumor and the possible long-term effects of hyperprolactinemia on bone mineralization and hypoestrogenism, particularly in the very young women.

Surgery frequently fails to entirely remove these large adenomas, although the degree of hyperprolactinemia is often reduced postoperatively [8] indicating that significant debulking of the tumor has occurred. This partial success, however, is far from satisfactory because of the possibility of tumor regrowth with time. Although precise figures in this regard are not available in the literature, this concern is probably justified by the fact that these large tumors may belong to the subgroup of pituitary adenomas with the highest replicative potential. In these patients with incomplete tumor removal, surgery should probably be followed by radiation therapy or long-term medical treatment with dopaminergic drugs.

The introduction of bromocriptine has made a major contribution to the treatment of large prolactin secreting tumors. Several reports have described dramatic reductions in tumor size with prompt resolution of symptoms, not infrequently occurring within days [26, 27]. These results are commonly achievable with modest doses of the drug (<7.5 mg/day) which are usually associated with good tolerability by the patient. The major problem with bromocriptine therapy is that rapid tumor regrowth frequently occurs upon discontinuation of the drug [28]. Consequently, the vast majority of patients are committed to indefinite therapy. A logical approach to treating this group of patients may be the sequential use of medical and surgical therapy. It is, in fact, possible that reduction of tumor size with bromocriptine may enhance the chances of complete removal of the adenoma by subsequent surgery. Limited data are available in the literature to support this hypothesis. Landolt et al. [29] observed that 3 of 6 patients with macroadenoma (diameter >10 mm) pretreated with bromocriptine were cured by surgery versus 10 of 48 patients treated with surgery alone. This difference was not significant and a larger number of patients needs to be studied. The same authors observed that pretreatment with bromocriptine may actually adversely affect the outcome of surgery in the case of microadenomas [29]. Only 8 of 24 patients (33%) were cured by sequential medical and surgical therapy versus 13/16 (81%) treated with transsphenoidal surgery alone (p<0.005). A subsequent report by Faglia et al. [30] did not support the view that previous bromocriptine worsens the success rate of surgery in microprolactinomas. These authors observed a similar cure rate in patients treated with bromocriptine followed by surgery (13/20, 65%) and in those treated with surgery alone (20/29, 69%). A major difference between these two studies is that, while in the former, bromocriptine was continued up to the time of surgery, in the latter it had been discontinued for 2–24 months (mean 8.4 months) prior to the operation. It is conceivable that bromocriptine may adversely affect the outcome of surgery by altering the consistency of the tumor and making its margins more indistinct. In any event, at present, it is advisable to withhold medical therapy for at least a few months before subjecting a patient with a microadenoma to transsphenoidal microsurgery.

In our opinion, the use of radiotherapy as a primary treatment of hyperprolactinemia has a limited role, despite claims to the contrary by some investigators [4]. A major drawback of radiation therapy is the considerable length of time, usually in terms of years, that it takes for the serum prolactin to normalize [4]. Such a delayed effect is unacceptable when fertility is desired, particularly in view of the fact that surgery or medical therapy can correct the hyperprolactinemia in a matter of days. Furthermore, radiation therapy is associated with a significant risk of development of hypopituitarism [3]. It is hard to justify this risk in young healthy women with a long life expectancy when this complication is rare with surgery, in experienced hands, and nonexistent with medical therapy.

Radiotherapy, however, continues to be a valuable treatment for preventing tumor growth in patients who are contemplating pregnancy [23], and for preventing or treating recurrent disease in patients who have had unsuccessful surgery for an aggressive tumor [31].

From this discussion, it appears that no one therapy is ideal for every patient. In our opinion, tumor size, desire for pregnancy, and age of the patient are of key importance in selecting the individual treatment. Because several forms of therapy are available for hyperprolactinemia, it is important that the patient is thoroughly informed of the potential benefits and limitations associated with each modality.

1.2 Growth hormone secreting tumors

As in the case of hyperprolactinemia, transsphenoidal microsurgery, radiation therapy and dopaminergic drugs are the alternatives available to the physician for the treatment of acromegaly. The considerations involved in the selection of the most appropriate therapy for an individual patient are, however, quite different.

It may be important at this point to mention some recent developments in our understanding of the pathophysiology of acromegaly. Until recently, the classical clinical manifestations of acromegaly, in association with elevated and glucose non-suppressible serum growth hormone levels were considered to be diagnostic of a pituitary growth hormone secreting tumor. Recently, there have been sporadic case reports of somatotroph hyperplasia induced by growth hormone releasing hormone ectopically secreted by a pancreatic tumor [32, 33]. Although this may be a rare cause of acromegaly, this possibility should be considered whenever a detailed radiologic evaluation fails to reveal a localized pituitary lesion. Obviously, the treatment of choice of this condition would be removal of the tumor secreting growth hormone releasing hormone.

When evaluating the therapeutic options for classic acromegaly due to a pituitary tumor, it is important to take into account the natural history of the disease. In contrast to hyperprolactinemia, growth hormone hypersecretion per se is associated with serious clinical sequelae. Significant morbidity and mortality derive from the development of diabetes mellitus, hypertension and cardiovascular complications in a significant fraction of acromegalic patients, which results in a shorter life span [34, 35]. Furthermore, disfigurement and morbidity result from the acral enlargement and arthritic manifestations secondary to growth hormone hypersecretion. At present, it is not known whether the growth pattern of growth hormone secreting tumors differs from that of prolactin-secreting adenomas. In any event, because of the serious clinical consequences of acromegaly mentioned above, therapy should be more aggressive than in the case of hyperprolactinemia.

Transsphenoidal microsurgery performed by an experienced neurosurgeon appears to be the treatment of choice for patients with small tumors. The results with this type of surgery reported by Arafah et al. [36] in their chapter clearly support this approach. Fifteen of their 17 patients without evidence of extrasellar extension at surgery were 'cured' of their disease after a median follow up of six years. Incidentally, it is worth emphasizing the usefulness of the postoperative dynamic studies of growth hormone secretion to identify those patients at risk of relapse [36]. A high degree of success of transsphenoidal microsurgery in correcting growth hormone hypersecretion in patients with intrasellar tumors has also been described by other investigators [2, 37]. All these reports have emphasized the success of surgery in selectively removing the growth hormone secreting adenomas while leaving intact, normal pituitary function.

Considerably less successful is the treatment of acromegaly due to tumors with extrasellar extension. Under these conditions, the probability of complete tumor removal markedly decreases, whereas the risk of development of hypopituitarism as a result of treatment increases. Transsphenoidal microsurgery can still be valuable since a small but significant fraction of patients can be cured by this modality of treatment alone [36]. In their chapter, Arafah et al. [36] recommend an aggressive surgical approach to the point of performing a total hypophysectomy whenever 'normal pituitary tissue could not be left intact without the risk of leaving tumor behind.' By doing this, they were able to cure two patients at the expense obviously of total hypopituitarism. While this approach cannot be justified in the case of hyperprolactinemia because of the benign nature of the disease, it may be acceptable in a selected group of patients with clinically active acromegly, particularly if fertility is not of concern. The alternative therapeutic approach in these patients with large tumors is to use radiotherapy as the primary treatment. This treatment modality, however, is also not ideal.

Conventional supervoltage radiation (4,000 rads) has also been found to be associated with insidious development of partial or total hypopituitarism over the years [3]. Furthermore, it may take up to 10 years before serum growth hormone becomes normal in 70% of patients [3]. Alternative forms of radiation therapy involving the use of proton beam or alpha particles in the attempt to deliver higher doses (up to 15,000 rads) are currently used in two centers in the United States [38, 39]. With this high-dosage method, radionecrosis is expected to occur sooner than after treatment from supervoltage sources. Surprisingly, it is disappointing to observe that it may still take years before normalization of growth hormone occurs in responding patients [38, 39]. Furthermore, with this method of high energy radiation, there is the risk of damage to surrounding structures resulting in a number of complications, particularly external ocular muscle palsy [38].

In any event, radiation therapy, either as a primary treatment or as a follow up therapy after surgery, has a much more prominent role in the management of growth hormone secreting tumors than in that of prolactinomas. This is essentially due to two reasons. First, the medical treatment of acromegaly is far less satisfactory than that of hyperprolactinemia (see below). Second, acromegaly needs to be treated more aggressively because of its significant associated complications.

Dopaminergic drugs such as bromocriptine, now widely used in the treatment of prolactin-secreting tumors, have a more limited role in the treatment of acromegaly. The inhibitory effect of bromocriptine on growth hormone secretion in patients with tumors has to be viewed as paradoxical, because the usual effect of dopamine agonists on growth hormone secretion in normal individuals is stimulatory [40]. Bromocriptine succeeds in totally normalizing serum growth hormone only in a small fraction of acromegalic patients, probably not exceeding 20% [41–43]. An additional 50% of patients show some lowering in their circulating growth hormone although not into the normal range, while the rest do not benefit at all from bromocriptine treatment. Interestingly, two studies have suggested that it may be possible to predict long-term response to bromocriptine in acromegaly by a fall in serum growth hormone after acute administration of the drug [41], or a rise following TRH administration [44]. These observations will have to be confirmed by other investigators before their clinical usefulness can be fully assessed.

Since in the vast majority of patients, bromocriptine only partially suppresses growth hormone, it is logical to ask whether a lower but not normal growth hormone results in any significant clinical benefit. Partial suppresion of serum growth hormone either as a result of surgery [36] or bromocriptine [41] has been found to produce symptomatic improvement such as reduction in soft tissue swelling and amelioration of glucose tolerance. The impact, however, of this partial improvement on the natural history of acromegaly and the progression of its complications remains unknown.

Finally, the success rate of bromocriptine in the reduction of tumor size in acromegaly is not fully established. Reports in the literature are somewhat conflicting in this regard with some studies showing no effect [45, 46] and others reporting more promising results [47]. Probably it is fair to summarize that the efficacy of bromocriptine in reducing the size of growth hormone secreting tumors is modest, definitely inferior to that observed in the treatment of prolactinomas.

On the basis of current knowledge, medical therapy with dopaminergic drugs cannot be advocated in general as the initial treatment of choice of acromegaly, particularly in the case of large extrasellar tumors posing a threat to surrounding structures. Bromocriptine, however, can be a valuable adjunct to surgery and radiation therapy in the treatment of selected patients.

2. Thyroid carcinoma

A wide range of opinion exists regarding the proper initial therapeutic approach for patients with well differentiated papillary and follicular carcinomas [48]. Thyroid cancer is rare, affecting only 37/1,000,000 population/year in the United States and relatively indolent (85–95% twenty year survival rates). Consequently, properly conducted clinical trials with randomization to various treatment groups, stratification of known risk factors, and prospective follow-up do not exist. In clinical areas where a paucity of data exist, fertile ground is present for development of major clinical controversies. Controversy regarding well differentiated thyroid cancer treatment centers upon two issues: 1) the extent of surgery necessary to cure patients, and 2) the use of radioactive iodine as adjuvant therapy prior to demonstration of tumor recurrence. One group of adherents, predominantly surgeons, feels that conservative surgery is curative and adjuvant therapy with radioactive iodine is unnecessary [49–54]. This approach spares patients the high risk of permanent hypoparathyroidism (i.e., 10–20%) and recurrent laryngeal nerve damage (i.e. 5–10%) which has been encountered following the performance of aggressive excisional surgery in previous studies. The other group of advocates, largely medical endocrinologists, feels that adjuvant radioiodine prevents disease recurrences and prolongs survival [55–59]. In order to utilize radioactive iodine in an adjuvant setting, more extensive surgery (i.e. near total thyroidectomy) is necessary to reduce the competition for radioactive iodine by normal thyroid tissue and to enhance uptake into residual thyroid carcinoma micrometastases.

In the absence of controlled trials, what principles can be used to guide the physican in the selection of appropriate therapy for individual patients. One concept is to treat high-risk patients with more aggressive methods and those at low risk with conservative approaches. In applying this strategy, it is important to know which patients are at high risk of death from thyroid cancer. The concepts developed in selecting patients with breast cancer for aggressive surgery and adjuvant chemotherapy can provide a conceptual framework for similar decisions regarding thyroid cancer. Major recent studies in the breast cancer field high-lighted important concepts regarding tumor biology and allowed identification of high-risk patients. Major predictors of risk in breast cancer include size of the primary tumor (T), presence of contiguous nodal involvement (N), presence of metastases (M) (i.e. the TNM system), degree of tumor differentiation, and age of the patient.

It is useful to examine whether these same factors can identify patients with thyroid cancer at high risk of dying from their disease. Mazzaferri recently demonstrated a good correlation between the diameter of the primary tumor (T) and percent of patients with tumor recurrence (Fig. 1) [55]. Buckwalter et al. found that patients with tumors <2.5 cm survive longer than those with larger lesions (Fig. 2) [53]. The size of the primary, then, does appear useful in identifying high-risk patients. The presence of distant metastases also imparts a poor prognosis in patients with thyroid cancer (Fig. 3) [53]. In contrast to breast cancer, however, local spread to contiguous lymph nodes may not be associated with a worse prognosis. Buckwalter's data (Fig. 3) as well as that of Cady (Table 1) [49, 60] and Mazzaferri support this contention [55, 61]. Only in patients >70 years of age (Fig. 4) does local nodal involvement indicate a poorer prognosis as with breast cancer [62]. The degree of tumor differentiation is also an important predictive factor in thyroid cancer. Poorly differentiated tumors behave more

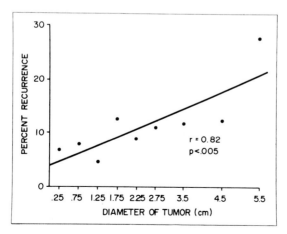

Figure 1. The direct correlation between diameter of the primary tumor and recurrence of tumor. Reprinted from the Study of Mazzaferri et al. [55].

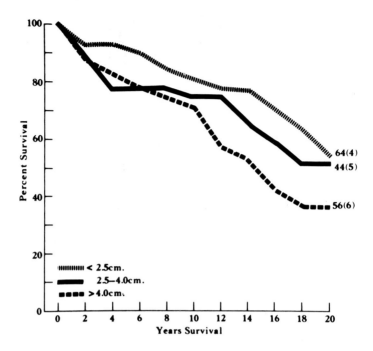

Figure 2. Size of primary lesions, survival curves. Reprinted from the study of Buckwalter et al. [53].

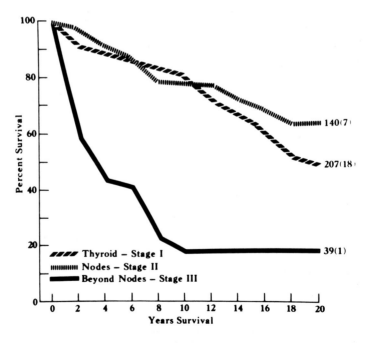

Figure 3. The stage of the disease survival curves. Reprinted from the study of Buckwalter et al. [53].

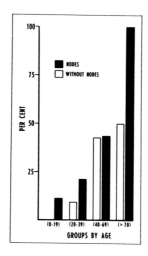

Figure 4. Significance of local nodal involvement in patients >70 years of age as opposed to those younger.

aggressively than well differentiated ones. Age, in contrast, has a different biologic significance when comparing breast with thyroid cancer. The biologic nature of differentiated thyroid tumors in older patients [53] is much more aggressive than in younger subjects (Fig. 5), whereas the converse is true for breast cancer. Local capsular invasion is an additional feature known to be important in thyroid cancer. Thus, infiltration through the thyroid capsule and its surrounding structures (Table 2), imparts a poor prognosis in thyroid cancer patients [61].

Table 1. Lahey Clinical Foundation: Differentiated thyroid carcinoma, 1941–1960; Relation of lymph node metastases to survival

Pathology	Negative nodes			1–3 Positive nodes			4–10 Positive nodes			>10 Positive nodes		
		Dead of disease			Dead of disease			Dead of disease			Dead of disease	
	No.	No.	%	No.	No.	%	No.	No.	%	No.	No.	%
Papillary and mixed	213	23	11	71	7	10	54	6	11	18	0	0
– Intrathyroid disease	84	4	5	48	2	4	32	4	13	9	0	0
– Extrathyroid disease	31	13	42	20	6	30	15	2	13	8	0	0
Follicular	136	37	27	11	2	18	9	1	11	4	0	0
– Intrathyroid disease	47	13	28	8	0	0	3	0	0	2	0	0
– Extrathyroid disease	13	9	69	3	2	67	6	1	17	2	0	0

Reproduced from Cady et al. Ann Surg, Nov. 1976 [60].

430

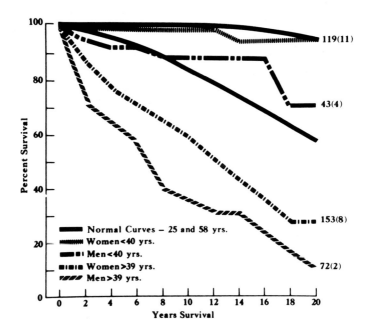

Figure 5. Age and sex survival curves. Reprinted from the study of Buckwalter et al. [53].

After establishing that a patient is at high risk of recurrence for thyroid cancer, it is logical to question whether adjuvant therapy for residual postoperative disease or micrometastases is an effective therapeutic approach. Two recent studies [55, 61] address this question in a large number of patients with papillary carcinoma of the thyroid. Mazzaferri et al. compared groups of patients receiving no adjuvant medical treatment (n = 30), adjuvant hormonal therapy in the form of thyroid hormone (n = 401) and adjuvant hormonal therapy plus radioactive iodine (n = 107) (Fig. 6). A major reduction in recurrence rate occurred in patients receiving thyroid hormone as adjuvant therapy and a further reduction was observed after I131 plus thyroid. A second study indicated a survival advantage as well (p<.05) for patients receiving I131 and thyroid hormone as adjuvant therapy compared to those given thyroid hormone alone [57]. This difference was

Table 2. Effect of local capsular invasion on prognosis

Status	% Recurrence	% Deaths from cancer
Absent	13.7 (75/548)	0.7 (4/548)
Present	39.1 (9/23)	7.1 (2/28)
	p<.001	p<.02

Adapted from the data of Mazzaferri et al. [55, 61].

only apparent if the patients were first subjected to a total (i.e., near-total) thyroidectomy. Neither studies were randomized or stratified and, thus, both were subject to major bias in patient selection. Nonetheless, in the Mazzaferri study [61], patients receiving radioactive iodine as adjuvant therapy had a trend toward more local tumor invasion, and therefore, were at higher risk than patients not receiving radioactive iodine. Taken together, these studies suggest that adjuvant radioactive iodine as well as adjuvant hormonal therapy may provide benefit to patients by delaying recurrences and prolonging survival.

If one accepts the fact that adjuvant therapy is efficacious, what risks are involved in choosing to give adjuvant radioactive iodine. The major risk is an associated one and involves the extent of surgery necessary rather than the radioactive iodine itself. In order to deliver sufficient radioiodine to the lesion, all normal thyroid tissue which competes with the cancer tissue for iodine uptake, must be removed. This necessitates exision of as much thyroid tissue as possible surgically. In practice, 'near total thyroidectomy' has resulted in permanent

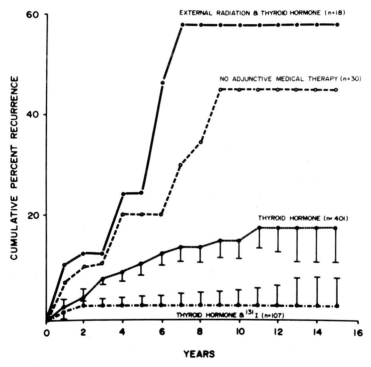

Figure 6. Cumulative recurrence rates for those in whom follow up was 1 year or longer divided according to the type of medical therapy used postoperatively. For those who had recurrences, there were no differences in the sex, mean age at presentation, clinical presentation, surgical findings, size of the primary lesion or extent of metastatic disease among the 4 medical therapy subgroups [61]. However, there was a trend towards more local tumor invasion and a greater number of cervical node metastases in the group treated with I^{131}. Reprinted from the study of Mazzaferri et al. [61].

hypoparathyroidism in 12–20% of patients and recurrent laryngeal nerve damage in another 7–10% in reported series [49, 53, 55, 57, 61]. This figure can probably be substantially lowered in the hands of highly experienced surgeons to a rate found by DeGroot et al. of 2/100 for hypoparathyroidism and 1/100 for recurrent laryngeal nerve damage in his last 100 patients treated with 'near total thyroidectomy' [63, 64]. Nonetheless, the chances of complications from near total thyroidectomy are much greater than from subtotal thyroidectomy, the preferred approach if one does not choose to administer adjuvant radioiodine.

Probably little morbidity is imparted from the use of adjuvant thyroid hormone therapy in patients with well differentiated thyroid cancer. Sufficient experience over several decades indicates that radioactive iodine therapy also presents minimal risks to the patient. Leukemia, permanent bone marrow suppression, or other major complications have been infrequently encountered, particularly in recent years [55, 57, 59, 61, 65].

Another consideration in selecting treatment approaches is the risk benefit ratio in individual patients. Very few patients with differentiated thyroid cancer actually die of their disease. Woolner et al. reported that cohorts with either occult (240 patients) or intrathyroidal papillary (348 patients) carcinoma of the thyroid experienced a similar survival rate as an age-matched control population when examined by life table analysis [50]. They could demonstrate reduced survival from thyroid cancer only in the small number (68) of patients with extrathyroidal tumors. This study has been criticized on several grounds [59]. Only one survival curve for controls is matched to 3 separate groups of cancer patients. Nine cancer-related deaths and 33 recurrences were identified in the intrathyroidal cancer group, a finding which must implicate a reduced survival at least for some patients. Finally, the control group of patients were not under as close medical supervision as the cancer patients and thus may have died from other treatable diseases more commonly than the thyroid cancer patients. Regardless of these critiques, this hallmark study clearly shows the relatively benign nature of differentiated thyroid cancer when it is confined to the thyroid gland.

One further question is also relevant in planning a treatment strategy. Is it more advantageous to use I131 in an adjuvant setting or should it be given only when residual or recurrent tumor can be demonstrated. No data are available on this point to our knowledge. The treatment implications of this question are major. Since only 30% of patients with papillary carcinoma experience tumor recurrence by 20 years after surgery when no adjuvant therapy is given, then by inference, 70% of patients undergoing near total thyroidectomy and radioactive iodine probably do not benefit from it because they have already been cured [55, 61]. If treatment at the time of recurrence proves to be as beneficial as in the adjuvant setting, then a substantial number of patients (approximately 70%) would be spared this aggressive adjuvant approach. The number of patients requiring treatment for recurrent disease would be even lower (approximately 20% at 20 years) if adjuvant thyroid hormone were given after subtotal thyroidectomy.

The various factors discussed above and the lack of controlled trials, have led to widely varying recommendations regarding adjuvant radioactive iodine in combination with near total thyroidectomy. In this volume (Chapter 5), Dr. Beierwaltes favors the use of adjuvant radioactive iodine whereas Dr. Harrison (Chapter 7) recommends a conservative surgical therapy without adjuvant radioactive iodine. Each of these author's opinions is supported by a cohort of investigators. The near-total thyroidectomy and adjuvant radioactive iodine approach is advocated by Mazzaferri, DeGroot, Robbins and Samaan [55, 57, 58, 61, 63] and a conservative surgical approach by Woolner and Behrs, Cady, Tollefson, Crile, Buckwalter and Thomas, among others [49–54]. The use of adjuvant thyroid hormone therapy, on the other hand, is favored by most investigators writing about this disease.

When controversy exists, the middle road often provides the more reasonable course [48]. In addition, use of concepts developed for the understanding of breast cancer treatment are probably appropriately applied to thyroid cancer. Taking this conceptual approach, we favor more aggressive therapy for high risk patients and a conservative approach for those with a lower risk. A graded series of indications for near total thyroidectomy and radioactive iodine treatment can then be developed (Table 3). With recurrent disease and distant metastases, patients have already declared themselves at high risk of dying of their disease and should be treated by completion of their thyroidectomy followed by radioactive iodine. This does not represent adjuvant treatment but reflects actual therapy for demonstrable lesions. A strong case can be made for adjuvant treatment of tumors >1.5 cm in size in patients >40 years of age because the risk of recurrence and death from tumor outweighs the hazards of treatment in this group. Patients under age 20 may also have a poorer prognosis [66] and perhaps should also be treated in this fashion. Another high risk group includes patients

Table 3. Selection of patients for total thyroidectomy and adjuvant radioactive iodine treatment

---

 I. Advanced disease (i.e., distant metastases)
  A. Presence of lesions which concentrate radioiodine
  B. Must complete thyroidectomy prior to I^{131}
 II. Adjuvant therapy (requires near total thyroidectomy)
  A. Definite indication
   1. tumor >1.5* cm in patients <20 or >40
   2. tumor of any size with capsular or extracapsular local invasion – all ages
  B. Probable indication
   1. tumor >1.5 cm in patient aged 20–40
  C. Doubtful indication
   1. tumor <1.5 cm in patient <20 or >40
  D. Not indicated
   1. tumor <1.5 cm in patient aged 20–40

---

* No agreement exists regarding the critical tumor size upon which to base these decisions. Varying recommendations include 1.0 cm [59], 1.5 cm [55], or large tumors [51].

with capsular or extracapsular local invasion. Patients with tumors >1.5 cm in diameter who are in the 20–40 age group could also be treated with near-total thyroidectomy and radioactive iodine treatment. This recommendation, however, would be debated by most investigators with a surgical as opposed to medical orientation. More general agreement exists that patients with tumors <1.5 cm, even if older than age 40, are best managed by subtotal thyroidectomy and adjuvant thyroid hormone treatment. These patients could be subjected to completion of their thyroidectomy and radioactive iodine upon demonstration of recurrent disease at a later time.

How are these recommendations altered in patients whose tumors occur following exposure to radiation in childhood or in patients with follicular as opposed to papillary cancers. We do not believe that these approaches should be changed in any way. No data are presently available to suggest that the subgroup of patients previously exposed to radiation behaves differently than those with spontaneous cancer. In addition, the differences in biologic aggressiveness of follicular cancer (differences which are not usually agreed upon) do not warrant major changes in approach based upon this concept.

The graded approach to treatment outlined above or other approaches will be the subject of continued debate until properly conducted randomized, stratified, controlled trials are completed. This will require an immense effort because of the time necessary to complete such trials (20–40 years) and the need to stratefy for numerous variables (i.e., age, size of tumor, age of patients, degree of differentiation, etc.). In the meantime, we believe that knowledge of tumor biology, consideration of risks and benefits will lead to proper patient selection for more aggressive treatment approaches.

References

1. Post KD, Biller BJ, Adelman LS, Molitch ME, Wolpert SM, Reichlin S: Selective transsphenoidal adenomectomy in women with galactorrhea-amenorrhea. J Am Med Assoc 242: 158–162, 1979.
2. Tucker HS-G, Grubb SR, Wigand JP, Watlington CO, Blackard WG, Becker DP: The treatment of acromegaly by transsphenoidal surgery. Arch Intern Med 140: 795–802, 1980.
3. Eastman RC, Gorden P, Roth J: Conventional supervoltage irradiation is an effective treatment for acromegaly. J Clin Endocrinol Metab 48: 931–940, 1979.
4. Grossman A, Cohen BL, Plowman N, Wass JAH, Jones A, Besser GM: Long-term effects of radiotherapy in patients with prolactin secreting pituitary adenomas. Program of the 65th Annual Meeting of the Endocrine Society, San Antonio, Texas, June, 1983 (Abstr 436), p 189.
5. Thorner MD, Besser GM: Bromocriptine treatment of hyperprolactinaemic hypogonadism. Acta Endocrinol (Suppl) (Copenh) 216: 131–146, 1978.
6. del Pozo E, Varga L, Wyss H, Tolis G, Friesen H, Wenner R, Vetter L, Uettwiler A: Clinical and hormonal response to bromocriptin (CB-154) in the galactorrhea syndromes. J Clin Endocrinol Metab 39: 18–26, 1974.
7. Kleinberg DL, Frantz AG: Human prolactin: measurement in plasma by in vitro bioassay. J Clin Invest 50: 1557–1568, 1971.

8. Arafah BM, Brodkey JS, Pearson OH: Prolactin secreting pituitary adenomas in women. In: Endocrine-Related Tumors I, Santen RJ, Manni A (eds), The Hague: Martinus-Nijhoff Publishers, 1984, pp 63–79.

9. Tolis G, Franks S: Physiology and pathology of prolactin secretion. In: Clinical Neuroendocrinology: A Pathophysiological Approach, Tolis G, Labrie F, Martin JB, Naftolin F (eds). New York: Raven Press, 1979, pp 291–317.

10. Post KD, Biller BJ, Adelman LS, Molitch ME, Wolpert SM, Reichlin S: Selective transsphenoidal adenomectomy in women with galactorrheaamenorrhea. J Am Med Assoc 242: 158–162, 1979.

11. Franks S, Murray MAF, Jequier AM, Steele SJ, Nabarro JDN, Jacobs HS: Incidence and significance of hyperprolactinaemia in women with amenorrhoea. Clin Endocrinol 4: 597–607, 1975.

12. Kleinberg DL, Noel GL, Frantz AG: Gaactorrhea: a study of 235 cases, including 48 with pituitary tumors. N Engl J Med 296: 589–600, 1977.

13. Hancock KW, Scott JS, Lamb JT, Gibson RM, Chapman C: Conservative management of pituitary prolactinomas: evidence for bromocriptine induced regression. Br J Obstet Gynecol 87: 523–529, 1980.

14. March CM, Kletzky OA, Davajan V, Teal J, Weiss M, Apuzzo ML, Marrs RP, Mishell DR Jr: Longitudinal evaluation of patients with untreated prolactin-secreting pituitary adenomas. Am J Obstet Gynecol 139: 835–844, 1981.

15. Burrow GN, Wortzman G, Rewcastle NB, Holgate RC, Kovacs K: Microadenomas of the pituitary and abnormal sellar tomograms in an unselected autopsy series. N Engl J Med 304: 156–158, 1981.

16. Randall S, Laing I, Chapman AJ, Shalet SM, Beardwell CG, Kelly WF, Davies D: Pregnancies in women with hyperprolactinaemia: obstetric and endocrinological management of 50 pregnancies in 37 women. Br J Obstet Gynecol 89: 20–23, 1982.

17. Klibanski A, Neer RM, Beitins IZ, Zervas NT, McArthur JW: Decreased bone density in hyperprolactinemic women. Med Intelligence 303: 1511–1514, 1980.

18. Schlechte JA, Sherman B, Martin R: Bone density in amenorrheic women with and without hyperprolactinemia. J Clin Endocrinol Metab 56: 1120–1123, 1983.

19. Robinson AG, Nelson PB: Prolactinomas in women: current therapies. Ann Int Med 99: 115–118, 1983.

20. Serri O, Rasio E, Beauregard H, Hardy J, Somma M: Recurrence of hyperprolactinemia after selective transsphenoidal adenomectomy in women with prolactinoma. N Engl J Med 309: 280–283, 1983.

21. Turkalj I, Braun P, Krupp P: Surveillance of bromocriptine in pregnancy. J Am Med Assoc 247: 1589–1591, 1982.

22. Gemzell C, Wang CF: Outcome of pregnancy in women with pituitary adenoma. Fertil Steril 31: 363–372, 1979.

23. Thorner MO, Edwards CRW, Charlesworth M, Dacie JE, Moult PJ, Rees LH, Jones AE, Besser GM: Pregnancy in patients presenting with hyperprolactinaemia. Br Med J 11: 771–774, 1979.

24. Dommerholt HBR, Assies J, Van Der Werf AFM: Growth of a prolactinoma during pregnancy: case report and review. Br J Obstet Gynecol 88: 62–70, 1981.

25. Bergh T, Nillius SJ, Wide L: Clinical course and outcome of pregnancies in amenorrhoeic women with hyperprolactinaemia and pituitary tumors. Br Med J 1: 875–880, 1978.

26. Thorner MO, Martin WH, Rogol AD, Morris JL, Perryman RL, Conway BP, Howards SS, Wolfman MG, MacLeod RM: Rapid regression of pituitary prolactinomas during bromocriptine treatment. J Clin Endocrinol Metab 51: 438–445, 1980.

27. Corenblum B, Hanley DA: Bromocriptine reduction of prolactinoma size. Fertil Steril 36: 716–719, 1981.

28. Thorner MO, Perryman RL, Rogol AD, Conway BP, MacLeod RM, Login IS, Morris JL: Rapid

changes of prolactinoma volume after withdrawal and reinstitution of bromocriptine. J Clin Endocrinol Metab 153: 480–483, 1981.

29. Landolt AM, Keller PJ, Froesch ER, Mueller J: Bromocriptine: Does it jeopardize the result of later surgery for prolactinomas. Lancet ii: 657–658, 1982.

30. Faglia G, Moriondo P, Travaglini P, Giovanelli MA: Influence of previous bromocriptine therapy on surgery for microprolactinoma. Lancet i: 133–134, 1983.

31. Sheline GE: Role of conventional radiation therapy in the treatment of functional pituitary tumors. In: Recent Advances in the Diagnosis and Treatment of Pituitary Tumors, Linfoot JA (ed). New York: Raven Press, 1979, p 442.

32. Thorner MO, Perryman RL, Cronin MJ, Rogol AD, Draznin M, Johanson A, Vale W, Horvath E, Kovacs K: Somatotroph hyperplasia: successful treatment of acromegaly by removal of a pancreatic islet tumor secreting a growth hormone-releasing factor. J Clin Invest 70: 965–977, 1982.

33. Guillemin R, Brazeau P, Bohlen P, Esch F, Ling N, Wehrenberg WB: Growth hormone-releasing factor from a human pancreatic tumor that caused acromegaly. Science 218: 585–587, 1982.

34. Evans HM, Briggs JH, Dixon JS: The physiology and chemistry of growth hormone. Acromegaly. In: The Pituitary Gland, Harris GW, Donovan BT (eds). Berkely and Los Angeles: University of California Press, 1966, p 439.

35. Wright AD, Hill DM, Lowry C, Fraser TR: Mortality in acromegaly. Q J Med 39: 1–16, 1970.

36. Arafah BM, Brodkey JS, Pearson OH: Acromegaly. In: Endocrine-Related Tumors 1, Santen RJ, A Manni (eds). The Hague: Martinus-Nijhoff Publishers, 1984, pp 45–61.

37. Atkinson RL, Becker DP, Martins AN, Schaaf M, Dimond RC, Wartofsky L, Earll JM: Acromegaly. Treatment by transsphenoidal microsurgery. J A Med Assoc 233: 1279–1283, 1975.

38. Kjellberg RN, Kliman B: A system for therapy of pituitary tumors: Proton or surgical therapy. In: Diagnosis and Treatment of Pituitary Tumors, Kohler PO, Ross GT (eds). Amsterdam: Excerpta Medica, 1973, pp 234–252.

39. Lawrence JH, Chong CY, Lyman JT: Treatment of pituitary tumors with heavy particles. In: Diagnosis and Treatment of Pituitary Tumors, Kohler PO, Ross GT (eds). Amsterdam: Excerpta Medica, 1973, pp 253–262.

40. Boyd AE, Lebovitz HE, Pfeiffer JB: Stimulation of human growth hormone secretion by L-dopa. N Engl J Med 238: 1425–1429, 1970.

41. Belforte L, Camanni F, Chiodini PG, Liuzzi A, Massara F, Molinatti GM, Muller EE, Silvestrini F: Long-term treatment with 2-Br-a-ergocryptine in acromegaly. Acta Endocrinol 85: 235–248, 1977.

42. Sachdev Y, Gomez-Pan A, Turnbridge WMG, Duns A, Weightman DR, Hall R, Goolamali SK: Bromocriptine therapy in acromegaly. Lancet 2: 1164–1167, 1975.

43. Moses AC, Molitch ME, Sawin CT, Jackson IMD, Biller BJ, Furlanetto R, Reichlin S: Bromocriptine therapy in acromegaly: Use in patients resistant to conventional therapy and effect on serum levels of somatomedin C. J Clin Endocrinol Metab 53: 752–758, 1981.

44. Schwinn G, Dirks H, McIntosh C, Kobberling J: Metabolic and clinical studies on patients with acromegaly treated with bromocriptine over 22 months. Eur J Clin Invest 7: 101–107, 1977.

45. Wass JAH, Moult PJ, Thorner MO, Dacie JE, Charlesworth M, Jones AE, Besser GM: Reduction of pituitary tumor size in patients with prolactinomas and acromegaly treated with bromocriptine with and without radiotherapy. Lancet 2: 66–69, 1979.

46. Chiodini PG, Liuzzi A, Cozzi R: Macroprolactinomas and GH secreting adenomas: medical treatment. In: Program of the International Symposium on Pituitary Hormones and Related Peptides, Motta M (ed). San Marino, 1981, 55 (abstr).

47. Wollesen F, Andersen T, Karle A: Size reduction of extrasellar pituitary tumors during bromocriptine treatment. Ann Intern Med 96: 281–286, 1982.

48. Leeper R: Controversies in the treatment thyroid cancer: The New York Memorial Hospital

approach. In: Thyroid Today, Vol 4, July/Aug, 1982.

49. Cady B, Sedgwick CE, Meissner WA, Wool MS, Salzman FA, Werber J: Risk factor analysis in differentiated thyroid cancer. Cancer 43: 810–820, 1979.

50. Woolner LB: Thyroid carcinoma: pathologic classification with data on prognosis. Semin Nucl Med 1: 481–502, 1971.

51. Wanebo HJ, Andrews W, Kaiser DL: Thyroid cancer: some basic considerations. Ca 33: 87–97, 1983.

52. Tollefsen HR, Shah JP, Huvos AG: Papillary carcinoma of the thyroid. Am J Surg 124: 468–472, 1972.

53. Buckwalter JA, Thomas CG Jr: Selection of surgical treatment for well differentiated thyroid carcinomas. Ann Surg 176: 565–578, 1972.

54. Crile G Jr: Changing end results in patients with papillary carcinoma of the thyroid. Surg. Gynec Obstet 71: 460–468, 1971.

55. Mazzaferri EL, Young RL, Oertel JE, Kemmerer WT, Page CP: Papillary thyroid carcinoma: the impact of therapy in 576 patients. Medicine 56: 171–196, 1977.

56. Young RL, Mazzaferri EL, Rahe AJ, Dorfman SG: Pure follicular thyroid carcinoma: Impact of therapy in 214 patients. J Nucl Med 21: 733–737, 1980.

57. Samaan NA, Maheshwari YK, Nader S, Hill CS Jr, Schultz PN, Haynie TP, Hickey RC, Clark RL, Goepfert H, Ibanez ML, Litton CE: Impact of therapy for differentiated carcinoma of the thyroid: an analysis of 706 cases. J Clin Endocrinol Metab 56: 1131–1138, 1983.

58. Schneider AB, Line BR, Goldman JM, Robbins J: Sequential serum thyroglobulin determinations, ^{131}I scans, and [131] uptakes after triiodothyronine withdrawal in patients with thyroid cancer. J Clin Endocrinol Metab 53: 1199–1206, 1981.

59. Beierwaltes WH: The treatment of thyroid carcinoma with radioactive iodine. Semin Nucl Med VIII: 79–94, 1978.

60. Cady B, Sedgwick CE, Meissner WA, Bookwalter JR, Romagosa V, Werber J: Changing clinical, pathologic, therapeutic, and survival patterns in differentiated thyroid carcinoma. Ann Surg 184: 541–553, 1976.

61. Mazzaferri EL, Young RL: Papillary thyroid carcinoma: A 10 year follow-up report of the impact of therapy in 576 patients. Am J Med 70: 511–518, 1981.

62. Harwood J, Clark OH, Dunphy JE: Significance of lymph node metastasis in differentiated thyroid cancer. Am J Surg 136: 107–112, 1978.

63. DeGroot LJ: Natural history and therapy of thyroid cancers. In: 35th Postgraduate Assembly of The Endocrine Society, Boston, MA, Oct 24–28, 1983, p 252–270.

64. Jacobs JK, Aland JW Jr, Ballinger JF: Total thyroidectomy. A review of 213 patients. Ann Surg 197: 542–549, 1983.

65. Pochin EE: Prospects from the treatment of thyroid carcinoma with radioiodine. Clin Radiol 18: 113–135, 1967.

66. Winship T, Rasvall RV: Thyroid carcinoma in childhood: Final report on a 20 year old study. Clin Proc Child Hosp 26: 327, 1970.

Index